Broadribb's
Introductory Pediatric Nursing

FIFTH EDITION

Broadribb's Introductory Pediatric Nursing

Margaret G. Marks, RN, BSNE

Former Instructor
Juniata-Mifflin Area Vocational Technical School
Lewistown, Pennsylvania

Lippincott
Philadelphia • New York

Acquisitions Editor: Jennifer Brogan
Developmental Editor: Danielle DiPalma
Coordinating Editorial Assistant: Susan V. Barta
Associate Managing Editor: Barbara Ryalls
Senior Production Manager: Helen Ewan
Senior Production Coordinator: Nannette Winski
Assistant Art Director: Kathy Kelley-Luedtke
Indexer: Michael Ferreira

Edition 5
Copyright © 1998 by Lippincott-Raven Publishers.
Copyright © 1994, 1983, 1973, 1967 by J. B. Lippincott Company

9   8   7   6   5   4   3   2   1

Library of Congress Cataloging in Publications Data

Marks, Margaret G.
    Broadribb's introductory pediatric nursing. — 5th ed. / Margaret
G. Marks.
        p.   cm.
    Includes bibliographical references and index.
    ISBN 0-397-55450-8 (alk. paper)
    1. Pediatric nursing.   I. Broadribb, Violet.   Introductory
pediatric nursing.   II. Title.
    [DNLM: 1. Pediatric Nursing.   WY 159 M3455b 1998]
RJ245.B764   1998
610.73'62—dc21
DNLM/DLC
for Library of Congress   97-24540
                                                                        CIP

Dedication

To April, Eddie, Shane, Chelsea and Jeffrey Carl-
the lights of my life—
with much love from their Honey,
and to their parents,
Jeff and Alice and Tracey and Randy,
my wonderful, supporting children.

Contributor

Judith Allender, RNC, MSN, EdD
Professor of Nursing
Department of Nursing
School of Health and Human Services
California State University
Fresno, California
Chapter 5: Community-Based Care of the Child

Reviewers

Karen Allen, PhD, RN
Associate Professor, Department of Psychiatry
Community Health and Adult Primary Care
University of Maryland at Baltimore School of Nursing
Baltimore, Maryland

H. Benoit, RN, BSN, MS
Faculty Coordinator
School of Health Sciences
Lafayette General Medical Center
Lafayette, Louisiana

Eileen Costa, LPN, RN
LPN Instructor
Sullivan County BOCES
Liberty, New York

Kay Gingerich, RN, BSN
Faculty Member
Parma School of Practical Nursing
Parma, Ohio

Constance J. Hirnle, MN, RN
Assistant Professor
Seattle University School of Nursing
Seattle, Washington

Bettyann Milliron, RNC
Instructor
Juniata-Mifflin Area Vocational Technical School
Lewistown, Pennsylvania

Patricia Laing-Arie, RN
Instructor, Program of Practical Nursing
Meridian Technology Center
Stillwater, Oklahoma

Kim Rawson, RNC, MSN
Instructor, Practical Nursing Department
Bishop State Community College, Southwest Campus
Mobile, Alabama

Betty E. Sims, MSN, RN
Instructor, Vocational Nursing Program
Bee County College
Beeville, Texas

Cheryl A. Smith, RNC, MSN
Nursing Supervisor
Dekalb County Board of Health
Decatur, Georgia

Melissa Vandeveer, C-PNT, PhD
Program Director of Graduate Nursing
University of Southern Indiana
Evansville, Indiana

Sheryl M. Zang, RN, MS
Instructor
College of Nursing
Health Science Center
State University of New York
Brooklyn, New York

Preface

We have been very pleased by the warm reception the fourth edition of **Broadribb's Introductory Pediatric Nursing** received. We felt that it was important to continue to make revisions in a timely manner. We have continued to stress the underlying philosophy of love and caring for children evident in the earlier editions.

Throughout this edition we continue to use nongender specific terminology or use "he or she" when necessary for clarity. We also have continued the use of family caregivers to recognize that many children live in families other than traditional two-parent family homes. Terminology referring to nurses continues to be nongender specific, to recognize there are many excellent nurses of either gender working with children in many different roles and a variety of settings. We have made a greater stress on broadening the cultural views of the text as we wish to recognize the wonderful cultural diversity of North America.

As a result of the changes in health care administration, community-based health care has become an even greater aspect of total health care. This has been a positive influence in caring for children since the child in the community is more easily viewed as part of a family, rather than a separate entity. Since more responsibility for caring for ill children has fallen on the family caregivers, the stress on teaching the child and family has continued with an emphasis on prevention. The nursing process has been used as the foundation for presenting nursing care. Implementation is presented in a narrative format to enable the discussion from which planning, goal setting, and implementation can be put into action.

We continue to strive to keep the readability of the text at a level with which the new student can be comfortable. In recognition of the limited time that the student has and the frustration that can result from having to turn to a dictionary or glossary for words that are unfamiliar, we have attempted to identify all possible unfamiliar terms and define them within the text. This increases the reading ease for the student, decreasing the time necessary to complete the assigned reading, and enhancing the understanding of the information.

Features

In an effort to provide the instructor and student with a text that is informative, exciting, and easy to use, we have incorporated a number of features throughout the text, many of which are included in each chapter. In this edition, we have added a stress on communication and interaction with children and caregivers. The principle features include:

- **Chapter Outlines**—Each chapter opens with an outline providing the reader with an overall view of the chapter's main topics and organization.
- **Key Terms**—A list of terms that may be unfamiliar to students and that are considered essential to the chapter's understanding appears at the beginning of each chapter. The first appearance in the chapter of each of these terms is in boldface type, with the definition included in the text. All key terms also are included in a glossary at the end of the text.
- **Student Objectives**—Measurable student-oriented objectives are included at the beginning of each chapter. These help to guide the student in recognizing the focus of the chapter and provide the instructor with guidance for evaluating the student's understanding of the information presented in the chapter.
- **Nursing Process**—The nursing process serves as an organizing structure for the discussion of nursing care for many of the health problems covered in the text. These provide the student with a foundation from which individualized nursing care plans can be developed. Each Nursing Process section includes nursing assessment, relevant nursing diagnoses, outcome identification and planning, implementation, outcome criteria and evaluation. Emphasis is placed on the importance of involving the child and family caregivers in the assessment process. We have selected NANDA-approved nursing diagnoses to represent appropriate concerns for a particular condition, but we do not attempt to include all diagnoses that could be identified. Outcome identification focuses on setting goals for the child. Outcome criteria and evaluation provide a goal for each nursing diagnosis and criterion to measure the successful accomplishment of that goal.
- **Nursing Care Plans**—Throughout the text Nursing Care Plans are presented to provide the student with a model to follow in using the information from the nursing process to develop specific nursing care plans. To make the care plans more meaningful, a scenario has been constructed for each one.

- **Family Teaching Boxes**—Information that the student can use in teaching family caregivers and children is presented in highlighted boxes ready for use.
- **Personal Glimpses**—Personal Glimpses are presented in every chapter. These are actual first-person naratives. The Glimpses help the student have a view of an experience a child or caregiver had in a given situation and their feelings about or during the incident. These are presented to enhance the student's understanding and appreciation of the feelings of others.
- **Communication Boxes**—We feel that communication is an important aspect of the foundation of caring for others. In a number of the nursing care chapters we have placed communication situations, with examples of effective and ineffective communications and the mechanisms which help or hinder in the given illustration.
- **Tables, Drawings, and Photographs**—These important aspects of the text have been updated and clarified with the addition of new material where appropriate.
- **Key Points**—We selected key points from the chapter to help the student focus on the important aspects of the given chapter. This provides a quick review of essential elements of the chapter.
- **Critical Thinking**—Critical thinking situations at the end of each chapter encourage the student to think about the chapter content in practical terms. These situations require the student to incorporate knowledge gained from the chapter and apply it to real-life problems. The instructor can also use them as a tool to stimulate class discussion.
- **Bibliography**—Each Bibliography contains references that the student can readily turn to for additional information on conditions discussed in the chapter.

Organization

The text is divided into four units to provide an orderly approach to the content. The basic approach to the study of health problems of children is organized within a framework of growth and development. Growth and development is presented for an age group, and the specific health problems that commonly affect that age group are discussed in the following chapter. This approach has been well received by nursing students and continues to provide a user-friendly approach to the study of nursing care of children.

Unit I, The Child, the Family, and Health Care, introduces the student in Chapter 1 to a brief history of pediatrics and pediatric nursing and the nursing process. Chapter 2 follows with a discussion of the family, its structure, and family factors that influence the growth and development of children. Concepts of growth and development are presented to provide a foundation for discussion in later chapters on growth and development. Chapter 3, Care of the Ill Child, presents physical care of the ill child, including general physical assessments, administration of medications and intravenous therapy. Chapter 4, Hospital-Based Care of the Child, presents the pediatric unit, infection control in the pediatric setting, admission and discharge, the child undergoing surgery, the hospital play program and safety in the hospital. Chapter 5, Community-Based Care of the Child, introduces community-based health care and discusses the various settings in the community through which health care is provided for the child.

Unit I provides an introduction to the care of children and pediatric nursing so that the student can function in a pediatric setting while completing the remainder of the course of study. This helps decrease the need to spend as many class hours preparing the student for the first days of pediatric nursing experience.

Unit II, A Child is Born, presents prenatal and new born nursing care. Chapter 6 covers prenatal growth and development including the influence of heredity and environment and parenthood education. Chapter 7 covers the normal newborn, daily care, and family interaction. Chapter 8 addresses the health problems of the high-risk newborn, including the premature infant. Chapter 9 covers the newborn with special needs and includes congenital anomalies, inborn errors of metabolism, and other congenital problems.

Unit III, A Child Grows, is organized by developmental stages, from infancy through adolescence. The even-numbered chapters cover growth and development of the designated age group and the odd-numbered chapters follow with health problems common to that age. Although many conditions are not limited to a specific age, they are included in the age group in which they most often occur. The nursing process and nursing care plans are integrated through this unit, as well as Personal Glimpses and Communication Boxes.

Unit IV, A Child in Crisis, focuses on several societal problems and their effect on children. Chapter 20 explores the impact that substance abuse in the family has on the child. The issues of child abuse, runaway children, latchkey children, children of divorces, and homeless children and families are also examined. Chapter 21 discusses the concerns that face the family of a child with a chronic illness. The impact on the family of caring for a child with a chronic illness and the nurse's role in assisting and supporting these families is presented. Chapter 22 concludes with the dying child. Included in this chapter is a teaching aid to help the nurse perform a self-examination of personal attitudes about death and dying as well as concrete guidelines to use when interacting with a grieving child or adult.

Throughout the text, family-centered care is stressed. Developmental enrichment and stimulation are stressed in the sections on nursing process. The basic premise of each child's self worth is fundamental in all of the nursing care presented.

Acknowledgments

I wish to thank the staff at Lippincott-Raven for their assistance in completing this fifth edition of **Broadribb's Introductory Pediatric Nursing.** I'm sure that many more have worked on this revision than I realize. However, there are several whom I particularly wish to thank. From the very first planning meeting with Jennifer Brogan, Sponsoring Editor, Danielle DiPalma, Developmental Editor, and Susan Barta, Editorial Assistant, I felt fortunate to have a supportive team working with me.

Most especially, I wish to thank Danielle DiPalma, who has been with me from the start of this edition as the developmental editor. Danielle has been patient and supportive and quietly listened to my rantings and ravings when I became frustrated. She has worked hard to arrange shoots for new photos and search for replacements where needed. Danielle was innovative in suggesting new features for the book. Danielle was always willing to work things out when we came to a time crunch. She truly made this revision work.

My former colleagues from Juniata-Mifflin Area Vo-Tech Practical Nursing Program continue to be supportive. Bettyann Milliron, who is now teaching the Maternal-Child Health course that I taught, has been very helpful with her keen eye for small glitches and helpful suggestions. I appreciate her continuing contact with me. Sylvia Swineford, the program's former coordinator, who retired at the same time I did, continues to offer me moral support.

I owe a great debt of gratitude to Ruth Anne Sieber for her generosity with her materials on children, death, and dying. Ruth Anne's experience as a pediatric nurse and a hospice nurse gave her the outstanding credentials to supply me with just what I needed to make the last chapter of the text a sensitive and warm treatment of a difficult but essential subject.

To my family and friends, I say "Thanks for your understanding and patience." They are getting used to me saying, "I've got to work on the book." My adult children are duly impressed by their Mom's apparent penchant for sitting in front of a computer playing with words. I also am grateful that I was able to use the Internet to explore for valid information. The Internet offers such a vast area to explore, and with care one can find many excellent pieces of information.

I also wish to show my appreciation to Wayne Memorial Hospital in Honesdale, Pennsylvania for hosting our 2 day photo shoot. Thanks to the staff, families and clients of the hospital for taking time out of your busy days, sharing your special moments, and welcoming us into your workplace and home. A special thanks to Donna Decker, Ellen Malloy, and Tammy Miller for making the photo shoot a reality.

I deeply appreciate Jennifer Brogan's support as sponsoring editor. She was always there in the background with an answer when I presented Danielle with a question. Susan Barta was always ready to send me any helpful items I needed. Others at Lippincott-Raven whom I wish to thank for contributing to the overall success of this edition include Barbara Ryalls, Project Editor, Helen Ewan, Production Manager, and many others whose names I do not know.

Contents

Chapter 18

Growth and Development of the Adolescent: 11 to 18 Years 392

Chapter 19

Health Problems of the Adolescent 408

Unit IV
A Child in Crisis 437

Chapter 20

The Child in a Stressed Family 439

Chapter 21

The Child With a Chronic Health Problem 454

Chapter 22

The Dying Child 465

Broadribb's
Introductory Pediatric Nursing

The Child,
the Family,
and Health Care

Chapter 1

The Nurse's Role in a Changing Child Health Care Environment

STUDENT OBJECTIVES

On completion of this chapter, the student will be able to:

1. State where the United States ranks compared with other developed countries in terms of infant mortality rate.
2. State two causes of the high rate of infant mortality in the United States.
3. Describe the post–World War I atmosphere in the care of children and its effect on those children.
4. List the five steps of the nursing process.
5. State who is involved in setting goals of nursing care for the child.
6. Compare observations indicating health or illness of an infant or young child.
7. Describe three additional useful observations of the older child.
8. List four categories of cultural attitudes that influence planning of care for the child.
9. Name one of the most important aspects of communication.
10. State the purpose of reflective statements when communicating with a caregiver or child.

KEY TERMS

actual nursing diagnoses	objective data
critical pathways	outcomes
dependent nursing actions	pediatric nurse practitioner
independent nursing	primary nursing
actions	risk nursing diagnoses
interdependent nursing	subjective data
actions	wellness nursing diagnoses
nursing process	

The nurse preparing to care for today's and tomorrow's children and families faces vastly different responsibilities and challenges than did the pediatric nurse of even a decade ago. Nurses and other health professionals are becoming increasingly concerned with much more than the care of sick children. Health teaching, prevention of illness, and promotion of optimal (most desirable or satisfactory) physical, developmental, and emotional health have become a significant part of contemporary nursing.

Scientific and technologic advances have reduced the incidence of communicable disease and have helped to control metabolic disorders such as diabetes. Much of health care takes place outside the hospital, at home or in schools, clinics, or physicians' offices. Prenatal diagnosis of birth defects, transfusions, and other treatments for the unborn fetus and improved life-support systems for premature infants are but a few examples of the rapid progress in child care.

Controversy continues to rage about choices in family planning. In January 1973, a Supreme Court decision declared abortion legal anywhere in the United States. In 1981, efforts were made to convince Congress that legislation should be passed to make all abortions illegal on the alleged grounds that the fetus is a person and therefore has the right to life. In the 1990s, bitter debate between "pro-life" and "pro-choice" groups is still raging and seems likely to continue for some years.

Tremendous sociologic changes have affected attitudes toward, and concepts in, child health. American society is largely suburban, with a population of highly mobile persons and families. The women's movement has focused new attention on the needs of families in which the mother works outside the home. Escalating divorce rates, changes in attitudes toward sexual roles, and general acceptance of unmarried mothers have increased the number of single-parent families. Many people have come to regard health care as a right, not a privilege, and expect fair value received for their investment. In addition, the demand for financial responsibility in health care has contributed to shortened hospital stays and alternative methods of health care delivery.

The reduction in the incidence of communicable and infectious diseases has made it possible to devote more attention to such critical problems as child abuse, learning and behavior disorders, developmental disabilities, and chronic illness. Research in these areas continues, and as these findings become available, nurses will be among the practitioners who will help translate this research into improved health care for children and families.

The ability of nurses to translate the relevant medical research into practice, however, is based on their understanding of the predictable but variable phases of a child's growth and development and their understanding of and sensitivity to the importance of family interactions.

CHANGING CONCEPTS IN CHILD HEALTH CARE

Child health care has evolved from a sideline of internal medicine to a specialty that focuses on the child and the child's family in health and illness, through all phases of development. Technologic advances account for many of the changes seen in the last 50 years, but sociologic changes—in particular, society's view of the child and the child's needs—have been just as important.

Institutional Care

Pediatrics is a relatively new medical specialty, developing only in the mid-1800s. In colonial times, epidemics were common and many children died in infancy or childhood. Families were large because so many children did not live to adulthood. Children were viewed as additional hands to help with the family farm chores. Children were often cared for by the adults in the family or by a neighbor who had a reputation of being able to care for the sick. In some cases, disease wiped out entire families. Native American children, usually cared for by medicine men, were exposed to new and fatal diseases. Children of slaves received only the care their slave owner cared to provide.

The first children's hospital opened in Philadelphia in 1855. Until that point in Western civilization, children were not considered important except as contributors to family income. If children were hospitalized, they were cared for in hospitals as adults were, often in the same bed.

Unfortunately, early institutions for children were notorious for their unsanitary conditions, neglect, and lack of proper infant nutrition. Well into the 19th century, mortality rates were commonly 50% to 100% among institutionalized children, whether in asylums or hospitals.

Arthur Jacobi, a Prussian-born physician, has been recognized as the father of pediatrics. Under his direction several New York hospitals opened pediatric units. He helped found the American Pediatric Society in 1888. During the early 1900s, a primary cause of death in children's institutions was the intractable diarrhea most of these children developed. Initiation of the simple practice of boiling milk and isolating children with septic conditions lowered the incidence of diarrhea. This practice of pasteurizing milk was instrumental in decreasing the rate of death in children.

After World War I, a period of strict asepsis began. Babies were placed in individual cubicles, and the nurses were strictly forbidden to pick up the children except when necessary. Crib sides were draped with clean sheets, leaving infants with nothing to do but stare at the ceiling. The importance of toys in a child's environment appears not to have been recognized; besides, it was thought that such objects could transmit infection. Parents were allowed to visit for half an hour or perhaps 1 hour each week. They were forbidden to pick up their children under penalty of having their visiting privileges taken away entirely.

Despite these precautions, the high infant mortality rates continued. One of the first people to suspect the cause was Joseph Brennaman, a physician at Children's Memorial Hospital, Chicago. In 1932, he suggested that the infants suffered from a lack of stimulation; other concerned child specialists became interested. In the 1940s, René Spitz published the results of studies that supported his contention that deprivation of maternal care caused a state of dazed stupor in an infant. He believed this condition could become irreversible if the child were not returned to the mother promptly. He termed this state "anaclitic depression." He also coined the term *hospitalism*, which he defined as "a vitiated condition of the body due to long confinement in the hospital" (*vitiated* means feeble or weak). Later, the term came to be used almost entirely to denote the harmful effects of institutional care on infants. Another physician, Bakwin, found that infants hospitalized for a long time actually developed physical symptoms, which he attributed to a lack of emotional stimulation and a lack of feeding satisfaction.

John Bowlby of London explored the subject of maternal deprivation thoroughly, working under the auspices of the World Health Organization. His 1951 study, which received worldwide attention, revealed the negative results of the separation of child and mother due to hospitalization. Bowlby's work, together with that of John Robertson, his associate, led to a reevaluation and liberalization of hospital visiting policies for children.

In the 1970s and 1980s, Marshall Klaus and John Kennell, physicians at Rainbow Babies and Children's Hospital, Cleveland, carried out important studies on the effect of the separation of newborns and parents. They established that this early separation may have long-term effects on family relationships and that offering the new family an opportunity to be together at birth, and for a significant period after birth, may provide benefits that last well into early childhood (Fig. 1-1). These findings also have helped to modify hospital policies.

Hospital regulations changed slowly, but gradually they began to reflect the needs of children and their families.

Figure 1-1
The mother, father, and infant son soon after birth.

Isolation practices have been relaxed for children who do not have infectious diseases; children are encouraged to ambulate as early as possible and to visit the playroom, where they can be with other children. Nurses at all levels who work with children are prepared to understand, value, and use play as a therapeutic tool in the daily care of children.

Family-Centered Care

Family-centered nursing is a new and broadened concept in the health care system of the United States. No longer are children treated merely as clinical cases, with attention given exclusively to their medical problems. Instead, health care providers recognize that children belong to a family, a community, and a particular way of life or culture, and their health is influenced by these and other factors (Fig. 1-2). Separating children from their background means that their needs are met only in a superficial manner, if at all. Even if nursing takes place entirely inside hospital walls, family-centered care pays attention to each child's unique emotional, developmental, social, and scholastic needs as well as physical ones. Family-centered nursing care also strives to help family members alleviate their fears and anxieties, cope and function normally, and understand the child's condition and their role in the healing process.

Regionalized Care

During the past several decades there has been a definite trend toward centralization and regionalization of pediatric services. Providing high-quality medical care in pediatrics necessitated moving the child to medical teaching centers with the best resources for diagnosis and treatment. To avoid duplication of services and equipment, and thus contributing to economic responsibility, the most intricate and expensive services and the most highly specialized personnel were made available in the centralized location: pe-

Figure 1-2
Internal and external factors that influence the health and
illness patterns of the child.

diatric neurologists, adolescent allergy specialists, pediatric oncologists, nurse play therapists, child psychiatrists, pediatric nurse practitioners, and clinical nurse specialists. Here are found geneticists, neonatal intensive care units, computed tomography scanners, burn care units, and other highly specialized equipment and units.

Regionalized care often takes the pediatric patient far from home. The family caregivers must travel a longer distance to visit than if the child were at the local suburban hospital. Family-centered care becomes even more important under these circumstances. Measures are always taken to keep the child's hospitalization as brief as possible, the child as ambulatory as possible, and the family as close as possible. For the child, separation from the family is traumatic and may actually retard recovery. Many of these regionalized centers (tertiary care hospitals) have accommodations where families may stay while their child is hospitalized.

Other Innovative Child Health Care Programs

Many pediatric hospitals have home care programs for children with chronic illness, such as leukemia, hemophilia, and cystic fibrosis. Between hospitalizations, the child's condition is monitored at home by the hospital's nurses, offering continuity of care.

Some pediatric heath care providers use **primary nursing**, a system whereby one nurse plans the total care for a child and directs the efforts of nurses on the other two shifts. The primary nurse is responsible for the child's care at all times and often makes home visits to the child after discharge and before readmission. In facilities where primary nursing is not practiced, a good procedure is to assign the same nurse to a child to provide stability in the child's care.

An approach somewhat similar to primary nursing, but with more concern and involvement with cost effectiveness and quality of care, is case management. Case management plans are multidisciplinary plans that include all aspects of and participants in the child's care. A nursing case manager is assigned to a child or group of children with similar conditions. Outcomes within specific time lines are established. These time lines have various names but are often called **critical pathways**. Regular documentation of care provides the opportunity for daily evaluation to determine where delays may be occurring so that appropriate adjustments in care can be made. Case management plans can also include home care of the child. Through case management, there is better coordination of care and less fragmentation, and this has led to increased family satisfaction.

Many children are now being cared for in health maintenance organizations (HMOs). HMOs are professional groups of physicians, laboratory service personnel, nurse practitioners, nurses, and consultants who care for the health of a family on a continuing basis and are geared toward health care and disease prevention. The family pays a set fee for total care; any necessary hospitalization is covered by that fee. The emphasis is on health and prevention, in contrast to the acute care, cure-oriented pediatric medical center.

In some private practices and in many clinic settings, the child is cared for by a **pediatric nurse practitioner**, a professional nurse prepared at the postbaccalaureate level to give primary health care to children and families. Pediatric nurse practitioners use pediatricians or family physicians as consultants but offer day-to-day assessment and care.

THE STATUS OF CHILD HEALTH

In the first half of the 20th century, many children died during or after childbirth or in early childhood as a result of disease, infections, or injuries. Technologic and socioeconomic changes have influenced the health care provided to children and also the health problems with which today's children are confronted. Communicable diseases of childhood and their complications are no longer a serious threat to the health of children. As the 20th century ends, health problems for children are focused much more on social concerns (Box 1-1). These issues are summarized below and will be discussed in full throughout the text.

Box 1-1. *Every Day in America the Following Occurrences Take Place*

	All U.S. Children	Black Children	White Children	Latino Children	Asian American Children	Native American Children
Children and youths under 25 die from HIV infection	3	1	1	—	—	—
Children and youths under 20 commit suicide	6	1	5	—	—	—
Children and youths under 20 are homicide victims	13	7	6	—	—	—
Children and youths under 20 are killed by guns	15	6	8	—	—	—
Children and youths under 20 die from accidental injuries	35	6	28	—	—	—
Babies die before their first birthday	95	31	61	12	1	1
Babies are born at very low birth weight (<3.5 lb)	144	55	84	18	—	7
Children and youths under 18 are arrested for drug offenses	255	108	144	—	2	1
Children and youths under 18 are arrested for alcohol-related offenses	318	19	290	—	2	7
Children and youths under 18 are arrested for violent crimes	327	165	157	—	4	2
Babies are born to mothers who had late or no prenatal care	564	175	358	167	20	12
Babies are born at low birth weight (<5.5 lb)	788	245	509	108	2	—
Babies are born to teenage mothers	1,388	420	954	302	23	22
Students drop out of high school each school day	2,217	444	1,689	333	—	—
Babies are born to mother who was not a high school graduate	2,582	541	45	953	78	39
Babies are born into poverty	2,699	723	1,811	753	—	—
Public school students are corporally punished each school day	3,086	1,198	1,639	210	7	32
Babies are born to unmarried mothers	3,356	1,257	1,978	689	61	60
Children and youths under 18 are arrested	5,504	1,547	3,802	—	96	59
Babies are born	11,137	1,846	8,772	1,762	412	108
Public school students are suspended each school day	13,076	4,404	6,674	1,644	216	137

Source: Children's Defense Fund, 1995
(Note: not all totals equal 100%)

Infants

Despite remarkable advances in many areas of maternal and child health, the maternal and infant mortality statistics are still grim. Infant mortality declined steadily in the 1960s and 1970s, but the 1980s saw a stall in that decline. In 1993, the United States ranked 18th and Canada ranked 10th in the rate of infant deaths among developed countries (Fig. 1-3). Of even greater concern is the fact that cities such as Washington DC, Philadelphia, and Detroit have twice the national infant mortality rate, making them infant mortality "disaster areas."[1]

Many factors may be associated with the high mortality rate and poor health of infants. Ample evidence indicates that low birth weight and late or nonexistent prenatal care are main factors in the poor rankings in infant mortality.[1] Other major factors that compromise the health of infants include congenital anomalies, sudden infant death syndrome, respiratory distress syndrome, and increasing rates of human immunodeficiency virus (HIV). Low birth weight

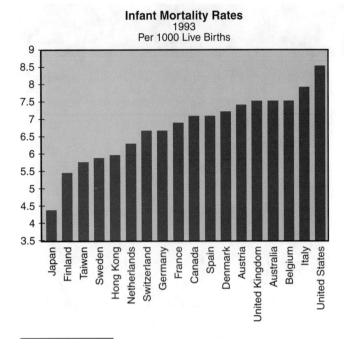

Figure 1-3
Adapted from Statistical Abstract of the United States, 1994.

and other causes of infant death and chronic illness are often linked to maternal factors such as lack of prenatal care, smoking, use of alcohol and illicit drugs, pregnancy before age 18 or after age 40, poor nutrition, lower socioeconomic status, lower educational levels, and environmental hazards. Both infant and maternal mortality rates are much higher among nonwhite populations, a fact that studies repeatedly attribute to lack of adequate prenatal care and an increased birth rate among women 15 to 19 years of age, a high-risk group (Fig. 1-4).

NATIONAL COMMISSION TO PREVENT INFANT MORTALITY

In 1986, Congress established the National Commission to Prevent Infant Mortality and charged it with the responsibility of creating a national strategic plan to reduce infant mortality and morbidity rates in the United States. The Commission's first report, in 1988, *Death Before Life: The Tragedy of Infant Mortality*, listed two primary objectives: to make the health of mothers and babies a national priority and to provide universal access to care for all pregnant women and children. The Commission concluded that educating the nation about the health needs of mothers and babies would cause a national response to the problem and that women would have to be given information and motivation to reduce infant mortality and morbidity rates. The Commission also stated that barriers of finances, geography, education, social position, behavior, and program administration problems must be eliminated to provide universal access to health care. In February 1990, the Commission published *Troubling Trends: The Health of the Next Generation*, which concluded that early prenatal care, along with smoking cessation, pregnancy planning, and

nutrition counseling and food supplementation, would result in heavier and healthier infants.

Children and Adolescents

Infectious diseases such as polio, diphtheria, scarlet fever, measles, and whooping cough once posed the greatest threat to children. However, today the largest risk to all children and adolescents is unintentional injury, most often the result of motor vehicle accidents.[2] Other unintentional injuries include drownings, falls, poisonings, and fires. The risks of injury-related death are being minimized through protection and safety measures by families, communities, and government agencies.

Developmental problems related to socioeconomic factors are on the rise, including mental retardation, learning disorders, emotional and behavioral problems, and speech and vision impairments. Lead poisoning appears to be a major threat to the child's developmental well-being. Although strict laws have minimized the amount of lead in gas, air, food, and industrial emissions, many children live and play in substandard housing areas where they are exposed to chipped lead-based paint, dust, and soil.

Other prevalent factors that affect the health of children include respiratory illness, violence toward children in the form of child abuse and neglect, homicide, suicide, cigarette smoking, alcohol and illicit drug use, risky sexual behavior, obesity, and lack of exercise.

Healthy living habits are established early in childhood. Many schools require antismoking, antidrug, health, nutri-

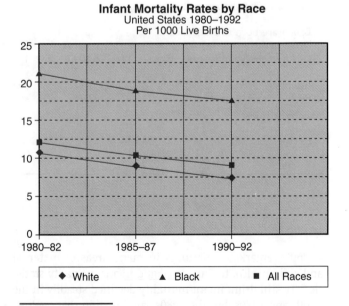

Figure 1-4
Source: *Health United States. 1994* on *Publications from the National Center for Health Statistics* CD-ROM Table 24. Centers for Disease Control and Prevention, National Center for Health Statistics.

TABLE 1-1. United States Goals for the Year 2000

Categories	Targeted for Reduction
Physical activity and fitness	Overweight among adolescents
Nutrition	Growth retardation among low-income children 5 years of age and younger
Tobacco	Start of cigarette smoking by children and youth
	Smoking during pregnancy
	Exposure of children ≤6 years of age to smoking in the home
	Smokeless tobacco use by adolescent and young adult males
Alcohol and other drugs	Alcohol-related accidents causing death
	Drug-related deaths
	Hospital visits resulting from drug abuse
Family planning	Number of pregnancies in females ≤17 years of age
	Number of unplanned pregnancies
	Number of infertile couples
Mental health and mental disorders	Suicides among 15- to 19-year-olds
	Suicide attempts among 14- to 17-year-olds
	Mental disorders in children and adolescents
Violent and abusive behavior	Homicides in 15- to 35-year-olds
	Violent deaths related to weapons
	Physical, sexual, and emotional abuse and neglect in children
	Spousal abuse against women
	Assault injuries in those older than 12 years of age
	Rape and attempted rape of women 12 to 34 years of age
Unintentional injuries	Drownings in children ≤4 years of age
	Death in home fires in children ≤4 years of age
	Poisonings in children ≤4 years of age
Environmental health	Asthma in children ≤14 years of age
	Mental retardation in school-age children
	Blood lead levels over 15 μg/dL in children ≤5 years of age
Oral health	Dental caries in children of all ages
Maternal and infant health	Infant mortality by ⅓
	Fetal death rate by ⅓
	Maternal death rate by ½
	Incidence of fetal alcohol syndrome
HIV infection	HIV infection in women giving birth to live-born infants
Sexually transmitted diseases	Incidence of:
	Gonorrhea in adolescents 15–19 years of age
	Chlamydia trachomatis infections
	Primary and secondary syphilis
	Congenital syphilis
	Genital herpes and genital warts
	Pelvic inflammatory disease
	Sexually transmitted hepatitis B
Immunization and infectious diseases	Diarrhea in children in child care centers
	Acute otitis media in children ≤4 years of age
Age-related objectives	Death rate for children and adolescents

Adapted from U.S. Department of Health and Human Services, Healthy people 2000. Washington DC: Public Health Service, 1990.

tion, physical, and sexual education. Many also provide immunization and screening programs. However, more and better educational and support programs for children, families, and communities are still needed to alleviate many child health problems and to provide children with adequate tools to make healthy living choices well into adulthood.

Healthy People 2000

In 1990, a national consortium of more than 300 organizations developed a set of objectives for the year 2000, *Healthy People 2000*. Prevention of illness, or health promotion, is the underlying goal of the objectives. States were encouraged to set their own objectives. Fifteen priority areas specifically affecting children were identified (Table 1-1). These objectives were reviewed in mid-decade, and although there has been encouraging progress in two thirds of the goals, much remains to be accomplished in the latter part of the decade. Nurses caring for children have a great responsibility to use these objectives as underlying guidelines in planning care.

THE NURSE'S CHANGING ROLE IN CHILD HEALTH CARE

The image of nursing has changed and the horizons and responsibilities have broadened tremendously in recent years. Child care now involves surveillance of growth and development, anticipatory guidance about maturational and common health problems, and teaching and follow-up about immunizations, as well as traditional health teaching, in addition to the treatment of disease and physical problems. The primary thrust of health care is toward prevention.

Nurses at all levels are legally accountable for their actions, assuming new responsibilities and accountability with every advance in education. Nurses practicing in any pediatric setting and at all levels must keep up to date with education and information on how to help their young patients and where to direct families for help when other resources are needed. When the nurse functions as a teacher, adviser, and resource person, it is important that the information and advice provided be correct, pertinent, and useful to the person in need.

As mentioned earlier, pediatric nurse practitioners have taken a significant place in caring for children. Some of these nurses specialize in school nursing or oncology, among other areas. In addition, clinical nurse specialists are nurses with advanced education prepared to provide care at any stage of illness or wellness.

In many settings, nurses can provide health education to both children and their families. Such teaching may be concerned with safety, nutrition, health habits, immunizations, dental care, healthy development, and discipline. Some of these settings include schools, home, and ambulatory settings. In schools, nurses have become much more than Band-Aid dispensers: they monitor well children, including their immunizations, and growth and development. School nurses often present or are consultants in classroom health education programs and often serve on committees that evaluate children with educational and social adjustment problems. For children with long-term or chronic illnesses, nurses can help provide care in the home. This home care often is part of a collaboration with other health care professionals. Ambulatory care settings help avoid separating the child from the family and provide

A Personal Glimpse

My Grandpa's eyes gave me my first vision of nursing. A Licensed Practical Nurse, he filled my head with hospital stories and my belly with chocolate milk. He saw people hurt by pain and fear, and he made them feel better. I wasn't much bigger than the children I saw, but I knew I wanted to make them feel better too. So, I went to nursing school, in the same hospital where I shared chocolate milk with Grandpa.

My pediatric nursing career started at graduation 25 years ago. Back then, the community pediatric unit was always filled to capacity. Outpatient and critical care services for children were minimal, so disorders ranged from the mild to the severe. Newborns through teens were treated for everything from mild diarrhea to significant trauma. But two things remained constant regardless of age or diagnosis—the pain and the fear.

Soon, helping sick children feel better was no longer enough. I realized early in my career that the best way to help was to prevent children from getting sick in the first place. So, I went back to school, through baccalaureate and masters' degrees, to become a Pediatric Nurse Practitioner. Seventeen years later, I still practice as a PNP in a rural community.

Changes in health care have put more emphasis on the various nonhospital settings, where most children receive care. Healthy children are less likely to become ill and more likely to become healthy adults. Prevention and health promotion are essential. They should be part of the care of all children (and adults!), including those who are hospitalized. I always take the time to teach the importance of immunizations, proper nutrition, growth and development. A little goes a long way, and there is tremendous satisfaction in knowing that I've helped to ease pain and fear before they have a chance to get started.

Mary

a less costly means of administering health care to children. The pediatric nurse plays an important role in ambulatory settings.

In addition, nurses are contributing to health care research that will help lead to more improvements in the care of children and their families.

Health teaching is one of the most important aspects of promoting wellness. Nurses are often in a position to do incidental teaching, as well as more organized formal teaching. Nurses must also be aware that they serve as role models to others in practicing good health habits. Some examples of possible teaching opportunities include those in a work environment, such as helping the child and family understand a diagnosis or proposed treatment, understanding medications, and providing teaching materials to children and families. In the community, the nurse can be an advocate for healthy living practices and policies or can serve as a volunteer in community organizations to promote healthy growth and development and anticipatory guidance. Nurses can become involved with their schools to offer knowledge and expertise in wellness practices. They should use every opportunity to contribute to and encourage healthy living practices.

Throughout this text, teaching opportunities are identified and teaching suggestions supplied. Nurses are encouraged to use these suggestions as a foundation for further teaching. During any teaching, however, the nurse must be alert to the ability of the child and the family to understand the material being presented. By using methods of feedback, questions and answers, and demonstrations when appropriate, the nurse can confirm that the information was understood. This also gives the nurse the opportunity to reinforce any areas of information that may still be weak. With experience, nurses can become very competent teachers.

THE NURSING PROCESS

The **nursing process** is a proven form of problem solving based on the scientific method. The nursing process consists of five components:

- Assessment
- Nursing diagnosis
- Outcome identification and planning
- Implementation
- Evaluation

Based on the data collected during the assessment, nursing diagnoses are determined, nursing care is planned and implemented, and the results are evaluated. The process does not end here but continues through reassessment, establishment of new diagnoses, additional plans, implementation, and evaluation until all the child's nursing problems are identified and dealt with (Fig. 1-5).

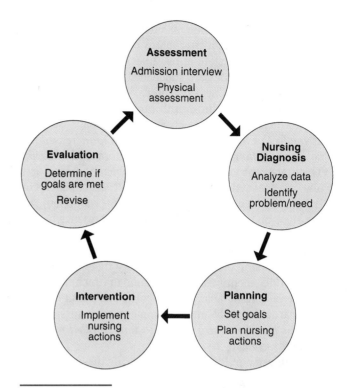

Figure 1-5
Diagram of the nursing process.

Assessment

Nursing assessment is a skill that must be practiced and perfected through study and experience. The nurse must be skilled in understanding the concepts of communication, both verbal and nonverbal; concepts of growth and development; anatomy, physiology, and pathophysiology; and the influence of cultural heritage and family social structure. The data collected during the assessment of the child and family form the basis of all nursing care of the child.

Assessment begins with the admission interview and physical assessment. During this phase, a relationship of trust begins to build between the nurse, the child, and the family caregivers. This relationship forms more quickly when the nurse is sensitive to the cultural background of the family. Careful listening and recording of **subjective data** (data spoken by the child or family) and careful observation and recording of **objective data** (observable by the nurse) are essential to obtain a complete picture.

Nursing Diagnosis

The process of determining a nursing diagnosis begins with the analysis of information (data) gathered during the assessment. A nursing diagnosis then may be made, based on actual or potential health problems that fall within the range of nursing practice. These diagnoses are not medical diagnoses but are based on the individual response to a disease process, condition, or situation. Nursing diagnoses change as the patient's responses change; therefore, they are in a continual state of reevaluation and modification.

Nursing diagnoses are subdivided into three types: actual, risk, and wellness diagnoses. **Actual nursing diagnoses** identify existing health problems. For example, a child who has asthma may have an actual diagnosis stated as *Ineffective Airway Clearance related to increased mucous production as evidenced by dyspnea and wheezing.* This statement identifies a health problem the child actually has (ineffective airway clearance), the factor that contributes to its cause (increased mucous production), and the signs and symptoms. Because of the presence of signs and symptoms of the child's inability to clear the airway effectively, this is an actual nursing diagnosis.

Risk nursing diagnoses, a category that became effective in 1992, identify health problems to which the patient is especially vulnerable. These identify patients at high risk for a particular problem. An example of a risk nursing diagnosis is *Risk for Injury related to uncontrolled muscular activity secondary to seizure.*

Wellness nursing diagnoses identify the potential of a person, family, or community to move from one level of wellness to a higher level. For example, a wellness diagnosis for a family adapting well to the birth of a second child might be *Potential for Enhanced Parenting.*

An approved list of nursing diagnoses was first published by the North American Nursing Diagnosis Association (NANDA) in 1973, and the list has been revised and expanded periodically since then. Currently, there are about 125 approved diagnoses.

Outcome Identification and Planning

To plan nursing care for the child, data must be collected (assessment) and analyzed (nursing diagnosis) and outcomes identified in cooperation with the child and family caregiver. These **outcomes** (goals) should be stated in measurable terms, with a specified time frame. For example, a short-term expected outcome for a child with asthma could be "Child demonstrates use of metered-dose inhaler within 2 days." The goal must be realistic and child-focused. After mutual goal setting has been accomplished, nursing actions are proposed. Although a number of possible diagnoses may be identified, the nurse must review them, rank them by urgency, and select those that require the most immediate attention.

After selecting the goals to accomplish first, the nurse must propose nursing interventions to achieve them. This is the planning aspect of the nursing process. These nursing interventions may be based on clinical experience, knowledge of the health problem, standards of care, standard care plans, or other resources. The interventions should be discussed with the child and family caregiver to determine if they are practical and workable. Proposed interventions are modified to fit the individual child. If standardized care plans are used, they must be individualized to reflect the child's age and developmental level, cog-

nitive level, and family, economic, and cultural influences. Expected outcomes are set with specific measurable criteria and time lines.

Implementation

Implementation is the process of putting the nursing care plan into action. These actions may be independent, dependent, or interdependent. **Independent nursing actions** are actions that may be performed based on the nurse's own clinical judgment—for example, initiating protective skin care for an area that might break down. **Dependent nursing actions** are actions that the nurse performs as a result of a physician's order, such as administering analgesics for pain. **Interdependent nursing actions** are actions that the nurse must work with other health team members to accomplish, such as meal planning with the dietary therapist and teaching breathing exercises with the respiratory therapist.

Evaluation

Evaluation is a vital part of the nursing process—it measures the success or failure of the nursing plan of care. Like assessment, evaluation is an ongoing process. Evaluation is achieved by determining if the identified outcomes have been met. The criteria of the nursing outcomes determine if the interventions were effective. If the goals have not been met in the specified time, or if implementation is unsuccessful, a particular intervention may need to be reassessed and revised. Possibly the outcome criterion is unrealistic and needs to be discarded or adjusted. The child and the family must be assessed to determine progress adequately. Both objective data (measurable) and subjective data (based on responses from the child and family) are used in the evaluation.

CRITICAL PATHWAYS

Concerns about cost containment, quality improvement, and managed care have led to a system of standard guidelines termed **critical pathways** in many facilities. Critical pathways are standard plans of care used to organize and monitor the care provided. They include all aspects of care, such as diagnostic tests, consultations, treatments, activities, procedures, teaching, and discharge planning (Fig. 1-6). Other names for clinical pathways are CareMap, collaborative care plans, case management plans, clinical paths, and multidisciplinary plans. To ensure success, the critical pathways must be a collaborative effort of all disciplines involved; all members of the health team must follow them.

The nursing process is part of the underlying framework of critical pathways. Nursing diagnoses and intermediate and discharge outcomes are necessary to avoid fragmenting care. Documentation of nursing interventions and outcomes is essential to the overall process. The nurse must thoroughly understand the nursing process to achieve ac-

Critical Path for Schoolager With Long-Leg Cast Postfracture

	DAY ONE	DAY TWO
Diagnostic Tests	CBC X-ray left leg	
Assessments	Establish baseline neurovascular status, then neurovascular checks every 2 hours Inspect cast Head, chest, and abdominal assessment for other injuries Assess skin integrity	Neurovascular checks every 4 hours Teach family neurovascular checks Inspect cast Teach family cast inspection Assess skin integrity Teach family skin integrity assessment
Diet	Diet as tolerated	Diet as tolerated Instruct on adding foods rich in protein
Activity	Elevated leg when lying or sitting Start non–weight-bearing crutch walking Initiate safety precautions	Elevated leg when lying or sitting Assess ability to use non–weight-bearing crutch walking for discharge Maintain safety precautions
Medications	Tylenol with codeine for pain as ordered	Tylenol with codeine for pain as ordered Tylenol for pain as ordered
Psychosocial	Assess developmental status Promote self-care (bathing, dressing, grooming, etc.) Provide diversional activities Assist in continuing school work Safety teaching	Instruct on diversional activities for home Instruct family on how to promote self-care Reinforce safety teaching
Discharge Planning	Teach cast care Teach crutch walking Arrange for home tutoring	Provide written instructions and obtain feedback on cast care Provide written instructions and obtain feedback on crutch walking Provide written instructions for home tutoring Include family and child in teaching Arrange for follow-up appointment.

Figure 1-6
A Critical Pathway is an abbreviated form of care plan used by the entire multidisciplinary team. It provides outcome-based guidelines for goal achievement within a designated length of stay.

countability when providing care in a setting where critical pathways are used.

OBSERVATION AND RECORDING

One of the most important parts of nursing care is continuous, careful observation of the patient's behavior and recording those observations in clear, specific terms. Nurses' notes often provide vital clues to a child's condition that health team members depend on for further diagnosis and treatment.

Observation of behavior should include the factors that influenced the behavior and how often the behavior is repeated. Physical behavior as well as emotional and intellec-

tual responses should be noted, considering the child's age and developmental level, the abnormal environment of the health care facility, and whether the child has been hospitalized previously or otherwise separated from family caregivers. It is important to note whether the behavior is consistent or unpredictable, and any apparent reasons for changed behavior.

The Infant

Characteristic behaviors of the healthy infant compared with behaviors that may indicate signs of illness are shown in Table 1-2. The nurse must be cautious when using the type of information shown in such a table, as occasional evidence of one or more of the behaviors may not be significant. Any instance of behavior indicating illness needs to be documented and further evaluated in light of the fre-

TABLE 1-2. Comparison of Observations of an Infant's Physical and Emotional Behavior

Observation	Healthy Activity	Behavior Indicating Illness*
Activity	Constantly active; some infants are more intense and curious than others	Lies quietly; little or no interest in surroundings; may stay in the same position
State of muscular tension	Muscular state is tense; grasp is tight, head is raised when prone, kicks are vigorous When supine, there is a space between the mattress and the infant's back	Lies relaxed with arms and legs straight and lax; makes no attempt to turn or raise head if placed in prone position; does not move about in crib
Constancy of reaction	Shows a constancy in reaction, does not regress in development; peppy and vigorous; interested in food; responds to caregiver's presence or voice	Not as peppy as usual; responds to discomfort and pain in apathetic manner; turns away from food that had once interested; turns head and cries instead of usual response
Behavior indicating pain	Appreciates being picked up Activity is not restlessness Shows activity in every part of body	Cries or protests when handled; seems to want to be left alone. May cry when picked up, but settles down after being held for a time, indicating something hurts when moved Turns head fretfully from side to side; pulls ear or rubs head; turns and rolls constantly, seemingly to try to get away from pain
Cry	Strong, vigorous cry	Weak, feeble cry or whimper High-pitched cry; shrill cry may indicate increased intracranial pressure
Skin color	Healthy tint to skin; nail beds and oral mucosa, conjunctivae, and tongue are reddish-pink	Light-skinned babies may show unusual pallor or blueness around the eyes and nose. All babies may have dark or cyanotic nail beds, pale oral mucosa, conjunctivae, and tongue.
Appetite or feeding pattern	Exhibits an eagerness and impatience to satisfy hunger	May show indifference toward formula; sucks half-heartedly; vomits feeding; habitually regurgitates. May exhibit discomfort after feeding
Bizarre behavior		Any behavior that differs from expected for level of development; unusually good, or passive, when in strange surroundings; responds with rejection to every overture, friendly or otherwise; extremely clinging, never satisfied with amount of attention received

* Any *one* manifestation in itself may not be significant. The important thing is whether this behavior is consistent with this particular child or is a change from previous behavior. The significance depends greatly on the constancy of the behavior.

quency of the behavior as well as the usual behavior of the infant. If the caregiver has indicated in the assessment interview or on further questioning that this behavior is not out of the ordinary for the infant, it may not be indicative of a problem.

The Older Child

Most of the observations in Table 1-2 are valid for the older child as well. In addition, there are a few different or more mature reactions that may indicate an unhealthy state.

COVERING UP FOR PAIN OR DISCOMFORT

Few children get any enjoyment from illness or hospitalization. Going home is usually the child's burning desire, and the child often goes to great lengths to cover up any discomfort. Observing when the child is unaware of being watched helps the nurse determine if the child is showing any signs of pain, such as limping, holding one side of the abdomen, and grimacing. Then the nurse should note what happens when the child realizes he or she is being watched.

Does the child straighten up and say, "I was just kidding around"? This is behavior that should be reported.

EXTREMES OF AGGRESSION OR PASSIVITY

How does this child behave? Is the child aggressive, resisting any and all advances and striking out against playmates or adults? Or is the child passive, accepting everything? Even more important, is this a change in behavior? To know the answers, the nurse must be consistently observant and record the child's behavior.

FAMILY CAREGIVERS

The nurse should get a feeling of the interaction between the child and family caregivers—how they interact may reflect their feelings toward each other. It also may reflect the caregivers' attitude to the situation of illness or to the care that the child is receiving. The behavior of family caregivers may offer insight into the condition of the child, particularly if the child's condition is related to ineffective parenting skills, neglect, or abuse.

COMMUNICATION

Although most people think of communication as an oral or written exchange of words, communication also includes the body language, facial expressions, voice intonations, and emotions behind the words that are exchanged between two or more people. One of the most important aspects of communication is listening to the other person. Listening is more than hearing. It includes "tuning in" to the other person, being sensitive to feelings, and concentrating on what the other person is trying to express. The nurse must be aware of underlying emotions and recognize the effect they have on the communication process. It is also important to clarify statements and feelings expressed by the child or caregiver. A reflective statement may indicate what the nurse believed was expressed. For instance, the nurse might say, "You are worried about Maria's loss of appetite." In this way the speaker may confirm or deny that the nurse has interpreted correctly. The pediatric nurse must be especially skilled in listening to communicate successfully with children and caregivers.

Listening

Listening to another person involves more than simply hearing words. *Attending* (giving the other person physical signs that you are listening) indicates to the speaker that you are listening. Eye contact, a posture of attention, and avoiding distractions are essential to attending. If the speaker feels the listener is not paying attention, all may be lost.

Following, the next step, means encouraging the speaker by staying out of his or her way. Do not stop the speaker by making judgmental statements, giving advice, or reassuring him or her. For instance, "Don't be so down in the dumps" is a judgmental statement that may cause the person to withdraw. "Get up and move around; things are bound to get better" is an example of advice that most often will turn the speaker off. "You're going to be fine before you know it" is an example of reassuring that does not help the person with the problem. A positive response that would be helpful instead of judgmental might be, "You look as though something is bothering you." This gives the person an opportunity to open up and indicates that the listener is tuned in. "Can you tell me what you see as your biggest problem?" gives the speaker encouragement to share his or her worries. "You look as though you feel that things are not going very well" is a description of what the person's body language message means to the listener and offers an invitation for the speaker to share what is on his or her mind.

On the other hand, remember that the speaker may not want to talk at that particular time. Respect those feelings.

In listening to another person, there may be times when the best response is silence to allow the speaker to have room to think and slowly express himself or herself. Observe the other person's body language and expressions and think about what they are communicating. Think about what the other person is saying instead of worrying about what response to give. Focus on the speaker and reflect what he or she has said. "You are worried about the pain you are having" appropriately reflects a speaker who has related that the pain comes and goes and radiates from here to there. This helps clarify that both people are talking about the same thing. "You are frustrated about the pace of your recovery" may help the speaker put his or her feelings into words. At the very least, the speaker can deny or agree that this is an accurate assessment of his or her feelings.

With children, it is often helpful to talk about how a doll, a teddy bear, or another toy is feeling. This enables the child to talk about the toy's fears, which accurately reflect the child's feelings. When the speaker (caregiver or child) uses a "feeling" word, it is helpful for the listener to rephrase what he or she believes the person is saying so that both are using the same frame of reference. For example, if the caregiver says "I'm scared," the nurse could respond, "You're worried about the outcome of your child's surgery." This gives the person an opportunity to affirm that the nurse understands or to clarify further what the concerns are.

Communicating with Children

Nurses are constantly communicating with patients, even though they may be unable to understand the words or respond. Infants evaluate actions, not realizing that nurses who handle them abruptly and hurriedly may be rushed or insecure; these small patients feel only that these nurses are frightening and unloving.

The child who is old enough to distinguish between people (generally after 6 months of age) tends to be frightened of strangers. Sudden, abrupt, or noisy approaches are almost certain to signal danger to the child. The child needs time to evaluate the situation while still secure in the familiar arms of the caregiver. The nurse should not rush the situation but allow time for the child to initiate the relationship. Often the conversation may be started through the child's doll or stuffed animal. The nurse may ask the toy's name and address the toy, or just call it "Dolly," "Teddy," "Puppy," or "Kitty" if the child will not reveal the name. The nurse also may ask the toy how it feels, referring to the part of the body that is the child's problem. For example, "Are you having trouble breathing today, Dolly?"

Distrust of strangers may last through the first 3 or 4 years of life. A casual approach with reluctant children is usually more effective. Children who show rejecting or aggressive behavior are putting up a defense against their own fears, and the behavior should be ignored unless it threatens the child's well-being or that of someone else.

Some nurses have difficulty accepting their own feelings while working with children. Each nurse brings personal feelings, fears, and conflicts to a new situation. Many nurses feel inadequate when beginning relationships with children. Nurses need to be willing to accept the fact that they are also human. A good nurse is self-accepting and self-confident but does not necessarily begin that way; this comes with maturity and insight.

When speaking with small or young children, the nurse should not stand over them and talk down to them but should get down on eye level with them (Fig. 1-7). The best plan is to speak in a slow, clear, positive voice, using simple words. Sentences should be short, and statements or questions should be expressed positively. Choices should be simple and offered only if a choice actually exists. Do not say, "Do you want to take your medicine now?" if there is no other option. Listen to the child's fears and worries; be honest in your answers.

The perceptions of young children are literal. For instance, if the nurse says, "This will only be a little bee sting," children actually visualize being stung by a bee, and that may be traumatic. As a result of this characteristic, the nurse must be careful to use positive explanations in terms that are familiar and nonthreatening to the child.

School-age children are interested in knowing what and why. Explanations that help them understand how equipment works are important to them. These children do not need a complex or detailed explanation; a simple response is best. Children of this age will ask more questions if their curiosity was not satisfied.

It may be challenging to communicate with adolescents. Young teenagers frequently waver between thinking like a child and thinking like an adult. Sometimes the adolescent does not want to reveal much if a parent is present. Teens may need to relate information that they do not wish others to know. A discussion about confidentiality may set the adolescent's concerns at ease. The adolescent needs to know that the nurse will listen attentively in an open-minded, nonjudgmental way.

The adolescent and the family may not view a problem in the same way. If this is the case, the problem may need to be defined more clearly so that an agreement may be reached, if possible. The nurse may be instrumental in assisting with the resolution of disagreements between the family and the adolescent.

Communicating with Family Caregivers

Routine conferences among the nursing staff, physicians, child-life workers, physical therapists, and other personnel concerned with children in the health care facility are helpful in gaining an understanding of child patients. A clearer picture of the child is obtained, his or her behavior is better understood, and an opportunity is presented to consider differing types of treatment and relationships. These outcomes may be rewarding to both the patient and the staff. When appropriate, the family caregivers may be invited to attend, and they may gain valuable insights and understanding. Some health care facilities prefer to hold parent group sessions. In either instance, it is most important that family caregivers are kept well informed about what is going on and what is being planned for their sick child (Fig. 1-8).

Much may be done to make the caregivers feel welcome and important. When a procedure is planned, the caregiver may be told what is going to happen and invited to help,

Figure 1-7
During a conversation with the child, the nurse gets down on eye level and uses easy, positive language. She also may include a favorite toy or doll in the conversation.

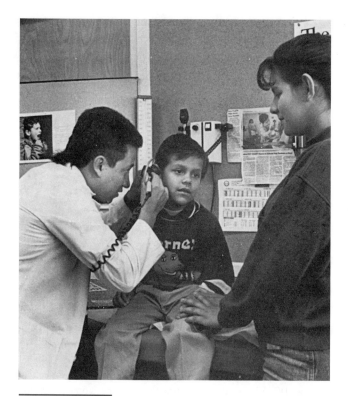

Figure 1-8
During a routine assessment or a more involved procedure, caregivers often find comfort in remaining close to the child and being well informed.

if practical. However, no caregiver who is reluctant to help with or observe a procedure should be urged to stay or made to feel it is a duty that should be fulfilled. Some caregivers are so anxious and apprehensive that they communicate their concern to the child rather than provide support. Attitudes from the caregiver may easily be conveyed to the child, sometimes causing negative reactions from the child. The nurse must be alert for any negative attitudes. Listening and communication skills are extremely important when working with the caregiver. Giving the caregiver time to discuss anxieties and concerns, exploring these problems with the caregiver, and demonstrating genuine caring and concern help ease these feelings. The nurse must remember that part of the nursing role is to be an ambassador of good will to the child and the family.

An older child may feel self-sufficient and may view the family caregiver's presence as being treated "like a baby." However, it is normal to regress during illness, and most children of any age appreciate the presence of a reassuring, self-controlled person during trying, uncomfortable times. The child needs to be able to trust the environment. If, as often happens, the child regresses in handling the overwhelming distress, the presence of a family caregiver may offer support.

Influences on Communication

Verbal and nonverbal communication styles may be influenced by several factors such as family, culture, community, religion, personality, and age. Varying styles of communication may cause conflict and misunderstanding among people. For example, one person may come from a family in which loud yelling is a loving form of self-expression. A second person may come from a family in which issues are calmly or stoically discussed. To the first person, the second person's lack of emotion about issues may seem uncaring. To the second person, the first person's emotional outbursts may seem aggressive and unkind. Another person may handle feelings by becoming quiet and uncommunicative; this, too is a communication style.

These are just a few of the many different styles of communication. The nurse does not need to know all these communication styles but should remember that differences exist. The nurse must first understand his or her own communication style. This helps the nurse realize his or her communication expectations and gain a sense of how he or she may be perceived by others. Only after self-understanding can the nurse distinguish differences in communication styles and understand the ways in which others are attempting to communicate.

■ KEY POINTS

- Many changes have taken place in the care of children in this century. Until the early part of the 20th century, children were treated as miniature adults and were expected to behave that way.

- Progress in medical science has advanced so rapidly and become so sophisticated that many children with chronic or serious conditions are cared for in regionalized centers, creating a need for caring for the family in a "home away from home" atmosphere.

- Healthy People 2000 sets goals for health care with a focus on prevention of illness as the nation approaches the year 2000.

- The role of the nurse has changed to include responsibilities of teacher, adviser, resource person, and researcher as well as caretaker.

- Although its infant mortality rate is improving, the United States still remains behind most of the other industrialized countries. A major cause of this is believed to be lack of or inadequate prenatal care.

- Pediatric nursing consists of preventive care of the well child as much as or more than care of the ill child.

- Nurses are caring for the health of children in many nontraditional settings, including schools, home, and ambulatory care units.

- The nursing process is essential in the problem-solving process necessary to plan nursing care.
- Listening includes really focusing on the speaker to determine what the speaker is trying to communicate.
- Communication with children and their families is a continuous process. The nurse must work to become a skilled communicator to meet the needs of children and their families.

? CRITICAL THINKING

1. Describe sociologic changes that have affected child health concepts and attitudes.
2. Discuss how children were cared for in institutions in the 19th and early 20th centuries. Then describe the hospital care of infants and children in the period immediately after World War I.
3. While working, you overhear an older nurse complaining about family caregivers "being underfoot so much and interfering with patient care." Describe how you would defend open visiting for family caregivers to this person.
4. Discuss contributions that the pediatric nurse can make to the health and care of children.
5. Describe critical pathways and their role in health care.
6. Kathi, a 5-year-old, has just returned from surgery. Her mother is nervously watching the IV line and asks you, "Is that IV running all right?" Give a response that is an example of reflective listening. Explain how reflective listening helps facilitate communication.
7. Vincent is trying to be a "tough" teenager after his football injury. He is scheduled for knee surgery. On entering his room, you notice his eyes are red. What will you say to establish effective communication with him? Role-play with another student as Vincent, or write a possible scenario.

REFERENCES

1. Chiles L. Troubling trends: The health of America's next generation. Washington DC: National Commission to Prevent Infant Mortality, 1990.
2. U.S. Department of Health and Human Services. Healthy People 2000 midcourse review and 1995 revisions. Washington DC: Public Health Service, 1995.

BIBLIOGRAPHY

Ahmann E. Family-centered care: Shifting orientation. Pediatr Nurs 20(2):113–117, 1994.
Broome ME. Advanced practice nursing—commentary on confronting the challenges. Pediatr Nurs 21(1):49–50, 1995.
Burns M, Thornam CB. Broadening the scope of nursing practice: Federal programs for children. Pediatr Nurs 19(6):546–552, 1993.
Cone TE Jr. History of American pediatrics. Boston: Little Brown, 1980.
Craven RF, Hirnle CJ. Fundamentals of nursing, 2d ed. Philadelphia: Lippincott-Raven, 1996.
Harper DC. Advanced nursing practice—changes on the horizon: An interview with Doreen C. Harper. Pediatr Nurs 21(1): 41–42, 1995.
Harvey B. New series of essays on pediatric history. Pediatrics 92(3):467–468, 1993.
Jackson PL. Advanced practice nursing—opportunities and challenges for PNPs. Pediatr Nurse 21(1):43–46, 1995.
Jost KE. Nursing standards for child development. MCN 21: 67–71, 1996.
Pillitteri A. Maternal and child health nursing, 2d ed. Philadelphia: JB Lippincott, 1995.
Totka JP. Exploring the boundaries of pediatric practice: Nurse stories related to relationships. Pediatr Nurs 22(3):191–196, 1996.
Wong DL. Whaley and Wong's nursing care of infants and children, 5th ed. St. Louis: Mosby, 1994.

Chapter 2

The Family and Child

THE FAMILY AS A SOCIAL UNIT
Family Function
Family Structure
Family Factors That Influence Children

CONCEPTS OF CHILD DEVELOPMENT
Sigmund Freud
Erik Erikson
Jean Piaget
Lawrence Kohlberg
Other Theorists

STUDENT OBJECTIVES

On completion of this chapter, the student will be able to:

1. Identify the primary purpose of the family in society.
2. List the functions of the family in relation to children.
3. Describe the process of socialization.
4. Describe how parents influence the psychological and emotional health of a child.
5. Name and discuss the two traditional kinds of family structure.
6. List four factors that have contributed to the growing number of single-parent families.
7. Describe three types of nontraditional families.
8. Describe how children are affected by family size and sibling order.
9. Explain how family relationships and communications are affected by working parents and other parental behaviors.
10. State three factors that influence the way that children react to divorce.
11. List and discuss the six stages of psychosexual development according to Freud.
12. Describe Erikson's theory of psychosocial development.
13. Name the eight stages of Erikson's psychosocial development, and list the developmental tasks in each.
14. Identify and describe the four stages of Piaget's theory of cognitive development.
15. Describe the first stage of the postconventional level of Kohlberg's theory, which usually occurs in adolescence.

KEY TERMS

archetypes	extended family
blended family	growth
cognitive development	id
cohabitation family	libido
communal family	nuclear family
cultural competency	single-parent family
development	socialization
developmental task	stepfamily
ego	sublimation
egocentric	superego

THE FAMILY AS A SOCIAL UNIT

The arrival of a baby alters forever the relationship of a couple and establishes a new social unit—a family—in which all members influence and are influenced by each other. Each subsequent child joining that family continues the process of reshaping the individual members and the family unit. In addition, family members are individually and collectively affected by the larger community around them.

Nursing care of children demands a solid understanding of normal patterns of growth and development—physical, psychological, social, and intellectual (cognitive)—and an awareness of the many factors that influence those patterns. It also demands an appreciation for the uniqueness of each child and each family. For nursing care to be complete and therefore as effective as possible, a child must be considered as a member of a family and a larger community.

Throughout history, family structure has evolved in response to ongoing social and economic changes. Today's families may only faintly resemble the nuclear families of 30 or 40 years ago, in which the father worked outside the home and the mother cared for the children. However, nuclear families in the 1950s and 1960s were far different from the farming families of centuries ago. It is estimated that in 60% to 70% of today's families with school-age children, only one parent lives at home. More than 50% of American women with a child younger than age 1 year work outside the home. Changes such as these create bigger demands on parents and have contributed to the growing demands on public institutions to fill the gaps. "Blended" families or stepfamilies have created other major changes in family structure and interactions within the family. Divorce, abandonment, and delayed childbearing are all contributing factors.

Family Function

The family is civilization's oldest and most basic social unit. The family's primary purpose is to ensure survival of the unit and its individual members and to continue the society and its knowledge, customs, values, and beliefs. It establishes a primary connection with a group responsible for a person until that person becomes independent. Although family structure varies among different cultures, its functions related to children are similar: providing physical care, educating and training children, and protecting children's psychological and emotional health.

PHYSICAL CARE

The family is responsible for meeting each child's basic needs for food, clothing, shelter, and protection from harm, including illness. The work necessary to meet these needs was once clearly divided between mother and father, with the mother providing total care for the child and the father providing the resources that made it possible. These attitudes have changed, so that in a two-parent family, each parent has an opportunity to share in the joys and trials of child care and other aspects of family living. In the single-parent family, all these responsibilities must be assumed by one person.

EDUCATION AND TRAINING

Within the family, a child learns the rules of the society and the culture in which the family lives: its language, values, ethics, and acceptable behaviors. This process, called **socialization**, is accomplished by training and education. The family teaches children acceptable ways of meeting physical needs, such as eating and elimination, and certain skills, such as dressing oneself. The family educates children about relationships with other people inside and outside the family. Children learn what is permitted and approved within their society and what is forbidden.

PSYCHOLOGICAL AND EMOTIONAL HEALTH

Research studies continue to support the importance of early parent–child relationships to emotional adjustment in later life. Even a few hours may constitute a critical period in the emotional bond between parent and child. Although the results of these studies are controversial, it is generally agreed that young children are highly sensitive to psychological influences, and those influences may have long-range effects, either positive or negative.

Within the family, children learn who they are and how their behavior affects other family members. Children observe and imitate the behavior of family members, learning quickly which behaviors are rewarded and which are punished. Participation in a family is a child's only rehearsal for parenthood. How parents treat the child has a powerful influence on how the child will treat future children. Studies have shown that many parents who abuse their children had been abused by their parents as children.

Family Structure

Various traditional and nontraditional family structures exist. The traditional structures that occur in many cultures are the nuclear family and the extended family. Nontraditional variations include the single-parent family, the communal family, the stepfamily, and the gay or lesbian family.

NUCLEAR FAMILY

The **nuclear family** is composed of a man, a woman, and their children (either biologic or adopted) who share a common household (Fig. 2-1). This was once the typical American family structure; now fewer than one third of families in the United States fit this pattern. The nuclear family is a more mobile and independent unit than an extended family but is often part of a network of related nuclear families within close geographic proximity.

EXTENDED FAMILY

Typical of agricultural societies, the **extended family** consists of one or more nuclear families plus other relatives, often crossing generations to include grandparents, aunts, uncles, and cousins. The needs of individual members are subordinate to the needs of the group, and children are considered an economic asset. Grandparents aid in child-rearing, and children learn respect for their elders by observing their parents' behavior toward the older generation.

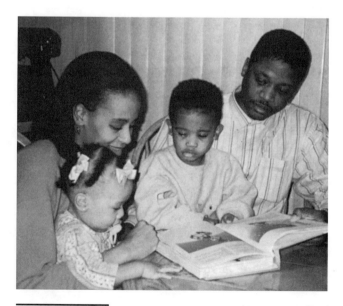

Figure 2-1

The nuclear family is an important and prominent type of family structure in American society. This nuclear family enjoys reading together.

A Personal Glimpse

Living with both my mother and grandmother definitely has its advantages. Even though I had a male figure around me while I was growing up, it wasn't really the same as having a father who would always be there. I lived with my aunt and her family, along with my mother and my grandmother. I had my uncle or cousin to turn to if I needed advice that my mother or my grandmother couldn't give me. However, my uncle wasn't always around, neither was my cousin, so a lot of my questions were left unanswered. Questions that I didn't think anybody else other than a man could answer. I learned a lot of things on my own, whether it was by experience or by asking somebody else.

Things are different now. It's only my mother, my grandmother, and myself. As I grow older, I'm finding that I can open up to the both of them a lot more. There is no reason to keep secrets. I can tell them anything and they understand. Actually, they are a lot more understanding than I thought they would be about certain things. Everyday I'm realizing that I can tell them anything.

People often ask me what it is like not knowing about my father. They ask me if I'm curious about my father. And I say, "Of course I'm curious. Who wouldn't be?" I also tell them that love is a lot stronger than curiosity. I love and care about my mother and grandmother more than anything in this world. No one father could ever give me as much love and devotion as the two of them give me. And I wouldn't give that up for anything.

Juan, age 15 years

SINGLE-PARENT FAMILY

Rising divorce rates, the women's movement, increasing acceptance of children born out of wedlock, and changes in adoption laws reflecting a more liberal attitude toward adoption have combined to produce a growing number of

single-parent families. About 23% of households in the United States are included in this category, and most are headed by women.[1] Although this family situation places a heavy burden on the parent, no conclusive evidence is available to show its effects on children. At some time in their lives, more than 50% of children in the United States may be part of a single-parent family.

COMMUNAL FAMILY

During the early 1960s, increasing numbers of young adults began to challenge the values and traditions of the American social system. One of the results of that challenge was the establishing of communal groups and collectives, or **communal families.** This alternative structure occurs in many settings and may favor either a primitive or a modern lifestyle. Members of a communal family share responsibility for homemaking and childrearing; all children are the collective responsibility of adult members. Not actually a new family structure, the communal family is a variation of the extended family. The number of communal family units has decreased in recent years.

GAY OR LESBIAN FAMILY

In the gay or lesbian family, two people of the same sex live together, bound by formal or informal commitment, with or without children. Children may be the result of a prior heterosexual mating or a product of the foster-child system, adoption, artificial insemination, or surrogacy. Although these families often face complex issues, including discrimination, studies of children in such families show that they are not harmed by membership in this type of family.[2] The children of a gay or lesbian family are no more likely to become homosexual than are children of heterosexual families.

STEPFAMILY OR BLENDED FAMILY

The **stepfamily** is made up of the custodial parent and children and a new spouse. As the divorce rate has climbed, the number of stepfamilies has increased. If both partners in the marriage bring children from a previous marriage into the household, the family is usually termed a **blended family.** The stress that remarriage of the custodial parent places on a child seems to depend in part on the child's age. Initially, there is an increase in the number of problems in children of all ages. However, younger children apparently can form an attachment to the new parent and accept that person in the parenting role better than do adolescents. Adolescents, already engaged in searching for identity and exploring their own sexuality, may view the presence of a nonbiologic parent as an intrusion. When children from each partner's former marriage are brought into the family, the incidence of problems increases. Second marriages often produce children of that union, which contributes to the adjustment problems of the family members. However,

remarriage may provide the stability of a two-parent family, which may offer additional resources for the child. Each family is unique and has its own set of challenges and advantages.

COHABITATION FAMILY

In the nuclear family, the parents are married; in the **cohabitation family,** the man and woman are not married. The children in this family may be children of earlier unions or they may be a result of this union. Although these families may be longlasting and may lead to marriage, they tend to be less stable, with relationships subject to change. This leads to insecurity for the children, especially when the adult members of the household change periodically.

Family Factors That Influence Children

FAMILY SIZE

The number of children in the family has a significant impact on family interactions. The smaller the family, the more time there is for individual attention to each child. Children in small families, particularly only children, often spend more time with adults and therefore relate better with them than with their peers. Only children tend to be more advanced in language development and intellectual achievement.

Understandably, a large family emphasizes the group more than the child. There is greater interdependence among these children and less dependence on the parents (Fig. 2-2). Less time is available for parental attention to each child.

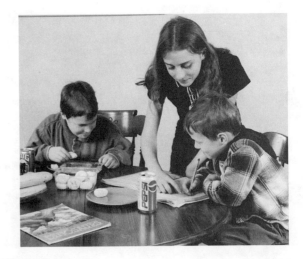

Figure 2-2

Children from large families learn to care for each other. Many older children are expected to help with homework and prepare afterschool snacks.

SIBLING ORDER AND SEX

Whether a child is the firstborn, a middle child, or the youngest also makes a difference in the child's relationships and behavior. Firstborn children command a great deal of attention from parents and grandparents and also are affected by their parents' inexperience, anxieties, and uncertainties. Often the parents' expectations for the oldest child are greater than for subsequent children. Generally, firstborn children are greater achievers than their siblings.

With second and subsequent children, parents tend to be more relaxed and permissive. These children are likely to be more relaxed and are slower to develop language skills. They often identify more with peers than with parents.

Sexual identity in relation to siblings also affects a child's development. Girls raised with older brothers tend to have more male-associated interests than girls raised with older sisters. Boys raised with older brothers tend to be more aggressive than boys who have older sisters.[3]

PARENTAL BEHAVIOR

Many factors have contributed to the change in the traditional mother-at-home, father-at-work image of the American family (Fig. 2-3). Sixty-five percent of American mothers of children younger than age 18 years work outside the home. Some mothers work because they are the family's only source of income, others because the family's economic status demands a second income, and still others because the woman's career is highly valued. More than half of all children between ages 3 and 5 years spend part of their day being cared for by someone other than their parent.

Many factors contribute to the trend for families to spend less time together. Both parents may work; the children participate in many school activities; family members watch television rather than talking together at mealtime, or eat fast food or individual meals without sitting down

Figure 2-3
In some American families, traditional roles are being reversed. The father cares for the children, while the mother is at work.

together as a family; there is emphasis on the acquisition of material goods rather than the development of relationships. All these factors contribute to a breakdown in family communication, and they are typical of many families. Their impact on today's children, the parents of tomorrow, is unknown.

DIVORCE

From 1970 to 1980, the number of divorces increased every year. Although there has been a slight decrease in this number in recent years, more than 1 million children younger than age 18 years have been involved in a divorce each year. Although obviously these children are affected, it is difficult to determine the exact extent of the damage. Children whose lives were seriously disrupted before a divorce may feel relieved, at least initially, when the situation is resolved. Others who were unaware of parental conflict and felt that their lives were happy may feel frightened and abandoned. All these emotions depend on the children involved, their ages, and the kind of care and relationships they experience with their parents after the divorce.

Children may go through many emotions when a divorce occurs. Feelings of grief, anger, rejection, and self-worthlessness are common. These emotions may follow the children for years, even into adulthood, even though they may understand the reason for the divorce. In addition, the parents, either custodial or noncustodial, may try to influence the child's thinking about the other parent, placing the child in an emotional trap. If the noncustodial parent does not keep in regular contact with the child, feelings of rejection may be overwhelming. The child often desperately wants a sign of that parent's continuing love.

CULTURE

Each child is the product of a family, a culture, and a community. In some cultures, family life is gentle, permissive, and loving; in others, unquestioning obedience is demanded and pain and hardship are to be stoically endured. The child may be from a cultural group that places a high value on children, giving them lots of attention from many relatives and friends, or the child may be from a group that has taught the child that from early childhood one must fend for oneself.

Health beliefs and practices of the family are also determined by culture. Respect for a child's cultural heritage and individuality is an essential part of nursing care. To plan culturally appropriate and acceptable care, nurses need to understand the health practices and lifestyle of families from various cultures. Rather than memorizing a list of generalized facts regarding different cultures, it is more useful for the nurse to develop **cultural competency**, the capacity to work effectively with people by integrating the elements of their culture into nursing care.[4] To develop cultural competency, the nurse must first understand cultural influences on his or her life. The nurse must recognize surface cultural influences (eg, language, food, clothing), as well as hidden cultural influences (eg, communication styles, beliefs, attitudes, values, perceptions). Then the nurse may recognize and accept the different attitudes, behaviors, and values of another person's culture.

Integrating cultural attitudes toward food, cleanliness, respect, and freedom are of utmost importance. The nurse must be especially sensitive to the fears of the child who is separated from his or her own culture for the first time and finds the food, language, people, and surroundings of the health care facility totally alien. Cultural competency promotes cooperation from the child and family and minimizes frustration. These factors are essential in restoring health so that the child may once again be a functioning part of the family and the community, whatever the cultural background.

CONCEPTS OF CHILD DEVELOPMENT

Growth and development refers to the total growth of the child from birth toward maturity. **Growth** is the physical increase in size and appearance of the body caused by increasing numbers of new cells. **Development** is the progressive change in the child's maturation. **Developmental tasks** are basic achievements associated with each stage of development. These tasks must be mastered to move successfully to the next developmental stage. Developmental tasks must be completed successfully at each stage for a person to achieve maturity.

How a helpless infant grows and develops into a fully functioning independent adult has fascinated scientists for years. Four pioneering researchers in this area whose theories are widely accepted are Sigmund Freud, Erik Erikson, Jean Piaget, and Lawrence Kohlberg (Table 2-1). Their theories present human development as a series of overlapping stages that occur in predictable patterns. These stages are only approximations of what is likely to happen in children at various ages, and each child's development may differ from these stages.

Sigmund Freud

Most modern psychologists base their understanding of children at least partly on the work of Sigmund Freud. His theories are concerned primarily with the **libido** (sexual drive or development). Although Freud did not study children, his work focused on childhood development as a cause of later conflict. Freud believed that a child who did not adequately resolve a particular stage of development would have a fixation (compulsion) that correlated with that stage. Freud described three levels of consciousness: the **id**, which controls physical need and instincts of the

body; the **ego**, the conscious self, which controls the pleasure principle of the id by delaying the instincts until an appropriate time; and the **superego**, the conscience or parental value system. These consciousness levels interact to check behavior and balance each other. The psychosexual stages in Freud's theory are the oral, anal, phallic, latency, and genital stages of development.

ORAL STAGE (AGES 0–2 YEARS)

The newborn first relates almost entirely to the mother (or someone taking a motherly role), and the first experiences with body satisfaction come through the mouth. This is true not only of sucking but also of making noises, crying, and breathing. It is through the mouth that the baby expresses needs and finds satisfaction and thus begins to make sense of the world.

ANAL STAGE (AGES 2–3 YEARS)

This stage is the child's first encounter with the serious need to learn self-control and to take responsibility. Toilet training looms large in the minds of many people as an important phase in childhood. Because elimination is one of the child's first experiences of creativity, it represents the beginnings of the desire to mold and control the environment—the "mudpie period" in the child's life.

The child has pride in the product created. Cleanliness and this natural pride do not always go together, so it may be necessary to help direct this pride and interest into more acceptable behaviors. Playing with such materials as modeling clay, crayons, and dough helps put the child's natural interests to good use, a process called **sublimation**.

PHALLIC (INFANT GENITAL) STAGE (AGES 3–6 YEARS)

It is only natural that interest moves to the genital area as a source of pride and curiosity. To the child's mind, this area constitutes the difference between boys and girls, a difference that the child is beginning to be aware of socially. The superego begins to develop during this stage, and by 10 years of age (the end of the latency stage), it is well established.

At about this time, a boy begins to take pride in being a male and a girl in being a female. In many families, a new brother or sister arrives at about this time, arousing the child's natural interest in human origins.

This stage is when the child begins to understand what it means to be a boy or a girl. The parents' reaction to the child's genital exploration may determine whether the child learns to feel satisfied with himself or herself as a sexual being or is laden with feelings of guilt and dissatisfaction throughout life.

Freud hypothesized that this awareness of genital differences leads to a time of conflict in the child's emotional relationships with parents. The conflict occurs between at-

TABLE 2-1. Comparative Summary of Theories of Freud, Erikson, Piaget, and Kohlberg

Age (years)	Stage	Freud (Psychosexual Development)	Erikson (Psychosocial Development)	Piaget (Intellectual Development)	Kohlberg (Moral Development)
1	Infancy	Oral Stage	Trust vs. Mistrust	Sensorimotor Phase	Stage 0—Do what pleases me
2–3	Toddlerhood	Anal Stage	Autonomy vs. Shame		Preconventional Level Stage 1—Avoid punishment
4–6	Preschool (early childhood)	Phallic (infant genital) Stage; Oedipal Stage	Initiative vs. Guilt	Preoperational Phase	Preconventional Level Stage 2—Do what benefits me
7–12	School-Age (middle childhood)	Latency Stage	Industry vs. Inferiority	Concrete Operational Phase	Conventional level Stage 3 (Age 7–10)—Avoid disapproval Stage 4 (Age 10–12)—Do duty, obey laws
13–18	Adolescence	Genital Stage (puberty)	Identity vs. Identity Confusion	Formal Operational Phase	Postconventional Level Stage 5 (Age 13)—Maintain respect of others Stage 6 (Age 15)—Implement personal principles

tachment to and imitation of the parent of the same sex and the appeal of the other parent. The boy who for years has depended on his mother for all his emotional and physical needs is now confronted by his desire to be a man (Oedipus complex). The girl, who has imitated her mother, now finds her father a real attraction (Electra complex). This is not only social but sexual; it is through contact with parents that the child learns to relate to the opposite sex. The child learns the interests, attitudes, concerns, and wishes of the opposite sex.

LATENCY STAGE (AGES 6–10 YEARS)

The latency stage is the time of primary schooling, when the child is preparing for adult life but must await maturity to exercise initiative in adult living. It is the time when the child's sense of moral responsibility (the superego) is built, based on what has been taught through the parents' words and actions.

When placed in an unfamiliar setting, children in this stage may become confused because they do not know what is expected of them. They need the sense of security that

comes from approval and praise and usually respond favorably to a brief explanation of "how we do things here."

GENITAL STAGE (AGES 11–13 YEARS)

Physical puberty is occurring at an increasingly early age, and social puberty occurs even earlier, largely due to the influence of sexual frankness on television and in movies and the print media. At puberty, all the child's earlier learning is concentrated on the powerful biologic drive, finding and relating to a mate. In earlier societies, mating and forming a family occurred at a young age. Our society delays mating for many years after puberty, creating a time of confusion and turmoil during which biologic readiness must take second place to educational and economic goals. This is a sensitive period when privacy is important and great uncertainty exists about relating to any members of the opposite sex.

Erik Erikson

Building on Freud's theories, Erikson described human psychosocial development as a series of tasks or crises. This development depends on a self-healing process within the

TABLE 2-2. Child and Parent Developmental Tasks According to Erikson

Developmental Level	Basic Task	Stage of Parental Development	Parental Task
Infant	Trust	Learning to recognize and interpret infant's cues	To interpret cues and respond positively to the infant's needs; hold, cuddle, and talk to infant
Toddler	Autonomy	Learning to accept child's need for self-mastery	To accept child's growing need for freedom while setting consistent, realistic limits; offer support and understanding when separation anxiety occurs
Preschooler	Initiative	Learning to allow child to explore surrounding environment	To allow independent development while modeling necessary standards; generously praise child's endeavors to build child's self-esteem
School-age	Industry	Learning to accept rejection without deserting	To accept child's successes and defeats, assuring child of acceptance to be there when needed without intruding unnecessarily
Adolescent	Identity	Learning to build a new life, supporting the emergence of the adolescent as a individual	To be available when adolescent feels need; provide examples of positive moral values, keep communication channels open; adjust to changing family roles and relationships during and after the adolescent's struggle to establish an identity

person that helps counterbalance the stresses created by natural and accidental crises. The self-healing process is delayed by any major crisis, such as hospitalization, which interrupts normal development. Interruptions may cause regression to an earlier stage, such as the older child who begins to wet the bed when hospitalized. Erikson commented that "children 'fall apart' repeatedly, and unlike Humpty Dumpty, grow together again," if they are given time and sympathy and are not interfered with.[5]

Erikson formulated a series of eight developmental tasks or crises, the first five of which pertain to children and youth. To present a complete view of Erikson's theory, all eight tasks are presented here. In each, the person must master the central problem before moving on to the next one. Each holds positive and negative counterparts, and each of the first five implies new developmental tasks for parents (Table 2-2).

TRUST VERSUS MISTRUST (AGES 0–1 YEAR)

The infant has no way to control the world other than crying for help and hoping for rescue. During the first year, the child learns whether the world can be trusted to give love and concern or only frustration, fear, and despair. The infant who is fed on demand learns to trust that cries communicating need will be answered. The baby fed according to the nurse or caregiver's schedule does not understand the importance of routine but only that these cries may go unanswered.

AUTONOMY VERSUS DOUBT AND SHAME (AGES 1–3 YEARS)

Even the smallest child wants to feel in control and needs to learn to perform tasks independently, even when this takes a long time or makes a mess. The toddler gains reassurance from self-feeding, from crawling or walking alone where it is safe, and from being free to handle materials and learn about things in the environment.

A toddler exploring the environment begins to explore and learn about his or her body, too. If caregivers react appropriately to this normal behavior, the child will gain self-respect and pride. If, however, they shame the child for responding to this natural curiosity, the belief that somehow the body is dirty, nasty, and bad may develop and remain.

INITIATIVE VERSUS GUILT (AGES 3–6 YEARS)

During this period, the child engages in active, assertive play. Steadily improving physical coordination and expanding social skills encourage "showing off" to gain adult attention and, the child hopes, approval. The preschool child, still self-centered, plays alone, although in the company of other children; interaction comes later. These children want to know what the rules are and enjoy "being good" and the adult approval that action gains. During this time, the child develops a conscience and accepts punishment for doing wrong because it relieves feelings of guilt.

Children in this phase of development generally do not have a concept of time and the changes it imposes on nursing shifts. Explaining that it is time for a nurse to go home to his or her own family may help an unhappy child realize that the nurse is not leaving because of any negative behavior of the child's. The child needs a familiar frame of reference to understand when something is going to happen. For example, the parent or caregiver may say, "I will be back when your lunch comes" or "I will be back when the cartoons come on TV."

INDUSTRY VERSUS INFERIORITY (AGES 6–12 YEARS)

Children begin to seek achievement in this phase. They learn to interact with others and, sometimes, to compete with them. They like activities they can follow through to completion and tangible results.

Competition is healthy as long as the standards are not so high that the child feels there is no chance of winning. Praise, not criticism, helps the child to build self-esteem and avoid feelings of inferiority. It is important to emphasize that everyone is a unique person and deserves to be appreciated for his or her own special qualities.

IDENTITY VERSUS IDENTITY CONFUSION (AGES 12–18 YEARS)

Adolescents are confronted by marked physical and emotional changes and the knowledge that soon they will be responsible for their own lives. The adolescent develops a sense of being an independent person with unique ideals and goals and may feel that parents, caregivers, and other adults refuse to grant that independence. Adolescents may break rules just to prove that they can. Stress, anxiety, and mood swings are typical of this phase. Relationships with peers are more important than ever.

INTIMACY VERSUS ISOLATION (EARLY ADULTHOOD)

This is the period during which the person tries to establish intimate personal relationships with friends and an intimate love relationship with one person. Difficulty in establishing intimacy results in feelings of isolation.

GENERATIVITY VERSUS SELF-ABSORPTION (YOUNG AND MIDDLE ADULTHOOD)

For many people, this phase means marriage and family, but for others it may mean fulfillment in some other way—a professional or business career or a religious vocation. The person who does not find this fulfillment becomes self-absorbed and ceases to develop socially.

EGO INTEGRITY VERSUS DESPAIR (OLD AGE)

This final phase is the least understood of all, for it means finding satisfaction with oneself, one's achievements, and one's present condition, without regret for the past or fear for the future.

Jean Piaget

Freud and Erikson studied psychosexual and psychosocial development; Piaget brought new insight into **cognitive** (intellectual) **development**—how a child learns and develops that quality called intelligence. He described intellectual development as a sequence of four principal stages, each made up of several substages.[6] All children move through these stages in the same order, but each moves at his or her own pace.

SENSORIMOTOR PHASE (AGES 0–2 YEARS)

The newborn behaves at a sensorimotor level linked entirely to desires for physical satisfaction. The newborn feels, hears, sees, tastes, and smells countless new things and moves in an apparently random way. Purposeful activities are controlled by reflexive responses to the environment. For example, while nursing, the newborn gazes intently at the mother's face, grasps her finger, smells the nipple, and tastes the milk, thus involving all senses.

As the infant grows, an understanding of cause and effect develops. When random arm motions strike the string of bells stretched across the crib, the newborn hears the sound that is made and eventually can manipulate the arms deliberately to make the bells ring.

In the same way, newborns cannot understand words or even the tone of voice, but only through hearing conversation directed to them can they pick out sounds and begin to understand. As the infant produces verbal noises, the responses of those nearby are encouraging and eventually help the infant learn to talk.

PREOPERATIONAL PHASE (AGES 2–7 YEARS)

The child in this phase of development is **egocentric**; that is, he or she cannot look at something from another's point of view. The child's interpretation of the world is from a self-centered point of view and in terms of what is seen, heard, or otherwise experienced directly.

This child has no concept of quantity; if it looks like more, it *is* more. Four ounces of juice poured into two glasses looks like more than four ounces in one glass. A sense of time is not yet developed, and thus the preschooler or early school-age child cannot always tell whether something happened a day ago, a week ago, or a year ago.

CONCRETE OPERATIONS (AGES 7–11 YEARS)

During this stage, children develop the ability to begin problem solving in a concrete, systematic way. They can classify and organize information about their environment, and they begin to understand that volume or weight may remain the same even though the appearance changes, unlike in the preoperational stage. These children can consider another's point of view and can deal simultaneously with more than one aspect of a situation.

FORMAL OPERATIONS (AGES 12–15 YEARS)

The adolescent is capable of dealing with ideas, abstract concepts described only in words or symbols. The person of this age begins to understand jokes based on double meanings and enjoys reading and discussing theories and philosophies. Adolescents can observe and then draw logical conclusions from their observations.

Lawrence Kohlberg

Each of the theorists focuses on one element in the development of children. Kohlberg's theory is about the development of moral reasoning in children. Moral development closely follows cognitive development because reasoning and abstract thinking (the ability to conceptualize an idea without physical representation) are necessary to make moral judgments. Kohlberg's theory is divided into three levels with two or three stages in each level.

PRECONVENTIONAL LEVEL (PREMORAL LEVEL)

During the first 2 years (stage 0), there is no moral sensitivity. This is a time of egocentricity; decisions are made with regard only to what pleases the child or makes him or her feel good, and what displeases or hurts the child. The child is not aware of how his or her behavior may affect others. The child simply reacts to pleasure with love and hurtful experiences with anger.

In stage 1, punishment and obedience orientation (ages 2–3 years), the child determines right or wrong by the physical consequence of a particular act. The child simply obeys the person in power with no understanding of the underlying moral principle. For children of this age, if they get punished for doing something, then it is wrong; if they do not get punished, it is right.

In stage 2, naïve instrumental self-indulgence (ages 4–7 years), the child views a specific act as right if it satisfies his or her needs. Children follow the rules to benefit themselves. They think, "I'll do something for you if you'll do something for me" and, on the other hand, "If you do something bad to me, I'll do something bad to you." This is basically the attitude of "an eye for an eye."

CONVENTIONAL LEVEL

As concrete operational thought develops, children can engage in moral reasoning. School-age children become aware of the feelings of others. Living up to expectations is a primary concern regardless of the consequences.

In stage 3, "good-boy" orientation (ages 7–10 years), being "nice" is very important. Children want to avoid a guilty conscience. Pleasing others is very important.

In stage 4, law and order orientation (ages 10–12 years), showing respect to others, obeying the rules, and maintaining social order is the desired behavior. "Right" is defined as something that finds favor with family, teachers, and friends. "Wrong" is symbolized by broken relationships.

POSTCONVENTIONAL LEVEL (PRINCIPLED LEVEL)

By adolescence, the child usually achieves Piaget's formal operational stage. For the postconventional level to be attained, the adolescent must have attained the formal operational stage. As a result, many persons do not reach this level.

In stage 5, social contract orientation (ages 13–18 years), personal standards and rights are defined by culturally accepted values. A person's rights must not be violated for the welfare of the group. The end no longer justifies the means. Laws are for mutual good, cooperation, and development.

Stage 6, personal principles, is not attained very frequently. The person who reaches this level does what he or she thinks is right without regard for legal restrictions, the cost to self, or the views of others. Because of this person's deep respect for life, he or she would not do anything that would intentionally harm him or herself or another.

Other Theorists

Freud, Erikson, Piaget, and Kohlberg are only four of the many researchers who have studied the development of children and families. During the 1940s and 1950s, Arnold Gesell studied many infants and talked with their parents concerning children's behavior. From his studies emerged a series of developmental landmarks that are still considered valid and the observation that children progress through a series of "easy" and "difficult" phases as they develop. For example, he labeled one period the "terrible twos," the time when a toddler begins to assert new mobility and coordination to gain parental attention, even if the attention is unfavorable. Knowing that these cycles are normal makes it easier for parents to cope.

Carl Jung's contribution to the study of child growth and development focused on the inner sequence of events that shape the personality. He emphasized that human development follows predetermined patterns called **archetypes**. These archetypes replace the instinctive behavior present in other animals. Interaction of the archetypes with the outside environment is evident throughout human life. For example, a normal child learns to suck, crawl, walk, and talk without any instruction, but the details of how the child does these things come from observation and imitation of others.

Jung believed that the first 3 years of a child's life are spent in coordinating experiences and learning to make a conscious personality, a distinct person who is separate from the rest of the environment. In the following years, the child learns to make sense of the environment by associating new discoveries to a general approach to the world. Dreams and nightmares help express developments of the personality that for some reason do not find a consciousoutlet.

Jung points out that what happens to a child is not so critical to the child's development as the responses to these happenings. A hospital experience may permanently scar a child's personality if the child's natural feeling of terror is overlooked. It may be accepted and even become a point of pride, however, if carried out in an atmosphere of assurance and support of the child's emotional concern and the need for love and acceptance.

The interaction between inner development and the environment is particularly clear in studies of young children who have been deprived in some way. John Bowlby's studies of children who were not held or loved and Bruno Bettelheim's studies of children given good physical care but little or no emotional satisfaction indicate how vital psychological interaction is.

In recent years, the theories of Erikson, Piaget, and Kohlberg have been criticized for being gender specific to males and culturally specific to Caucasians. In response, several theorists have conducted research on the growth and development of females and varying ethnic groups. Most notably, Carol Gilligan researched the moral development of males and females, and Patricia Green sought to construct a "truly universal theory of development through the empirical and theoretical understanding of cultural diversity."[7]

■ KEY POINTS

- The family is the basic social unit. It provides for survival and teaches the knowledge, customs, values, and beliefs of the family's culture.

- Mobility, changing attitudes about children born out of wedlock and about divorce, women working outside the home, and changes in adoption laws have all contributed to an increase in single-parent families.

- Family size and the child's birth position in the family affect the child's development.

- A child's growth and development follows a pattern that is similar for all children.

- Erikson's theory of psychosocial development sets out tasks that the child must successfully complete before going on to the next stage.

- Cognitive and moral development flow along together because reasoning is necessary for more advanced moral development.

 CRITICAL THINKING

1. Describe changes in family structure that have occurred since the middle of the 20th century.
2. Freud's latency stage, Erikson's industry stage, Piaget's concrete operational stage, and Kohlberg's conventional level all involve the early elementary years. Compare the four psychologists' interpretations of these stages, pointing out similarities.
3. The developmental task identified by Erikson for the first stage of life is trust. Discuss why successful accomplishment of this task is essential to the person's future happiness and adjustment.
4. Ask your classmates how many children there were in their family as they grew up, the sex of their siblings, and where they ranked in birth order. Ask them how they believe these factors affected their development and academic success. Ask for concrete examples of why they feel this way.
5. Using this information, present a written or oral discussion of the conclusions you could make about the effect that sibling number, birth order, and sex had on the development of a given group of people.

REFERENCES

1. United States Bureau of Census. Statistical abstract of the United States: 1990, 110th ed. Washington DC: Superintendent of Documents, 1990.
2. Gottman J. Children of gay and lesbian parents. In Bozett FW, Sussman M, eds. Homosexuality and family relations. New York: Harrington Park, 1990.
3. Craig G. Human development, 6th ed. Englewood Cliffs, NJ: Prentice-Hall, 1992.
4. Snow C. Cultural sensitivity workshop. Philadelphia: Nationality Service Council, United Way, 1996.
5. Erikson EH, Senn MJE. Symposium on the healthy personality. New York: Macy Foundation, 1958.
6. Piaget J. The language and thought of the child. Cleveland: World Publishing, 1967.
7. Cocking RR, Greenfield PM, eds. Cross-cultural roots of minority child development. Hillside, NJ: Lawrence Erlbaum Associates, 1994.

BIBLIOGRAPHY

Bowlby J. Attachment. New York: Basic Books, 1969.
Erikson EH. Childhood and society, 2d ed. New York: Norton, 1963.
Gilligan C. In a different voice. Cambridge, Mass.: Howard University Press, 1982.
Kalman N, Waughfield CG. Mental health concepts, 2d ed. Albany: Delmar, 1987.
Schuster C, Ashburn S. The process of human development, 3d ed. Philadelphia: JB Lippincott, 1992.
Wadsworth BJ. Piaget's theory of cognitive and affective development. New York: Longman, 1984.

Chapter 3

Care of the Ill Child

PHYSICAL CARE OF THE ILL CHILD
Assessment of Vital Signs and Growth
Assessment of Cardiovascular and Respiratory Status
Neurologic Assessment
Regulation of Body Temperature
Therapeutic Application of Cold
Therapeutic Application of Heat
Assisting With Diagnostic and Treatment Procedures

MEDICATION ADMINISTRATION
Computing Dosages

Oral Medication
Intramuscular Medication
Other Routes of Medication Administration

INTRAVENOUS THERAPY
Fundamentals of Fluid Balance
Intravenous Fluid Administration
Intravenous Medication
Intravenous Sites
Infusion Control

STUDENT OBJECTIVES

On completion of this chapter, the student will be able to:

1. List the types of patients on whom a rectal temperature should not be taken.
2. Identify the five types of respiratory retractions and the location of each.
3. Name four methods of obtaining blood pressure.
4. State the purpose of pulse oximetry.
5. Identify the purpose of using the Glasgow coma scale for neurologic assessment.
6. List four methods of reducing fever in a child.
7. Identify four ways that pathogens are transmitted, and give an example of each.
8. Identify the role that handwashing plays in infection control.
9. Identify the five "rights" of medication administration.
10. Identify the muscle preferred for intramuscular injections in the infant.
11. State the reason that a pediatric intravenous set-up has a burette chamber in the line.

KEY TERMS

acid–base balance	hyperalimentation
acidosis	induration
alkalosis	interstitial fluid
azotemia	intracellular fluid
body surface area method	intravascular fluid
electrolytes	total parenteral nutrition
extracellular fluid	tympanic membrane sensor
extravasation	West nomogram
homeostasis	

Caring for children in a pediatric setting varies greatly from caring for adults. The nurse must know the growth and development characteristics of each age level, understand the relationship of children and their caregivers, and know the modifications of nursing procedures that are necessary in caring for children. Most important, the nurse must remember that children should never be viewed as "miniature adults." Every procedure, including assessment of temperature and pulse, fever reduction, medication administration, and preparation for surgery, requires a keen awareness of the specific needs of the child undergoing the procedure.

PHYSICAL CARE OF THE ILL CHILD

Physical care of the ill child requires a wide variety of nursing skills and includes ongoing and continuous assessment of vital signs and specific system functioning, regulation of body temperature, therapeutic application of heat and cold, and assistance in medical procedures and diagnostic tests. Understanding and respecting a child's developmental age and stage, as described in Chapter 2, is an essential component of all these skills. Using this information, the nurse can tailor procedures and teaching to meet the needs of these young patients and their families.

Assessment of Vital Signs and Growth

Assessment of the child's vital signs is an essential part of the admission procedure. The results of the initial assessment serve as a baseline for determining the child's progress.

TEMPERATURE

The method of measuring a child's temperature commonly is set by the policy of the pediatric unit. The temperature can be measured by oral, rectal, axillary, or tympanic method. Temperatures are recorded in Celsius or Fahren-

heit according to the policy of the health care facility. Any deviation from the normal range of temperature should be reported. Temperatures vary with the method by which they are taken; thus, it is important to record the route of temperature measurement along with the measured temperature.

Mercury or electronic thermometers may be used to measure temperature by the oral, rectal, and axillary routes. Electronic thermometers have oral and rectal probes. The nurse should be careful to select the correct probe when using the thermometer. In pediatrics, oral temperatures usually are taken only on children older than 4 to 6 years of age who are conscious and cooperative. Oral thermometers should be placed in the side of the child's mouth. The child should not be left unattended while any temperature is being taken (Fig. 3-1).

Rectal temperatures commonly are measured in infants and children younger than 4 to 6 years of age. They are not desirable in the newborn because of the danger of irritation to the rectal mucosa. When a rectal temperature is taken, the bulb end should be lubricated with a water-soluble lubricant. The infant is placed in a prone position, the buttocks are gently separated with one hand, and the thermometer is inserted gently about ¼" to ½" into the rectum. If any resistance is felt, the nurse should remove the thermometer immediately, take the temperature by some other method, and notify the physician about the resistance. The nurse must keep one hand on the child's buttocks and the other on the thermometer during the entire time the rectal thermometer is in place. A mercury thermometer is left in place for 3 or 4 minutes. An electronic thermometer is removed as soon as it signals that the temperature has been recorded.

Axillary temperatures are taken on newborns and on infants and children with diarrhea, or when a rectal temperature is contraindicated. When taking an axillary tem-

Figure 3-1
The nurse stays with the child while she takes his temperature with an electronic oral thermometer.

Figure 3-2
Taking an axillary temperature on a newborn.

TABLE 3-1. Normal Pulse Ranges in Children (bpm)

Age	Normal Range	Average
0–24 hr	70–170 bpm	120 bpm
1–7 d	100–180 bpm	140 bpm
1 mo	110–188 bpm	160 bpm
1 mo–1 y	80–180 bpm	120–130 bpm
2 y	80–140 bpm	110 bpm
4 y	80–120 bpm	100 bpm
6 y	70–115 bpm	100 bpm
10 y	70–110 bpm	90 bpm
12–14 y	60–110 bpm	85–90 bpm
14–18 y	50–95 bpm	70–75 bpm

bpm, beats per minute

perature on an infant or child, the nurse must be certain to place the bulb of the thermometer well into the armpit, bringing the child's arm down close to the body (Fig. 3-2). The nurse must check to see that there is skin-to-skin contact and that no clothing is in the way. The thermometer is left in place for 10 minutes or until the electronic thermometer signals.

Tympanic membrane sensors have been adopted by an increasing number of facilities (Fig. 3-3). The tympanic thermometer records the temperature rapidly (registering in about 2 seconds) and is noninvasive, causing little disturbance to the child. A temperature often can be obtained without awakening a sleeping infant or child. Tympanic thermometers are used according to the manufacturer's directions and the facility's policy. A disposable speculum is used for each child.

PULSE

Counting an apical rate is the preferred method to determine the pulse in an infant or young child. The nurse should try to accomplish this while the child is quiet. Approaching the child in a soothing, calm, quiet manner is helpful. The apical pulse should be counted before the child is disturbed for other procedures. A child can be held on the caregiver's lap for security for the full minute that the pulse is counted. The stethoscope is placed between the child's left nipple and sternum. A radial pulse may be taken on an older child. This pulse may be counted for 30 seconds and multiplied by two. If the pulse is unusual in quality, rate, or rhythm, it should be counted for a full minute. Any rate that deviates from the normal rate should be reported. Pulse rates vary with age, from 100 to 180 beats per minute for a neonate (birth to 30 days old) to 50 to 95 beats per minute for the 14- to 18-year-old adolescent (Table 3-1).

RESPIRATIONS

Respirations of an infant or young child also must be counted during a quiet time. The child can be observed while lying or sitting quietly. Infants are abdominal breathers; therefore, the movement of the infant's abdomen is observed to count respirations. The older child's chest can be observed much as an adult's would be. The infant's respirations must be counted for a full minute because of normal irregularity. The chest of the infant or young child must be observed for retractions that indicate respiratory

Figure 3-3
Today many facilities use a tympanic thermometer sensor to take the child's temperature.

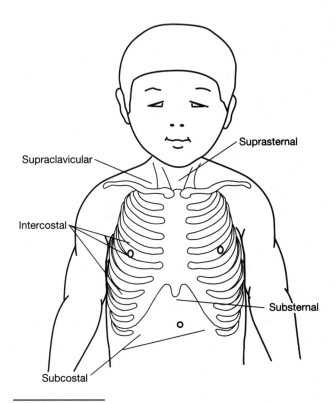

Figure 3-4
Sites of respiratory retraction.

For any method of measuring blood pressure, allow the child to handle the equipment. Use terminology appropriate to the child's age. A preschool or young school-age child may want to use equipment to take the blood pressure of a doll or stuffed animal.

Auscultation

1. Place the correct size of cuff on the infant's or child's bare arm.
2. Locate the artery by palpating the antecubital fossa.
3. Inflate the cuff until radial pulse disappears, or about 30 mmHg above expected systolic reading.
4. Place stethoscope lightly over the artery and slowly release air until pulse is heard.
5. Record readings as in adults.

Palpation

1. Follow steps 1 and 2 above.
2. Keep the palpating finger over the artery and inflate the cuff as above.
3. The point at which the pulse is felt is recorded as the systolic pressure.

Doppler

1. Obtain the monitor, dual air hose, and proper cuff size.
2. If monitor is not on a mobile stand, be certain that it is placed on a firm surface.
3. Plug in monitor (unless battery-operated) and attach dual hose, if necessary.
4. Attach appropriate-size blood-pressure cuff and wrap around child's limb.
5. Turn power switch on. Record the reading.

Flush

(Used for newborns or small infants)

1. Apply cuff to distal limb (if arm, outer edge is at wrist; if leg, outer edge is at ankle).
2. Wrap extremity distal to cuff with elastic bandage.
3. Inflate cuff to 150–200 mmHg and remove elastic bandage.
4. Lower cuff pressure 5 mmHg and leave at that level 3–4 seconds. Repeat until flush appears in blanched limb.
5. Repeat at least twice to confirm reading. This is recorded as the mean arterial pressure.

distress (Fig. 3-4). Retractions are noted as substernal (below the sternum), subcostal (below the ribs), intercostal (between the ribs), suprasternal (above the sternum), or supraclavicular (above the clavicle).

BLOOD PRESSURE

For children 3 years of age and older, blood-pressure monitoring is part of a routine physical assessment. Children of any age who are admitted to the health care facility should have an admission blood pressure taken. Obtaining a blood-pressure measurement in an infant or small child is difficult, but equipment of the proper size helps ease the problem. The cuff should be wide enough to cover about two thirds of the upper arm and long enough to encircle the upper arm without overlapping. The blood pressure can be taken by the auscultation, palpation, Doppler, or flush method (Box 3-1). The Doppler method is used with increasing frequency to monitor pediatric blood pressure, but the cuff still must be the correct size. Normal blood-pressure values gradually increase from infancy through adolescence (Table 3-2).

WEIGHT AND HEIGHT

The child's weight and height are helpful indicators of growth and development. Weight and height should be measured and recorded each time the child has a routine physical examination and at other health care visits. These

measurements must be charted and compared with norms for the child's age (see Appendix B). This process gives a good picture of how the child is progressing; however, the size of other family members and the child's illnesses, general nutritional status, and developmental milestones also must be considered.

The infant or child should be weighed at the same time each day, on the same scales, wearing the same amount of clothing. An infant is weighed naked, with no shirt or diaper. The nurse must keep a hand within 1″ of the infant at all times to be ready to protect the infant from injury. The scale is covered with a fresh paper towel or clean sheet of paper as a means of infection control. An older infant

TABLE 3-2. Normal Blood-Pressure Ranges (mmHg)

Age	Systolic	Diastolic
Newborn–12 hr (<1,000 g)	39–59	16–36
Newborn–12 hr (3,000 g)	50–70	24–45
Newborn–96 hr (3,000 g)	60–90	20–60
Infant	74–100	50–70
Toddler	80–112	50–80
Preschooler	82–110	50–78
School-age	84–120	54–80
Adolescent	94–140	62–88

may sit up on the scale, but the nurse must still keep a hand ready to protect the infant from injury. A child who can stand alone steadily is weighed on platform-type scales. The child should be weighed without shoes; if weighed daily in the health care facility, he or she must be weighed at the same time and in the same clothing. Bed scales may be used if the child cannot get out of bed. Weights are recorded in grams and kilograms or pounds and ounces.

The child who can stand is usually measured for height at the same time. The standing scales have an adjustable measuring device that may be used. An infant is measured while lying on a flat surface. Usually, examining tables have a measuring device mounted along the side of the table. The infant is measured flat with knees held flat to the table. Height is recorded in centimeters or inches according to the practice of the health care facility; the nurse must know which measuring system is used.

Assessment of Cardiovascular and Respiratory Status

Various monitors are used to measure cardiovascular and respiratory status in infants and children. Noninvasive methods are preferred when possible. The following are several noninvasive monitors that may be used.

PULSE OXIMETRY

Pulse oximetry measures the oxygen saturation of arterial hemoglobin. The probe of the oximetry unit can be taped to the toe or finger or clipped on the earlobe (Fig. 3-5). It is changed at least every 4 hours to prevent skin irritation. In an infant, the foot may be used. The site should be checked every 2 hours to ensure that the probe is secure and tissue perfusion is adequate. Alarms can be set to sound when oxygen saturation decreases lower than a predetermined limit. At the beginning of each shift and after transport of the patient, the nurse must check that alarms are accurately set and have not been inadvertently changed. This is true for all types of monitors.

APNEA MONITOR

An apnea monitor detects the infant's respiratory movement. Electrodes or a belt are placed on the infant's chest where the greatest amount of respiratory movement is detected and are attached to the monitor by a cable. An alarm is set to sound when the infant does not breathe for a predetermined number of seconds. These monitors can be used in a hospital setting and often are used in the home for an infant who is at risk for apnea or who has a tracheostomy. Family caregivers are taught to stimulate the infant when the monitor sounds and to perform cardiopulmonary resuscitation if the infant does not begin breathing.

CARDIOPULMONARY MONITOR

Cardiac monitors assess cardiac and respiratory function. Many of these monitors have a visual display of the cardiac and respiratory actions. Electrodes must be placed properly to obtain accurate readings of the cardiac and pulmonary systems. The skin is cleansed with alcohol to remove oil, dirt, lotions, and powder. Alarms are set to maximum and minimum settings above and below the child's resting rates. The electrode sites must be checked every 2 hours to detect any skin redness or irritation and to determine that the electrodes are secure. The child's cardiac and respiratory status must be checked immediately when the alarm sounds (Fig. 3-6).

Neurologic Assessment

Increased intracranial pressure often is caused by a head injury. It also may be caused by certain metabolic conditions, such as diabetes mellitus, or by drug ingestion, severe hemorrhage, dehydration, and seizures. To determine the level of the child's neurologic functioning, the nurse must perform a neurologic assessment. The most frequently used neurologic assessment tool is the Glasgow coma scale. The use of a standard scale for testing permits

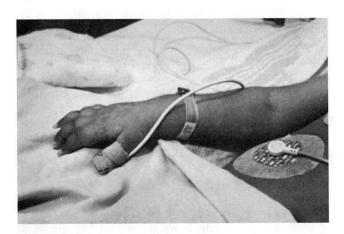

Figure 3-5
Pulse oximetry sensor taped to infant's thumb.

Figure 3-6
It is important for the nurse to frequently check the cardiopulmonary monitor, settings, and electrode sites.

the comparison of results from one time to another and from one examiner to another. Neurologic assessment is performed every 1 or 2 hours to observe for significant changes (Fig. 3-7).

Regulation of Body Temperature

Significant alterations in body temperature can have severe consequences for children. "Normal" body temperature varies from 98.6°F (37°C) orally to 100.4°F (38°C) rectally. The body temperature generally should be maintained below 101°F (38.3°C) orally or 102°F (38.9°C) rectally, although the health care facility or physician may set lower limits. Excess coverings should be removed from the child with fever to permit additional cooling through evaporation. Methods used to reduce fever are:

- Giving a tepid sponge bath
- Maintaining hydration (encouraging fluids)
- Administering acetaminophen
- Using a hypothermia pad or blanket

Sponge baths and hypothermia treatments should not be maintained for longer than 20 to 30 minutes at one time. Otherwise, vasoconstriction occurs, resulting in further increases in the child's core temperature. Because many children have a fever but do not need hospitalization, family caregivers need instructions on fever reduction (Box 3-2).

TEPID SPONGE BATH

When a sponge bath is administered, only tepid water should be used. Ice or alcohol should never be added to the water. Extreme cooling may be a shock to the immature

nervous system, and alcohol may be absorbed through the skin or the fumes can be inhaled, further complicating the child's problems. The child should not be permitted to shiver because the process of shivering raises the temperature. The temperature, pulse, and respiration measurements are taken at the beginning of the procedure. Extra washcloths are needed to place in the axilla and groin. Long, gentle strokes are used during the procedure, starting from the head and working down the body, exposing only one part of the body at a time. A tub bath may be given unless contraindicated by the child's condition. The sponge bath is continued for 20 to 30 minutes but should be stopped if the child begins to shiver. After the bath, the child is dried and can be dressed in light pajamas or covered lightly with a sheet. The temperature is taken 30 minutes after the bath is completed. If the temperature is not falling, the procedure may need to be repeated. Documentation includes the time the procedure was started, the length of the bath, the initial temperature, the temperature taken 30 minutes after the procedure, and the child's reaction to the procedure.

Therapeutic Application of Cold

In addition to reducing body temperature, the local application of cold also may help prevent swelling, control hemorrhage, and provide an anesthetic effect. Intervals of about 20 minutes are recommended, both for dry cold (ice bag and commercial instant-cold preparation) and moist cold (compress, soak, and bath) treatments. Dry cold applications should be covered lightly to protect the child's skin from direct contact. Because cold decreases circulation, prolonged chilling may result in frostbite and gangrene. The child's skin must be inspected before and after the cold application to detect skin redness or irritation. Documentation includes the application, the beginning time, the length of time, and the condition of the skin before and after the application.

Detailed instructions for the therapeutic application of cold and heat may be obtained in the procedures manual of each facility and from manufacturers of commercial devices.

Therapeutic Application of Heat

The local application of heat increases circulation by vasodilation and promotes muscle relaxation, thereby relieving pain and congestion. It also speeds the formation and drainage of superficial abscesses.

Artificial heat should never be applied to the skin of a child without a physician's order. Tissue damage can occur, particularly in fair-skinned people or those who have suffered sensory loss or impaired circulation. Children should be closely monitored, and none should receive heat treatments longer than 30 minutes at a time unless specifically ordered by the physician.

GLASGOW COMA SCALES			MODIFIED COMA SCALE FOR INFANTS		
ACTIVITY	BEST RESPONSE		ACTIVITY	BEST RESPONSE	
Eye Opening	Spontaneous	4	Eye Opening	Spontaneous	4
	To speech	3		To speech	3
	To pain	2		To pain	2
	None	1		None	1
Verbal	Oriented	5	Verbal	Coos, babbles	5
	Confused	4		Irritable	4
	Inappropriate words	3		Cries to pain	3
	Nonspecific sounds	2		Moans to pain	2
	None	1		None	1
Motor	Follows commands	6	Motor	Normal spontaneous movements	6
	Localizes pain	5		Withdraws to touch	5
	Withdraws to pain	4		Withdraws to pain	4
	Abnormal flexion	3		Abnormal flexion	3
	Extend	2		Abnormal extension	2
	None	1		None	1

PUPIL SIZE:

6mm ● 5mm ● 4mm ●
3mm ● 2mm ● 1mm ·

REACTION: N−normal, S−sluggish, F−fixed

		PUPIL SIZE		PUPIL REACTION		EXTREMITY MOVEMENT/ RESPONSE				GLASGOW COMA SCALE			VITAL SIGNS		
DATE	TIME	R	L	R	L	RA	LA	RL	LL	VERBAL RESP.	MOTOR RESP.	EYE OPENING	BP	PULSE	RESP.

GUIDE TO NEUROLOGIC EVALUATION

Pupils

Pupils should be examined in dim light
1. Compare each pupil with the size chart and record pupil size.
2. Use a bright flashlight to check the reaction of each pupil. Hold the flashlight to the outer aspect of the eye. While watching the pupil, turn the flashlight on and bring it directly over the pupil. Record the reaction. Repeat for the other eye. Report if either pupil is fixed or dilated.

Extremities
1. Observe the child for quality and strength of muscle tone in each upper extremity. Have child squeeze nurse's hand. Have child raise arms. Ask child to turn palms up, then palms down. Infant is observed for movement and position of arms when stroked or lightly pinched.
2. The child should be able to move each leg on command, and push against nurse's hands with each foot. Infant is observed for movement of legs and feet when stroked or lightly pinched.
3. Score the extremities using the motor scale appropriate for age (below).

Glasgow Coma Scale

Assess each response according to age

Eye opening
4 Opens eyes spontaneously when approached
3 Opens eyes to spoken or shouted speech
2 Opens eyes only to painful stimuli (nail bed pressure)
1 Does not open eyes in response to pain

Verbal
5 Oriented to time, place, person; infant responds by cooing and babbling, recognizes parent
4 Talks, not oriented to time, place, person; infant irritable, doesn't recognize parent
3 Words senseless, unintelligible; infant cries in response to pain
2 Responds with moaning and groaning, no intelligible words; infant moans to pain
1 No response

Motor
6 Responds to commands; infant smiles, responds
5 Tries to remove painful stimuli with hands; infant withdraws from touch
4 Attempts to withdraw from painful stimuli; infant withdraws from pain source
3 Flexes arms at elbows and wrists in response to pain (decorticate rigidity)
2 Extends arms at elbows in response to pain (cerebrate rigidity)
1 No motor response to pain

Check infant's fontanelle for bulging and record results

Figure 3-7
Neurologic flow sheet and neurologic evaluation guide.

Box 3-2. *Home Care Guide for Fever Reduction*

1. Temperature for sponging bath should begin with warm water and gradually be lowered to 98.6°F (37°C) so that child becomes used to the cool water.
2. Do not place child in a tub for the bath if it may be difficult to hold him or her securely.
3. Sponge for no longer than 30 minutes.
4. If tub is used, gently dribble water over child's body.
5. If child is in bed, uncover only one body part at a time. Use long strokes, and place extra washcloths in armpits and groin.
6. Never use alcohol in sponge bath.
7. Never use ice in the water for sponging.
8. Stop if child begins to shiver. Shivering raises body temperature.
9. When finished, dry child by gently rubbing skin to increase circulation.
10. When done, do not overdress or heavily cover child. Diaper, light sheet, or light pajamas are sufficient.
11. Do not repeat unless temperature is elevated and skin is warm.
12. Encourage child to drink fluids.
13. Keep room environment cool.
14. Use acetaminophen or other antipyretic according to directions of physician. Do not give aspirin.
15. Wait for 30 minutes to take temperature again.
16. Call physician at once if child's temperature is 105°F (40.6°C) or higher.
17. Call physician if child has history of febrile seizures.

Moist heat produces faster results than does dry heat and is usually applied in the form of a warm compress or soak. Towels should not be warmed in the microwave, as the microwave may unevenly heat them and in turn they may burn the child.

Dry heat may be applied by means of an electric heating pad, a K-pad (a unit that circulates warm water through plastic-enclosed tubing), or a hot water bottle. Many children have been burned because of improper use of hot water bottles; therefore, these devices are not recommended. Electric heating pads and K-pads should be covered with a pillowcase, towel, or stockinette. As with the application of cold, documentation includes the application, the beginning time, the length of time, and the condition of the skin before and after the application.

Assisting With Diagnostic and Treatment Procedures

Many procedures in highly technologic health care facilities may be frightening and painful to children. The nurse can be an important source of comfort to children who must undergo these procedures, even though it is difficult to assist with or perform procedures that cause pain. The child who is old enough to understand the purpose of the procedure and the expected benefit must have the procedure explained; he or she should be encouraged to ask questions and should be given complete answers. Infants can be soothed and comforted only before and after the procedure.

The nurse caring for toddlers has a greater opportunity to explain procedures than when caring for infants, but at best the nurse will be only imperfectly understood. Even when toddlers grasp the words, they have little meaning. The reality is the pain that occurs.

Sometimes children's interest can be diverted so that they may forget their fear. They must be allowed to cry if necessary, and they should always be listened to and have their questions answered. It takes maturity and experience on the nurse's part to know exactly which questions are stalling techniques and which call for firmness and action. Children need someone to take charge in a kind, firm manner that tells them the decision is not in their hands. They are too young to take this responsibility for themselves.

Nurses have conflicting feelings about the merit of giving some reward after a treatment. Careful thought is necessary. Children given a lollipop or a small toy after an uncomfortable procedure tend to remember the experience as not totally bad. This has nothing to do with their behavior. It is not a reward for being brave or good or big; it is simply a part of the entire treatment. The unpleasant part is mitigated by the pleasant. An older person's reward is contemplating the improvement in health the procedure may provide, but the child does not have sufficient reasoning ability to understand future benefits.

BLOOD TESTS

Blood tests are part of almost every hospitalization experience. Although the specimens usually are obtained by laboratory personnel or a physician, the nurse must be familiar with the general procedure to explain it to the child. The nurse may be asked to help restrain the child during the procedure. Blood specimens are obtained either by pricking the heel, great toe, earlobe, or finger or by venipuncture. In infants, the jugular or scalp veins are most commonly used; sometimes the femoral vein is used (Fig. 3-8). In older children, the veins in the arm are used.

URINE TESTS

Equipment needed to obtain a urine specimen is assembled, including sterile water, soap or antiseptic solution, sterile cotton balls or gauze squares, urine collector, specimen container, and nonsterile gloves. The procedure is explained to the child who is old enough to comprehend. The infant or child is positioned so that the genitalia are exposed. The nurse washes his or her hands, puts on gloves, and cleanses the genitalia. On the male patient, the tip of the penis is wiped with a soapy cotton ball, followed by a rinse with a cotton ball saturated with sterile water. In the female patient, the labia majora are cleansed front to back,

Figure 3-8
(A) Position of infant for jugular venipuncture. (B) Position of infant for femoral venipuncture.

using one cotton ball for each wipe. The labia minora are then exposed and cleansed in the same fashion. The area is rinsed with a cotton ball saturated with sterile water. The male or female genitalia are permitted to air-dry. The paper backing is removed from the urine collection container, and the adhesive surface is applied over the penis in the male and the vulva in the female. The child may be diapered. The nurse completes the procedure with careful handwashing. The specimen may be sent to the laboratory in the plastic collection container or in a specimen container preferred by the laboratory. Appropriate documentation includes the time of specimen collection, the amount and color of the urine, the test to be performed, and the condition of the perineal area.

Occasionally, children must be catheterized to obtain a specimen. An older child may be able to cooperate in the collection of a midstream specimen, if needed.

STOOL TESTS

Stool specimens are tested for various reasons, including the presence of occult blood, ova and parasites, bacteria, glucose, or excess fat. The nurse puts on gloves and collects these specimens from a diaper or bedpan using a tongue blade and places them in clean specimen containers. Stool specimens must not be contaminated with urine, and they must be labeled and delivered to the laboratory promptly. Documentation includes the time the specimen is collected, the color, amount, consistency, and odor of the stool, the test to be performed, and the skin condition.

CEREBROSPINAL FLUID TESTS

When analysis of cerebrospinal fluid is necessary, a lumbar puncture is performed. During this procedure, the nurse must restrain the child in the position shown in Figure

3-9 until the procedure is completed. The nurse holds the child's hands with the hand that has passed under the child's lower extremities and holds the child snugly against his or her chest. This position enlarges the intervertebral spaces for easier access with the aspiration needle. Children undergoing this procedure may be too young to understand the nurse's explanation. The nurse should tell the child, however, that it is important to hold still and the child will

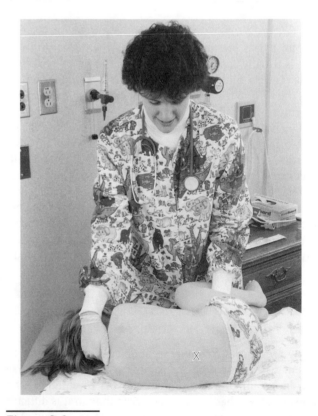

Figure 3-9
Position of child for lumbar puncture.

have help to do this. The lumbar puncture is performed with strict asepsis. A sterile dressing is applied when the procedure is complete. The child must remain quiet for 1 hour after the procedure. Vital signs, level of consciousness, and motor activity should be monitored frequently for several hours after the procedure.

MEDICATION ADMINISTRATION

Caring for children who are ill challenges every nurse to function at the highest level of professional competence. Giving medications is one of the most important nursing responsibilities, calling for accuracy, precision, and considerable psychological skill. Basic to administering medications to a person of any age are the following five "rights" of medication administration:

- The right patient—check the identification bracelet *each* time a medication is given to confirm identification of the patient.
- The right drug—check the drug label to confirm it is the correct drug. Do not use a drug that is not clearly labeled. Check the expiration date of the drug.
- The right dose—always double-check the dose when in doubt. Question the order if it is unclear. Have another qualified person double-check any time a divided dosage is to be given, or for insulin, digoxin, and other agents governed by the policy of the facility. Use drug references or check with a physician or pharmacist for the appropriateness of the dose. Orders must be questioned *before* the drug is given.
- The right route—give the drug only by the route indicated. Question the order if it is unclear or confusing.
- The right time—administering a drug at the correct time helps maintain the desired blood level of the drug.

Administering medications to children is much more complex than these guidelines indicate. Accurate administration of medications to children is especially critical because of the variable responses to drugs that children have as a result of immature body systems. The nurse must understand the factors that influence or alter how the child absorbs, metabolizes, and excretes the medication and any allergies that the child has. The nurse is responsible for the administration of medications and therefore is legally liable for errors of medication.

Nine rules to guide the nurse in administering medications are presented in Box 3-3. The nurse should evaluate each child from a developmental point of view to administer medications successfully. Understanding, planning, and implementing nursing care that considers the child's developmental level and coping mechanisms contribute to administering medications with minimal trauma to the child (Table 3-3).

Box 3-3. *Nine Rules of Medication Administration in Children*

1. Never give a child a choice of whether to receive medicine. The medication is ordered and is necessary for recovery, therefore there is no choice to be made.
2. Do give choices that allow the child some control over the situation, such as the kind of juice or the number of bandages.
3. Never lie. Do not tell a child that an injection will not hurt.
4. Keep explanations simple and brief. Use words that the child will comprehend.
5. Assure the child that it is all right to be afraid and that it is OK to cry.
6. Do not talk in front of the child as though he or she were not there. Include the child in the conversation when talking to family caregivers.
7. Be positive in approaching the child. Be firm and assertive when explaining to the child what will happen.
8. Keep the time between explanation and execution to a minimum. The younger the child, the shorter the time should be.
   Keep the explanation simple.
   Preparations such as setting up an injection, solutions, or instrument trays should be done out of the child's sight.
9. Obtain cooperation from family caregivers. They may be able to calm a frightened child, persuade the child to take the medication, and achieve cooperation for care.

A Personal Glimpse

I have been sick so many times that I don't know which one to write about. When I had hapetitis [sic], I was very sick for a very long time. I missed a lot of school. I had to get blood tests, urine tests, and medications all the time, and I slept a lot, because I felt tired all the time. Every time I had to get a blood test I would cry because I didn't want to go. After a very long time, I got well enough to go back to school, but I couldn't play any gym games or activities because I couldn't get hit in my belly.

Justin, age 9 years

TABLE 3-3. Developmental Considerations in Medication Administration

Age	Behaviors	Nursing Actions
Birth–3 mo	Reaches randomly toward mouth and has a strong reflex to grasp objects	The infant's hands must be held to prevent spilling of medications.
	Poor head control	The infant's head must be supported while medications are being given.
	Tongue movement may force medication out of mouth	A syringe or dropper should be placed along the side of the mouth.
	Sucks as a reflex with stimulation	Use this natural sucking desire by placing oral medications into a nipple and administering in that manner.
	Stops sucking when full	Administer medications before feeding when infant is hungry. Be aware that some medications' absorption is affected by food.
	Responds to tactile stimulations	The likelihood that the medication is taken will increase if the infant is held in a feeding position.
3–12 mo	Begins to develop fine muscle control and advances from sitting to crawling	Medication must be kept out of reach to avoid accidental ingestion.
	Tongue may protrude when swallowing	Administer medication with a syringe.
	Responds to tactile stimuli	Physical comfort (holding) given after a medication is helpful.
12–30 mo	Advances from independent walking to running without falling	Allow the toddler to choose position for taking medication.
	Advances from messy self-feeding to proficient feeding with minimal spilling	Allow the toddler to take medicine from a cup or spoon.
	Has voluntary tongue control. Begins to drink from a cup	Disguise medication in a small amount of food to decrease incidence of spitting out medication.
	Develops second molars	Chewable tablets may be an alternative.
	Exhibits independence and self-assertiveness	Allow as much freedom as possible. Use games to gain confidence. Use a consistent, firm approach. Give immediate praise for cooperation.
30 mo–6 y	Responds to sense of time and simple direction	Give directions to "Drink this now" and "Open your mouth."
	Responds to and participates in routines of daily living	Involve the family caregivers and include the toddler in medicine routines.
	Expresses feelings easily	Allow for expression through play.
	Knows full name	Ask the child his or her name before giving medicine.
	Is easily influenced by others when responding to new foods or tastes	Approach the child in a calm, positive manner when giving medications.
	Has a good sense of time and a tolerance of frustration	Use correct immediate rewards for the young child and delayed gratification for the older child.
	Enjoys making decisions	Give choices when possible.
	Has many fantasies; has fear of mutilation	Give simple explanations. Stress that the medication is not being given because the child is bad.
	Is more coordinated	Can hold cup and may be able to master pill-taking.
	Begins to lose teeth	Chewable tablets may be inappropriate because of loose teeth.

(continued)

TABLE 3-3. Developmental Considerations in Medication Administration *(Continued)*

Age	Behaviors	Nursing Actions
6–12 y	Strives for independence	Give acceptable choices. Respect the need for regression during hospitalization.
	Has concern for bodily mutilation	Give reassurance that medication, especially injectables, will not cause harm. Reinforce that medications should be taken only when given by nurse or family caregiver.
	Can tell time	Include the child in daily schedule of medication. Make the child a poster of medications and time due so he or she can be involved in care.
	Is concerned with body image and privacy	Provide private area for administration of medication, especially injections.
	Peer support and interaction are important	Allow child to share experiences with others.
12+ years	Strives for independence	Write a contract with the adolescent, spelling out expectations for self-medication.
	Can understand abstract theories	Explain why medications are given and how they work.
	Decisions are influenced by peers	Encourage teens to talk with their peers in a support group. Work with teens to plan medication schedule around their activities. Differentiate pill-taking from drug-taking.
	Questions authority figures	Be honest and provide medication information in writing.
	Is concerned with sex and sexuality	Explain relation between illness, medications, and sexuality. For example, emphasize, "This medication will not react with your birth-control pills."

Computing Dosages

Commercial unit-dose packaging often does not include dosages for children, so the nurse must calculate the correct dosage. The most reliable formula to calculate dosages is the **body surface area (BSA) method**. The **West nomogram**, commonly used to calculate BSA, is a graph with several scales arranged so that when two values are known, the third can be plotted by drawing a line with a straightedge (Fig. 3-10). The child's weight is marked on the right scale, the height on the left scale. A straightedge is used to draw a line between the two marks. The point at which it crosses the column labeled *SA* (surface area) is the BSA expressed in square meters (m²). The average adult BSA is 1.7 m²; thus, the formula to calculate the appropriate dosage for a child is

$$\text{Estimated child's dose} = \frac{\text{Child's BSA (m}^2)}{1.7 \text{ (Adult BSA)}}$$
$$\times \text{ Adult dose}$$

For example, a child is 37″ (95 cm) tall and weighs 34 lb (15.5 kg). The usual adult dose of the medication is 500 mg. Place and hold one end of a straightedge on the first column at 37″ and move it so that it lines up with 34 lb in the far right column. On the SA column, the straightedge falls across 0.64 (m²). You are ready to do the calculation

$$\frac{0.64}{1.7} = 0.38$$

You now know that the child's BSA is 0.38 that of the average adult. You are ready to calculate the child's dose by multiplying 0.38 times 500 mg:

$$0.38 \times 500 = 190$$

The child's dose is 190 mg.

CALCULATING FRACTIONAL DOSAGE

It may be necessary to calculate a fractional dosage when full-strength drugs must be diluted to achieve the concentration ordered by the physician. The simplest way to determine the amount needed of a full-strength drug is to divide the desired strength (the dose ordered) by the strength of the drug on hand. The required fraction of the standard amount is then given. The formula is

$$\frac{\text{Dose desired}}{\text{Dose on hand}} \times \text{Quantity (diluent)}$$
$$= \text{Amount to be given}$$

HEIGHT		SURFACE AREA	WEIGHT	
feet	centimeters	in square meters	pounds	kilograms

Figure 3-10

West nomogram for estimating surface area of infants and young children. To determine the body surface area, draw a straight line between the point representing the child's height on the left scale to the child's weight on the right scale. The point at which this line intersects the middle scale is the child's body surface area in square meters.

For example, elixir of phenobarbital contains 20 mg of phenobarbital in each 5 mL of the elixir. If the order reads "elixir of phenobarbital 4 mg PO," the desired dose (dose ordered) is 4 mg and the dose on hand is 20 mg/5 mL. The problem is set up as follows:

$$\frac{4 \text{ mg}}{20 \text{ mg}} \times 5 \qquad \frac{1}{5} \times 5 = 1$$

The correct dose is 1 mL.

(Because this medication is in elixir form, it should be well diluted with water before giving it to a child, as discussed later.)

After computing the dosage, the nurse should *always* have the computation checked by another staff person qualified to give medication, or someone in the department who is delegated for this purpose. Errors are easy to make and easy to overlook. A second person should do the computation separately, then both results should be compared.

ERRORS IN MEDICATIONS

Medication errors can occur because nurses are human and not perfect. To admit an error is often difficult, especially if there has been carelessness concerning the rules. A person may be strongly tempted to adopt a "wait and see" attitude, which is the gravest error of all. Nurses must accept responsibility for their own actions. Serious consequences for the child may be avoided if a mistake is disclosed promptly.

Oral Medication

Small babies are not too particular about the taste of food if they are hungry. Almost anything liquid may be sucked through a nipple, including liquid medicines, unless it is bitter. Medications that are available in syrup or fruit-flavored suspensions are easily administered this way. Another method of administering oral medications is to drop them slowly into the baby's mouth with a plastic medicine dropper or oral syringe (Fig. 3-11).

Figure 3-11

An oral syringe may be used to administer pediatric oral medications.

Elixirs contain alcohol and are apt to cause choking unless they are diluted. Syrups and suspensions are thick and may need dilution to ensure that the child gets the full dose. Always check with the pharmacist before diluting any medication.

When a child is old enough to swallow a pill, make sure that the pill is actually swallowed. When asked to open their mouths, children usually cooperate so well and open so wide that their tonsils can be inspected. While the mouth is open, the nurse can look under the tongue. Chewable tablets work well for the preschool child.

It usually is best to give medicine in solution form to a small child. Tablets, if used, must be dissolved in water. Do not use orange juice for a solvent unless specifically ordered to do so—the child may always associate the taste of orange juice with the unpleasant medicine. If the medicine is bitter, honey or corn syrup may disguise the taste. The child may develop a dislike for corn syrup, but that is not as important as a lifelong dislike of orange juice.

There is little excuse for restraining a small child and forcing a medication down the child's throat. The child can always have the last word and bring it up again. The danger of aspiration is real. Of even greater importance are the antagonism and helplessness built up in the child by such a procedure. A child's sense of dignity must be respected as much as that of an adult. Refer to Table 3-3 to review the developmental characteristics to be considered at each age.

Intramuscular Medication

Children have the same fear of needles as do adults. Inexperienced nurses are reluctant to hurt children and often cause the pain they are trying to prevent by inserting

the needle slowly. A swift, sure thrust and insertion is the best way to minimize pain, but the nurse must stay calm and sure and be prepared for the child's squirming. It is best to have a second nurse help hold the child if he or she is younger than school age or if this is his or her first injection.

Injections should be given to a child in the treatment room rather than in bed or in the playroom. The bed and playroom should be "safe" places for the child. The nurse may have a ready Band-Aid to cover the injection site. This technique prevents young children from worrying that they might "leak out" of the hole, and the bandage serves as a badge of courage or bravery for the older child.

Figures 3-12 through 3-15 illustrate each intramuscular injection site and how to locate them. Table 3-4 describes each of these sites, how to locate them, and the suggested needle size and amount of medication.

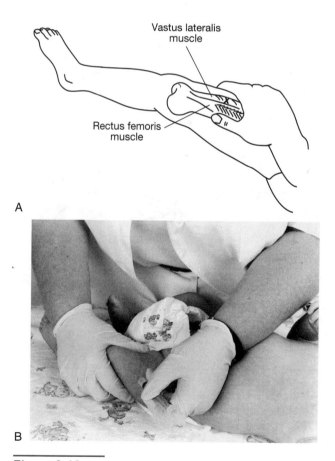

Figure 3-12

(A) Vastus lateralis muscle. (B) Intramuscular injection into the vastus lateralis—note the angle of the needle and syringe.

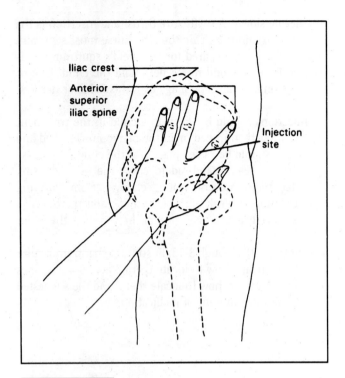

Figure 3-13
Locating the ventrogluteal intramuscular injection site.

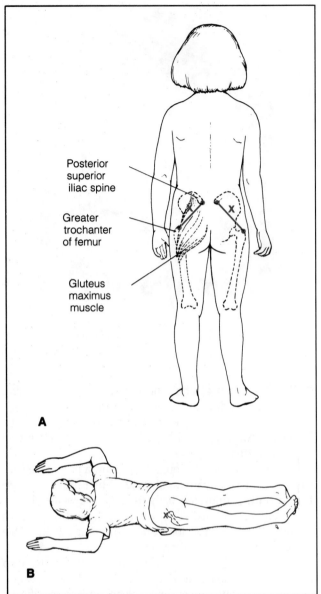

Figure 3-15
(A) Locating the gluteus intramuscular injection site. (B) Child in position for gluteus intramuscular injection. Site marked by X.

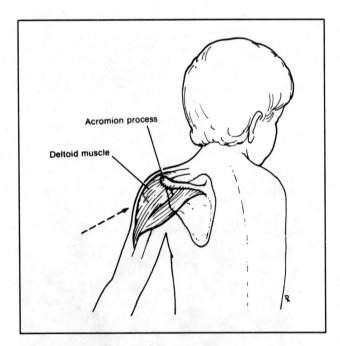

Figure 3-14
Location of deltoid intramuscular injection site. Site marked by X.

TABLE 3-4. Intramuscular Injection Sites

Muscle Site	Needle Size	Maximum Amount	Procedures
Vastus lateralis (Fig. 3-12)	Infant: 25 gauge, ⅝″ or 23 gauge, 1″ Older: 22 gauge, 1″ to 1.5″	1 mL 2 mL	This main thigh muscle is used almost exclusively in infants for intramuscular injections but is used frequently in children of all ages. Locate the trochanter (hip joint) and knee as landmarks. Select a site midway between these landmarks, using the lateral aspect. Inject at a 90° angle, or a 45° angle, directing the needle toward the knee.
Ventrogluteal (Fig. 3-13)	Assess child's muscle mass, and choose from those listed for the ventrogluteal. 22–25 gauge, ⅝″ to 1″	Infant: ½–¾ mL Toddler: 1 mL School-age and older: 1½–2 mL	With thumb facing the front of the child, place forefinger on the anterior superior iliac spine, middle finger on the iliac crest with the palm centered over the greater trochanter. Inject at a 90° angle below the iliac crest within the triangle defined. No important nerves are in this area.
Deltoid (Fig. 3-14)	Not recommended for infants Older: 22–25 gauge, 0.5″ to 1″	Small muscle limits amount to ½–1 mL	Expose entire arm. Locate the acromion process at the top of the arm. Give the injection in the densest part of the muscle, below the acromion process and above the armpit. Not recommended for repeated injections. Can be used for one-time immunizations. Angle needle slightly toward the shoulder.
Gluteal (Fig. 3-15)	This site is not recommended in children who have not been walking for at least 1 y. 20–25 gauge, 0.5° to 1.5″	Not recommended for infant or toddler School-age and older: 1½–2 mL	Because of the location of the sciatic nerve, use of this site is discouraged in younger children. Place child on abdomen, with toes pointing in; this relaxes the gluteus. Locate the posterior superior iliac crest and the greater trochanter of the femur. Draw an imaginary line between the two. Give the injection above and to the outside of this line. The needle should be inserted at a 90° angle.

Other Routes of Medication Administration

The principles of administering medications by other routes are much the same as those for adults, with a few variations. Eye, ear, and nose drops should be warmed to room temperature before being administered. The infant or young child may need to be restrained for safe administration. This restraint may be accomplished with a mummy restraint or the assistance of a second person. The nurse must realize that these are invasive procedures and that the young child may be resistant. Approaching the child with patience, explanations, and praise for cooperation helps gain the child's cooperation. Documentation must be completed after the administration of any medication.

EYE DROPS OR OINTMENT

The child is placed in a supine position. To instill the drops, the lower lid is pulled down to form a pocket, and the solution is dropped into the pocket. The eye is held shut briefly, if possible, to help distribute the medication to the conjunctiva. Ointment is applied from the inner to the outer canthus, with care not to touch the eye with the tip of the dropper or tube.

NOSE DROPS

Before nose drops are instilled, the nostrils should be wiped free of mucus. For instillation, an infant may be held in the nurse's arms with the head tilted over the arm. For a toddler or older child, the head may be placed over a pillow

Figure 3-16
Positioning for ear drops. The pinna is pulled up and back.

while the child is lying flat. The infant or child should maintain the position for at least 1 minute to ensure distribution of the medication.

EAR DROPS

The infant or young child is placed in a side-lying position with the affected ear up. In an infant or toddler, the pinna (the outer part of the ear) is pulled *down* and back to straighten the ear canal. In a child older than 3 years of age, the pinna is pulled *up* and back, as with adults, to straighten the canal (Fig. 3-16). After instillation of the drops, the area in front of the ear may be gently massaged. The child should be kept in a position with the affected ear up for 5 to 10 minutes. A cotton pledget may be loosely inserted into the ear to prevent leakage of medication, but care should be taken to avoid blocking drainage from the ear.

RECTAL MEDICATIONS

For the administration of rectal medications, the child is placed in a side-lying position, and the nurse must wear gloves or a finger cot. The suppository is lubricated and then inserted into the rectum, followed by a finger, up to the first knuckle joint. The little finger should be used for insertion in infants. After the insertion of the suppository, the buttocks must be held tightly together for 1 or 2 minutes until the child's urge to expel the suppository passes.

INTRAVENOUS THERAPY

Fluids and medications are often administered intravenously (IV) to infants and children. Planning nursing care for the child receiving IV therapy requires knowledge of the physiology of fluids and electrolytes as well as the child's developmental level and an understanding of the emotional aspects of IV therapy for children. Intravenous therapy is commonly administered in the pediatric patient for the following reasons:

- To maintain fluid and electrolyte balance
- To administer antibiotic therapy
- To provide nutritional support
- To administer chemotherapy or anticancer drugs
- To administer pain medication

Candidates for IV therapy include children who have poor gastrointestinal absorption caused by diarrhea, vomiting, and dehydration; those who need a high serum concentration of a drug; those who have resistant infections that require IV medications; those with emergency problems; and those who need continuous pain relief.

Fundamentals of Fluid Balance

Maintenance of fluid balance in the body tissues is essential to health. Severe imbalance, when uncorrected, causes death, as in patients with serious dehydration resulting from severe diarrhea or vomiting or from the loss of fluids in extensive burns. The fundamental concepts of fluid and electrolyte balance in body tissue are reviewed briefly to help the student understand the importance of adequate fluid therapy for the sick child.

WATER

A continuous supply of water is necessary for life. At birth, water accounts for about 77% of body weight. This proportion decreases to the adult level of about 60% between ages 1 and 2 years.

In health, the body's water requirement is met through the normal intake of fluids and foods. Intake is regulated by the person's thirst and hunger. Normal body losses of fluid occur through the lungs (breathing) and the skin (sweating) and in the urine and feces. In the normal state of health, intake and output amounts balance each other, and the body is said to be in a state of **homeostasis** (a uniform state). Homeostasis signifies biologically the dynamic equilibrium of the healthy organism. This balance is achieved by appropriate shifts in fluid and electrolytes across the cellular membrane and by elimination of the end products of metabolism and excess electrolytes.

Body water, which contains electrolytes, is situated within the cells, in the spaces between the cells, and in the plasma and blood. Imbalance (failure to maintain homeostasis) may be the result of some pathologic process in the body. Some of the disorders associated with imbalance are pyloric stenosis, high fever, persistent or severe diarrhea and vomiting, and extensive burns. Retention of fluid may occur through impaired kidney action or altered metabolism.

COMMUNICATIONS BOX

Three-year-old Nickie must have an intramuscular injection. He is crying and protesting loudly.

INEFFECTIVE COMMUNICATION

Nurse: Nickie, I have to give you an injection to help make you better.

Nickie: No! Get away from me!

Nurse: Oh, come on, Nickie! Show me what a big boy you can be.

Nickie: (Protesting even louder) No! I hate you! I don't want a shot!

Nurse: You have to have it, Nickie. Turn over so we can get it over with.

Nickie: No!! (Kicking)

Nurse: I'll have to have Miss Jones hold you down so I can give it to you. It's only going to feel like a little sting.

Nickie: Shots hurt a lot. I want my Mommy.

Nurse: No, I'll just have Miss Jones help hold you still. Your mother can wait out in the hall.

Nickie: I want my Mommy!

Nurse: Just wait till we finish here and she can come back in.

(The injection is accomplished with two nurses holding Nickie while he loudly protests.)

In this scenario, the nurse larges Nickie to be a big boy. The nurse does not acknowledge his fears or offer him any sense of control. The nurse even refuses to let Nickie have his mother for consolation.

EFFECTIVE COMMUNICATION

Nurse: Nickie, I have to give you an injection to help make you better.

Nickie: No! Get away from me!

Nurse: Getting an injection is scary for you. You are afraid it's going to hurt.

Nickie: Yes! Get away!

Nurse: It will hurt a little when it goes in, but I'll be very quick about it, and we can put a bandage on it when we are finished.

Nickie: But I don't want it. (Beginning to quiet a little)

Nurse: I know. You can choose which hip to use. How would it be if you hold the bandage for me till we're finished?

Nickie: Well, OK, but I want Mommy to hold my hand.

Nurse: Sure, and I'll need you to help me by lying very still while Miss Jones helps you keep your legs still. Can you count to ten for me while I give it to you?

Nickie: OK.

In this scenario, the nurse acknowledges Nickie's feelings of fear and pain. The nurse lets him know that she will listen to him and offers him some control by allowing him to choose the site and hold the bandage. The nurse also agrees to his request for his mother. The nurse admits the injection may be painful, but suggests ways to reduce the pain.

Intracellular Fluid Intracellular fluid is contained within the body cells. Nearly half the volume of body water in the infant is intracellular. Intracellular fluid accounts for about 40% of body weight in both infants and adults. Each cell must be supplied with oxygen and nutrients to keep the body healthy. In addition, the body's water and salt levels must be kept constant within narrow parameters.

Cells are surrounded by a semipermeable membrane that retains protein and other large constituents within the cell. Water, certain salts and minerals, nutrients, and oxygen enter the cell through this membrane. Waste prod-ucts and useful substances produced within the cell are excreted or secreted into the surrounding spaces.

Extracellular Fluid Extracellular fluid is situated outside the cells. It may be **interstitial fluid** (situated within the spaces or gaps of body tissue) or **intravascular fluid** (situated within the blood vessels or blood plasma). Blood plasma contains protein within the walls of the blood vessels and water and mineral salts that flow freely from the vascular system into the surrounding tissues.

Interstitial fluid (also called intercellular or tissue fluid) has a composition similar to plasma except that it contains almost no protein. This reservoir of fluid outside the body cells decreases or increases easily in response to disease. An increase in interstitial fluid results in edema. Dehydration depletes this fluid before the intracellular and plasma supplies are affected.

In the infant, about 25% to 35% of body weight is due to interstitial fluid. In the adult, interstitial fluid accounts for only about 15% of body weight (Fig. 3-17). Infants and children become dehydrated much more quickly than do adults. In part, this dehydration occurs because of a greater fluid exchange caused by the rapid metabolic activity associated with infants' growth and because of the relatively larger ratio of skin surface area to body fluid volume, which is two or three times that of adults.

Because of these factors, the infant who is taking in no fluid loses an amount of body fluid equal to the extracellular volume in about 5 days, or twice as rapidly as does the adult. The infant's relatively larger volume of extracellular fluid may be designed to compensate partially for this greater loss.

ELECTROLYTES

Electrolytes are chemical compounds (minerals) that break down into ions when placed in water. An ion is an atom having a positive or a negative electrical charge. Important electrolytes in body fluids are sodium (Na^+), potassium (K^+), magnesium (Mg^{++}), calcium (Ca^{++}), chloride (Cl^-), phosphate (PO_4^{---}), and bicarbonate (HCO_3^-). Electrolytes have the important function of maintaining acid–base balance. Each water compartment of the body has its own normal electrolyte composition.

ACID–BASE BALANCE

Acid–base balance is a state of equilibrium between the acidity and the alkalinity of body fluids. The acidity of a solution is determined by the concentration of hydrogen (H^+) ions. Acidity is expressed by the symbol pH. Neutral fluids have a pH of 7.0, acid fluids lower than 7.0, and alkaline fluids higher than 7.0. Normally, body fluids are slightly alkaline. Internal body fluids have a pH of 7.35 to 7.45. Body excretions, however, are products of metabolism and become acid; the normal pH of urine, for example, is 5.5 to 6.5.

Defects in the acid–base balance result either in **acidosis** (excessive acidity of body fluids) or **alkalosis** (excessive alkalinity of body fluids). Acidosis may occur in conditions such as diabetes, kidney failure, and diarrhea. Hypochloremic alkalosis may occur in pyloric stenosis because of the decrease in chloride concentration and increase in carbon dioxide.

In normal health, the fluid and electrolyte balance is maintained through the intake of a well-balanced diet. The kidneys play an important part in regulating concentrations of electrolytes in the various fluid compartments. In illness, the balance may be disturbed because of excessive losses of certain electrolytes. Replacement of these minerals is necessary to restore health and maintain life. When the infant or child can take sufficient fluids orally, that is the preferred route, but often it is necessary to administer fluids IV.

Intravenous Fluid Administration

Intravenous fluids are administered to provide water, electrolytes, and nutrients that the child needs. **Total parenteral nutrition** (TPN), chemotherapy, and blood products also are administered IV. Total parenteral nutrition, often called **hyperalimentation**, is the administration of dextrose, lipids, amino acids, electrolytes, vitamins, minerals, and trace elements into the circulatory system to meet the nutritional needs of a child whose needs cannot be met through the gastrointestinal tract.

These solutions often are given through a central venous line. Medications are not given by the central venous line but must be given through a peripheral site. A central venous line passes directly into the subclavian vein through the jugular or subclavian vein. The line is inserted by surgical technique. Caring for a child with a central venous line calls for skilled nursing care because of the danger of complications such as contamination, thrombosis, dislodgement of the catheter, and **extravasation** (fluid escap-

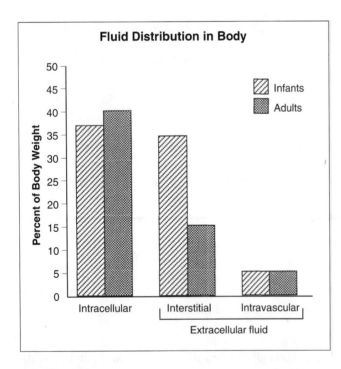

Figure 3-17

Graph indicating distribution of fluid in body compartments. Comparison between the infant and adult fluid distribution in body compartments shows that the adult total is about 60% of body weight, but the infant total is more than 70% of body weight.

ing into surrounding tissue). The infant or child must be closely monitored for hyperglycemia, dehydration, or **azotemia** (nitrogen-containing compounds in the blood).

Peripheral vein hyperalimentation may be used on a short-term basis. Extra care must be taken to avoid infiltration because tissue sloughing may be severe.

For long-term administration of TPN, a venous access device such as a Hickman or Broviac catheter may be inserted into the jugular or subclavian vein in a surgical procedure under anesthesia. These catheters may exit through a tunnel in the subcutaneous tissue on the right chest. Children can be discharged from the hospital on TPN therapy after family caregivers have been instructed in the care of the device, thus reducing hospitalization time and expense.

Dressing changes are routinely performed on the external site of a central venous device. This is a sterile procedure, and the nurse must have adequate space to place the equipment and must wear sterile gloves to use sterile forceps. All application is done in a circular motion, working from the insertion site to the outer edge in a "clean-to-dirty" fashion. A commonly used procedure begins with cleaning the skin with acetone, followed by tincture of iodine for its antibacterial action, and finishing with alcohol to clean off the iodine to prevent skin irritation. Topical antimicrobial ointment (bacitracin) is applied to the insertion site, followed by two small gauze sponges. The skin around these small sponges is sprayed with tincture of benzoin to toughen the skin. When the skin is dry, a large dressing is placed over the site and the edges are securely taped. Documentation includes the dressing change and skin condition, including redness, swelling, drainage, irritation, and any unusual reaction.

Intravenous Medication

Intravenous medications often are administered to pediatric patients. Some drugs must be administered IV to be effective, and in some patients the quick response gained from IV administration is important. Delivering medications IV is actually less traumatic than administering multiple intramuscular injections. Extra caution is necessary to observe for irritation of small pediatric veins from irritating medications. The nurse must double-check the medication label before hanging the IV fluid bottle to ensure that the medication is correct for the correct patient, that it is being administered at the correct time, and that it is not outdated.

Intravenous Sites

Site selection in the pediatric patient varies with the child's age. The best site in infants and toddlers is the scalp because there is an abundant supply of superficial veins. Other sites include the hand, the foot, and the antecubital fossa. When a scalp vein is used, the infant's hair is shaved over a small area (family caregivers can be reassured that the infant's hair will grow back quickly). An inverted medicine cup, or a paper cup with the bottom cut out, is often taped over the site to protect it. The needle is stabilized with U-shaped taping, and a loop of the tubing is taped so that if the child pulls on the tubing, the loop will absorb the pull and the site will remain intact. The older infant's hands may need to be restrained. This restraint may be accomplished by pinning the shirt sleeves to the bed or diapers.

If a site in the hand, foot, or arm is used, the limb should be stabilized on a board before insertion is attempted. These sites restrict the child's movement much more than the scalp site, so they are less desirable (Fig. 3-18).

The use of a plastic cannula or winged small-vein needle has reduced the need for surgical cutdowns. In a surgical cutdown, a small incision is made, usually in the foot or hand, providing access to a vein. The cutdown procedure is performed by a physician under sterile conditions.

Older children may be permitted some choice of site, if possible. The child should be involved in all aspects of the procedure within age-appropriate capabilities. The preschool child often can cooperate if given adequate explanation. Play therapy in preparation for IV therapy may be helpful. Honesty is essential with children of any age. The older school-age child and adolescent may have many questions that should be answered at their level of understanding. Family caregivers also need explanations and should be included in the preparation for the procedure. By their presence and reassurance, family caregivers may provide the emotional support the child needs and may help the child remain calm throughout the procedure.

In preparation for starting an IV line, the nurse must collect all the equipment that may be needed, including the IV tubing, any extension tubing that may be needed, the container of solution, the equipment to stabilize the site, a tourniquet, cleansing supplies such as povidone-iodine or alcohol swabs, sterile gauze, adhesive tape, cling roll gauze, an IV pole, an infusion pump or controller,

Figure 3-18
The infant on intravenous therapy rests snugly in the nurse's arm. Note the peripheral site and padded board to stabilize the hand and arm.

and a plastic cannula or winged small-vein needle, usually between a 21-gauge and 25-gauge size (depending on the child's size).

Only nurses skilled in the procedure should start an IV infusion in children. An unskilled nurse should not attempt the procedure unless under the direct supervision of a person skilled in pediatric IV administration. It is sometimes difficult to gain access to children's small veins, and they may easily be "blown." Venipuncture requires practice and expertise. The staff nurse may serve as the child's advocate when the physician or IV nurse comes to start an infusion. The staff nurse who has cared for the child has the child's confidence and knows the child's preferences.

Infusion Control

Numerous IV infusion pumps are suitable for pediatric use. The rate of infusion for infants and children must be carefully monitored. The IV drip rate must be slow for the small child to avoid overloading the circulation and inducing cardiac failure. Various adapting devices are available that decrease the size of the drop to a "mini" or "micro" drop of 1/50 or 1/60 mL, thus delivering 50 or 60 minidrops or microdrops per milliliter rather than the 15 drops per milliliter of a regular set (Fig. 3-19). Many IV sets also contain a control chamber (or burette) that contains 100 to 150 mL of fluid and is designed to deliver controlled volumes of fluid, avoiding the accidental entrance of too great a volume of fluid into the child's system.

Regardless of the control systems and safeguards, the

Figure 3-19
Secondary administration through a volume control set.

child and the IV infusion should be monitored as frequently as every hour. The IV site must be checked to see that it is intact and observed for redness, pain, **induration** (hardness), rate of flow, moisture at the site, and swelling. Documentation is done on an IV flow sheet on which is recorded the rate of flow, the amount in the bottle, the amount in the burette, the amount infused, and the condition of the site.

For the administration of an IV medication, a heparin lock may be used. This method allows the child more freedom and frees him or her from IV tubing between medication administrations. The veins on the back of the hand are often used for heparin lock insertion. Medication is administered through the lock, and when the administration is completed, the needle and tubing are removed and the heparin lock is flushed. A self-healing rubber stopper closes the heparin lock so that it does not leak between administrations. This method also may be used for a child who must have frequent blood samples drawn. The heparin lock is flushed every 4 to 8 hours with saline or heparin, according to the facility's procedure.

■ KEY POINTS

■ When administering physical care to an ill child, the nurse calls on a wide variety of skills that must be modified to meet the growth and developmental level of the child.

■ Although assessing vital signs may seem like a routine procedure, the nurse must use good judgment in selecting the means to measure each vital sign. The nurse also must document the vital signs promptly and accurately.

■ The nurse must become skilled at performing the neurologic assessment tool, which is instrumental in evaluating the child's neurologic functioning.

■ When teaching a family caregiver methods to relieve an elevated temperature in a child, the nurse must be certain to include safety measures.

■ The five "rights" of medication administration are basic to administering medications to anyone, but administering medications to children is much more complex because of their immature body systems and varying sizes.

■ The nurse should always have another person check his or her computations of drug dosage before administering it to a child.

■ Administration of IV fluids requires careful observation of the child's appearance, vital signs, intake and output, and rate of flow of the fluid, since the child's fluid balance can fluctuate very rapidly.

■ Intravenous infusion sites must be monitored to avoid infiltration and tissue damage.

CRITICAL THINKING

1. Tell step by step how you would take vital signs on a young infant. Explain the order in which you would do them and why.
2. Three-year-old Denise has a fever of 104.4°F (40.2°C). You must give her a sponge bath. Describe exactly what you would do. Include all explanations to the child.
3. Five-year-old Jason dashed into the street and was hit by the side of a passing car. He has been admitted with possible head injuries. What is one of your primary concerns? What nursing care will he need? Describe this care.
4. Catlin weighs 28.5 lb (13 kg) and measures 35.5″ (90 cm). Find her BSA using the West nomogram. Calculate the dose of a medication for her if the adult dosage is 750 mg.
5. Describe how you would approach each of the following children when giving oral medications and intramuscular medications.
   a. 6-month-old Kristi
   b. 18-month-old Jared
   c. 3-year-old Sarah
   d. 4.5-year-old Miguel
   e. 8-year-old Nicole
   f. 16-year-old Jon
6. Identify each of the intramuscular injection sites, state how to locate each of the sites, and name the landmarks used.

BIBLIOGRAPHY

Baird SC, White NE, Basinger M. Can you rely on tympanic thermometers? RN 55(8):48–51, 1992.

Castiglia PT, Harbin RE. Child health care: Process and practice. Philadelphia: JB Lippincott, 1992.

Danek GD, Noris EM. Pediatric IV catheters: Efficacy of saline flush. Pediatr Nurs 18(2):111–113, 1992.

Gildea JH. When fever becomes an enemy. Pediatr Nurs 18(2): 165–167, 1992.

Pillitteri A. Maternal and child health nursing, 2d ed. Philadelphia: JB Lippincott, 1995.

Skale N. Manual of pediatric nursing procedures. Philadelphia: JB Lippincott, 1992.

Thompson V. An IV therapy teaching tool for children. Pediatr Nurse 20(4):351–355, 1994.

Wong DL. Whaley and Wong's nursing care of infants and children, 5th ed. St. Louis: Mosby, 1995.

Care of the Hospitalized Child

STUDENT OBJECTIVES

On completion of this chapter, the student will be able to:

1. List nine possible influences on the family's response to a child's illness.
2. Explain the family caregivers' role in preparing a child for hospitalization.
3. Describe the benefits of rooming-in.
4. State the role that handwashing plays in infection control.
5. Identify four ways that pathogens are transmitted, and give an example of each.
6. Describe how the nurse can help ease the feelings of isolation a child may have when segregated by transmission-based precautions.
7. Identify and differentiate the three stages of response to separation seen in the young child.
8. Describe how a preadmission visit differs from an open house program.
9. State how the caregiver may be involved in the child's admission physical.
10. Discuss the need for written discharge instructions for the caregiver.
11. State how family members should react to the postdischarge child during this period of adjustment.
12. Describe how health professionals can help the adjustment of the child scheduled for surgery.
13. Discuss variations in preoperative preparation for children, including skin, gastrointestinal, urinary, and medication preparation.
14. Identify behavioral characteristics that may indicate that an infant or a young child is having pain.
15. State how a nasogastric tube is measured to determine how far it is inserted.
16. Tell why stomach contents are aspirated before a gastric tube feeding and what to do with the aspirated contents.
17. Discuss the purpose of a hospital play program.
18. Describe therapeutic use for puppets.
19. State how stress affects the frequency of accidents and how this relates to hospitalization of a child.
20. List safety measures to consider when using restraints.

KEY TERMS

anuria	mummy restraint
child-life program	papoose board
clove hitch restraint	patient-controlled analgesia
elbow restraint	play therapy
gastrostomy tube	rooming-in
gavage feedings	therapeutic play

Hospitalization may cause anxiety and stress at any age. Fear of the unknown is always threatening. The child who faces hospitalization is no exception. Children are often too young to understand what is happening or are afraid to ask questions. Short hospital stays are more frequent, but even during a short stay the child is often apprehensive. In addition, the child may pick up on the fears of family caregivers, and these negative emotions may hinder the child's progress.

The child's family suffers stress for a number of reasons. The cause of the illness, its treatment, guilt about the illness, past experiences of illness and hospitalization, disruption in family life, the threat to the child's long-term health, cultural or religious influences, coping methods within the family, and financial impact of the hospitalization all may affect how the family responds to the child's illness. Although these are concerns of the family and not specifically the child, they nevertheless influence how the child feels. Children are tuned in to the feelings and emotions of their caregivers.

The child's developmental level also plays an important role in determining how he or she handles the stress of illness and hospitalization. The nurse who understands the child's developmental needs may significantly improve the child's hospital stay and overall recovery. Many hospitals have a **child-life program** to make hospitalization less threatening for children and their parents. These programs are usually under the direction of a child-life specialist whose background is in psychology and early childhood development. This person works with nurses, physicians, and other health team members to help them meet the developmental, emotional, and intellectual needs of hospitalized children. The child-life specialist also works with students interested in child health care to help further their education. Sometimes, however, the best way to ease the stress of hospitalization is to ensure the child has been well prepared for the hospital experience.

THE PEDIATRIC HOSPITAL SETTING

Early Childhood Education About Hospitals

Hospitals are part of the child's community, just as police and fire departments are. When the child is capable of un-

derstanding the basic functions of these community resources and the people who staff them, it is time for an explanation. Some hospitals have open house programs for well children on a monthly or biweekly basis. Children may attend with parents or caregivers or in an organized community or school group. A room is set aside where children can handle equipment (Fig. 4-1), try out call bells, try on masks and gowns, have their blood pressure taken to feel the squeeze of the blood-pressure cuff, and see a hospital pediatric bed and compare it with their bed at home. Hospital staff members explain simple procedures and answer children's questions. A tour of the pediatric department, including the playroom, may be offered. Some hospitals have puppet shows or show slides or videos about admission and care. Child-life specialists, nurses, and volunteers help with these orientation programs.

Families are encouraged to help children develop a positive attitude about hospitals, beginning at an early age. The family should avoid negative attitudes about hospitals. Young children need to know that the hospital is more than a place where "mommies go to get babies." But it is also important to avoid fostering the view of the hospital as a place where people go to die. This is a particular concern if the child knows someone who died in the hospital. A careful explanation of the person's illness and simple, honest answers to questions about the death are necessary.

Figure 4-1
A nurse helps children learn what to expect from hospitalization during a prehospital program.

The Pediatric Unit Atmosphere

An effort by pediatric units and hospitals to create friendly, warm surroundings for children has produced many attractive, colorful pediatric settings. Walls are colorful, often decorated with murals, wallpaper, photos, and paintings specifically designed for children. Furniture is attractive, appropriate in size, and designed with safety in mind. Curtains and drapes are often coordinated with wall coverings in appealing colors or designs.

The staff members of the pediatric unit often wear colored smocks, colorful sweatshirts, or printed scrub suits. Research has shown that children react with greatest anxiety toward the traditional white uniform. Children often are encouraged to wear their own clothing during the day. Colorful printed pajamas are provided for children who need to wear hospital clothing.

Treatments are not performed in the child's room but in a treatment room. Using a separate room to perform procedures promotes the concept that the child's bed is a "safe" place. All treatments, with no exceptions, should be performed in the treatment room to reassure the child.

A playroom or play area is a vital part of all pediatric units. The playroom should be a place that is safe from any kind of procedures. Some hospitals provide a person trained in therapeutic play to coordinate and direct the play activities.

Most pediatric settings provide **rooming-in** facilities and encourage parents or family caregivers to visit as frequently as possible (Fig. 4-2). This approach helps minimize the separation anxiety of the young child, in particular. Caregivers are involved in much of the young child's care, providing comfort and reassurance to the child. Many pediatric

A Personal Glimpse

Hi my name is Jenni. I am 15 years old and would like to tell you about my experience in the hospital.

I am an asthmatic. I have been since my early childhood because of alergies to many things. Whenever I get a cold, it sometimes agrivates my asthma. I recently had an episode where I needed to be hospitalized because of an asthma attack.

I don't like hospitals. I could not wait until I was released. The IV hurt and needed to be put back in. The nurse had dry, scaly hands. It looked like she worked on a farm and then came to work at the hospital. The food was not too great either—not like Pizza Hut or McDonalds.

The person that made the hold ordeal tolerable was the respiratory therapist. I needed regular nebulizer treatments and it was a dream when he came into the room. Yes, he was good looking but what made the difference was his personality and sense of humor. It makes a big difference when it seems as if the staff person wants to be there and really cares rather than being cared by someone who is there just because it's a job and can't wait until the shift ends.

Jenni, age 15 years

units use primary nursing assignments so that the same nurse is with a child as much as possible. This approach gives the nurse the opportunity to establish a trusting relationship with the child.

Planning meals that include the child's favorite foods, within the limitations of any special dietary restrictions, may perk up a flagging appetite. In addition, when space permits, several children may eat together at a small table. Younger children should be seated in high chairs or other suitable seats. Meals should be served out of bed, if possible, and in a pleasant atmosphere. Some pediatric units use the playroom to serve meals to ambulatory children.

Pediatric Intensive Care Units

A child's admission to a pediatric intensive care unit (PICU) may be overwhelming for both the child and the family, especially if the admission is unexpected. Highly technical

Figure 4-2
Rooming-in helps alleviate separation anxiety for both the child and caregiver.

equipment, bright lights, and the crisis atmosphere may be frightening. Visiting may be restricted. Many stressors are present to increase the effect on the child and the family. Great care should be taken by PICU nurses to prepare the family for how the child will look when they first visit. The family should be given a schedule of visiting hours so that they may plan to visit when permitted. Visiting hours should be flexible enough to accommodate the best interests of the child. The family should be encouraged to bring in a special doll or toy of the child's to provide comfort and security. The child's developmental level must be assessed so that appropriate explanations and reassurances may be provided before and during procedures. Positive reinforcements, such as stickers and small badges, may provide a symbol of courage. The nurse also needs to interpret technical information for family members. The nurse should promote the relationship between the family caregiver and the child as much as possible. The caregiver should be encouraged to touch and talk to the child. The caregiver may hold and rock the child, if possible; if not, he or she can comfort the child by caressing and stroking.

Infection Control in the Pediatric Setting

Infection control is important in the pediatric setting. The child who is ill may be especially vulnerable to pathogenic (disease-carrying) microorganisms. Precautions must be taken to protect the children, families, and personnel. Microorganisms are spread by contact (direct, indirect, or droplet), vehicle (food, water, blood, or contaminated products), airborne (dust particles in the air), or vector (mosquitoes, vermin) means of transmission. Each type of microorganism is transmitted in a specific way; thus, precautions are tailored to prevent the spread of microorganisms of that specific type.

In January 1996, the Centers for Disease Control and Prevention and the Hospital Infection Control Practices Advisory Committee published new guidelines for isolation practices in hospitals. The guidelines were revised to include two levels of precautions, standard precautions and transmission-based precautions.

Standard precautions blend the primary characteristics of universal precautions and body substance isolation. Standard precautions apply to blood, all body fluids, secretions, and excretions except sweat, nonintact skin, and mucous membranes. Standard precautions are geared toward reducing the risk of transmission of microorganisms from recognized or unrecognized sources of infection in hospitals. Standard precautions are used in the care of all patients.

Transmission-based precautions pertain to patients documented or suspected to have highly transmissible or other pathogens that require additional precautions beyond those covered under standard precautions. Transmission-based precautions include three types: airborne precautions, droplet precautions, and contact precautions. They may need to be combined to cover certain diseases. The new infection control guidelines are presented in the Guidelines for Standard and Transmission-Based Precautions on the last page of this book. See the Nursing care plan for the child segregated for transmission-based precaution.

Handwashing is the cornerstone of all infection control. The nurse *must* wash his or her hands conscientiously between seeing each patient, even when gloves are worn for a procedure.

The child who is segregated by transmission-based precautions is subject to social isolation. Feelings of loneliness and depression are common. Every effort must be made to help reduce these feelings. The child must not think that being in a room alone is a punishment. The nurse can arrange to spend extra time in the room when performing treatments and procedures. While in the room, the nurse might read a story, play a game, or just talk with the child rather than going quickly in and out of the room.

Family caregivers should be encouraged to spend time with the child. The nurse might help them with gowning and other precaution procedures that are necessary so that they become more comfortable in the situation. Caregivers may need to have the precaution measures reviewed, including handwashing, gowning, and masking as necessary. The nurse may encourage the family to bring the child's favorite dolls, stuffed animals, or toys. Most of these items can be sterilized after use. For the older child, electronic toys may help provide stimulation to ease the loneliness. The child should be encouraged to make phone calls to friends or family members to keep up social contacts. For the school-age child, family caregivers might be encouraged to contact the child's teacher so that classmates can send cards and other school items to keep the child involved. If the child's room has a window, move the bed so the child can see outside.

If masks or gloves are part of the necessary precautions, the child may experience even greater feelings of isolation. The nurse should allow the child to see his or her face before putting on the mask, so that the nurse is easily identified. Gloves prevent the child from experiencing skin-to-skin contact, and the nurse should talk to the child to draw out any feelings the child has about this. Explaining, at the child's level of understanding, why gloves are necessary may help the child accept them. Gowns on the staff are generally not upsetting to the child, but the child may be bothered by the fact that caregivers must wear gowns. If this is the case, a careful explanation should help the child accept this. No matter what precautions are necessary, the nurse should always be alert to the child's loneliness and sadness and should be prepared to meet these needs.

Importance of Caregiver Participation

Research has shown that separating young children from their family caregivers, especially during times of stress, may have damaging effects. Young children have no con-

Nursing Care Plan
for the Child Placed on Transmission-Based Precautions

Tanya is a five year old who has a highly infectious illness resulting from an airborne microorganism. She is placed on Airborne Transmission-Based Precautions.

NURSING DIAGNOSIS

Risk for Social Isolation related to transmission-based precautions

GOAL: *Social contact will be encouraged.*

OUTCOME CRITERIA

- Tanya interacts with nursing staff and family
- Tanya visits with friends via telephone

Nursing Interventions	Rationale
Identify ways in which Tanya can communicate with staff, family, and friends.	Frequent contact with family and staff helps to decrease the child's feeling of isolation.
Facilitate the use of telephone for Tanya to talk with friends.	Use of the telephone helps Tanya feel connected with her friends.
Suggest family caregivers ask Tanya's preschool friends to send notes and drawings.	Notes, photos, and drawings are concrete signs to Tanya that her friends are thinking of her. It helps her stay in touch with her preschool.

NURSING DIAGNOSIS

Diversional Activity Deficit related to monotomy of restrictions

GOAL: *Tanya will be engaged in age-appropriate sensory stimulation*

OUTCOME CRITERIA

- Tanya participates in age-appropriate activities
- Tanya approaches planned activities with enthusiasm

Nursing Interventions	Rationale
Gather a collection of age appropriate books, puzzles and games. Consult with play therapist if available.	A variety of appropriate activities provide diversion and entertainment without boredom.
Encourage family caregivers to engage Tanya in activities she enjoys. Audiotapes can be made for (or by) playmates.	Family caregivers can use visiting time to help alleviate the monotony of isolation. Audiotapes make friends seem closer.
Plan nursing care to include time for reading or playing a game with Tanya.	Activities with a variety of persons (besides family caregivers) is welcome to the child.
Encourage physical exercise within the restrictions of Tanya's condition.	Physical activity helps to improve circulation and feelings of well-being.

(continued)

Nursing Care Plan (*Continued*)
for the Child Placed on Transmission-Based Precautions

NURSING DIAGNOSIS

Powerlessness related to separation resulting from required precautions

GOAL: *Tanya will have control over some aspects of her situation*

OUTCOME CRITERIA

• Tanya makes choices about some of her daily routine
• Tanya's family caregivers and the staff keep their promises to her about planned activities

Nursing Interventions	Rationale
Include Tanya in planning for daily activities such as bath routine, food choices, timing of meals and snacks, and other flexible activities.	Tanya will feel she has some control over her life if she is included in ways where she can have a choice.
Maintain the schedule after making the plan.	Keeping the schedule reinforces for Tanya that she really does have some control.
Plan a special activity with Tanya each day and keep your promise.	When Tanya can depend on the word of those in control she is reassured about her own value.

cept of time, so separation from their primary caregivers is especially difficult for them to understand. Three characteristic stages of response to the separation have been identified: protest, despair, and denial. During the first stage (protest), the young child cries, often refusing to be comforted by others and constantly seeking the primary caregiver in every sight and sound. When the caregiver does not appear, the child enters the second stage—despair—and becomes apathetic and listless. Health care personnel often interpret this as a sign that the child is accepting the situation, but this is not the case; the child has given up.

In the third stage—denial—the child begins taking interest in the surroundings and appears to accept the situation. However, the damage is revealed when the caregivers do visit: the child often turns away from them, showing distrust and rejection. It may take a long time before the child accepts them again, and even then remnants of the damage linger. The child may always have a memory of being abandoned at the hospital. Childhood impressions have a deep effect, regardless of how mistaken they may be.

Rooming-in helps remove the hurt and depression of the young hospitalized child. Although separation from primary caregivers is thought to cause the greatest upset in children younger than 5 years of age, all ages of children should be considered when setting up a rooming-in system.

One advantage of rooming-in is the measure of security the child feels as a result of the caregiver's care and attention. The primary caregiver may participate in bathing, dressing, and feeding, preparing the child for bed, and pro-

viding recreational activities. However, this system should not be used to relieve staff shortage. If treatments are to be continued at home, rooming-in creates an excellent opportunity for the caregiver to observe and practice before leaving the hospital.

Rules should be clearly understood before admission, and facilities for caregivers should be clearly explained. The hospital may provide a folding cot or reclining chair in the child's room. Provision for meals should be explained to the caregiver.

The nursing staff should be careful to avoid creating a situation in which they appear to be expecting the primary caregivers to perform as health care technicians. The basic role of the primary caregiver is to provide security and stability to the child.

Many pediatric units also have recognized the importance of allowing siblings to visit the ill child. This policy provides benefits to both the ill child and the sibling. The sibling at home may be imagining a much more serious illness than is actually the case. Visiting policies usually require that a family adult accompanies and is responsible for the child and that the visiting period is not too long. There also should be a policy requiring that the visiting sibling does not have a cold or other contagious illness and is up to date in immunizations.

The nursing staff also should be aware of the caregiver's needs. The caregiver needs to be encouraged to leave for meals or a break or to go home, if possible, for a shower and rest. The child may be given a possession of the caregiver's to help reassure him or her that the caregiver will return. Some hospitals have established a program in which family caregivers are given pagers so that they can leave the immediate area of the child's room or waiting area but can be quickly paged to return if needed. This gives the family freedom with the reassurance that they can be easily contacted. This is particularly useful during periods when the caregivers must wait for procedures, surgery, or other activities to take place.

ADMISSION AND DISCHARGE PLANNING

Although admission may be a frightening experience, the child feels in much better control of the situation if the person taking the child to the hospital has explained where they are going and why and has answered questions truthfully. When the caregiver and the child arrive on the nursing unit, they should be greeted in a warm, friendly manner and taken to the child's room or to a room set aside specifically for the admission procedure. The caregiver and the child need to be oriented to the child's room, the nursing unit, and regulations (Box 4-1).

Planned Admissions

Preadmission preparation may make the experience less threatening and the adjustment to admission as smooth as possible. Children who are candidates for admission to

Box 4-1. Guidelines to Orient Child to Pediatric Unit

1. Introduce the primary nurse.
2. Orient to the child's room:
   a. Demonstrate bed, bed controls, side rails
   b. Demonstrate call light
   c. Demonstrate television; include cost, if any
   d. Show bathroom facilities
   e. Explain telephone and rules that apply
3. Introduce to roommate(s); include families.
4. Give directions to or show "special" rooms:
   a. Playroom—rules that apply, hours available, toys or equipment that may be taken to child's room
   b. Treatment room—explain purpose
   c. Unit kitchen—rules that apply
   d. Other special rooms
5. Explain pediatric rules—give written rules if available:
   a. Visiting hours, who may visit
   b. Mealtimes, rules about bringing in food
   c. Bedtimes, naptimes, or quiet time
   d. Rooming in arrangements
6. Daily routines:
   a. Vital signs routine
   b. Bath routine
   c. Other routines
7. Guidelines for involvement of family caregiver

Figure 4-3
The child who is going to have surgery may act out the procedure on a doll, thereby reducing some of her fear.

the hospital may attend open house programs or other special programs that are more detailed and specifically related to their upcoming experience. It is important for family caregivers and siblings to attend the preadmission tour along with the future patient to reduce anxiety in all family members.

During the preadmission visit, children may be given surgical masks, caps, and shoe covers and the opportunity to "operate" on a doll or other stuffed toy specifically designed for teaching purposes (Fig. 4-3). Many hospitals have developed special coloring books to help prepare children for tonsillectomy or other specific surgical procedures. These books are given to children during the preadmission visit or sent to children at home before admission. Questions may be answered and anxieties explored during the visit. Children and their families often are hesitant to ask questions or express feelings; the staff must be sensitive to this problem, discussing common questions and feelings. Children are told that some things will hurt but that doctors and nurses will do everything they can to make the hurt go away. Honesty must be a keynote to any program of this kind. The preadmission orientation staff also must be sensitive to cultural and language differences and make adjustments whenever appropriate.

Emergency Admissions

Emergencies leave little time for explanation. The emergency itself is frightening to the child and the family, and the need for treatment is urgent. Even though a caregiver tries to act calm and composed, the child often may sense the anxiety. If the hospital is still a great unknown, it will only add to the child's fear and panic. If the child has even a basic understanding about hospitals and what happens there, the emergency may seem a little less frightening.

In an emergency, physical needs assume priority over emotional needs. The presence, when possible, of a family caregiver who can conceal his or her own fear often is comforting to the child; however, the child may be angry that the caregiver does not prevent invasive procedures from being performed. Sometimes, however, it is impossible for the caregiver to stay with the child. A staff member may use this time to collect information about the child from the family member. This helps the family member to feel involved in the child's care.

Emergency department nurses must be sensitive to the needs of the child and the family. Recognizing the child's cognitive level and how it affects the child's reactions is important. In addition, the staff must explain procedures and conduct themselves in a caring, calm manner to reassure both the child and the family.

The Admission Interview

An admission interview is conducted as soon as possible after the child has been admitted. A quiet, private place is desirable, where interruptions and noise are minimized. The caregiver and the nurse should be comfortably seated, and the child should be included. The nurse should be introduced to the caregiver and the child and should address each of them by name. The admission questionnaire should ask for the child's nickname, feeding habits, food likes and dislikes, allergies, sleeping schedule, toilet-training status, and any special words the child uses or understands to indicate needs or desires, such as words used for urinating and bowel movements. Figure 4-4 provides an example of an assessment form that may be used during this interview.

Rather than simply asking the caregiver to fill out a form, the nurse may ask the questions and write down the answers, gaining the opportunity to observe the reactions of the child and the caregiver as they interact with each other and answer the questions. In addition, this eases the problem of the caregiver who cannot read or write. The nurse must be nonjudgmental, being careful not to indicate disapproval by verbal or nonverbal responses. The child's comments should be listened to attentively, and the child should be made to feel important in the interview.

The reason for the child's admission is the primary concern of the caregiver. While gathering information about the child's physical condition, the nurse also must allow the caregiver to express concerns and anxieties. The caregiver needs to answer the nurse's questions about the problem, including the child's symptoms, how long the symptoms have been present, a description of the symptoms and their intensity and frequency, and treatments up to this time. The nurse should ask the questions in a way that encourages the caregiver to be specific. The nurse also should ask the caregiver about any other concerns regarding the child.

Questions concerning the child's social and family history are important. The nurse should preface these questions with an explanation that the answers will help in caring for the child. Useful information includes:

- The child's primary caregiver
- Other adults in the home
- Siblings in the family, including names the child calls them
- Type of housing the child lives in
- In the case of separation or divorce, the person who has custody of the child and whether this affects who may visit the child
- Whether the child sleeps alone or with others
- Pets in the household
- Favorite toys and types of play
- If all adults work outside of the home, what the child care arrangements are

Through careful questioning, the interviewer tries to determine what the family's previous experience with hospitals and health care providers has been. It is also important to ascertain how much the caregiver and the child understand about the child's condition and their expectations of this hospitalization, what support systems are available when the child returns home, and any disturbing or threatening concerns on the part of the caregiver or the child. These findings, in addition to a careful history and physical assessment, form the basis for the patient's total plan of care while hospitalized.

During the interview, an identification bracelet is placed on the child's wrist. If the child has allergies, an allergy bracelet must be placed on the wrist as well. The child must be prepared for even this simple procedure with an explanation of why it is necessary.

The nurse who receives the child on the pediatric unit should be friendly and casual, remembering that even a well-informed child may be shy and suspicious of excessive friendliness. The child who reacts with fear to well-meaning advances and clings to the caregiver is telling the nurse to go more slowly with the acquaintance process. Children who know that the caregiver may stay with them are more quickly put at ease.

The Admission Physical Assessment

After the child has been oriented to the new surroundings, perhaps clinging to the family caregiver's hand or carrying a favorite toy or blanket, the caregiver may undress the child for the physical examination. This procedure may be familiar from previous health care visits. If comfortable with helping, the caregiver may take a young child's temperature and help obtain the urine specimen. Arrange-

PEDIATRIC NURSING ASSESSMENT FORM

1. Name _____ Date/Time of Admission _____ Via _____
2. Birth Date _____ Information obtained from: _____ Relationship to child _____
3. Child's legal guardian: _____ Child's Nickname: _____

VITAL SIGNS	Temp	Apical Pulse	Radial Pulse	Respirations	BP	Height	Weight	Head Circum

CURRENT CHIEF COMPLAINT/DIAGNOSIS:
Symptoms and Duration

Child's/Caregivers' Understanding of Condition:

PREVIOUS ILLNESS/INJURIES/DIAGNOSIS:
Illness, Symptoms, and Duration

Injuries or Surgery:

Anesthesia Complications?

Allergies and Reactions:	Immunizations	Dates:	Exposure to Infectious Disease	Date
	DPT (DT)		(chicken pox, measles, etc.)	
	Oral Polio			
	Hepatitis B			
	Hib (type)			
	MMR (measles, mumps, rubella)			
	TB skin test Result			

Medications: Name:	Dose	Frequency	Time of Last Dose

Child's reaction to previous hospitalizations: _____

Special fears of child about hospitalization? _____

Family History: (Check all that apply—indicate relationship to child)

_____ Cancer _____   _____ Seizures _____   _____ TB _____
_____ Heart disease _____   _____ Asthma _____   _____ Anesthesia complications _____
_____ Allergy _____   _____ Smoking _____   _____ Other (specify) _____
_____ Diabetes _____   _____ Hypertension _____

Figure 4-4

A sample pediatric nursing assessment form.

Living Facilities (check)

_____ House _____ Apartment _____ Trailer _____ Steps to travel?_____

Who does child live with? _____

Names, ages, of siblings in home_____

Names, ages of other children in home _____

Other persons in home _____

Special interests, toys, games, hobbies: _____
_____

Security object:_____ Was it brought to hospital? _____

Bowel/Bladder Habits:

Toilet Training(if applicable)

			Terms Used for:
Started	_____ Yes	_____ No	Bowel Movement _____ Urination _____
Completed	_____ Yes	_____ No	

Diapers:

Frequency of BM _____ Color _____ Consistency _____

Does child have problems with diarrhea or constipation?_____

| Day | _____ Yes | _____ No |
| Night | _____ Yes | _____ No |

Does child have urinary frequency, burning, discomfort: _____ Yes _____ No

Potty Chair:	_____ Yes	_____ No
Toilet:	_____ Yes	_____ No
Bedwetter:	_____ Yes	_____ No

If yes, please explain:_____
_____
_____

Patterns of:

Sleep/rest:

Bedtime_____ Wakeup _____

Nap ____ Yes ____ No — When? _____

Activity:

Does infant roll over? _____

Does child stand/walk? _____

Does child climb? _____

Does child dress self? _____

Does child go up and down stairs? _____

Does child talk in formed sentences? _____

Eating Habits:

Does child: Feed self _____ Yes ____ No

Does child need help to eat? _____

Food and beverage:

Likes:_____

_____

Dislikes: _____

_____

Usual appetite? _____

Appetite now? _____

Last time child had food or beverage: _____

Items brought to hospital:

Glasses	_____ Yes	_____ No
Contacts	_____ Yes	_____ No
Hearing Aid	_____ Yes	_____ No
Dentures	_____ Yes	_____ No
Braces	_____ Yes	_____ No
Retainer	_____ Yes	_____ No

Special bottle _____ Yes _____ No

Own pacifier _____ Yes _____ No

Does child smoke or drink alcoholic beverages? _____ Yes _____ No

If yes, please give details _____
_____

Does child use street drugs? _____ Yes _____ No

If yes, please give details_____
_____

Other behavior habits of the child (Please check)

Thumbsucking _____ ; Nailbiting _____ ; Headbanging _____

Rituals (Explain) _____
_____

Disposition (Describe)_____
_____

Skin Assessment:

_____ Jaundice _____ Cyanosis _____ Pallor _____ Redness

_____ Cool _____ Warm _____ Clammy _____ Dry

_____ Normal appearance

Describe: (Location and character)

Rash _____

Abrasions _____

Lacerations _____

Contusions _____

Respiratory Assessment:

____ Clear ____ Stridor ____ Rales (___moist, ___ dry) ____ Wheezing

____ Rhonchi ____ Retractions (type) _____

____ Coughing, Sneezing ____ Nasal Discharge (describe) _____

Child/Caregiver oriented to unit? _____ Yes _____ No; understanding verbalized by child _____, caregiver _____

Reviewed safety measures with child _____, caregiver _____; understanding verbalized by child _____, caregiver _____

Additional information nursing staff should know:

Figure 4-4

(continued)

ments should be made so that the caregiver also may be present, if possible, for tests or examinations that need to be performed. The nurse completes a baseline assessment of height, weight, blood pressure, temperature, pulse, and respiration. Included in this initial assessment is an inspection of the child's body. All observations are recorded. The nurse carefully documents any finding that is not within normal limits, describing in detail any unusual findings.

The nurse conducts or assists in conducting a complete physical assessment, with special attention to any symptoms that the caregiver has identified. The nurse's primary role in this complete assessment may be to support the child. All the information gathered is used to plan the care of the child.

Discharge Planning

Planning for discharge and care of the child at home begins early in the hospital experience. Nurses and other health team members must assess the level of understanding of the child and family and their ability to learn about the child's condition and about the care that will be necessary after the child goes home. Giving medications, using special equipment, and enforcing necessary restrictions must be discussed with the person who will be the primary caregiver and with one other person, if possible. It is necessary to provide specific, written instructions for reference at home; the anxiety and strangeness of hospitalization often limit the amount of information retained from teaching sessions. The nurse must be certain the caregiver can understand the written materials, too. If the treatment necessary at home appears too complex for the caregiver to manage, it may be helpful to arrange for a visiting nurse to assist for a period after the child is sent home.

Shortly before the child is discharged from the hospital, a conference may be arranged to review information and procedures with which the family caregivers must become familiar. This conference may or may not include the child, depending on his or her age and cognitive level. Questions and concerns must be dealt with honestly, and a resource should be offered for questions that arise after discharge, perhaps a telephone number the caregiver can call.

The return home may be a difficult period of adjustment for the entire family. The preschool child may be aloof at first, followed by a period of clinging, demanding behavior. Other behaviors such as regression, temper tantrums, excessive attachment to a toy or blanket, night waking, and nightmares may demonstrate fear of another separation. The older child may demonstrate anger or jealousy of siblings. The family may be advised to encourage positive behavior and avoid making the child the center of attention because of the illness. Discipline should be firm, loving, and consistent. The child may express feelings verbally or in play activities. The family may be reassured that this is not unusual.

THE CHILD UNDERGOING SURGERY

Surgery frightens most adults, even though they understand why it is necessary and how it helps correct their health problem. Young children do not have this understanding and may become frightened of even a minor surgical procedure. Older children and adolescents are capable of understanding the need for surgery and what it will accomplish, if they are properly prepared.

Many health care facilities have outpatient surgery facilities (surgicenters) that are used for minor procedures and permit the patient to return home the day of the operation. These facilities reduce or eliminate the separation of parents and children, one of the most stressful factors in surgery for infants and young children. Whether admitted for less than 1 day or for several weeks, the child who has surgery needs sympathetic and thorough preoperative and postoperative care. When the child is too young to benefit from preoperative teaching, explanations should be directed to family caregivers to help relieve their anxiety and to prepare them to participate in the child's care after surgery.

Preoperative Care

Specific physical and psychological preparation of the child and the family varies according to the type of surgery planned. General aspects of care include patient teaching, skin preparation, preparation of the gastrointestinal and urinary systems, and preoperative medication.

PATIENT TEACHING

The child admitted for planned surgery probably has had some preadmission preparation by the physician and family caregivers. Many families, however, have an unclear understanding of the surgery and what it involves, or they may be too anxious to be helpful. The health professionals involved in the child's care must determine how much the child knows and is capable of learning, help correct any misunderstandings, and explain the preparation for surgery and what the surgery will "fix," as well as how the child will feel after surgery. This preparation must be based on the child's age, developmental level, previous experiences, and caregiver support. All explanations should be clear and honest, expressed in terms the child and the family caregivers can understand. Questions should be encouraged to ensure all information is understood correctly. If possible, preoperative teaching should be conducted in short sessions rather than trying to discuss everything at once.

Therapeutic play, discussed later in this chapter, is useful in preparing the child for surgery. Identifying the area of the body to be operated on with drawings helps the child have a better understanding of what is going to happen.

Children need to be prepared for standard preoperative tests and procedures, such as radiographs and blood and urine tests. Nurses may explain the reason for withholding food and fluids before surgery so children do not feel they are being neglected or punished when others receive meal trays.

Children sometimes interpret surgery as punishment and should be reassured that they did not cause the condition. They also fear mutilation or death and must be able to explore those feelings, recognizing them as acceptable fears. Children deserve careful explanation that the physician is going to repair only the affected body part.

It is important to emphasize that the child will not feel anything during surgery because of the special sleep that anesthesia causes. Describing the postanesthesia care unit (PACU or wake-up room) and any tubes, bandages, or appliances that will be in place after surgery lets the child know what to expect. If possible, the child should be able to see and handle the anesthesia mask (if this is the method to be used) and equipment that will be part of the postoperative experience.

Role playing, adjusted to the child's age and understanding, is helpful. This approach may include a trip on a stretcher, pretending to go to surgery. The nurse or play leader can pretend to be the patient, if the child makes such a request.

The older child or adolescent may have a greater interest in the surgery itself, what is wrong and why, how the repair is done, and the expected postoperative results. Models of a child's internal organs, or individual organs such as a heart, are useful for demonstration, or the patient may be involved in making the drawing.

A child needs to understand that several people will be involved in preoperative, surgical, and postoperative care. If possible, staff members from the anesthesia department and the operating room, recovery room, or the ICU should visit the child preoperatively. Explaining what the people will be wearing (caps, masks, and gloves) and what equipment will be used (including bright lights) helps make the operating room experience less frightening. A preoperative tour of the ICU or PACU is also helpful.

Most patients experience postoperative pain, and children should be prepared for this experience. They also need to know when they may expect to be allowed to have fluids and food after surgery.

Children should be taught to practice coughing and deep-breathing exercises. Deep-breathing practice may be done with games that encourage blowing. Teaching children to splint the operative site with a pillow helps reassure them that the sutures will not break and let the wound open.

Children should be told where their family will be during and after surgery, and every effort should be made to minimize separation. Family caregivers should be encouraged to be present when the child leaves for the operating room.

SKIN PREPARATION

Depending on the type of surgery, skin preparation may include a tub bath or shower and certainly includes special cleaning and inspection of the operative site. If shaving is needed as part of the preparation, it usually is performed in the operating room. If fingers or toes are involved, the nails are carefully trimmed. The operative site may be painted with a special antiseptic solution as an extra precaution against infection, depending on the physician's orders and the procedures of the hospital.

GASTROINTESTINAL AND URINARY SYSTEM PREPARATION

The surgeon may order a cleansing enema the night before surgery. An enema is an intrusive procedure and must be explained to the child before it is given. If old enough, the child should understand the reason for the enema.

Children usually receive nothing by mouth (NPO) 4 to 12 hours before surgery because food or fluids in the stomach may cause vomiting and aspiration, particularly during general anesthesia. The child should be told that food and drink are being withheld to prevent an upset stomach. The NPO period varies according to the child's age; infants become dehydrated more rapidly than older children and thus require a shorter NPO period before surgery. Pediatric NPO orders should be accompanied by an intravenous (IV) fluid initiation order. Loose teeth are also a potential hazard and should be counted and recorded according to hospital policy.

In some instances, urinary catheterization may be performed preoperatively, but usually it is done while the child is in the operating room. The catheter is often removed immediately after surgery but can be left in place for several hours or days. Children who are not catheterized before surgery should be encouraged to void before the administration of preoperative medication.

PREOPERATIVE MEDICATION

Depending on the physician's order, preoperative medications usually are given in two stages: a sedative is administered about 1.5 to 2 hours before surgery, and an analgesic–atropine mixture may be administered immediately before the patient leaves for the operating room. When the sedative has been given, the lights should be dimmed and noise minimized to help the child relax and rest. Family caregivers and the child should be aware that atropine can cause a blotchy rash and a flushed face.

Preoperative medication should be brought to the child's room when it is time for administration. At that time, the child is told that it is time for medication and that another nurse has come along to help the child hold still. Medication should be administered carefully and quickly because delays only increase the child's anxiety.

If hospital regulations permit, family caregivers should accompany the child to the operating room and wait until the child is anesthetized. If this is impossible, the nurse who has been caring for the child can go along to the operating room and introduce the child to personnel there.

Postoperative Care

During the immediate postoperative period, the child is cared for in the PACU or the surgical ICU. Meanwhile, the room in the pediatric unit should be prepared with appropriate equipment for the child's return. Depending on the type of surgery performed, it may be necessary to have suctioning, resuscitation, or other equipment at the bedside.

When the child has been returned to the room, nursing care focuses on careful observation for any signs or symptoms of complications: shock, hemorrhage, or respiratory distress. Vital signs are monitored according to postoperative orders and recorded. The child is kept warm with blankets as needed. Dressings, IV apparatus, urinary catheters, and any other appliances are noted and observed. An IV flow sheet is begun that documents the type of fluid, the amount of fluid to be absorbed, the rate of flow, any additive medications, the site, and the appearance and condition of the site. The IV flow sheet may be separate or incorporated into a general flow sheet for the pediatric patient. The first voiding is an important milestone in the child's postoperative progress because it indicates the adequacy of blood flow; it should be noted, recorded, and reported. Any irrita-

tion or burning also should be noted, and the physician should be notified if **anuria** (absence of urine) persists longer than 6 hours.

Postoperative orders may provide for ice chips or clear liquids to prevent dehydration; these may be administered with a spoon or in a small medicine cup. Frequent repositioning is necessary to prevent skin breakdown, orthostatic pneumonia, and decreased circulation. Coughing, deep breathing, and position changes are performed at least every 2 hours.

PAIN MANAGEMENT

Pain is a concern of postoperative patients in any age group. Most adult patients can verbally express the pain they feel and request relief. However, infants and young children cannot adequately express themselves and need help to tell where or how great the pain is. Longstanding beliefs that children do not have the same amount of pain that adults have, or that they tolerate pain better than adults, have contributed to the undermedication of infants and children in pain. Recent research has shown that children do experience pain as keenly as adults.

The nurse must be alert to indications of pain, especially in young patients. Careful assessment is necessary, noting changes in behavior such as rigidity, thrashing, facial expressions, loud crying or screaming, flexion of knees (indicating abdominal pain), restlessness, and irritability. Physiologic changes, such as increased pulse rate and blood pressure, sweating palms, dilated pupils, flushed or moist skin, and loss of appetite, also may indicate pain. Some children may try to hide pain because they fear an injection

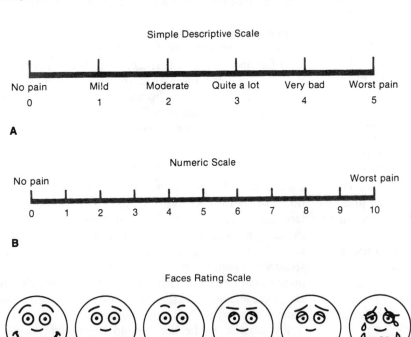

Figure 4-5

Pain scales: (A) Simple descriptive scale; (B) Numeric scale; (C) Faces rating scale.

Figure 4-6
(A) PCA pump. (B) Distraction supplements pain control while child is using PCA.

or because they are afraid that admitting to pain will increase the time they have to stay in the hospital.

Various tools have been devised to help children express the amount of pain they feel and allow nurses to measure the effectiveness of pain management efforts. These tools include the faces scale, the numeric scale, descriptive scales, and the color scale. The first three scales are useful primarily with children 7 years of age and older (Fig. 4-5). To use the color scale, the young child is given crayons ranging from yellow to red or black. Yellow represents no pain, and the darkest color (or red) represents the most pain. The child selects the color that represents the amount of pain felt.

Pain medication may be administered orally, by routine intramuscular or IV routes, or by **patient-controlled analgesia**, a programmed IV infusion of narcotic analgesia that the child may control within set limits (Fig. 4-6). A low-level dose of analgesia may be administered, with the child able to administer a bolus as needed. Patient-controlled analgesia may be used for children 7 years of age or older who have no cognitive impairment and undergo a careful evaluation. Intramuscular injections are avoided, if possible. Vital signs must be monitored, and the child's level of consciousness must be documented frequently, following the standards of the facility.

Comfort measures should be used along with the administration of analgesics. The child is encouraged to become involved in activities that may provide distraction. Such activities must be appropriate for the child's age, level of development, and interests. No child should be allowed to suffer pain unnecessarily. Appropriate nonpharmacologic comfort measures may include position changes, massage, distraction, play, heat or cold application, soothing touch, talk, coddling and affection.

SURGICAL DRESSINGS

Postoperative care includes close observation of any dressings for signs of drainage or hemorrhage and reinforcing or changing dressings as ordered. Wet dressings can in-

crease the possibility of contamination; clean, dry dressings increase the child's comfort. If there is no physician's order to change the dressing, the nurse is expected to reinforce the moist original dressing by covering it with a dry dressing and taping the second dressing in place. If bloody drainage is present, the nurse should draw around the outline of the drainage with a marker and mark it with the time and date. In this way the amount of additional drainage can be assessed when the dressings are inspected later.

Supplies needed for changing dressings vary according to the wound site and the physician's orders, which specify the sterile or antiseptic technique to be used. Detailed procedures for these techniques and the supplies to be used can be found in the facility's procedures manual.

As with all procedures, the nurse must explain to the child what will be done and why before beginning the dressing change. Some dressing changes are painful; if so, the child should be told that it will hurt and should be praised for behavior that shows courage and cooperation.

PATIENT TEACHING

Postoperative patient teaching is as important as preoperative teaching. Some explanations and instructions given earlier must be repeated during postoperative care because the child's earlier anxiety may have prevented thorough understanding. Now that tubes, restraints, and dressings are part of the child's reality, they need to be discussed again: why they are important and how they affect the child's activities.

Family caregivers want to know how they can help care for the child and what limitations are placed on the child's activity. If caregivers know what to expect and how to aid in their child's recovery, they will be cooperative during the postoperative period.

As the child recuperates, the caregivers and child should be encouraged to share their feelings about the surgery, any changes in body image, and their expectations for recovery and rehabilitation.

When the sutures are removed, the nurse should reas-

Figure 4-7
Incorporating the entire family into the teaching process increases learning effectiveness © Kathy Sloane.

sure the child that the opening has healed and the child's insides will not fall out, a common fear.

Before the child is discharged from the hospital, teaching focuses on home care, use of any special equipment or appliances, medications, diet, restrictions on activities, and therapeutic exercise (Fig. 4-7). Caregivers should demonstrate the procedures or repeat information so the nurse can determine if learning has occurred. The nursing process is used to assess the needs of the child and the family to plan appropriate postoperative care and teaching.

GAVAGE FEEDING

Sometimes infants or children who have had surgery are too weak to take adequate food and fluid by mouth and must receive nourishment by means of gavage feedings. **Gavage feedings** provide nourishment directly through a tube passed into the stomach. This procedure is particularly appropriate in infants. If gavage feedings are not well tolerated, the nurse should report it and await alternate orders from the physician.

Whether the tube is inserted nasally or orally, the measurement is the same: from the tip of the child's nose to the earlobe and down to the tip of the sternum (Fig. 4-8). This length may be marked on the tube with tape or a marking pen. The end of the tube to be inserted should be lubricated with sterile water or water-soluble lubricating jelly, *never* an oily substance because of the danger of oil aspiration into the lungs.

To prepare the child for gavage feeding, elevate the head and place a rolled-up diaper behind the neck. Turn the head and align the body to the right.

After the tube is inserted, its position is verified by aspirating stomach contents or by inserting 1 to 5 mL of air (using a syringe with an adapter) and listening with a stethoscope. If the tube is properly placed, gurgling or growling sounds are heard as air enters the stomach. If stomach contents are aspirated, these should be measured and re-

placed and, in a very small infant, subtracted from the amount ordered for that particular feeding.

The nurse may hold the tube in place if it is going to be removed immediately after the feeding. If the tube is left in position for further use, it should be secured with tape (Fig. 4-9). The correct position must be verified before each feeding.

The feeding syringe is inserted into the tube, and its plunger is pushed gently to start the flow of formula, which has been warmed to room temperature. The plunger is then removed, and the feeding is allowed to flow by gravity only. The entire feeding should take 15 to 20 minutes, after which the infant must be burped and positioned on the right side for at least 1 hour to prevent regurgitation and aspiration.

The type and amount of contents aspirated by the nurse, the amount of formula fed, the infant's tolerance for the procedure, and the positioning of the infant after completion should be recorded on the chart. The feeding tube and any leftover formula should be discarded at the completion of the procedure.

GASTROSTOMY FEEDING

Children who must receive tube feedings over a long period may have a **gastrostomy tube** surgically inserted through the abdominal wall into the stomach. This procedure is performed under general anesthesia. It also is used in children who have obstructions or surgical repairs in the mouth, pharynx, esophagus, or cardiac sphincter of the stomach or who are respirator-dependent.

The surgeon inserts a catheter (plain, Foley, or mushroom [Pezzer] catheter with the tip removed) that is left unclamped and connected to gravity drainage for 24 hours. Meticulous care of the wound site is necessary to prevent

Xyphoid process

Figure 4-8
Measurement of tubing for nasogastric tube insertion.

Figure 4-9
Nasogastric tube taped to infant's cheek.

infection and irritation. Until the area has healed, it must be covered with a sterile dressing. Ointment, Stomadhesive, or other skin preparations may be ordered for application to the site. The child may need to be restrained to prevent pulling on the catheter, which may cause leakage of caustic gastric juices.

Procedures for positioning and feeding the child with a gastrostomy tube are similar to those for gavage feedings. The residual stomach contents are aspirated, measured, and replaced at the beginning of the procedure. The child's head and shoulders are elevated during the feeding. After each feeding, the child is placed on the right side or in Fowler's position.

When regular oral feedings are resumed, the tube is surgically removed, and the opening usually closes spontaneously.

For long-term gastrostomy feedings, a gastrostomy button may be inserted. Among the advantages of buttons are that they are more desirable cosmetically, are simple to care for, and cause less skin irritation.

THE HOSPITAL PLAY PROGRAM

Play is the business of children and a principal way in which they learn, grow, develop, and act out feelings and problems. Playing is a normal activity, and the more it can be part of hospital care, the more normal and more comfortable this environment becomes.

Play helps children come to terms with the hurts, anxi-

eties, and separation that hospitalization brings. In the hospital playroom children may express frustrations, hostilities, and aggressions through play without the fear of being scolded by the nursing staff. Children who keep these negative emotions bottled up suffer much greater damage than those who are allowed to let them out where they may be handled constructively. Children must feel secure enough in the situation to express negative emotions without fear of disapproval.

Children must not be allowed to harm themselves or others, however. Although it is important to express feelings, acceptable or not, unlimited permissiveness is as harmful as excessive strictness. Children rely on adults to guide them and set limits for behavior because this means the adults care about them. When disapproval is necessary, it is important to make it clear that the child's action is being disapproved, not the child.

The Hospital Play Environment

An organized and well-planned play area is of considerable importance in the overall care of the hospitalized child (Fig. 4-10). The play area should be large enough to accommodate cribs, wheelchairs, IV poles, and children in casts. It should provide a variety of play materials suitable for the ages and needs of all children. The child chooses the toy and the kind of play needed or desired; thus, the selection and kind of play may usually be left unstructured. However, all children should participate, and none should be ignored by the play leaders.

Adolescents should have a separate recreation room or area, if possible. Ideally, this is an area where adolescents may gather to talk, play pool or table tennis, and drink soft drinks (if permitted) and eat snacks. Tables and chairs should be provided to encourage interaction among the adolescents. Television with a videocassette tape player, computer games, and shuffle board are also desirable. These activities should be in an area away from young chil-

Figure 4-10
Children in a hospital playroom.

dren. Rules may be clearly spelled out and posted. If adolescents must share the same recreation area with younger children, the area should be referred to as the "activity center" rather than the "playroom."

Although a well-equipped playroom is of major importance in any pediatric department, some children cannot be brought to the playroom, or some play programs may be cut due to cost-containment efforts. In these situations, nurses must be creative in providing play opportunities for children. Children may act out their fantasies and emotions in their own crib or bed if materials are brought to them and someone (a nurse or student volunteer) is available to give them the support and attention needed. Children in isolation may be given play material, providing infection control precautions are strictly followed.

Therapeutic Play

The nurse should understand the difference between play therapy and therapeutic play. **Play therapy** is a technique of psychoanalysis that psychiatrists or psychiatric nurse clinicians use to uncover a disturbed child's underlying thoughts, feelings, and motivations to help understand them better. **Therapeutic play** is a play technique that may be used by play therapists, nurses, child-life specialists, or trained volunteers to help the child express feelings, fears, and concerns.

The play leader should be alert to the needs of the child who is afraid to act independently as a result of strict home discipline. Even normally sociable children may carry their fears of the hospital environment into the playroom. It could be some time before timid, fearful, or nonassertive children feel free enough to take advantage of the play opportunities. Too much enthusiasm on the part of the play leader in trying to get the child to participate may defeat the purpose and make the child withdraw. The leader must decide carefully whether to initiate an activity for a child or let the child advance at a self-set pace.

Often, other children provide the best incentive by doing something interesting, so that the timid child forgets his or her apprehensions and tries it, or a child says, "Come and help me with this," and soon the other child becomes involved. A fearful child trusts a peer before trusting an adult, who represents authority. Naturally, this fact does not mean the child's presence should be ignored. The leader shows the child around the playroom, indicating that the children are free to play with whatever they wish and that the leader is there to answer questions and to help when a child wishes help.

When group play is initiated, the leader may invite the timid child to participate but should not insist. The leader must give the child time to adjust and gain confidence.

Play Material

Play material should be chosen with safety in mind; for instance, no sharp edges and no small parts that can be swallowed or aspirated. Toys and equipment should be in-spected regularly for broken parts or sharp edges. Constant supervision of children while they are playing is necessary for safety.

One important function of a playroom is that it gives opportunities for the child to dramatize hospital experiences. One section of the playroom containing hospital equipment, miniature or real, gives the child an opportunity to act out feelings about the hospital environment and treatments. Stethoscopes, simulated thermometers, stretchers, wheelchairs, examining tables, instruments, bandages, and other medical and hospital equipment are useful for this purpose.

Dolls or puppets dressed to represent the people with whom the child comes in contact daily—boy, girl, and infant, as well as adult family members, nurses, physicians, therapists, and other personnel—should be available. Hospital scrub suits, scrub caps, isolation-type gowns, masks, or other types of uniforms may be provided for children to use in acting out their hospital experiences. These simulated hospitals also serve an educational purpose: they may help a child who is to have surgery, tests, or special treatments to understand the procedures and why they are done.

Other useful materials include clay, paints, markers, crayons, stamps, stickers, sand art, cut-out books, construction paper, puzzles, building sets, and board games. Tricycles, small sliding boards, and seesaws may be fun for children who can be more physically active. Books for all age groups are also important.

Sometimes only a little imagination is needed to initiate an interesting play time. Table 4-1 suggests activities for various age levels, most of which may be played in the child's room. These are especially useful for the child who cannot go to the playroom.

Puppets play an important part in the children's department. The use of hand puppets does much to orient or reassure a hospitalized child. The doctor or nurse puppet on the play leader's hand answers questions (and discusses feelings) that the puppet on the child's hand has asked. A child often finds it easier to express feelings, fears, and questions through a puppet than to verbalize them directly. A ready sense of magic can let the child make believe that the puppet is really expressing things that he or she hesitates to ask (Fig. 4-11).

Ambulatory Play Facilities

Pediatric ambulatory departments are busy places. Due to growing knowledge of childhood diseases and their treatment, more children can be treated as outpatients, allowing them to live at home. Because they must also be treated as children, a properly equipped and adequately staffed playroom is needed in a pediatric ambulatory setting.

Many children with serious but chronic diseases become frequent visitors to the ambulatory department. Having a playroom is enjoyable and also helpful to children who are

TABLE 4-1. Games and Activities Using Materials Available on a Nursing Unit

Age	Activity
Infant	Make a mobile from roller gauze and tongue blades to hang over a crib.
	Ask the pharmacy or central supply for different-size boxes to use for put-in, take-out toys. (Do not use round vials from pharmacy; if accidentally aspirated, these can completely occlude the airway.)
	Blow up a glove as a balloon; draw a smiling face on it with a marker.
	Play "Patty Cake," "So Big," "Peek-a-Boo."
Toddler	Ask central supply for boxes to use as blocks for stacking.
	Tie roller gauze to a tissue box for a pull toy.
	Sing or recite familiar nursery rhymes such as "Peter, Peter, Pumpkin Eater."
Preschool	Play "Simon Says" or "Mother, May I?"
	Draw a picture of a dog; ask child to close eyes; add an additional feature to the dog; ask the child to guess the added part, and repeat until a full picture is drawn.
	Make a puppet from a lunch bag or draw a face on your hand with a marker.
	Cut out a picture from a nursing journal (or draw a picture); cut it into large puzzle pieces.
	Pour breakfast cereal into a basin; furnish boxes to pour and spoons to dig.
	Furnish chart paper and a Magic Marker for coloring.
	Make modeling clay from 1 cup salt, $\frac{1}{2}$ cup flour, $\frac{1}{2}$ cup water from diet kitchen.
	Play "Ring-Around-the-Rosey" or "London Bridge."
School-age	Play "I Spy" or charades.
	Make a deck of cards to play "Go Fish" or "Old Maid"; invent cards such as Nicholas Nurse, Doctor Dolittle, Irene Intern, Polly Patient.
	Play "Hangman."
	Furnish scale or table paper and a Magic Marker for a huge drawing or sign.
	Hide an object in the room and have child look for it (have child name places for you to look if child cannot be out of bed).
Adolescent	Color squares on a chart form to make a checkerboard.
	Have adolescent make a deck of cards to use for "Hearts" or "Rummy."
	Compete to see how many words the adolescent can make from the letters in the child's name.
	Compete to guess whether the next person to enter room will be a man or woman, next car to go by window will be red or black, and so forth.
	Compete to see who can name the most episodes of the television shows "Star Trek" or "The Brady Bunch."

From Pillitteri A. Maternal and child health. Philadelphia: JB Lippincott, 1992.

to undergo medical procedures, which may be frightening to the unprepared child. Play workers have an excellent opportunity to help an anxious child work through fears. Toys should be durable and easily cleaned. They should not require a specific time commitment so that children may leave when called for examination. They should also allow for both individual and group play. A play house, for instance, allows children to use their imaginations and incorporate one another in and out of the play as they arrive and leave for their appointments.

Some children who have become engrossed in a play project may resent having to leave when called for examination. The child may be assured that the project may be finished after the treatment if the family caregiver is willing

Figure 4-11
A puppet play group led by a pediatric nurse oncologist allows children to talk about what it's like to be in the hospital. Group sessions inform children that others have similar feelings.

or able to take the time. If for any reason a child must be left in the playroom without the caregiver, name bands or name tags should be available, particularly for a new child or one unfamiliar to the staff.

SAFETY

Safety is an essential aspect of pediatric nursing care. Accidents occur more often when people are in stressful situations, and infants, children, and their caregivers experience additional stress when a child is hospitalized. They are removed from a familiar home environment, faced with anxieties and fear, and must adjust to an unfamiliar schedule. The pediatric nurse must have safety in mind at all times, consciously assessing every situation for accident potential.

The environment should meet all the safety standards appropriate for other areas of the facility, including good lighting, dry floors with no obstacles that may cause falls, electrical equipment checked for hazards, safe bath and shower facilities, and beds in low position for ambulatory patients.

The child's age and developmental level must be considered. Toddlers are explorers whose developmental task is to develop autonomy. Toddlers love to put small objects into equally small openings, whether the opening is in their body, the oxygen tent, or elsewhere in the pediatric unit. Careful observation may prevent the toddler from having access to small objects, eliminating some of the dangers. Toddlers are also often climbers and must be protected from climbing and falling. Toddlers and preschoolers must be watched to protect them from danger. Nurses also must encourage family members to keep the crib sides up when not directly caring for the infant in the crib. One unguarded

moment may mean a fall out of a crib. Box 4-2 presents a summary of pediatric safety precautions.

Restraints

Restraints often are needed to protect a child from injury during a procedure or an examination or to ensure the infant's or child's safety and comfort. Restraints should never be used as a form of punishment. When possible, restraining by hand is the best method. However, mechanical restraints must be used to secure a child during IV infusions, to protect a surgical site from injury, such as cleft lip and cleft palate, or when restraint by hand is impractical.

Various types of restraints may be used. A **mummy restraint** is used for an infant or small child during a procedure (Fig. 4-12). This device is a snug wrap that is effective when performing a scalp venipuncture, inserting a nasogastric tube, or performing other procedures that involve only the head or neck. A **papoose board** is used with toddlers or preschoolers.

Clove hitch restraints are used to secure an arm or leg, most often when a child is receiving an IV infusion. The restraint is made of soft cloth formed in a figure eight. Padding under the restraint is desirable if the child puts any pull on it. The site should be checked and loosened at least every 2 hours. Commercial restraints also are available for this purpose.

Elbow restraints often are made of muslin that has two layers. Pockets wide enough to fit tongue depressors are placed vertically the width of the fabric. The top flap folds over to close the pockets. The restraint is wrapped around the child's arm and tied securely, preventing the child from bending the elbow. Care must be taken that the elbow restraints fit the child properly. They should not be too high under the axillae. They may be pinned to the child's shirt to keep them from slipping.

Jacket restraints are used to secure the child from climbing out of bed or a chair or to keep the child in a horizontal position. The restraint must be the correct size for the child. A child in a jacket restraint should be checked frequently to prevent him or her from slipping and choking on the neck of the jacket. Ties must be secure to the bed frame, not the sides, so that the jacket is not pulled when the sides are put up and down.

Whatever the type of restraint, caution is essential. Close and conscientious observation is a necessary part of nursing care. The nurse also must be alert to concerns of the family when the child is in restraints. Explanations about the need for restraints help the family understand and be cooperative. The caregiver may wish to restrain the child physically to prevent use of restraints, and this action is often possible. Each situation must be judged individually.

Box 4-2. *Safety Precautions for Pediatric Units*

1. Cover electrical outlets.
2. Keep floor dry and free of clutter.
3. Use tape or Velcro closures when possible.
4. Always close safety pins when not in use.
5. Inspect toys (child's or hospital's) for loose or small parts, sharp edges, dangerous cords, or other hazards.
6. Do not permit friction toys where oxygen is in use.
7. Do not leave child unattended in high chair.
8. Keep crib sides up all the way, except when caring for child.
9. If the crib side is down, keep hand firmly on infant at all times.
10. Use crib with top if child stands or climbs.
11. Always check temperature of bath water to prevent burns.
12. Never leave infant or child unattended in bath water.
13. Keep beds of ambulatory children locked in low position.
14. Turn off motor of electric bed if young children might have access to controls.
15. Always use safety belts or straps for children in infant seats, feeding chairs, strollers, wheelchairs, or stretchers.
16. Use restraints only when necessary.
17. When restraints are used, remove and check for skin integrity, circulation, and correct application at least every hour or two.
18. Never tie a restraint to the crib side; tie to bed frame only.
19. Keep medications securely locked in designated area; children should never be permitted in this area.
20. Set limits and enforce them consistently; do not let children get out of control.
21. Place needles and syringes in sharps containers; make sure children have no access to these containers.
22. Always pick up any equipment after a procedure.
23. Never leave scissors or other sharp instruments within child's reach.
24. Do not allow sleepy family caregivers to hold a sleeping child as they may fall asleep and drop the child.

Figure 4-12
(A) Mummy restraint. (B) Papoose board. (C) Clove hitch restraint. (D) Elbow restraint. (E) Jacket restraint.

■ KEY POINTS

- Many factors affect the way the family reacts to hospitalization of the child. These factors may place great stress on the child and the family.

- Preadmission education helps prepare the child for the event. Nevertheless, many anxieties persist. An emergency admission of the child may be especially traumatic for both the child and the family.

- Liberal visiting policies, encouraging family caregivers to stay with young children, and sibling visits help decrease the stress of hospitalization.

- Conscientious handwashing is the cornerstone of infection control. Standard precautions are applied to all patients of every age and diagnosis.

- The family caregiver is an vital participant in the care of an ill child and should be included in planning of nursing care.

- The admission interview sets the stage for the hospitalization, providing information that helps the health care team give the best possible care to the child and help him or her adjust to the hospitalization.

- Discharge planning includes teaching the child and the family about care needed after discharge from the hospital. Discharge teaching should include written and verbal instructions; the nurse must be certain that instructions are fully understood.

- Play is fundamental to the care of children. Therapeutic play offers the child the opportunity to express anger and fear in a safe environment. Expressing these emotions is beneficial to the child. Adolescents need a special area where they may enjoy activities suited to their age.

- Safety is an essential aspect of pediatric care. Children must be protected from hazards. Understanding the growth and development levels of each age group helps the nurse be alert to possible dangers for each child.

- When restraints are necessary, care must be taken to protect the child from injury by regular, careful observation.

? CRITICAL THINKING

1. Your neighbor's daughter, 3-year-old Angela, is going to be admitted to the pediatric unit for tests and possible surgery. Describe how you will help her mother prepare her for this event.

2. Edgar, the 4-year-old son of migrant workers, is hurt in a farming accident. You are working in the emergency department when he is brought in for treatment. His grandmother, who speaks little English, is with him. Design a plan of care that will help both the child and his grandmother.

3. On a playground, you hear a child's caregiver say, "If you don't stop that, you're going to hurt yourself and end up in the hospital!" Explain how you feel about this. Describe how you would like to respond if you could.

4. Plan an orientation visit for a group of preschoolers from a nursery school. Check and use what is available in the pediatric unit where you have your clinical experience.

5. Discuss how rooming-in can be helpful in discharge planning.

6. Design an ideal teen activity room. List all furniture and equipment you would have, and state the use(s) for each.

BIBLIOGRAPHY

Ashenberg MD, Lambert SA, Maier NP, McAliley LG. Easing the wait: Development of a pager program for families. Pediatr Nurs 22:103–107, 1996.

Austin JK. Assessment of coping mechanisms used by parents and children with chronic illness. MCN 15:98–102, 1990.

Byrnes K. Conducting the pediatric health history: A guide. Pediatr Nurs 22:135–137, 1996.

Greenberg LA. Teaching children who are learning disabled about illness and hospitalization. MCN 16:260–263, 1991.

Howe CJ. A new standard of care for pediatric pain management. MCN 18:325–329, 1993.

Johnson A, Lindschau A. Staff attitudes toward parent participation in the care of children who are hospitalized. Pediatr Nurs 22: 99–102, 1996.

Meyer D. Children's responses to nursing attire. Pediatr Nurs 18: 157–160, 1992.

Pillitteri A. Maternal and child health nursing, 2d ed. Philadelphia: JB Lippincott, 1995.

Rosenblum RK. Developing a pediatric patient-family education program. 20(4):359–362, 1994.

Summers KH. Providing for play in the care of children. Pediatr Nurs 18:266–267, 1992.

Thomas DO. Assessing children—it's different. RN 59(4):38–44, 1996.

Vessey JA, Farley JA, Risom LR. Iatrogenic developmental effects of pediatric intensive care. Pediatr Nurs 18:229–232, 1992.

Wong D. Whaley and Wong's nursing care of infants and children, 5th ed. St. Louis: Mosby, 1995.

Chapter 5

Care of the Child in the Community

HEALTH CARE SHIFT FROM HOSPITAL TO COMMUNITY
Community-Based Nursing
Community Care Settings for the Child
CARING FOR THE CHILD IN THE COMMUNITY
The Nursing Process
Communication
Teaching

Case Management
Client Advocacy
THE CHALLENGE OF COMMUNITY-BASED NURSING
The Unique Aspects of Community-Based Nursing
Issues Facing Children and Families
Rewards of Community-Based Nursing

STUDENT OBJECTIVES

On completion of this chapter, the student will be able to:

1. Identify the focus of community-based nursing.
2. Describe advantages of community-based health care for the child and family.
3. Identify community settings where children are cared for.
4. List conditions of infants or children that may be treated in home care settings.
5. Differentiate between primary, secondary, and tertiary prevention. Give an example of each.
6. Describe at least five community-based nursing settings.
7. Discuss what information a nurse needs to teach a group of children successfully.
8. Describe how child advocacy helps children in community-based health care.
9. Identify and explain the unique characteristics of community-based nursing.

KEY TERMS

case management	primary prevention
child advocacy	secondary prevention
community-based nursing	tertiary prevention

HEALTH CARE SHIFT FROM HOSPITAL TO COMMUNITY

In the last century, health care has gone through a number of changes. The sophisticated health care currently available is extremely expensive and has strained health care funding to a point where other approaches to health care have become necessary. This need for change has led to the emergence of community-based health care and a stress on wellness and preventive health care.

The shift to community-based health care has been a positive factor in the care of children. The child is no longer viewed simply as a person with an illness, but rather as a child who is a member of a family from a certain community with deep-seated cultural values and social customs (Fig. 5-1). Learning about the child's community and then using that knowledge improves the level of care the child receives. In the community, the child can also receive preventive care and wellness teaching not usually available in the hospital setting unless one is ill.

Community-Based Nursing

Community-based nursing focuses on prevention and is directed toward persons and families within a community. The goals are to help them meet their health care needs

Figure 5-1
Native American children celebrate a festive social custom with their family.

and to maintain continuity of care as they move through the various health care settings available to them. The role of the nurse who works in the community is different from that of the hospital nurse. Generally, the nurse in the community focuses on **primary prevention** (the level of prevention that includes teaching regarding safety, diet, rest, exercise, and disease prevention through immunizations), emphasizing the role of teacher and client advocate. Examples of primary prevention are a drug education program given by a school nurse to a fourth-grade class, and family health teaching about home safety practices for a toddler given by a nurse in a well-baby clinic.

In some community settings, the nurse's role focuses on **secondary prevention** (the level of prevention that focuses on early diagnosis and initiation of treatment). Such settings are clinics, home care nursing, and schools. The nurse participates in screening measures such as height, weight, hearing, and vision. During child assessments and follow-up, a health history and other assessments are conducted, including vital signs, blood work, and other diagnostic tests as ordered by the health care practitioner. One example of secondary prevention is the identification by a school nurse of a child with pediculosis (head lice). The school nurse would contact the child's family caregivers and provide instructions on the care of the child and other family members to eliminate the infestation.

Another example of secondary prevention is the identification by a community clinic nurse of a child who is underweight and possibly anemic. The nurse works with the family caregiver to review the family's dietary habits and nutritional state. This would help determine if the problem is limited to this child or if other family members are also malnourished, and if there is lack of knowledge or inadequate means. After finding these answers, the nurse can help the family caregiver provide better nutrition for the child and other family members as needed.

Tertiary prevention (prevention focusing on rehabilitation and teaching to prevent further injury or illness) occurs in special settings for high-risk infants and children, special intervention programs, group homes, and selected outpatient settings focusing on rehabilitation, such as orthopedic clinics. Tertiary prevention can be illustrated by the example of a young rural family with a child who has spina bifida and needs to be catheterized several times a day. The child is seen regularly at a specialized clinic at a major medical center. The family has no insurance, and the cost of catheters has become just one more item they feel they cannot handle. The nurse helps the family explore additional resources for financial help—perhaps an organization that will help fund their trips to the clinic for regular appointments—and also finds a source to cover the costs of catheters and other incidental expenses.

Such a broad selection of settings and roles places the nurse in a remarkable situation. Children are seen in settings that are familiar to them (homes, schools, or community centers). In the community setting, the child's caregivers can more freely make choices—for instance, welcoming the nurse into their home, following a medication regimen—than in the hospital, which may be perceived as a strange territory. Although involved in direct care, the nurse in the community spends a great part of his or her time as a communicator, teacher, administrator, and manager.

Community Care Settings for the Child

Care for children is provided in a wide variety of community settings. Some provide primarily wellness care; others provide specialized care for children with a particular diagnosis or condition. These include outpatient settings, home care, schools, camps, community centers, parishes, intervention programs, and group homes.

OUTPATIENT SETTINGS

Outpatient settings for children are varied, and as the health care delivery system continues to move into the community, more will be developed. Outpatient settings are organized according to who offers the services and who pays for them. Public (tax-supported) outpatient clinics may be an extension of a hospital's services or may be sponsored by a regional, county, or city health department. Private (based on fees charged) clinics are owned and operated by corporations or individuals and operate for a profit. A third system is the growing network of health maintenance organizations (HMOs). Some HMO plans charge a small co-payment for each visit. However, under the HMO system, the family is not free to choose the specialty care the child may receive. The child's primary physician determines what, if any, specialized care is needed and who will administer that care.

Clinic services are based on the needs of the community. Examples include a well-baby clinic offered by the county health department, an orthopedic clinic offered by a regional children's hospital, or a pediatric clinic of an HMO. Infants, children, and caregivers use the clinics for education, anticipatory guidance, immunizations, diagnosis, treatment, and rehabilitation.

A specialty clinic focuses on one aspect of an infant's or child's well-being—for instance, dentistry, oncology, sickle cell anemia, or HIV/AIDS. Some health department clinics specialize in high-risk infants born to drug-addicted mothers, children of parents with a history of child abuse, or low-birth weight infants. Nurses in these clinics devote much of their efforts to parental education and guidance as well as follow-up services for the child.

HOME HEALTH CARE

Infants, children, and their families make up a significant proportion of the home health care population. Shortened acute care stays have contributed to the increasing number of children cared for by home nurses. Children are often more comfortable in familiar home surroundings (Fig. 5-2). Children and infants can be successfully treated for many conditions at home, where they and their caregivers are more comfortable and where they can receive the love and attention of family members. The child's caregivers feel more confident about performing treatments and procedures when they have the guidance of the home nurse. Common conditions for which an infant or child may receive home care services include:

- Phototherapy for elevated bilirubin levels
- Intravenous antibiotic therapy for systemic infections
- Postoperative care
- Chronic conditions such as asthma, sickle cell anemia, cystic fibrosis, HIV/AIDS, and leukemia and other cancers
- Respirator-dependent children
- Reconstructive or corrective surgery for congenital malformations
- Corrective orthopedic surgery.

Other home health care team members may include a physical therapist, speech therapist, occupational therapist, home schooling teacher, home health aide, primary health care provider (physician or nurse practitioner), and social worker. Members of the team vary with the child's health needs.

SCHOOLS AND CAMPS

Health care has been practiced for many years in schools and camps, but the role of health care professionals in these settings has expanded (Fig. 5-3).

The school nurse may be responsible for classroom teaching, health screenings, immunizations, first aid for injured children, care of ill children, medication adminis-

Figure 5-2
During a visit by the nurse, the child is comforted by the familiar surroundings of his home.

Figure 5-3
The school nurse cares for a young girl who injured her knee on the playground. In addition to first aid, the school nurse's duties include counseling, health education, and health promotion.

tration, assisting with sports physicals, and identifying children with problems and recommending programs for them. Classroom teaching can cover personal hygiene, sex education, substance abuse, safety, and emotional health, geared for each grade level. Many mainstreamed children have chronic health problems that need daily supervision or care—for example, a child with spina bifida who needs to be catheterized several times during the day, or a diabetic child who needs to perform glucose monitoring and administer insulin during school hours.

Health records are maintained on each child. Some schools have school-based clinics that provide routine dental care, school and sports physicals, follow-up of students identified in routine vision, hearing, scoliosis, tuberculosis, or other screenings, and follow-up on immunizations.

Children learn to know the school nurse over a number of years and usually establish a comfortable, friendly relationship. This relationship often aids the nurse in helping the child solve his or her health problems.

The camp nurse knows the child for a much briefer time, but many camp nurses establish warm relationships with the children in their care. Camp nurses provide first aid for campers and staff, maintain health records, teach first aid and cardiopulmonary resuscitation, offer relevant health education, maintain an infirmary for ill campers, and dispense tender loving care to homesick children.

At camps for children with special needs, the campers' health care needs determine the type of nursing care required. For example, at a camp for diabetic children, the nurse may teach self-administration of insulin and the many aspects of diabetic care. Other camps may cater to children with developmental delays, physical challenges,

A Personal Glimpse

The clinic is where you go when you're on the public access card and cannot afford real insurance. You hardly see the same doctor twice. A lot are interns working out their internship.

My baby was about 2 months old when he developed a bumpy rash on the crown of his head. I took him to the clinic because it was spreading and I didn't know what it could be. A doctor, who I could hardly understand, was on duty. This was the same doctor that told me I had chickenpox when I was pregnant (I didn't). He looked at the rash and looked at me very strange, then said, "This looks similar to a rash connected to HIV." He requested a test for AIDS! You cannot know the thoughts that go through your head. How? Where? Who? Why? Then I remembered that I had been tested when I first found out I was pregnant and it was negative. Since Jack, the baby's father, and I had not been with anyone else, I knew there must be another reason for this rash.

That doctor never took a sample to test or asked another doctor to come in and look at the rash. I took little Tommy home and started to use an ointment I'd heard about on his head every day for about a month. The rash went away and I've changed clinics since—like they're not all really the same. You get what you pay for.

Michelle

or chronic illness, such as asthma or cystic fibrosis. Others have specific purposes, such as weight control or behavior management. In each of these settings, the nurse provides basic health care, with individualized health teaching based on the camp population. Each type of camping brings its own challenges and rewards; the benefits to the children and their families are often exceptional.

COMMUNITY CENTERS, PARISHES, INTERVENTION PROGRAMS

Community centers and parishes provide care relevant to a particular community. Parish centers may be sponsored by a church, synagogue, or other religious group as an outreach program. The services offered by these centers are designed to meet the needs of the community. For example, in areas with many homeless persons, centers may provide basic health care and nutrition. These centers may also provide food, clothing, money, or other resources. Other centers may provide child care classes for new mothers or young families.

Some communities offer walk-in or residential clinics for special purposes—for instance, teen pregnancy, alcohol and drug abuse, nutritional guidance, and family violence. Other specialized clinics offer programs on HIV/AIDS, cancer, and mental health, provide maternal and well-baby care, and offer day care services for children or the elderly.

Many communities also have services provided by volunteer community service organizations such as the Lions, Rotary Club, Shriners, or Kiwanis. Some of these organizations have specific goals—for instance, the Shriners sponsor clinics for children with orthopedic problems.

In any community center, there are people who can benefit from the services of health care professionals. Often the health services focus on education and other primary prevention practices. Nurses can help design safety, exercise, and nutrition programs, provide basic immunization services, conduct parenting classes, organize crisis intervention programs for youth and teens, and help organize health fairs. The health care staff may be paid or may work on a volunteer basis, or there may be a combination of paid and volunteer staff.

Many services can be provided to smaller groups of infants and children with special needs. Such intervention programs may be supported by federal or state funds and offered through the school district or private associations for developmentally delayed, physically challenged, or emotionally disturbed children. The interventions are often multidisciplinary, consisting of a team of professionals who work together to meet the multiple needs of the child.

Professional teams may consist of a teacher, psychologist, neurologist, physical therapist, social worker, physician, and nurse. The most important members of the team are the family caregivers and the child, and it is essential to include them in planning meetings and program intervention development. The nurse's role as a team member involves interpreting diagnoses or medical orders to other team members and the family, teaching the family how to manage a medically fragile child, and integrating the family into intervention programs effectively.

RESIDENTIAL PROGRAMS

Residential programs, often called group homes, provide services for a number of health needs. Those geared primarily to children include chemical dependency treatment centers and homes for children with mental or emotional health needs, pregnant adolescents, and abused children. These homes vary in size and setup according to the children's needs.

Depending on the number of children a home serves, the nurse may be contracted to provide specific services. The nurse may work for the local health department or for a corporation that owns several group homes. For example, in a home with six children with minimal disabilities, the nurse may visit every 2 weeks to meet with and educate the staff, update health records, and provide immunizations. This may be all the health care service the home requires to maintain its group home license.

Homes that serve many children or that serve children with very complex needs may need to have nurses 24 hours a day. Often this is required by licensing standards (in addition to meeting the health care needs of the children). Some homes hire a multidisciplinary team of health care practitioners that may include nurses, medical social workers, psychologists, physical, speech, or occupational therapists, special education teachers, home health aides or attendants, and physicians. Not all the team members provide services to group homes on a full-time basis.

CARING FOR THE CHILD IN THE COMMUNITY

The nursing process serves as the foundation of nursing care for the child in the community just as it does for the child in a health care facility. Communication with the child and family is essential. Teaching is a fundamental part of community-based care because of the emphasis on health promotion and preventive health care. Case management is necessary to direct the child's care and determine the progress of that care through the health care system.

The Nursing Process

Although the family of the child in a health care facility is important, in the community setting the family takes on even greater importance. Understanding the structure of the family and the roles and functions of family members is vital to caring for the child in the community (see Chap. 2; for a review of the nursing process, see Chap. 1).

In the initial family assessment interview, the nurse determines how various family members affect the child and his or her condition. The nurse may obtain additional information by picking up on cues in the child's environment. After the assessment is completed, the information is analyzed and the family's needs and strengths are identified. Nursing diagnoses are then determined, and planning proceeds with the development of expected outcomes related specifically to the child. The expected outcomes are mutually set with the family to encourage family interaction and cooperation. In the community setting, the family is much more directly involved in providing care for the child; thus, their compliance is essential to the success of that care. Interventions are initiated based on the expected outcomes. Family teaching is key (Fig. 5-4). As the interventions are performed, the results are documented and evaluated, and the ongoing cycle of the nursing process continues.

Communication

Positive, effective communication is fundamental to the nursing process and the care of the child in the community. The principles of communication, both verbal and nonverbal, are covered in Chapter 1. Establishing rapport with the child and the family, understanding and appropriately responding to cultural practices, and being sensitive to the needs of the child and family all require good communication skills.

Teaching

Teaching is one of the most important facets of nursing care. Health teaching is very important to health promotion in community-based care. In many settings, health care of the child involves the teaching of small groups—for instance, the child, family caregivers, older siblings, or members of the extended family. However, teaching need not be limited to family members or the child's immediate surroundings. Depending on the setting and the child's age, the nurse may teach large groups of children and families on various topics that focus on primary prevention.

Figure 5-4
Teaching plays a major role in community-based nursing. Here a young woman is taught infant care by the home care nurse involved in home care.

To teach a group successfully, the nurse must know the needs of the target population and must have basic teaching skills and strategies and appropriate resources. If the nurse is familiar with the children, he or she already has some important information, such as their age, educational level, ethnic and gender mix, language barriers, and any previous teaching the group has had on the subject. If asked to teach an unfamiliar group, the nurse can ask the group leader for this information to help develop an appropriate teaching plan. The nurse should review growth and developmental principles to identify the appropriate level of information, learning activities, and average attention span. Additional information includes any teaching resources that are available, the size of the group, the seating arrangements, and other advantages or restrictions of the environment. For instance, the nurse may want to find out:

- Are the chairs movable for small-group discussions?
- Is there a VCR to show a video?
- Can the children go outside?
- Will a lot of noise disturb others in the building?
- Will the classroom teacher or teacher's aide be in attendance?

Being prepared makes all the difference between a successful and an unsuccessful group teaching experience.

Case Management

Case management (a systematic process that ensures that a client's multiple health and service needs are met) may be a formal or an informal process. In some community-based agencies, case management is formalized. In these systems, the contact with the client is predetermined by the agency or insurer who pays for the health care services. In other settings, the nurse may determine the follow-up that is needed and either provides the needed services or assists with referrals to obtain them.

If case management is formalized, nursing services are paid for by the insurer. The case manager's role is clearly outlined, with care plans, protocols, and limits to service determined by the insurer. In community agencies where nursing services are part of the overall services (for instance, schools or group homes), the intensity of follow-up is determined by the philosophy of the agency, the resources available, and the nurse's perception of the role and his or her individual skills.

Client Advocacy

Client advocacy is speaking or acting on behalf of others to help them gain greater independence and to make the health care delivery system more responsive and relevant to their needs. The nurse working in a community setting often can develop longer relationships with children and their families because of the continuous nature of client contact in outpatient, school, or other settings. This addi-

COMMUNICATIONS BOX

At a neighborhood clinic, a mother rushes in with her young child in her arms. She is upset and unsure of herself. A nurse is at the desk.

INEFFECTIVE COMMUNICATION

Nurse: Can I help you?

Mother: (Anxiously) My baby is sick.

Nurse: Just have a seat in the waiting area and we'll call you. (Handing her a clipboard with papers attached) Fill this out while you wait.

Mother: (Nervously goes to seat. Cradles baby in arms.)

After 45 minutes, the nurse calls the mother.

Nurse: Have a seat here while we go over your information. (Looking at clipboard) You haven't filled any of this out.

Mother: No, I . . . I was busy with the baby.

Nurse: I don't have time to fill all of these out with everyone. Can you read this?

Mother: (Very softly) I left my glasses at home.

Nurse: Oh, all right, but you better remember your glasses after this. You need to do these papers yourself.

During this interview, the nurse has been centered on his/her own concerns and does not read any of the mother's concerns or clues. The nurse does not ask what is wrong with the baby, so the nurse has no real idea if the baby can safely wait or not. The nurse hands the mother the clipboard to fill out without trying to find out if that is something the mother can do. When the mother came back with the unanswered questionnaire, the nurse was abrupt and was not sensitive to the mother's possible inability to read. The nurse was not tuned in to the mother's needs.

EFFECTIVE COMMUNICATION

Nurse: Can I help you?

Mother: (Anxiously) My baby is sick.

Nurse: How has the baby been acting?

Mother: She's been really fussy. She hasn't been able to sleep at night and she has been spitting up a lot.

Nurse: Has she had any fever?

Mother: I don't know. I don't have a thermometer.

Nurse: Have a seat in the waiting area and I'll call you as soon as possible. Do you think you will be able to fill out these information papers?

Mother: I don't know if I can with the baby and all.

Nurse: No problem. I'll call you as soon as possible to help you fill out these papers.

Mother: Thank you.

The nurse in this instance initially gave the mother an opportunity to tell how her baby is. This helps the nurse decide if they can wait for attention. After hearing the mother's response about the thermometer, the nurse suspects she may not be able to read. For this reason she gives the mother a nonthreatening reason to say that she wouldn't be able to fill out the papers. When the mother accepts that offer, the nurse reassures her that this is fine. The mother's self-respect remains intact and the mother is grateful. The nurse throughout this interview has picked up on clues of behavior and responses to determine this mother's circumstances.

tional contact time allows the nurse to discover broader health and welfare issues. Example of interventions include:

- Teaching a family about the services for which their child is eligible
- Identifying inexpensive or free transportation services to medical appointments
- Making the several phone calls necessary to establish

eligibility for and to acquire special equipment needed by a physically challenged child.

Examples of child advocacy are limitless and include health and social welfare services that intertwine in ways that cannot be managed by families alone. One example is assistance with referrals and acquisition of needed resources. As a member of a team of health care professionals, the nurse assists with the referral process. This process

Figure 5-5
A nurse advocate can help the child enter a school lunch program so that the child's nutritional needs are met.

focuses on getting the child to the services needed or obtaining the resources needed. Actions taken are geared toward improving the child's health or quality of life. The nurse must be knowledgeable about community resources, contact persons, and the details of appropriate applications and other documentation that may be required (Fig. 5-5).

THE CHALLENGE OF COMMUNITY-BASED NURSING

There are several differences between caring for children in a hospital or clinic and caring for them in community settings. Community-based work requires a different set of skills.

The Unique Aspects of Community-Based Nursing

Community-based nursing practice is more autonomous. The nurse must be self-reliant to be successful. There may be few other health care practitioners, and even those may be physically distant. To provide children and families with high-quality care, the nurse must have well-developed assessment and decision-making skills.

Community practice also tends to be more holistic. The child is viewed as an integrated whole—mind, body, and spirit, interacting with the environment. The effects of the child's health on family functioning, the impact on the child's educational progress, the multiple services the family and child need to improve the quality of life: are all considered by the nurse in the community.

A final difference is the focus on wellness. Some community settings have a population of children with an illness or diagnosis in common, such as cerebral palsy or

diabetes. Working with these children involves managing their disease or limitations, but with a wellness focus. For instance, the focus might be on how the child with cerebral palsy can be included comfortably within the regular classroom or how the diabetic teenager can juggle sports, eating out, and slumber parties.

In most areas where the community nurse works, the focus is on wellness. The children are basically well but may be going through growth and developmental crises. The nurse intervenes with children and family members to ease the transition from one stage to another. Anticipatory guidance can be given to family caregivers and preventive health practices can be stressed. Teaching health-promotion practices to children is another activity of primary importance.

Issues Facing Children and Families

Nurses who work in the community begin to see and interact with the other issues facing children and their families. Caregiving activities in the community combine the uniqueness of the community setting with the knowledge the nurse gains from seeing the child in his or her own environment.

Poverty is a major issue and one that affects all aspects of recovery and response to care. A lack of resources takes its toll on children's health and hinders compliance in many families. Services and resources may be inaccessible because of cost, location, lack of public or private transportation or the cost of transportation, or neighborhood safety; the family may see such services as unnecessary. Poverty, lack of information, questionable decisions about priorities, and deficient coping skills affect the health of children in significant ways, and the results are often seen in the emergency department or the acute care beds of children's units.

The community nurse must explore these issues with the family caregivers. When a family does not follow up with an orthopedic appointment for a new cast application on the legs of a 6-month-old infant, what factors influenced their decision? When a family caregiver saves half of the antibiotic suspension for another child in the family with similar symptoms, what motivates this decision? When a single parent keeps a physically disabled and developmentally delayed 9-year-old son at home in one room of the apartment, what types of caregiving services and information might be of benefit?

Rewards of Community-Based Nursing

Individual clients do not change as much in community-based settings. The clinic nurse may see the same family for different problems over many years. The camp or school nurse watches children grow and gets to know siblings and families over many years. A group home nurse works intensely with a group of developmentally disabled children, learning to know each one and rejoicing in their small triumphs.

For the community nurse, rewards come slowly and in different ways. For 4 months, a school nurse may diligently work with a child and family and a community service organization to obtain a pair of glasses for the child. This nurse may feel rewarded when the child no longer comes into the nurse's office at school with headaches and is doing better in class work. The camp nurse may help a homesick new camper design a way to stay in touch with his or her parents and may encourage the camper to participate in camp activities. This nurse may also find reward when the camper returns each season. The nurse in a group home for teenage foster children with behavioral problems may help the teens develop a theater group that presents plays on safe sex and responsible teen dating to other group homes, high school classes, or community service organizations. This nurse may find reward after a year of work with the teens, when they write the scripts, build the sets independently, and declare that they enjoy the theater group more than any other activity in the residence. This nurse may also find a deeper reward when he or she realizes that as a result of the theater group, there are fewer behavioral problems and the teens' self-esteem is high.

Community nurses work in many ways to prevent unnecessary hospitalization. Health problems that could have been prevented leave the nurse wondering why they were not prevented—for instance, an auto accident involving a child not appropriately secured in a car seat, a toddler with a scalded face from grabbing a tablecloth and spilling a cup of coffee, a child who almost drowned in a backyard pool, an infant who fails to thrive because the parents do not know that infants need specific amounts of formula, or a pregnant teen who did not have safe sex. The community nurse helps families develop the skills and knowledge they need to make decisions that affect their lives and those of other family members. In this way, families can learn and practice preventive health care. With a focus on wellness, the community nurse provides a service that eventually improves the health of the entire community.

■ KEY POINTS

■ Community-based health care focuses on wellness and prevention and is directed toward helping persons and families meet their health care needs.

■ Community nurses focus on primary prevention, followed by secondary prevention.

■ The community offers many settings where children are

cared for. Some focus on wellness care, others on specialized care for children with specific diagnoses.

■ Shortened acute care stays have increased the number of children and families cared for by home nurses.

■ School nurses provide classroom health teaching, perform health screenings, offer first aid to injured children, care for children who become ill in school, administer medications, care for mainstreamed children with chronic conditions, serve on professional panels, assist with sports physicals, and keep health records.

■ In any community health care setting, the family and the child are the most important members of the health care team.

■ Communication is one of the most important aspects of community health care.

■ To establish rapport, the community nurse must understand and respond appropriately to cultural practices of community members.

■ Community nurses spend much of their time teaching, on a one-to-one basis or with a family, a small group, or a large group. The nurse must assess each audience and gear the teaching appropriately.

? CRITICAL THINKING

1. Survey your community and make a list of community-based health care providers. Find out how each is funded. Identify those settings that provide health care for children. Evaluate your community's health care needs to determine if the available services meet those needs.

2. Identify strengths you believe a community nurse need. Compare your nursing skills with these strengths, being as realistic as possible. Determine if your strengths meet those needed.

3. Select a community-based setting and outline the services a nurse in that setting should ideally provide. Include the resources needed to provide the services.

4. You are making a home visit to the Smith family because their newborn infant needs home phototherapy treatment for 3 to 5 days. You find 6-year-old Samantha ill with bronchitis. Both parents smoke. Outline a teaching plan for these caregivers regarding the health of their family.

5. Mrs. Perez, a second-grade teacher, asks you to teach a unit on personal hygiene to her class. Identify the information you will need from Mrs. Perez. Describe how you will present the lesson to these children.

6. You are a camp nurse at an overnight scout camp. When Doug, a 10-year-old camper who is diabetic, comes to the infirmary to obtain his insulin for self-administration, you notice reddened areas on his abdomen and

thighs, apparently at injection sites. What would you wish to teach him? How might you approach him without making him feel defensive?

BIBLIOGRAPHY

Children's Defense Fund. The state of America's children 1991. Washington DC, 1991.

Corby R. Assessing child abuse in community health nursing. Imprint 39(2), 77–78, 1992.

Hunt R, Zurek EL. Introduction to community-based nursing. Philadelphia: Lippincott-Raven, 1997.

Karp RJ, ed. Malnourished children in the United States: Caught in the cycle of poverty. New York: Springer, 1993.

Malloy C. Children and poverty: America's future at risk. Pediatr Nurs 18(6), 553–557, 1992.

National Safety Council. Accident facts. Chicago, 1990.

Novello AC, Degraw C, Kleinman DV. Healthy children ready to learn: An essential collaboration between health and education. Public Health Reports 107(1), 3–10, 1992.

Proctor ST. Guidelines for a model school nursing services program. Scarborough, ME: National Association of School Nurses, 1990.

Spradley BW, Allender JA. Community health nursing: Concepts and practice. Philadelphia: Lippincott-Raven, 1996.

Stanhope M, Knollmueller RN. Public and community health nurse's consultant: A health promotion guide. St. Louis: Mosby, 1997.

Wong DL. Whaley and Wong's nursing care of infants and children, 5th ed. St. Louis: Mosby–Year Book, 1995.

A Child Is Born

Chapter 6

The Prenatal Period

PRENATAL GROWTH AND DEVELOPMENT
Gestation
Genetic Influences
Environmental Influences

EDUCATION FOR PARENTHOOD
Prenatal Care
Prepared Childbirth

STUDENT OBJECTIVES

On completion of this chapter, the student will be able to:

1. Define the vocabulary terms listed in the key terms section.
2. Identify the three stages of prenatal development that occur during the first 8 weeks after conception.
3. State three pieces of information that can be obtained from an amniocentesis.
4. State how many pairs of chromosomes there are in each human cell.
5. List the kind of information that a karyotype can provide.
6. Describe how the sex of the child is determined at the time of conception.
7. Draw a diagram illustrating the inheritance of an autosomal recessive inheritance in which both parents are carriers of the disease. Explain the pattern.
8. List three primary goals of genetic counseling.
9. Identify the factors that may create problems for the pregnant teenager.
10. State the primary dietary goal for the pregnant woman.
11. List three maternal habits that may be harmful to the fetus.
12. Describe the danger that rubella presents for the fetus, and discuss preventive procedures.
13. Name three types of childbirth preparation.

KEY TERMS

amniocentesis	genotype
amniotic sac	gestation
autosomal dominant trait	growth
autosomal recessive trait	heterozygous
autosome	homozygous
centromere	karyotype
chromosome	mutation
conception	organogenesis
differentiation	placenta
dominant gene	recessive gene
embryo	sex chromosome
fertilization	teratogen
fetus	trimester
genes	umbilical cord
genetic code	viability
genetic counseling	zygote

From the moment of conception until full maturity, human life proceeds in an orderly pattern of growth and development. This pattern and the person that results from it are shaped by various factors that precede and follow conception. Genetic influences help determine a child's physical and intellectual characteristics, as do environmental influences. Once conception has occurred, a child's genetic heritage does not change. The environment can be altered, however, with either positive or negative effects on the child and the family. Fortunately, a great deal of knowledge is now available to prospective parents to help them provide a favorable environment in which their child may grow and develop.

PRENATAL GROWTH AND DEVELOPMENT

Conception occurs when a sperm cell reaches and penetrates an ovum. This process, also called **fertilization**, produces a fertilized ovum, or **zygote**. During the first 10 days to 2 weeks of life, the zygote becomes implanted in the lining of the uterus. Once implanted, the growing organism is referred to as an **embryo**. After it acquires a human likeness, usually about the eighth week of life, it is termed a **fetus**.

At no other time in a person's life is growth more rapid than during the intrauterine period. The microscopic zygote increases in size more than 200 billion times during the 9 months before birth. Two distinct but related processes take place during the transformation of zygote to infant: growth and differentiation. **Growth** is the result of cell division and is marked by an increase in size and weight. **Differentiation** changes the dividing cells, creating specialized tissues necessary to form an organized, coordinated person.

Gestation

Gestation is the period between conception and birth. The normal time required for a child to grow from a single cell to a newborn infant is 9 calendar months, 10 lunar months, or 40 weeks (Fig. 6-1). A baby born before the sixth month is considered at risk and may not survive, even with the special life-support systems available in modern intensive care nurseries. The age of **viability** is the earliest gestational age at which a fetus can survive outside the uterine

Figure 6-1

Growth of the ovum, embryo, and fetus during the early weeks of pregnancy.

environment. At one time the age of viability was considered to be 28 weeks, but technology has improved to such a degree that many states prepare a birth certificate for a fetus of 500 grams or more or a gestation of 20 weeks. Deviation in the gestational age of newborn babies is normal, but the closer the infant comes to the full 9 months' gestation, the greater the chances are for a healthy neonatal period.

TRIMESTERS

Gestation is divided into **trimesters** (periods of 3 months). In the first trimester, **organogenesis**, the process by which cells differentiate into major organ systems, occurs. It commences shortly after conception and is almost complete by the end of the eighth week. Even the 4-week-old embryo shows evidence of beginning organs and organ systems (Fig. 6-2). After the eighth week of life, the major changes are the growth and development of organs and organ systems. The first trimester is the time when the fetus is most vulnerable to any hazard in the intrauterine environment.

The second trimester is a period of continuing growth and development. All reflexes are present by the end of the fourth month, except for functional respiration and vocal response. All nerve cells are present by the fifth month, although they are not functionally mature.

If circumstances cause premature birth during the third trimester, the child has developed sufficiently to survive, assuming that constant, expert care is provided. During this last trimester, the fetus stores iron for postnatal use and develops subcutaneous fat, which enables it to begin independent life. Figure 6-3 summarizes the month-by-month growth and development of the fetus.

INTRAUTERINE DEVELOPMENT

The child develops within the protection of a fluid environment surrounded by the **amniotic sac**. This strong translucent membrane is large and elastic enough to permit the fetus to move about and turn at will during most of its intrauterine life. The amniotic sac usually contains about 1,000 mL of amniotic fluid, a clear, neutral to slightly alkaline (pH 7.0–7.25) liquid. This fluid protects the fetus from direct impact on the mother's abdomen, separates the fetus from the membranes, aids symmetric growth and development, helps maintain a constant body temperature by preventing heat loss, provides oral fluid for the fetus, and acts as an excretion collection system.

Ultrasound examination is a noninvasive procedure commonly performed during pregnancy. Through the use of high-frequency sound waves directed toward the uterus, a visual image is formed on a monitor. Intrauterine pregnancy can be verified. Fetal breathing, cardiac action, and movement may be seen. Fetal measurements may be made, multiple fetuses identified, and excessive or inadequate amounts of amniotic fluid noted. Early identification of problems such as polycystic kidneys, limb abnormalities,

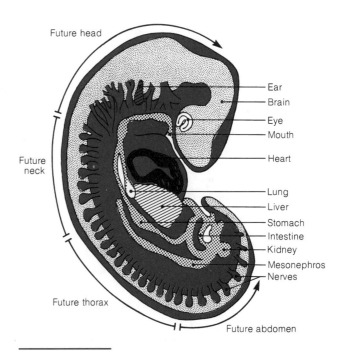

Figure 6-2
Four-week-old embryo.

hydrocephalus, intestinal obstructions, and myelomeningocele is possible.

Analysis of amniotic fluid through **amniocentesis** reveals much about the fetus, including sex, state of health, and maturity. A sample of amniotic fluid is withdrawn for early diagnosis of possible disorders, such as chromosomal abnormalities, blood disorders, and respiratory problems. Performed under local anesthesia, the procedure is done by inserting a needle through the abdominal and uterine walls into the amniotic sac and withdrawing a small amount of fluid (10–20 mL) through a syringe. Although amniocentesis carries a slight risk to the mother and fetus, it is recommended when the mother is older than 35 years of age or when there is a known risk to the fetus of inheriting a serious genetic defect. Later in pregnancy, this test also may be used to determine fetal lung and kidney maturity before early cesarean delivery or induction of labor.

During intrauterine development, the **placenta** links the fetus to the mother. This organ performs four functions for the developing fetus: respiration, nutrition, excretion, and protection. The placenta is a reddish, disk-shaped organ connected to the fetus by the **umbilical cord** (Fig. 6-4). Blood from the placenta brings food, oxygen, hormones, and protective antibodies to the fetus by way of the umbilical vein. The umbilical arteries carry deoxygenated fetal blood and waste products back to the placenta. The placenta normally emerges soon after delivery of the baby (hence the term *afterbirth*).

Many drugs, viruses, and infections cross the placental barrier from the mother to the fetus. These hazards to the

Fetal Development

1st Lunar Month

The fetus is 0.75 cm to 1 cm in length.

Trophoblasts embed in decidua.

Chorionic villi form.

Foundations for nervous system, genitourinary system, skin, bones, and lungs are formed.

Buds of arms and legs begin to form.

Rudiments of eyes, ears, and nose appear.

4 weeks

2nd Lunar Month

The fetus is 2.5 cm in length and weighs 4 g.

Fetus is markedly bent.

Head is disproportionately large, owing to brain development.

Sex differentiation begins.

Centers of bone begin to ossify.

8 weeks

3rd Lunar Month

The fetus is 7 cm to 9 cm in length and weighs 28 g.

Fingers and toes are distinct.

Placenta is complete.

Fetal circulation is complete.

12 weeks

4th Lunar Month

The fetus is 10 cm to 17 cm in length and weighs 55 g to 120 g.

Sex is differentiated.

Rudimentary kidneys secrete urine.

Heartbeat is present.

Nasal septum and palate close.

16 weeks

5th Lunar Month

The fetus is 25 cm in length and weighs 223 g.

Lanugo covers entire body.

Fetal movements are felt by mother.

Heart sounds are perceptible by auscultation.

20 weeks

6th Lunar Month

The fetus is 28 cm to 36 cm in length and weighs 680 g.

Skin appears wrinkled.

Vernix caseosa appears.

Eyebrows and fingernails develop.

24 weeks

7th Lunar Month

The fetus is 35 cm to 38 cm in length and weighs 1200 g.

Skin is red.

Pupillary membrane disappears from eyes.

The fetus has an excellent chance of survival.

28 weeks

8th Lunar Month

The fetus is 38 cm to 43 cm in length and weighs 2.7 kg.

Fetus is viable.

Eyelids open.

Fingerprints are set.

Vigorous fetal movement occurs.

32 weeks

9th Lunar Month

The fetus is 42 cm to 49 cm in length and weighs 1900 g to 2700 g.

Face and body have a loose wrinkled appearance because of subcutaneous fat deposit.

Lanugo disappears.

Amniotic fluid decreases.

36 weeks

10th Lunar Month

The fetus is 48 cm to 52 cm in length and weighs 3000 g.

Skin is smooth.

Eyes are uniformly slate colored.

Bones of skull are ossified and nearly together at sutures.

40 weeks

Figure 6-3
Critical stages of fetal development.

Figure 6-4
Left, the maternal surface of the placenta is rough and irregular. *Right,* the fetal surface is smooth and shiny.

developing fetus are discussed in the section on environmental influences.

Genetic Influences

The science of genetics studies the ways in which normal and abnormal traits are transmitted from one generation to the next. The basic principles of genetics were discovered in 1865 by an Austrian monk named Gregor Mendel through his experimentation with common garden peas. Only in the 20th century have Mendel's principles been rediscovered and employed in science and medicine.

Before Mendel's time it was believed that the characteristics of parents were blended in their children. Mendel's experiments proved that this blending does not occur; rather, each parent's individual characteristics can reappear unchanged in later generations.

All living organisms are composed of living cells that contain all the material necessary for the maintenance and propagation of the particular species. Each cell contains a number of small bodies called **chromosomes.** Chromosomes are threadlike structures that occur in pairs; each pair is attached at the center by a **centromere.** Threaded along these chromosomes are **genes,** the units that carry genetic instructions from one generation to another. Like chromosomes, genes also occur in pairs. The instructions they carry are called the **genetic code,** the blueprint for the development of the individual organism. Each person's unique set of genes is called his or her **genotype.**

Each human cell contains 46 chromosomes, consisting of 23 essentially identical or homologous pairs. One member of each pair is contributed by the father and one by the mother to the single cell formed by the union of sperm and egg at conception, which determines the sex and inherited traits of the new organism.

Twenty-two of these pairs are alike in the male and the female and are called **autosomes.** The remaining pair is a pair of **sex chromosomes,** which differ in the male and the female. When the form or number of autosomes is altered, birth defects or abnormalities result.

KARYOTYPES

Modern technology has made it possible to photograph the nuclei of human cells and enlarge them to show the chromosomes. The chromosomes are cut from the photographs, matched in pairs, and grouped. The resulting picture is a **karyotype** and is used to locate chromosomal malformations and translocations (the change in position of a segment of chromosome to another location on the chromosome or to another chromosome). Karyotypes of normal chromosomes are properly paired (Fig. 6-5). In some abnormal conditions, translocations occur. In other conditions, such as trisomy 21 (Down syndrome), three chromosomes occur in the 21 or 22 position (Fig. 6-6), producing a total of 47 chromosomes instead of the normal 46.

Figure 6-5
Arrangement of normal chromosomes into a standard karyotype.

Figure 6-6
Karyotype showing trisomy 21. Note three chromosomes in the 21 position.

DETERMINATION OF SEX

All egg cells from the female carry a pair of female chromosomes called the X chromosomes. Sperm cells, however, carry one X (female) and one Y (male) chromosome. It appears to be a matter of chance whether the egg, which always has an X chromosome, is fertilized by a sperm carrying an X chromosome or by one carrying a Y chromosome. In the former instance, the offspring is a girl. The Y chromosome is dominant over the X, so that if the Y enters into the union, the result is always a male child. Thus, it is the father's sex cell that determines the child's sex (Fig. 6-7).

Cells reproduce by division; each parent cell produces two daughter cells, each of which in turn produces two new cells. In this manner, the single cell produced by the union of the sperm and the ovum eventually multiplies to produce an infant.

DETERMINATION OF INHERITED TRAITS

The ultramicroscopic bodies called genes carry genetic instruction from one generation to another with mathematic regularity. Any gene can be altered, however, by mutation or chromosomal rearrangement. **Mutation** in a gene means that a fundamental change has taken place in its structure, resulting in the transmission of a trait different from that normally carried by the particular gene. Much remains to be learned about the causes of mutations, most of which result in undesirable traits.

When the two members of a pair of genes carry the same genetic instructions, the person carrying these genes is

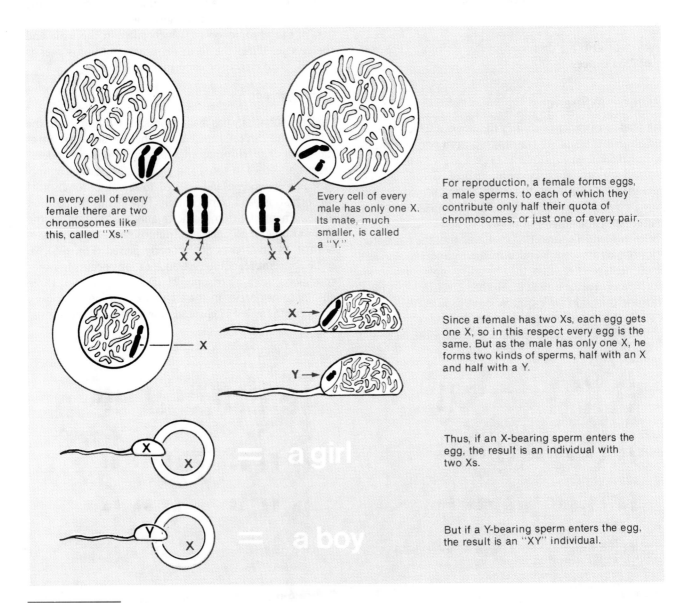

Figure 6-7
Sex is determined at the time sperm and ovum unite.

said to be **homozygous** for that particular trait. When each member of a pair of genes carries different instructions, the person is **heterozygous** for the trait. One member of a heterozygous pair of genes is the **dominant gene** (one that is expressed in only one of a chromosome pair). Thus, a trait or condition appearing in a heterozygous person is called an **autosomal dominant trait.** Huntington's disease, neurofibromatosis, and osteogenesis imperfecta are examples of dominantly inherited diseases (Fig. 6-8).

A gene carrying different information for the same trait that is not expressed (eg, blue eyes versus brown eyes) is called a **recessive gene.** A recessive gene is detectable only when present on both chromosomes. Inheritance patterns for **autosomal recessive traits** are shown in Figure 6-9. However, if both parents express the recessive trait, all their children will have the same trait or condition because each parent must have two genes for the trait, and the children cannot possibly escape inheriting two also. Some examples of recessively inherited diseases are thalassemia and cystic fibrosis.

GENETIC COUNSELING

Knowledge about genetics and the causes of specific birth defects continues to increase rapidly. One of the benefits of this increased knowledge is **genetic counseling.** Couples concerned about transmitting a specific disease to their children may consult a genetic counselor for screening and counseling. The counselor, a geneticist, studies the family history of both partners and may perform tissue analysis to determine chromosome patterns. This counseling is particularly important to people who may think they are carriers of hereditary disorders such as Tay-Sachs disease and sickle cell anemia. It is also helpful to people whose family

history includes one or more members who are mentally retarded.

Genetic counseling has four primary goals:

- To identify malformations and diseases that can be transmitted genetically and determine the probability of their recurrence

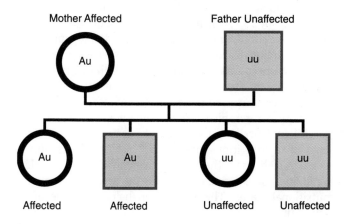

Figure 6-8
Autosomal dominant pattern inheritance. The affected mother has one gene for the trait (A) and one which does not carry the trait (u). As a result, the mother has the trait. The father has no genes for the trait (u). Two of the children will be affected by the trait and two will be unaffected. The two unaffected children will not carry the trait to their children.

Figure 6-9
Autosomal recessive pattern inheritance. **(A)** Both parents carriers—ratio of one patient, two carriers, one free from disease. **(B)** One patient—one parent free from disease, all children carriers—no clinical disease. **(C)** One parent carrier, one parent has disease—ratio of two children with disease, two carriers.

- To help couples make informed choices about reproduction
- To identify potential problems for the fetus or neonate and to ensure early diagnosis and management
- Ultimately, to reduce the number of children born with hereditary disorders.

Health professionals can provide only information and support; the final decision about whether to have a child remains with one or both members of the couple.

Environmental Influences

Although we know that genetic material furnishes the building blocks for a new person, the old controversy concerning the importance of heredity versus environment ("nature versus nurture") has lost its significance, at least in relation to intrauterine life. Current knowledge indicates that heredity and environment influence and modify each other.

Because the mother's body is the environment for the developing fetus, nothing is more important to the successful outcome of a pregnancy than the mother's health, both physical and emotional. Although it is no longer believed that a mother who attends art exhibitions will have a child who appreciates art, for instance, it is known that some of her reactions influence the child. Emotions such as fear and anxiety cause epinephrine to be released into the bloodstream, which passes through the placenta to the fetus, triggering a physical reaction similar to the mother's. There is growing evidence that extreme, prolonged stress in the mother may interfere with the supply of blood to the fetus, which may have an effect on the unborn child or lead to preterm labor.

MATERNAL AGE

Statistics indicate that the most favorable time for a woman to bear children is between 20 and 34 years of age. Mothers younger than 20 years of age experience difficulties such as excessive weight gain, toxemia, and prolonged labor more often than do older mothers. Teenage pregnancies produce infants of low birth weight, increasing the risk of neonatal morbidity and mortality. In addition to the physical problems encountered by teenage mothers, emotional and financial complications often occur. A young adolescent still has growing and maturing of her own to do. Issues of independence versus dependency of an unborn child or infant may result in resentment. This resentment may be reflected in neglect of her own health and, later, in neglect or abuse of the infant. Very young couples often are limited in their earning capacity, and the added expense of a baby places further burdens on an already strained financial situation.

The unmarried teenage mother presents special problems. She often has no one to support her emotionally or financially or anyone with whom to share the wondrous changes that are happening in her body. She may deny the need for or find it difficult to obtain the prenatal care and advice necessary for a normal birth and healthy development of the infant. Should she decide to give up her baby for adoption, she needs counseling and guidance to rebuild her changed life. Nurses who care for these young women must do so in a supportive, nonjudgmental manner so as not to contribute to their guilt and emotional insecurity.

An increasing number of women are delaying childbearing to the later part of their reproductive years. It was once thought that women who became mothers after 35 years of age would be subject to a host of pregnancy complications. But with early prenatal care, the older primigravida is not likely to experience more complications than her younger counterpart, aside from a slightly greater chance of hypertension, varicosities, and hemorrhoids. However, older women do have a greater likelihood of bearing children with Down syndrome or other congenital anomalies. For instance, the incidence of Down syndrome is five times as great for mothers older than 35 years of age as for those aged 30; however, currently only 20% of infants with Down syndrome are born to mothers older than 35, possibly because of early prenatal diagnosis and intervention.

MATERNAL NUTRITION

The unborn child has a comfortable nutritional arrangement with the mother. In general, a prospective mother who follows a sensible diet and augments it correctly to fit the needs of the fetus provides adequately for both herself and her child. The primary goal should be optimal growth and development of the fetus. A weight gain of 25 to 35 lb is considered desirable. During the first part of pregnancy, women 23 years of age and up need about 2,300 calories/day. The pregnant girl younger than 15 years of age should have an intake of 2,700 calories/day to fulfill both her own and her baby's growth needs. The pregnant woman's caloric intake should include nutritious foods and ample liquids, including six to eight glasses of water each day.

Women need more protein, iron, vitamins A, B, C, and D, and calcium during pregnancy. The infant needs to receive sufficient iron to build up an iron store for the first few months after birth. The pregnant adolescent needs careful guidance because she may be accustomed to eating a lot of nonnutritious "fast foods." Table 6-1 lists nutritional guidelines for the pregnant woman. Box 6-1 provides a nutrition questionnaire to assess the pregnant woman's nutritional status. These tools can help the nurse offer sound nutritional teaching and guidance so that the pregnant woman can provide her unborn baby with adequate nourishment.

MATERNAL INFECTIONS

Maternal infections pose distinct hazards for the unborn child. One example is maternal rubella (German measles). Although a mild disease in adults, rubella produces a high

TABLE 6-1. Daily Food Guide for Pregnancy

Food Group	Pregnancy	
	Adult Woman	Adolescent
Milk, yogurt, cheese	3 or 4 servings	4 or 5 servings
Meat and meat substitutes	5–6 oz	6–7 oz
Fruits	2–4 servings	2–4 servings
Vitamin C-rich	1 or 2 servings	1 or 2 servings
Vegetables	3–5 servings	3–5 servings
Vitamin A-rich	1 serving	1 serving
Bread, cereals, rice, pasta	6–11 servings	6–11 servings
Fats, oils, sweets	To meet caloric needs	To meet caloric needs

percentage of congenital malformations in the fetus when the mother is infected during the first trimester. Congenital cataracts, deafness, mental retardation, and congenital heart disease are abnormalities commonly resulting from this virus.

A live-virus rubella vaccine is used to vaccinate young children; this has markedly reduced the incidence of rubella in pregnant women and thus the number of newborns affected by the virus. In addition, newly pregnant mothers are tested for rubella titer during their early prenatal examinations, and those inadequately protected are given the rubella vaccine after delivery to protect subsequent pregnancies. The vaccine must not be administered to a pregnant woman, so caution must be used when giving the vaccine to adolescent girls and women of childbearing age.

Another virus encountered with increasing frequency is herpes simplex virus, hominis type 2. A primary first-episode infection during the first trimester may result in serious congenital anomalies. A recurrence during pregnancy is not as harmful, but if vaginal lesions are present at the time of delivery, a cesarean delivery is necessary to prevent the newborn from a possibly fatal direct exposure to the virus. In addition, babies born to mothers with untreated syphilis may be born with congenital syphilis.

Of increasing concern is the human immunodeficiency virus (HIV), which may be transmitted to the unborn children of infected mothers. Infants who are HIV positive usually have no major symptoms when born but develop symptoms of acquired immunodeficiency syndrome (AIDS) within the first 24 months of life. At present, there is no cure for AIDS, and these children ultimately die from complications of the disease.

TERATOGENS

As mentioned earlier, the placenta makes possible the transfer of food and oxygen from the mother to the fetus, but the placenta is not selective in the materials trans-

ferred. Therefore, many illicit, prescribed, or over-the-counter drugs taken by the mother also reach the fetus and can produce birth defects. Drugs taken by the pregnant woman that are known to disrupt prenatal growth processes are called **teratogens** (from the Latin *terato*, meaning monster, and *genesis*, meaning birth). The effect of a teratogen depends on when it enters the fetal system and in what stages of differentiation the various organs and organ systems are at that time. Generally, the fetus is most vulnerable to teratogens during the first trimester.

Alcohol Alcohol consumption per capita has decreased since 1980 in the United States, although a National Institute of Drug Addiction survey indicates that about one in six pregnant women drink during pregnancy.[1] Use of alcohol has been shown to cause permanent damage to the fetus. No safe amount of alcohol consumption has been determined because the degree of toxicity is controlled by the ability of the mother's liver to detoxify the alcohol. Ingestion of alcohol during pregnancy may retard fetal growth and produce fetal alcohol syndrome, characterized by a flat facial profile, short eye slits, a smaller brain with mental retardation, poor coordination, and irritability as infants and hyperactivity as children. Every woman of childbearing age must understand the damage that her use of alcohol and other drugs may inflict on her unborn child, because the most serious damage can occur during the first 4 weeks of life, before pregnancy is suspected.

Smoking A survey conducted by the National Institute of Drug Addiction found that a little over 20% of pregnant women smoke cigarettes at some time during pregnancy.[2] Smoking during pregnancy retards the growth of the fetus, reduces birth weight by an average of 200 g, and doubles the chance that the baby will be low birth weight. The rate of fetal and infant death is 25% to 50% higher among women who smoke during pregnancy than among those who do not. Women who stop smoking in the first 3 or 4 months of pregnancy and abstain for the rest of

Box 6-1. *Nutrition Questionnaire*

What your eat and the lifestyle choices you make can affect your present and future nutrition and health. Your nutrition can also have an important effect on your baby's health. Please answer these questions by circling the answers that apply.

Eating Behavior

1. Are you frequently bothered by any of the following? (Circle all that apply)

   Nausea   Vomiting   Heartburn   Constipation

2. Do you skip meals at least three times a week?   No   Yes

3. Do you try to limit the amount or kind of food you eat to control your weight?   No   Yes

4. Are you on a special diet now?   No   Yes

5. Do you avoid any foods for health or religious reasons?   No   Yes

Food Resources

6. Do you have a working stove?   No   Yes
   Do you have a working refrigerator?   No   Yes

7. Do you sometimes run out of food before you are able to buy more?   No   Yes

8. Can you afford to eat the way you should?   No   Yes

9. Are you receiving any food assistance now?   No   Yes
   (circle all that apply):

Food Stamps	School Breakfast	School lunch
WIC	Donated food/ commodities	CSFP*

   Food from a food pantry, soup kitchen, or food bank

10. Do you feel you need help in obtaining food?   No   Yes

Food and Drink

11. Which of these did you drink yesterday? (circle all that apply):

Soft drinks	Coffee	Tea	Fruit drink
Orange juice	Grapefruit juice	Other juices	Milk
Kool-Aid®	Beer	Wine	Alcoholic drinks
Water	Other beverages (list)		

12. Which of these foods did you eat yesterday? (circle all that apply):

Cheese	Pizza	Macaroni and cheese
Yogurt	Cereal with milk	

    Other foods made with cheese (such as tacos, enchiladas, lasagna, cheeseburgers)

Corn	Potatoes	Sweet potatoes	Green Salad
Carrots	Collard greens	Spinach	Turnip greens
Broccoli	Green beans	Green peas	Other vegetables
Apples	Bananas	Berries	Grapefruit
Melon	Oranges	Peaches	Other fruit
Meat	Fish	Chicken	Eggs
Peanut butter	Nuts	Seeds	Dried beans
Cold cuts	Hot dog	Bacon	Sausage
Cake	Cookies	Doughnut	Pastry
Chips	French fries		

    Other deep-fried foods such as fried chicken or egg rolls

Bread	Rolls	Rice	Cereal
Noodles	Spaghetti	Tortillas	

    Were any of these whole grain?   No   Yes

13. Is the way you ate yesterday the way you usually eat?   No   Yes

Lifestyles

14. Do you exercise for at least 30 minutes on a regular basis (3 times a week or more)?   No   Yes

15. Do you ever smoke cigarettes or use smokeless tobacco?   No   Yes

16. Do you ever drink beer, wine, liquor, or any other alcoholic beverages?   No   Yes

17. Which of these do you take? (circle all that apply):

    Prescribed drugs or medications

    Any over-the-counter products (such as aspirin, Tylenol®, antacids, or vitamins)

    Street drugs (such as marijuana, speed, downers, crack, or heroin)

*Commodity Supplemental Food Program
(National Academy of Sciences Institute of Medicine, Food and Nutrition Board, Committee on Nutritional Status During Pregnancy and Lactation, Subcommittee for a Clinical Application Guide. Nutrition during pregnancy and lactation: an implementation guide. Washington, DC: National Academy Press, 1992:7–8.)

pregnancy give birth to babies of normal weight, as do women who stop smoking before they become pregnant. Simply reducing the number of cigarettes smoked, however, provides little benefit, if any; only stopping completely can reverse the risks.[3]

Many organizations provide educational materials that point out the hazards of smoking during pregnancy and help people to quit. Among these groups are the National Foundation of the March of Dimes and the American Lung Association.

Prescription and Over-the-Counter Medications Certain medications taken by the mother during the first 12 weeks of pregnancy may produce structural changes in the embryo. The thalidomide tragedy of the 1960s focused international attention on this problem. This drug, a sedative and tranquilizer, had been used widely in Germany and other parts of Europe for only a few years when its teratogenic effects became apparent. In Germany alone, more than 4,000 children were born with severe malformations of the extremities (phocomelia or amyelia) as well as abnormalities of the face, heart, and viscera. Bendectin, a drug prescribed in the 1970s and early 1980s for morning sickness, was also thought to have teratogenic effects and as a result was taken off the market.

Some hormones also may cause fetal abnormalities. Because they are often administered as drugs, in addition to being present in both mother and fetus, the increased supply may cause a harmful imbalance or interaction with other drugs. Diethylstilbestrol (DES) is a drug that was given in large doses to many pregnant women from the 1940s through the 1960s to prevent abortion. When the offspring of these women reached young adulthood, the girls had an increased risk for vaginal cancer and the men experienced infertility caused by sperm changes.

Pharmaceutical companies must conduct research on drugs before their approval by the Food and Drug Administration for general use. Drugs are classified by the degree of teratogenic risk; however, new information sometimes reveals that a drug formerly thought safe may have effects not known earlier. A pregnant woman should ask her physician's advice before taking *any* medication, even those she has been accustomed to taking, including aspirin. Caution is the best policy when medications are involved.

Cocaine, Heroin, and Other Illicit Drugs Cocaine is the leading illicit drug in the United States. With the advent of crack, an inexpensive form of cocaine, drug use has increased among all socioeconomic groups. The resulting increase in infants affected adversely has reached 11%, or 375,000, each year nationwide.[4] This drug use results in many new challenges in the care of infants. Figure 6-10 illustrates the amount of drug use in racial and ethnic groups in the United States.

The effects of cocaine on the circulatory system of the mother cause constriction of the uterine blood vessels, thus creating complications such as first-trimester abortion, premature delivery, premature placental separation, intrauterine growth retardation, and numerous congenital abnormalities.

Other illicit drugs that affect the fetus include heroin, phencyclidine piperidine (PCP), and narcotics, such as meperidine (Demerol). Most of these cause intrauterine growth retardation, passive addiction, and possible neurologic impairment. Although methadone is a prescribed drug (used for the treatment of heroin addiction), it also falls into this group of drugs because it is a synthetic drug

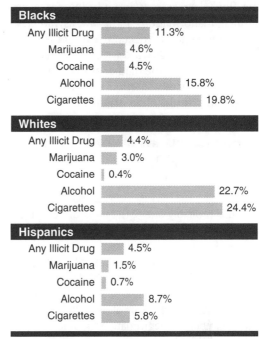

Drug Use During Pregnancy*
Among Racial and Ethnic Groups

Blacks	
Any Illicit Drug	11.3%
Marijuana	4.6%
Cocaine	4.5%
Alcohol	15.8%
Cigarettes	19.8%

Whites	
Any Illicit Drug	4.4%
Marijuana	3.0%
Cocaine	0.4%
Alcohol	22.7%
Cigarettes	24.4%

Hispanics	
Any Illicit Drug	4.5%
Marijuana	1.5%
Cocaine	0.7%
Alcohol	8.7%
Cigarettes	5.8%

*Percent of American women who gave birth in 1992 and used drugs during pregnancy

Figure 6-10
Drug use during pregnancy among racial and ethnic groups. Adapted from Mathias, R: NIDA survey provides first national data on drug use during pregnancy. NIDA Notes V, 10 Jan/Feb 1995. National Institute on Drug Abuse/National Institute of Health, Bethesda, Md.

with many of the same properties as heroin and morphine and affects the fetus adversely.

Radiation Since the atomic bombs fell on Hiroshima and Nagasaki, Japan, over 50 years ago, evidence has clearly shown that radiation causes genetic mutation and birth defects. Irradiation of the abdomen of a pregnant woman may arrest embryonic development and cause malformations. Natural background radiation, occupational exposure, and diagnostic or therapeutic procedures are a few sources of irradiation. Because the most sensitive period of organogenesis begins within a week or two after conception, radiographic examination of the abdomen of any woman of childbearing age should be done only during the first 2 weeks after a regular menstrual period.

Mechanical Factors Moving freely within the fluid of the amniotic sac, the fetus is protected from physical trauma. During the latter part of pregnancy, however, the fetus may be large enough to crowd the uterine cavity. This may result in certain positional abnormalities such as metatarsus varus (clubfoot), torticollis, and dislocation of the hip. Occasionally, bands of amniotic tissue can constrict fetal limbs and inhibit growth. If the production of amniotic fluid decreases as intrauterine space becomes more limited, malformations of the jaw, asymmetry of the head, and compression marks on the body may result. Although the fetus is safeguarded within the uterus, its protection is not perfect. If the mother suffers severe abdominal trauma, spontaneous abortion, or premature delivery, a disabling injury to the child may result.

EDUCATION FOR PARENTHOOD

Parenthood is probably one of the most difficult tasks anyone can assume, and its difficulties are more complex than ever before. Even in our "affluent" society, the United States still has a high infant mortality rate, a large number of mentally retarded infants and children, a continuing breakdown in family structure, many culturally deprived families, increasing neglect or abuse of children, and an increasing number of illegitimate pregnancies. Education for parenthood thus becomes a primary need.

Much of the education for parenthood focuses on prenatal care of the mother and on the mechanics of the birth process. These topics are paramount concerns because they are the foundation from which the child grows. However, complete education for parenthood must be an ongoing venture, helping parents cope with children at all stages of development. Nurses are providing more of that education as they assume an increasingly important role in the care of children and families.

Prenatal Care

Proper prenatal care is the best method to protect the health of the mother and her infant. Ideally, prenatal visits to the physician, nurse midwife, or clinic should begin soon after the woman's last menstrual period. For a normal pregnancy, these visits should be monthly until the 32nd week, every 2 weeks until the 36th week, and weekly thereafter until delivery. Visits may be more frequent in a high-risk pregnancy.

In prenatal care, the goals for the health care provider are to ensure that the pregnancy is proceeding normally, to answer questions and discuss concerns of the patient and family, and to teach parenting skills. Continuing care permits diagnosis of any maternal health problems that existed before the pregnancy or that develop during gestation and monitoring of the growth and health of the fetus.

PRENATAL CLINICS

Those in greatest need of prenatal care and other preparation for parenthood often have the least awareness about the need for or the availability of such services. National

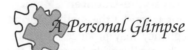

A Personal Glimpse

I attended labor classes with my wife during her first pregnancy. The sessions were held in the midwife's office at night. The classes consisted of lectures, review material, movies, exercises, and lots of discussion regarding the upcoming event. Overall, I felt the classes were very informative since they gave me a clearer picture of what my role as husband and coach would be during labor and delivery. They also helped my wife identify what key things she should be concentrating on—a very important point, considering how overwhelming a first pregnancy can be.

As a husband, one of the hardest things to come to terms with is a feeling of helplessness, particularly during labor and delivery. The classes helped me by explaining the stages of labor and their effect on my wife, when I should get my wife to the hospital, what the delivery would be like, and how I could help her deal with the pains of childbirth. Before the classes, my perception of the delivery process was similar to my father's—"take your wife to the delivery room, pace outside, wait till the baby is born, go out, buy cigars, and drink to celebrate." By understanding what my wife was going through, I was able to feel more comfortable in my role so that I could more fully support her. When our first daughter was born, I was glad that I had a role, albeit a small one, in delivering her to the world.

Larry

attention has been directed toward the importance of locating and assisting women in the high-risk pregnancy group. These are women in particular need of prenatal care because of socioeconomic factors, poor health, history of previous difficulties in childbirth, and lack of knowledge of prenatal development.

Particular attention has been focused on providing adequate prenatal clinics. A prenatal clinic is inadequate if it cannot serve the population for which it is intended. An adequate prenatal clinic should be located in the area where it is needed. The amount of money and time involved in reaching a clinic that is far away discourages early and regular attendance. A clinic is inadequate if it is too small or understaffed. Women are not likely to attend if they have to wait hours for attention that is often routine, impersonal, and inadequate.

Successful clinics need adequately trained personnel representing the various disciplines involved in healthy childbearing. Competent obstetricians and registered nurses are necessary. Nutritionists, social workers, and family counselors should be readily available for consultation. An atmosphere of caring, interest, and support is essential for a successful clinic.

Prepared Childbirth

Pregnancy affects more than the prospective mother; it touches the lives of the father-to-be, other children in the family, grandparents, and other relatives. Although it is often a time of joyous anticipation, pregnancy holds potential problems for everyone involved. "Pregnancy is more than simply a biologic event; it is a time of crisis for those involved, a time when identities are changing and new roles are being explored."[5] Each person reacts in a unique way, based on his or her needs and interpretations of the event.

Preparation for childbirth includes consideration of total family involvement, particularly the father-to-be. He should be included in as much of the prenatal activity as possible, especially classes about prenatal care and hygiene, fetal development, and the mechanics of birth. These classes are offered by many healthcare facilities and other groups in most communities.

Classes also have been developed specifically for pregnant teenagers, including the father whenever possible. Sibling and grandparent classes also are offered by many healthcare facilities. The emphasis on a family-centered experience is the primary concern of most childbirth educators.

NATURAL CHILDBIRTH

Never has more knowledge about pregnancy, labor, and birth been available to prospective parents. Many couples have taken advantage of this information and have come to regard pregnancy and birth as natural rather than pathologic processes. These couples often choose "natural" childbirth (birth unassisted by maternal anesthesia) because they are aware that no drug can be considered completely safe for the unborn baby. They attend classes that emphasize the Lamaze or other prepared childbirth methods, including pain control through proper breathing. The father or another support person learns how to coach the mother during labor and how to support the mother's emotional and physical needs throughout pregnancy (Fig. 6-11). These classes offer couples the opportunity to share experiences, emotions, and concerns with each other as well as with the instructor. Two of the principal organizations fostering these kinds of prenatal

Figure 6-11
This couple is practicing some of the breathing and coaching skills taught in childbirth preparation class.

education programs are the International Childbirth Education Association and the American Society for Psychoprophylaxis in Obstetrics.

Although the couple may opt for natural childbirth, in the end some woman may need an analgesic or an epidural to ease the pain of childbirth, or some partners may be unable to participate. The nurse can offer support to these couples and convey to them that they are not failures.

CESAREAN BIRTH

Not all women have the option of natural childbirth or even a vaginal delivery in the traditional delivery room. Certain maternal problems, such as a contracted pelvis, a weak or defective uterine scar, preeclampsia, eclampsia, placental disorders, difficult labor, cephalopelvic disproportion, pelvic tumors, gonorrhea, and herpes type 2 infections, necessitate cesarean delivery (delivery of the infant through a uterine incision). Some of these problems may be apparent early in the pregnancy, and the couple is therefore aware that cesarean delivery will be needed. This couple has as great a need for educational preparation for their particular birth experience as does the couple planning natural childbirth. Classes for these parents are being offered by most hospitals and often are taught by women who have experienced cesarean delivery.

When cesarean delivery is performed as an emergency procedure due to fetal or maternal distress, there is little time to prepare the couple psychologically. However, most childbirth preparation classes cover this possibility. In some hospitals, the father may not be permitted in the operating room to witness the birth unless he has attended cesarean birth preparation classes. This policy may lead to feelings of inadequacy and disappointment for the mother and feelings of exclusion for the father. This couple needs postdelivery counseling and reassurance to be sure they understand and accept the reason for the cesarean delivery.

■ KEY POINTS

■ The sex and genetic makeup of the baby-to-be are established at conception.

■ From zygote to embryo to fetus to newborn, the infant is shaped by the interaction of genetic and environmental influences.

■ A knowledgeable mother who conscientiously cares for herself during pregnancy increases her probability of producing a healthy newborn.

■ Parenthood is a great responsibility; couples can begin preparing for it by attending childbirth classes.

? CRITICAL THINKING

1. Laurie, the 15-year-old daughter of your cousin, has just confided to you that she thinks she is pregnant. Describe the guidance you would give her and the rationale for it.
2. Laurie's pregnancy has been confirmed. Her knowledge of anatomy and physiology is weak. Discuss what would you teach her about the growth and development of her fetus, starting with conception.
3. Laurie says she hopes the baby is a boy. Develop the response you will make to help her understand the sex determination of the fetus.
4. Explain what you would tell Laurie about the impact of her age on the pregnancy. Discuss the health teaching you would want to give Laurie concerning a) nutrition, b) drugs, and c) smoking.
5. Explore the types of prenatal classes available in your area.
6. Your 38-year-old neighbor is thinking about having a baby. Discuss what you might tell her about the hazards of pregnancy in women over 35 years of age.

REFERENCES

1. Mathias R. NIDA Notes, January/February, 1995.
2. Ibid
3. Educator update: It still pays to quit smoking now. Childbirth Instructor 1:6, 1991.
4. Jacques JT, Snyder N. Newborn victims of addiction. RN 4:47, 1991.
5. Colman AD, Colman LL. Pregnancy: The psychological experience. New York: Herder and Herder, 1971.

BIBLIOGRAPHY

Eschleman MM. Introductory nutrition and diet therapy, 3d ed. Philadelphia: Lippincott-Raven, 1996.

Lowdermilk DL, Perry SE, Bobak IM. Maternity and women's health care, 6th ed. St. Louis: CV Mosby, 1997.

Olds SB, London ML, Ladewig PW. Maternal-newborn nursing, 5th ed. Menlo Park, CA: Addison-Wesley, 1996.

Pillitteri A. Maternal and child health nursing, 2d ed. Philadelphia: JB Lippincott, 1995.

Reeder SJ, Martin LL Koniak D. Maternity nursing, 18th ed. Philadelphia: Lippincott-Raven, 1997.

Schuster C, Ashburn S. The process of human development, 3d ed. Philadelphia: JB Lippincott, 1992.

Wong D. Whaley and Wong's nursing care of infants and children, 5th ed. St. Louis: Mosby, 1995.

Chapter 7

The Normal Newborn

TRANSITION PERIOD
Respiration Begins
Circulation Changes
CARE IN THE DELIVERY ROOM
Apgar Score
Cord Care
Eye Care
Identification
Prevention of Heat Loss
Observation and Documentation
**PHYSIOLOGIC CHARACTERISTICS
OF THE NEWBORN**
Head and Skull
Chest
Bony Structure
Body Temperature
Respiratory System
Circulatory System
Gastrointestinal Tract
Genitourinary Tract
Nervous System: Reflexes

Special Senses
Skin
NEWBORN–PARENT BEHAVIOR
Newborn Activity
Mother–Infant Interaction
Father–Infant Interaction
**CARE IN THE NEWBORN NURSERY
OR THE MOTHER'S ROOM**
Mother–Baby Nursing
Admission to Nursery
Routine Nursing Care
Newborn Screening
NEWBORN FEEDING
Breast-Feeding
Formula Feeding
TEACHING THE NEW PARENT
FAMILY ADJUSTMENT
The Parents' Adjustment
The Infant's Adjustment
The Sibling's Adjustment

STUDENT OBJECTIVES

On completion of this chapter, the student will be able to:

1. Describe how a newborn is assessed at birth for a patent airway.
2. Discuss the circulatory changes that take place at birth.
3. Describe molding of the head, and explain why it occurs.
4. Explain the Apgar scoring system.
5. Identify the reason for eye care at birth, and name three effective medications.
6. Describe the common means of identification of the neonate in the delivery room.
7. List three reasons why the newborn regulates body heat poorly.
8. List four mechanisms of heat loss in the newborn, and give an example of each.
9. State the average weight and length of a newborn.
10. List three advantages and three disadvantages of circumcision.
11. Describe the general appearance of the newborn's a) head, b) skin, and c) genitalia.
12. Describe six normal neonatal reflexes.
13. Explain physiologic jaundice (icterus neonatorum).
14. State seven advantages of breast-feeding.
15. Explain the need for vitamin K in the newborn.
16. List two metabolic conditions for which newborns are screened in most states.
17. List four purposes of the newborn bath.

KEY TERMS

acrocyanosis	milia
areola	mongolian spots
Babinski reflex	Moro reflex
bonding	mother–baby nursing
caput succedaneum	mutual gazing
cavernous hemangioma	neonate
cephalhematoma	palmar grasp reflex
circumcision	petechiae
colostrum	phimosis
conduction	physiologic jaundice
convection	pseudomenses
cradle cap	pseudostrabismus
ductus arteriosus	radiation
ductus venosus	regurgitation
en face position	rooting reflex
erythema toxicum	smegma
evaporation	startle reflex
fontanelle	step reflex
foramen ovale	sucking reflex
forceps marks	suture
gag reflex	tonic neck reflex
lanugo	vascular nevus
meconium	vernix caseosa

Birth is hard work for the mother and the baby; therefore, calling it labor is accurate. As the uterus prepares for birth, the infant is slowly squeezed against the bony areas of the mother's pelvis and movement is restricted. Uterine contractions propel the infant down, into, and around through the birth canal, with the head serving as a dilator. The head pushes repeatedly against the mother's perineum before finally emerging.

After 9 months in the warm, dark security of the uterus, the newborn suddenly enters a strange, bright, cooler world. Is it any wonder that a cry is forthcoming? The cry fulfills a biologic need: by drawing air into the lungs with the first breath, the breathing process is initiated, which is one big step for the infant toward maintaining life.

Although totally helpless in comparison with other baby mammals, the human infant is physically equipped to survive outside the uterus—to regulate temperature, eat, sleep, and respond to certain stimuli—provided that someone else is ready to meet all his or her needs.

The newborn is also ready to develop social relationships, usually beginning with the parents. Research has shown that the first hour after birth is critically important to future family relationships. Hospitals and birthing centers have responded to this knowledge and to parents' requests by providing settings in which the father may be fully involved with the birthing experience.

TRANSITION PERIOD

The transition period from intrauterine life to extrauterine existence is a period of instability. During the first 24 hours of life, the infant is highly vulnerable and needs intensive observation because this is when many of the physiologic adjustments required for extrauterine life are completed (Table 7-1).

Respiration Begins

Secretions of mucus and amniotic fluid fill the newborn's nose and mouth. As soon as the head is delivered, the secretions should be suctioned gently with a bulb syringe, first from the mouth and then from the nose (Fig. 7-1). After delivery is completed, the **neonate** (a newborn in the first 28 days of life) should be held for a few seconds with the head lower than the body to facilitate drainage.

Failure to breathe within 1 minute after birth is an indication that some method of resuscitation is needed. Complications during labor often indicate possible respiratory problems at birth. Signs of respiratory distress include delayed respiration or irregular, gasping breath, sternal retractions, and cyanosis. Factors that add to the potential for respiratory complications include fetal distress, meconium-stained amniotic fluid, maternal medical complications (such as diabetes, hypertension, and cesarean birth), prematurity, and postmaturity.

In the event of airway obstruction after secretions are cleared from the nose and mouth, gentle stimulation, such as rubbing the infant's back, may be helpful. If further measures are required, suctioning may be necessary.

Figure 7-1
A bulb syringe is used to suction mucus from the newborn's nose and mouth.

TABLE 7-1.   Comparison of Physiologic Changes Between Fetal and Neonatal Life

Area of Change	Fetal Period	Neonatal Period
Environmental	Warm, stable, watery, fluid absorber of shock; stable temperature, twilight lighting; minimal sensory stimulations	Bright, noisy, dry atmosphere; temperature changes, much sensory stimulation
Circulatory	Ductus venosus—arterialized blood from umbilical vein goes to inferior vena cava	Ductus venosus becomes occluded and is known as the *ligamentum venosum.* Anatomic closure completed at end of 2 months.
	Ductus arteriosus—blood from right ventricle bypasses lung into descending aorta	Ductus arteriosus becomes occluded and is known as the *ligamentum arteriosum.* Functional closure within 3–4 days; anatomic closure completed by 3 weeks.
	Foramen ovale—permits major portion of oxygenated blood entering the heart to go directly from the right atrium to the left atrium, left ventricle, and out the ascending aorta	Foramen ovale closes, but closure is reversible for several days. Pulmonary circulation increases and more blood is returned from the lung to the left atrium.
Umbilical blood supply	Oxygenated blood travels to fetus by way of the umbilical vein and returns to placenta via the umbilical arteries	Placental circulation ceases when cord is tied. Umbilical vein becomes obliterated.
Blood composition	High numbers of red blood cells and high hemoglobin level necessary to provide adequate oxygenation in utero	Decrease in red blood cells and hemoglobin levels during first day of life
Respiratory	Respiratory movements begin during 4th month of fetal life. Amniotic fluid moves in and out of lungs as result of these movements. Lungs are collapsed; oxygenation is via placental circulation.	Lungs start to expand at first breath; full expansion takes several days. Placental oxygenation ceases with severance of umbilical cord.
Neurologic	Fetus responds to stimulation as a whole. Neurologic activity seen at about 8 weeks' gestation; isolated muscular reactions seen in response to stimulation. By 9 weeks, swimming motions and some spontaneous movements are present. By 13–14 weeks, movement may be perceptible to mother.	Infant responds to stimulation by certain discrete reflexes, such as rooting, plantar, and Moro reflexes.

When respirations are delayed or depressed, the use of an Ambu bag may be helpful. Measures used to relieve serious respiratory problems are intubation, oxygen, and mouth-to-mouth resuscitation. These measures require the serious attention of the physician, the anesthesiologist, and the obstetric team. Infants manifesting severe distress are transferred to the neonatal intensive care unit (NICU).

Circulation Changes

During fetal life, the lungs are inactive, requiring only a small amount of blood to nourish their tissues. Blood is circulated through the umbilical arteries to the placenta, where waste products and carbon dioxide are exchanged for nutrients. The blood then is returned to the fetus through the umbilical vein.

At birth, the umbilical cord is cut and the infant establishes an independent system. Certain fetal circulatory bypasses, such as the ductus arteriosus, the foramen ovale, and the ductus venosus, are no longer necessary after birth. They close and atrophy gradually through the first weeks of life (Fig. 7-2).

The **foramen ovale** (an opening between the right and left atria) closes with the first breath, but the closure is reversible for the first few days of life, with fusion of tissue taking 6 to 8 weeks. The **ductus arteriosus** (the prenatal blood vessel between the pulmonary artery and the aorta) closes functionally within 3 or 4 days, but the **ductus venosus** (the prenatal blood vessel between the umbilical vein and the inferior vena cava) does not achieve complete closure until the end of the second month of life.

The cord stump is examined immediately after being cut to determine the presence of one vein and two arteries. If only one artery is present, the newborn must be further examined for congenital defects of the internal organs.

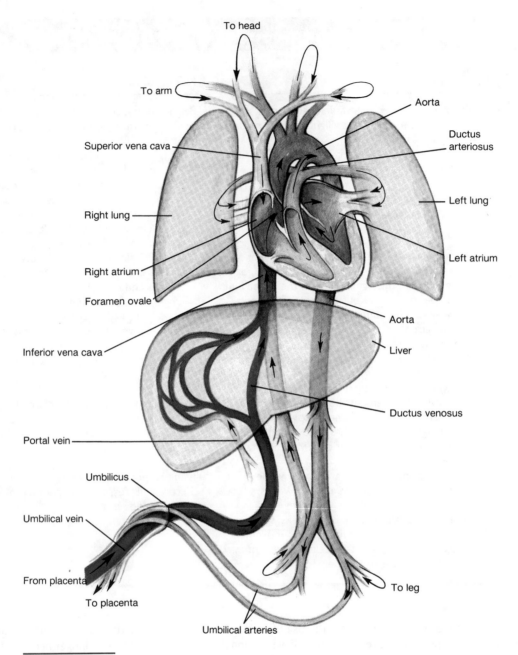

To head

To arm

Superior vena cava

Right lung

Right atrium

Foramen ovale

Inferior vena cava

Portal vein

Umbilicus

Umbilical vein

From placenta

To placenta

Umbilical arteries

Aorta

Ductus arteriosus

Left lung

Left atrium

Aorta

Liver

Ductus venosus

To leg

Figure 7-2
Fetal circulation.

CARE IN THE DELIVERY ROOM

The first few minutes of life are a critical period in which the immediate needs of establishing and maintaining an open airway and keeping the newborn warm take priority. The newborn's condition is assessed by means of Apgar scoring at 1 and 5 minutes of life. Identification of the newborn and eye care also are completed shortly after birth.

Apgar Score

Within 1 minute after birth, and again at 5 minutes, the general condition of all infants should be assessed according to the Apgar scoring method introduced by the physician Virginia Apgar in 1958 (Table 7-2). The infant is given a score of 0, 1, or 2 for each of five specific signs: heart rate, respiratory rate, muscle tone, reflex irritability, and color. A score of 10 indicates that the infant is in the best possible condition. A score of 7 to 9 is considered good and usually requires no special treatment. A score of 4 to 6

TABLE 7-2. Apgar Scoring Chart

Sign	0	1	2	1 min	5 min
Heart rate (beats/min)	Absent	<100	>100	—	—
Respiratory rate (breaths/min)	Absent	Slow, irregular	Good, crying	—	—
Muscle tone	Limp	Some flexion of extremities	Active motion	—	—
Reflex irritability					
Response to catheter in nostril	No response	Grimace	Cough or sneeze	—	—
or					
Slap to sole of foot	No response	Grimace	Cry and withdrawal of foot	—	—
Color	Blue, pale	Body pink, extremities blue	Completely pink	—	—

Developed by Dr. Virginia Apgar.

indicates a moderately depressed neonate who needs close observation. A score lower than 4 indicates the need for immediate attention and treatment as well as careful and continuous observation in the NICU.

The Apgar score is documented in the infant's chart for immediate availability. It serves as a reliable index of the condition at birth and as an important guide for subsequent care.

Cord Care

Shortly after birth, the umbilical cord is clamped with two clamps and then cut between the two clamps. Some physicians and nurse midwives encourage the father to perform this cutting to involve him in the birth process and to enhance the symbolism of freeing the newborn from the uterus and accepting responsibility for the infant's care. The end attached to the infant is clamped with a cord clamp or tied; the maternal clamp is then released. The cord appears to contain no nerve endings; neither the mother nor the infant shows any discomfort when it is cut. The stump is left without a dressing and should be inspected daily until it falls off. The stump may be treated with an antiseptic agent, which also may encourage it to dry. The stump is usually dry enough in 24 hours that the clamp may be removed.

Eye Care

Prophylactic eye treatment against gonococcal ophthalmia neonatorum is mandatory in the United States. Because gonorrhea in a woman may be asymptomatic, this disease was once a frequent cause of neonatal blindness, infecting the infant during passage through the birth canal of the infected mother.

The drugs approved for instillation into the eyes of the neonate are erythromycin 0.5% ophthalmic ointment in single-use tubes, tetracycline 1% ointment, and 1% silver nitrate solution. Erythromycin is believed to be more effective against *Chlamydia* infections, so many facilities use it. Another advantage of the ointment is that it does not cause the chemical conjunctivitis common with silver nitrate solution. However, silver nitrate, the older method, is more economical, and some facilities continue to use it.

Because of the sensitive parent–infant attachment, or **bonding**, period during the early hours after birth, some authorities recommend waiting 1 hour before instilling eye medication. Some state health codes, however, require instillation "immediately" after birth. Additional studies are needed to provide more conclusive evidence on the need for immediate treatment versus the value of uninterrupted bonding during the first hour of life.

Before the medication is administered, the infant's eyelids should be cleansed with sterile cotton moistened in sterile water. A separate pledget should be used for each eye, sponging from the nose outward until all blood or mucus is removed.

Next, the infant's eyes should be opened, one at a time, using gentle pressure on the upper and lower lids. One or two drops of solution or a 0.25″ ribbon of ointment should be applied per eye onto the conjunctival sac, never onto the cornea. If silver nitrate is used, the eyelids are held open for 30 to 60 seconds to allow the solution to flow from the inner to the outer aspect of the eye.

Formerly, the practice was to flush the eyes with sterile water or sterile saline solution after the instillation of silver nitrate. This practice has been discontinued because studies showed that the rinse did not reduce conjunctival irritation and may have diluted the effectiveness of the prophylactic eye drops. Parents should be warned that eye irritation may occur in the next 24 hours, with swelling and drainage, if silver nitrate is used.

Identification

Before the infant is transferred from the delivery room or the birthing room, identification bracelets with identical numbers are placed on the mother's wrist and the baby's wrist and ankle. In some hospitals, handprints or footprints are also taken and become part of the infant's chart, sometimes with the addition of the mother's right index fingerprint.

Prevention of Heat Loss

From a stable intrauterine temperature of 98.6°F (37°C), the wet neonate emerges into a world almost 30°F cooler. With an immature temperature-regulating system, a proportionately large body surface area relative to weight, a larger surface area for size than an adult's, and just a thin layer of subcutaneous fat, the neonate is subject to heat loss at birth. Unable to regulate body temperature by shivering, the neonate exposed to cool air kicks and cries, thereby increasing the metabolic rate and oxygen consumption, which may lead to metabolic acidosis. Conversely, in an overheated environment, the newborn has difficulty dispersing heat and may suffer from hyperthermia.

Newborns may lose heat through four processes: evaporation, radiation, conduction, and convection. **Evaporation** is heat loss through conversion of a liquid to a vapor. To prevent the rapid loss of heat from evaporation of the amniotic fluid, the infant must be dried rapidly and gently with a warm towel and placed into a warm environment. In settings where skin-to-skin contact between the infant and the mother is encouraged, an overhead radiant warmer may be used to reduce heat loss. Some hospitals and birthing rooms use stockinette caps on neonates because so much heat is lost through the neonate's wet head. If the infant is not placed skin-to-skin with the mother, a soft, warm blanket is used to wrap the newborn, who is either given to the mother to hold or placed in a warm crib or infant warmer.

Heat loss through **radiation** is the transfer of body heat to cooler solid objects that are not in direct contact with the infant. The temperature of the surrounding air has no effect on heat loss through radiation; therefore, the infant should not be examined until he or she is moved as far as possible from the walls of the delivery room, which tend to be colder than the air.

Conduction heat loss occurs when the neonate's skin is in direct contact with a cooler solid object. To avoid this, the infant should be placed on a padded surface and should be insulated with clothes and blankets.

Convection heat loss is similar to conduction but is increased by moving air currents. Transporting the infant in a crib with solid sides reduces convection heat loss.

Observation and Documentation

During this critical transition period, close observation of the infant is essential. In addition to the Apgar score, the nurse records the exact time of birth, the skin condition, the quality of the infant's cry, the presence of any congenital anomalies or evidence of birth injuries, and the type of forceps (if any) used to extract the infant. Weight and length of the infant are noted before transfer from the delivery room or immediately on admission to the nursery. The first urination and defecation must be noted and recorded; usually this happens after transfer to the nursery or the mother's room. Failure to urinate during the first 24 hours or to defecate during the first 36 hours may indicate a serious problem.

PHYSIOLOGIC CHARACTERISTICS OF THE NEWBORN

About 95% of newborns born at term weigh 5.5 to 10 lb (2.5 to 4.6 kg) and measure 18″ to 23″ (45 to 55 cm) long. Normal head circumference is about 12″ to 14″ (33 to 35 cm). The crown-to-rump measurement is about equal to the head circumference.

Head and Skull

The six bones of the newborn's skull are not united but can mold and overlap to permit the large head to pass through the birth canal. These bones are divided by narrow bands of connective tissue called **sutures**. At the juncture of these bones are small spaces called **fontanelles**. At birth, the two palpable fontanelles, or soft spots, are the anterior fontanelle at the juncture of the frontal and parietal bones and the posterior fontanelle at the juncture of the parietal and occipital bones (Fig. 7-3).

During delivery, the head is molded along the suture lines and may appear asymmetric or elongated (Fig. 7-4). Usually, normal shape is assumed after a few days. The sections of the bony skull calcify and join during the first months of life. The posterior (triangle-shaped) fontanelle closes in about 1.5 to 3 months of life; the anterior (diamond-shaped) fontanelle closes between 12 and 18 months.

The brain is covered with a tough membrane, making it difficult to injure the child's head through the fontanelles by ordinary handling. Mothers need to be reassured that the baby's scalp may be washed with soap and water (*not* baby oil) over these areas without harm. Ordinary cleansing may be helpful to prevent **cradle cap** (seborrheic dermatitis), an accumulation of oil, serum, and dirt that often forms on an infant's scalp.

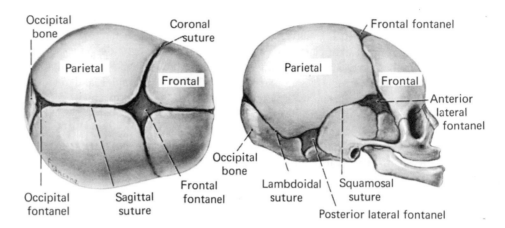

Figure 7-3
Infant skull showing fontanelles and cranial sutures.

Chest

The chest of the newborn has a smaller circumference than the head. The breasts of both male and female newborns may be engorged as a result of maternal estrogens in the bloodstream, and a pale, milky fluid (witches' milk) may be secreted. This condition disappears within 4 to 6 weeks. Meanwhile, the breasts should be handled gently and not manipulated in any way.

Bony Structure

The arms and legs of the newborn are short in comparison with the trunk. Prenatal development proceeds in a cephalocaudal (head-to-toe) progression and in a proximal (nearest to center) to distal (remote) sequence (Fig. 7-5). This means that the head and trunk are well developed, but the distal areas (arms, hands, legs, and feet) develop later. Development always proceeds from the general to the specific (for instance, gross muscle control comes before fine muscle control).

Body Temperature

At delivery, the infant's body temperature is generally the same as the mother's, but it drops rapidly after entering the cooler environment. As mentioned earlier, a warm, stable

Figure 7-4
Molding: the head of this newborn is elongated due to the pressure of passage through the birth canal.

Figure 7-5
Arrows indicate the cephalocaudal and proximodistal progress of infant development.

environment is necessary until the neonate has adjusted to independent living. In the delivery room, the infant is usually wrapped in a warm blanket or placed in a heated crib. Body temperature varies after birth according to the environment, with a range of 97.5° to 98.6°F (36.4° to 37°C), due to the immature nervous system. It usually stabilizes in a few days. Normal newborn axillary temperature, after stabilization, varies from 96.8° to 99°F (36° to 37.2°C).

The newborn's temperature may be taken by rectum, axilla, or tympanic membrane. In most newborn nurseries, the first temperature is taken rectally to determine the patency of the anal opening. There may be a shallow opening in the anus, however, with the rectum ending in a blind pouch. In this instance, the ability to insert a thermometer into the rectum does not signify a patent rectum. When a temperature is measured rectally, care must be taken to insert the thermometer only just beyond the bulb of the thermometer. Axillary and tympanic temperatures are obtained using the procedure outlined in Chapter 3.

Respiratory System

The first and most important task of the neonate is to oxygenate the red blood cells; this occurs with the first cry. Although respiratory movements appear in fetal life, there is no *functional* respiration before birth. Breathing in the healthy newborn is quiet and shallow, and variations in rate and rhythm are normal. In normal infants, the rate may vary from 20 to 100 breaths per minute, according to whether the infant is sleeping or awake, crying, lying passively, or vigorously moving the arms and legs. Because the rate fluctuates rapidly, the respirations should be counted for a full minute. Persistent rates greater than 60 or less than 30 breaths per minute should be called to the physician's attention because this may indicate cardiac or pulmonary difficulty. Sternal retractions are considered abnormal and also should be reported.

The newborn's breathing is diaphragmatic (abdominal); therefore, respirations may be counted most easily by watching the rise and fall of the abdomen rather than the chest. Parents should be informed of this characteristic to prevent any alarm about what may seem to them to be abnormal breathing.

Circulatory System

The changes that occur in the circulatory system at birth are primarily due to oxygenating the blood through the pulmonary system and to discarding the placenta, umbilical vein, and arteries. Shortly after birth, the blood flows through the infant's circulatory system in the same manner as that of an adult. **Acrocyanosis** (cyanosis of the hands and feet) is common and occurs because of the immature peripheral circulatory system. When the infant cries, however, the skin becomes rosy red.

At birth, the infant's heart rate may reach 180 beats per minute, then decrease to 100 to 120. Usually by the second day of life, the pulse is 90 to 160, depending on whether the infant is asleep or awake and active. Blood pressure is difficult to measure in the newborn unless it is taken with specialized equipment using ultrasonography, such as a Doppler and an oscillometer. An initial blood-pressure measurement should be taken, however, to provide a baseline and to alert the staff to any cardiac problems.

Gastrointestinal Tract

The gastrointestinal tract is functional at birth, and within 8 to 24 hours, **meconium** (a sticky, greenish-black substance composed of bile, mucus, cellular waste, intestinal secretions, fat, hair, and other materials swallowed during fetal life, together with amniotic fluid) usually is passed. The time of the first stool should be recorded to confirm anal patency. If no stool is passed during the first 24 hours after birth, the physician should be notified because some obstruction may exist in the intestinal tract.

The neonate can digest the fat, protein, and carbohydrates in breast milk or in a modified formula. **Regurgitation**, spitting up of small quantities of milk, occurs rather easily in the young infant and is different from vomiting. It may be caused by an air bubble in the infant's stomach, too-rapid nursing, or overfeeding.

Vomiting differs from regurgitation in that an appreciable amount of fluid is expelled. Although this also may result from rapid feeding or inadequate burping, frequent or persistent vomiting may signal an abnormal condition and should be reported to the physician.

The neonate hiccups easily; this is most likely caused by feeding too rapidly. However, hiccupping does occur in fetal life. Burping the infant to bring up swallowed air or nursing for another minute usually controls the hiccups. In any instance, they eventually stop without treatment.

Genitourinary Tract

The kidneys secrete urine before birth, and some urine collects in the bladder after birth. A record of the first urination is important to confirm adequate kidney function and the absence of severe constrictions somewhere in the urinary system.

The male testes are usually descended into the scrotum at birth, but occasionally one or both are in the process of descending or remain in the abdomen. These testes usually descend spontaneously during the first year of life.

In the newborn, the prepuce of the penis is normally tight. **Phimosis**, or adherence of the foreskin to the glans penis, is normal in early infancy. Forceful retraction should not be attempted. The foreskin usually becomes retractable by 3 years of age. If minor irritations develop, cleansing with soap and water is all that is needed. One danger of forceful retraction of the foreskin during early infancy is that the elastic fibers at the tip of the foreskin may tear and bleed. The result will be that the foreskin heals by scarring, perhaps making circumcision necessary later.

TABLE 7-3. Advantages and Disadvantages of Neonatal Circumcision

Advantages	Disadvantages

Prevention of
    Penile cancer
    Inflammation of glans and prepuce
    Complications of later
        circumcision
Possible decrease of
    Urinary tract infections in males
    Sexually transmitted disease
Preserves male body image
    (to be same as circumcised father
    or peers when older)
	Complications of
	    Hemorrhage
	    Infection
	    Dehiscence
	    Meatitis from loss of protective foreskin
	    Adhesions
	    Concealed penis
	    Urethral fistula
	    Meatal stenosis
	Pain at time of procedure

In 1975, the American Academy of Pediatrics opposed the routine **circumcision** (surgical removal of all or part of the prepuce, or foreskin, of the penis) of the newborn, stating that there is no sound medical reason for the procedure and that good personal hygiene is adequate without surgical risk. The Academy changed its position in 1989, stating that circumcision for the newborn has potential medical advantages and benefits as well as disadvantages and risks. Today, the controversy over circumcision continues. Parents should be thoroughly informed by the physician about both the risks and benefits of the procedure (Table 7-3). Circumcision of the newborn is performed frequently for religious reasons, most notably by those of the Jewish faith. Circumcision prevents the accumulation of the secretions collectively called **smegma**. If the foreskin of the newborn is so tight that it obstructs the urinary system, circumcision is performed at once.

In the female neonate, the labia are prominent due to the effect of the mother's estrogens during intrauterine life. The infant may have a slight red-tinged vaginal discharge called **pseudomenses**, which results from a decline in the hormonal level compared with the higher concentration in the maternal hormone environment. Unless the mother understands why this happens, she may become alarmed. She should be told that although it does not appear in all newborn females, it is a natural manifestation resulting from hormonal transfer and will disappear in a few days. It should be emphasized that this discharge is not due to any trauma or infection.

Nervous System: Reflexes

The neonate exhibits several normal reflexes triggered by an immature nervous system. Research indicates that infants follow their reflexes for the first 3 months of life. For example, all newborns smile, even if they are blind, and all infants tightly grasp objects placed in their palms. Most of

the reflexes disappear during the first year of life. Infants should be tested for the most common ones because their absence may indicate a disturbance in the nervous system.

The **rooting reflex**, present at birth, is seen when the cheek is stroked and the infant responds by turning the head toward that side (Fig. 7-6). Thus, when the mother or the nurse places a hand on the infant's cheek to turn the head toward the breast, the infant turns instead toward the person's hand.

The **sucking reflex** is so well developed at birth that personnel in the delivery room are often startled by the loud sucking noises coming from the newborn's crib.

The **gag reflex** is present at birth and continues throughout life. Any stimulation of the posterior pharynx by food, suction, or passage of a tube causes gagging.

Pressure on the palms of the hands or soles of the feet

Figure 7-6
The rooting reflex is elicited when the newborn's cheek is stroked.

Figure 7-7
Grasp reflex present in all normal newborns is sufficiently strong to lift them from the examining table.

Figure 7-8
Step, or dance, reflex simulates walking when infant is held so that the sole of the foot touches examining table.

near the base of the digits causes flexion of hands and toes. The **palmar grasp reflex** is so strong in a healthy infant that the infant can be lifted off the examining table (Fig. 7-7). The palmar grasp reflex diminishes after 3 months; the plantar grasp reflex but it persists until 9 to 12 months of age.

When the lateral plantar surface is stroked, the toes flare open. Called the **Babinski** (or plantar) **reflex**, this reaction usually disappears by the end of the first year.

Until 6 weeks of age, most normal infants, when held in an upright position, make stepping movements (Fig. 7-8). This movement is called the **step** (or dance) **reflex**.

Any sudden jarring or abrupt change in equilibrium elicits the **Moro reflex** in the normal newborn. It consists primarily of abduction and extension of the arms. All digits extend except the index finger and the thumb, which are flexed to form a C shape (Fig. 7-9). If the response is not immediate, bilateral, and symmetric, injury to the brachial plexus, the humerus, or the clavicle may be present. Persistence of this reflex after 6 months of age may indicate brain damage.

Similar to the Moro reflex, the **startle reflex** follows any loud noise and consists of abduction of the arms and flexion of the elbows. Unlike the Moro reflex, the hands remain clenched. Absence of this reflex may indicate hearing impairment.

Not always apparent during the first weeks of life, the **tonic neck reflex**, also called the fencing reflex, may be observed when the infant lies on the back, with the head turned to one side, the arm and leg on the same side extended, and the opposite arm flexed as if in a fencing position (Fig. 7-10). Usually, this reflex disappears between 3 and 4 months of age.

Special Senses

SIGHT

Research has shown that the unborn baby can distinguish light from dark and at birth can see. The rod cells in the retina of the eyes, which are responsible for light perception, are functional at birth; however, the retina, the newborn's special organ of visual perception, is not fully developed until about 16 weeks of age. The neonate's head turns

Figure 7-9
Moro reflex is elicited by sudden jarring or change in equilibrium. Arms abduct at the shoulder and extend at the elbow. All digits extend except the index finger and the thumb, which curve into a C-shape.

Figure 7-10
Tonic neck reflex is present when the infant lies on his or her back with the head turned to one side, with the arm and leg on the same side extended and the arm on the opposite side flexed.

toward a light, and the neonate blinks and closes his or her eyes at a bright light. The infant follows a bright moving object momentarily, but fixation of coordination comes much later. The nerves and muscles that control focusing and coordination are not completely developed until the sixth month, accounting for the cross-eyed look (**pseudostrabismus**) that babies sporadically show. Parents have no cause for alarm if their infant's eyes are not coordinated in their movements occasionally, but if lack of focusing remains at 4 months, the pediatrician should be alerted.

Most dark-skinned infants have brown eyes at birth, whereas most light-skinned newborn's eyes are slate gray or dark blue. Tears are produced constantly at birth but are completely disposed of through the nasolacrimal duct until about 2 or 3 months of age, when tear production increases. Newborns have about 20/500 vision, compared with a normal-seeing adult's vision of 20/20. This means that most distant objects appear very fuzzy. Close vision is much better, and the infant can see most of the features of a human face clearly at a distance of 7" to 15" (17–38 cm). This is one reason why the **en face position** (the caregiver and the infant establish eye contact in the same vertical plane) is so important to parent–infant attachment immediately after birth.

HEARING

A newborn stops crying momentarily at the sound of a soothing voice and is startled and cries at a loud noise. By the age of 3 days, the infant can distinguish the mother's voice from that of other females. The sense of hearing certainly contributes to the infant's emotional reactions to fear and to comforting. It is not known exactly how early the infant hears soft voices and other faint sounds, but infants 2 or 3 days old stop crying momentarily when talked to soothingly.

SMELL

The sense of smell is not highly developed at birth, but research has shown that the newborn infant does turn toward the mother's breast because of the smell of breast milk. A neonate can differentiate the smell of his or her mother's breast milk from that of other females. Strong smells also bring about reaction, and a newborn turns away from smells such as vinegar and alcohol.

TASTE

Because much of taste depends on the sense of smell, the infant's sense of taste is probably not highly developed at birth. Some studies have shown, however, that breathing, sucking, and swallowing patterns are different when infants are fed formula than when they are fed breast milk. In addition, neonates have produced the expected reaction of distaste for sour or bitter solutions and pleasure at a sweet solution. They definitely prefer glucose and water over unflavored (sterile) water.

TOUCH

Sensitivity to touch is present from birth, particularly in the lips and tongue. The sense of pain is also present at birth, but like adults infants vary in their sensitivity to pain. Newborns react to painful pinpricks. Sensitivity appears to increase during the first few days of life as part of individual development. The infant cries lustily when suffering gastrointestinal discomfort.

Skin

NORMAL APPEARANCE

Sluggish peripheral circulation and vasomotor instability are manifested in the deep-red color the infant acquires when crying, as well as in the pale hands and feet of many newborns. The skin is usually red to dark pink in white newborns. African American newborns have reddish-brown skin, and Hispanic infants have an olive or yellowish tint to the skin. The skin should feel elastic when picked up between the examiner's fingers.

Fine, downy hair called **lanugo** covers the skin of the fetus. It is usually not present in a full-term infant but may be seen on a premature infant.

A greasy, cheeselike substance called **vernix caseosa** protects the skin during fetal life. Vernix caseosa is a mixture of oil and water containing cells flaked from the skin and fatty substances secreted by the sebaceous glands. At birth, vernix may cover the skin or remain only in the folds of the skin. In most hospitals, not all of the vernix is removed with the first bath, but it is left on as a protective agent. It eventually is absorbed or rubs off.

SKIN BLEMISHES

Newborns may have various temporary skin blemishes. One of the most common is a **vascular nevus** ("strawberry mark"). A nevus is a circumscribed new growth of the skin of congenital origin; it may be either vascular or nonvascular. The strawberry mark is a slightly raised, bright-red collection of blood vessels that does not blanch completely on pressure. It may be present at birth or may appear during the first 6 months of life. This blemish may enlarge during the first 6 months of life, but eventually when it ceases to grow, fibrosis replaces the capillaries and the lesion shrinks. Treatment is not usually indicated because most of these marks regress and disappear by 10 years of age. If the lesion is so large as to cause emotional trauma in the child, the physician may suggest removal.

Erythema toxicum (fine rash of the newborn) may appear over the trunk, back, abdomen, and buttocks. It appears in about 24 hours and disappears in several days. It is not infectious and needs no treatment.

Vascular nevi sometimes are present in **cavernous hemangiomas**, subcutaneous collections of blood vessels with bluish overlying skin. Although these lesions are benign tumors, they may become so large and extensive as to interfere with the functions of the body part on which they appear. Small hemangiomas ("stork bites") often are seen on the eyelids or the back of the neck. They disappear within 6 to 12 months without treatment. In infants of African, Mediterranean, Native American, or Asian descent, **mongolian spots** (areas of bluish-black pigmentation resembling bruises) may be seen, most often over the sacral or gluteal region. They usually fade within a year or two.

Milia are pearly white cysts appearing on the face in about 40% of newborns. They are usually retention cysts of sebaceous glands or hair follicles and disappear in a few weeks without treatment.

Petechiae are small bluish-purple spots caused by tiny broken capillaries. They may be seen on the face as a result of excess pressure on the head during a rapid or difficult delivery. They disappear in a day or so.

Forceps marks may be noticeable on the infant's face if forceps were used during delivery. These marks ordinarily disappear in a day or two. After a difficult delivery, bruises and edema may be present on the head or scalp, or on the buttocks and the genitalia after a breech delivery. Although these gradually clear up without treatment, such bruises may be distressing to the parents, who may not understand the relative insignificance of these marks. The nurse may carefully and simply explain that they are minor bruises and will fade quickly.

Occasionally, the infant's head is misshapen by its passage through the birth canal. The mother is naturally distressed and needs to know that this is temporary and is

Figure 7-11
Cephalhematoma of left parietal hemisphere.

caused by the head's inability to accommodate to the narrow passage. The head acquires a normal rounded shape in a few days.

Caput succedaneum is an edematous swelling of the soft tissues of the scalp caused by prolonged pressure of the occiput against the cervix during labor and delivery. The edema disappears in a few days. **Cephalhematoma** is a collection of blood between the periosteum and the skull (Fig. 7-11). The swelling of the overlying scalp usually is not visible until several hours after birth. This swelling also may frighten the caregivers, who may think some injury has occurred. The edema of caput succedaneum may spread across the scalp, but the swelling of cephalhematoma is contained by the periosteum and cannot cross suture lines. Most cephalhematomas are reabsorbed within 2 weeks to 3 months, depending on their size. Because the only serious complication may be the introduction of infection, aspiration, incision, or any other treatment is contraindicated.

Physiologic jaundice (icterus neonatorum) occurs in many newborns and has no medical significance. It is believed to result from the breakdown of fetal red blood cells. It must, however, be carefully observed and reported in an effort to distinguish it from a serious jaundice condition. A simple heel stick may be done by the nursing staff to perform a microbilirubin examination. This study may confirm or rule out an elevated bilirubin level. Physiologic jaundice, with yellowing of the skin, does not appear until after the second day of life, which may be after the newborn

A Personal Glimpse

When my daughter was born, she was jaundiced, but her bilirubin level was not high enough to put her under the "lights." The doctors wanted to monitor her with heel prick blood tests twice a day. In between the tests at the hospital, I was to go home and put her in the sunlight (unfortunately, it was overcast all that week) and nurse her as much as possible. They said that would help. Each time she was tested, we waited at the hospital an hour for the test results, only to find that the level went up a little, but not enough to put her under the lights. We did this twice a day for 5 days, back and forth to the hospital. I was stressed out from listening to my infant wail at the heel pricks, having my sleep interrupted every 2 hours to nurse her, and crashing postpartum hormones. Add to that the trips back and forth and I was a mess. On the fourth day, after they jabbed my baby's heel once again and once again she wailed in pain, I burst into tears and said that maybe she wasn't fighting off the jaundice because of me—because my breasts were not making enough milk. The nurse got very firm and said, "Lift up your blouse." I did and we both looked down on my more-than-ample breasts. She said, "You have more than enough milk for that baby." We both laughed.

Nancy

goes home. Caregivers should be advised to report to the physician any jaundice appearing during the first 3 days.

NEWBORN–PARENT BEHAVIOR

Newborn Activity

The healthy newborn, if placed face down, lifts or turns the head to one side to clear the airway. The infant exercises in uncoordinated, random movements, involving the entire body in the activity. The muscles are taut, and it is difficult to extend the extremities manually. The infant momentarily ceases activity at the sound of a nearby voice.

The newborn may sneeze to clear the nasal passages, yawn, hiccup, stretch, blink, and cough. The fetus learned to suck and swallow during intrauterine life.

The infant's only way of expressing tension from hunger, cold, pain, or other discomfort is by crying. Prompt comforting and attention to the infant's needs usually restores composure and alleviates the discomfort. It is often with these first moments of comforting and soothing that the parent–child attachment process begins.

Mother–Infant Interaction

Even though infant and mother have been physically inseparable for 9 months, their emotional togetherness and the beginning of mutual love and attachment start after delivery, ideally in the first few hours. Many babies are alert for a short time after delivery, offering a good opportunity for sensory contact with the mother.

Research indicates that early attachment activities have a significant effect on the long-term parent–child relationship. This does not mean that early attachment guarantees a satisfactory lifetime relationship or that lack of opportunity for early attachment seriously threatens the family's chances for a strong relationship. It simply means that the family relationship is given the best possible start if the mother, the father, and the infant are together during this early period in their new life as a family.

Touch is a highly significant part of the attachment process. Many hospitals and birthing rooms offer the opportunity for skin-to-skin contact between the mother and the infant (and sometimes the father and the infant). Shortly after delivery, the nude infant may be placed on the mother's abdomen and chest and held to the mother's breast if the mother plans to breast-feed (Fig. 7-12). Touching

Figure 7-12
Immediate bonding between the mother, partner or father, and infant should be encouraged whenever possible.

provides warmth, comfort, and a sense of security, all vital for the vulnerable newborn.

Studies have shown that the mother is likely to follow a predictable pattern of touching her new baby, first using only the fingertips to touch the extremities, then gradually moving her fingers over the infant's entire body, and finally using her entire hand to massage the trunk of the body. Next, she tries to reposition herself and the baby in the en face position. This is also referred to as **mutual gazing**. The attachment process is affected by many factors, among them the mother's physical and emotional condition after labor, the infant's condition and behavior, and the comparison of the real infant with the fantasy infant the mother has imagined since she became aware of her pregnancy. The mother who had a difficult labor or heavy sedation may not be alert enough to participate effectively. If the infant has a problem that requires immediate transfer to the special care nursery or NICU, there will be no time for early attachment.

Every woman during her pregnancy imagines what her baby will look like, how he or she will act, what the child will eventually accomplish, and how she and others in the family will be affected by this new person. This imaginary baby is likely to be different from the real infant she meets soon after delivery. At first sight, the infant seldom resembles the chubby, well-formed baby pictured by the world in general. The head is large in proportion to the body and may be misshapen by the birth process. Blood and vernix still cling to the body, and the neonate probably is crying. Is this the baby the mother has dreamed about and planned for? The newborn may appear completely self-centered, displeased over this abrupt introduction to the world. Such a first impression may summon feelings of guilt in the mother that she does not feel the expected gush of love and tenderness. If the baby is quiet and passive and she had imagined an awake, alert, active child, she may be disappointed, giving less attention and stimulation than she would to an infant who more closely resembles the imagined child.

Both parents must understand that each infant is unique, with individual characteristics and potential. Studies have shown that pointing out to parents their child's unique characteristics may help develop a more positive attitude, reduce feeding and sleeping problems, and bring about greater activity and alertness in the infant.

One widely used guide for assessing neonatal activity is the Brazelton Neonatal Behavioral Assessment Scale (Fig. 7-13). Special training is necessary to use the test. The Brazelton criteria also help the parents tune in to their baby and learn more about this budding personality and how their responses affect their adjustment to each other.

Father–Infant Interaction

Fathers who are involved during pregnancy, delivery, and the postpartum period develop an attachment as strong as that of the mother.[1] The father's attachment behavior is

---

BRAZELTON SCALE CRITERIA

1. Response decrement to light
2. Response decrement to rattle
3. Response decrement to bell
4. Response decrement to pinprick
5. Orientation response—inanimate visual
6. Orientation response—inanimate auditory
7. Orientation—animate visual
8. Orientation—animate auditory
9. Orientation—animate-visual and auditory
10. Alertness
11. General tonus
12. Motor maturity
13. Pull-to-sit
14. Cuddliness
15. Defensive movements
16. Consolability with intervention
17. Peak of excitement
18. Rapidity of buildup
19. Irritability (to aversive stimuli: uncover, undress, pull-to-sit, prone, pinprick, TNR, Moro, defensive reaction)
20. Activity
21. Tremulousness
22. Amount of startle during exam
23. Lability of skin color
24. Lability of states
25. Self-quieting activity
26. Hand to mouth facility
27. Smiles

Figure 7-13
Brazelton Neonatal Behavioral Assessment Scale.

similar to the mother's: touching, holding the infant in the en face position, observing the beauty of the child (particularly any features that resemble the father), and expressing feelings of elation and satisfaction (Fig. 7-14). Many fathers indicate that they want to share the responsibility of raising the baby.

Some cultures dictate that men not show emotion; thus, some fathers may need encouragement to express their feelings about their infant. Nurses should reinforce any positive attachment behavior displayed by either parent and should show, whenever necessary, the soothing effect of cuddling, stroking, rocking, and talking to the baby.

CARE IN THE NEWBORN NURSERY OR THE MOTHER'S ROOM

After a careful assessment of the newborn has been made and the family has had time together, the infant is transferred either to the newborn nursery or to the mother's

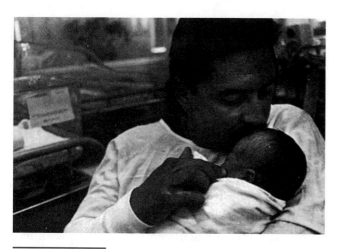

Figure 7-14
In the nursery, the father has an excellent opportunity to explore and interact with his new daughter.

room. Many maternity units have a receiving or recovery nursery in which the infant is cared for and carefully watched for the first hours of life. Other units may set aside part of the general newborn nursery as a receiving area.

Premature infants are transferred to a premature unit or the NICU. In the NICU, infants with serious congenital anomalies or birth defects also receive special care. Infants of diabetic mothers may be placed in the specialized unit because they must be carefully observed, even though they are generally large for gestational age. Often, newborns with serious problems who are born in smaller hospitals or birthing centers may need to be transferred to a tertiary hospital where they can receive intensive, specialized care.

Every maternity unit must have a way to segregate infants who have been exposed to any sort of infection before, during, or after birth. Infants born outside the hospital or infants born to mothers whose membranes were ruptured longer than 24 hours are kept in segregation to protect the other newborns in the nursery.

Mother–Baby Nursing

Many hospitals offer mothers **mother–baby nursing**. In mother–baby nursing, postpartum and nursery nurses are cross-educated so that one nurse cares for both the mother and the infant. After the infant's condition has stabilized, the infant's bassinet is kept beside the mother, who participates in caring for her newborn while being carefully guided and taught by the nurse. Some hospitals have labor–delivery–recovery–postpartum (LDRP) suites into which the mother is initially admitted. Labor and delivery occur in this suite, and the mother and infant stay there for the entire hospitalization. Nurses who staff these units are educated and skilled in providing nursing care throughout labor, delivery, recovery, and the postpartum period, including care of the newborn. LDRP suites and mother–baby nursing offer the following advantages that were found desirable with rooming-in:

- Provides maximum opportunity for maternal–infant interaction while the mother and the newborn are still in the care of maternity personnel
- Fosters infant feeding on a permissive (demand) schedule
- Offers a fine opportunity to teach the mother, father, or other support persons about infant care and allows supervised experience in infant care
- Allows siblings and grandparents to visit in privacy
- Reduces the incidence of cross-infection.

Admission to Nursery

On admission, the infant's identification is verified, the Apgar score is reported, the cord stump is inspected, and the delivery room record is reviewed. The infant is placed on the side in a bassinet or isolette to facilitate mucous drainage from the nose and mouth. In many facilities, vitamin K is administered at this time (if it was not given in the delivery room) to prevent hemorrhage and promote clotting. The neonate usually cannot produce adequate vitamin K because the intestine of the newborn is sterile and the flora needed to help produce vitamin K in the body is unavailable. Vitamin K is administered intramuscularly in the vastus lateralis. By the second week of life, after the infant has ingested food and normal flora is produced, the infant manufactures sufficient vitamin K.

Until the newborn is given his or her first bath, the nurse must wear gloves for protection from blood and body fluids during any contact with the neonate. The infant's temperature is taken, the vital signs are assessed, and then the infant is allowed to rest. Bathing, weighing, and dressing may be postponed until the infant's condition and temperature are stabilized. However, close observations are made and vital signs are assessed at 15- to 30-minute intervals (Fig. 7-15). The nursery temperature should be about 75°F (24°C), and the humidity should be lower than 50%. The neonate is bundled to maintain body heat; if necessary, additional external heat may be used in the form of heat lamps or warmers. When stable, the infant may be weighed, sponge-bathed, and dressed.

Routine Nursing Care

Newborns are highly susceptible to infection. Removed from the protection of the uterus, they have not developed any defenses against disease; therefore, particular attention to hygiene is essential when the infant is handled. Except for weighing, all care, including bathing, examinations, and taking temperatures, is given inside the bassinet. The nursery scale should be covered with a disposable liner or paper towel that is discarded after each infant is weighed. The scale is sprayed or wiped with a germicidal, fungicidal

Figure 7-15
The newborn's respiratory rate is evaluated periodically after admission to the nursery.

solution and freshly covered before the next infant is put on the scale.

HANDWASHING

The most important precaution is handwashing before handling any infant. This principle applies to anyone handling a newborn, including nurses, physicians, laboratory personnel, and parents.

Before entering the nursery, wristwatches, rings, and bracelets should be removed. After entering the handwashing area, the area under the fingernails should be cleaned with an orangewood stick. The hands should be washed with disposable sponge brushes under running water, using an antiseptic preparation. The area between the fingers, the palms, the backs of the hands, and the wrists and arms up to the elbows should be washed with circular motions for 3 minutes. The hands and lower arms should be rinsed and dried with a paper towel. The faucet should be turned off with a paper towel. Between handling babies, staff should wash thoroughly for 30 seconds. In most obstetric units, attendants must wear scrub gowns or suits. Anyone suffering from a respiratory condition, intestinal upset, skin rash or cuts, elevated temperature, or any sign of illness should not enter the nursery or participate in the care of infants.

Caregivers should be taught to use a thorough handwashing technique after toileting and before handling her baby. Fathers, siblings, grandparents, or other visitors who are in the room when the baby is in the mother's room should put on long-sleeved gowns over their clothing. An area where these persons may wash, with appropriate brushes, antiseptic solution, and paper towels as well as clean gowns, should be available in the room. Directions for handwashing and putting on gowns should be displayed prominently.

BATHING

Daily sponge baths are given using warm water and, if needed, a bland soap. Cleansing proceeds from the head down. If the scalp needs cleansing, it should be washed with water and soap and then rinsed with a washcloth, taking care not to get water in the infant's eyes.

A mild soap may be used in cleansing the infant. Some nurseries prefer to use "dry" skin care, in which only the head, face, and body folds are cleansed with cotton balls moistened with sterile water, leaving the rest of the skin untouched unless it is very dirty. The diaper area is cleansed after each bowel movement. In some nurseries, complete sponge baths are given every other day instead of daily.

An antiseptic is applied to the stump of the cord each day. The stump should be inspected for infection daily while the infant is undressed. The stump may be painted with an antiseptic or cleansed several times a day with 70% alcohol to prevent infection and promote drying. The stump is exposed to the air to allow it to dry. The diaper should be turned down and the shirt turned up so that the cord is not closely covered.

If the infant has been circumcised, the penis should be checked for bleeding. Sterile gauze with sterile petroleum jelly may be applied to the area. The caregivers may be taught to apply Vaseline or other recommended ointment to the surgical site with each diaper change for about 2 weeks until healing is complete. Retraction of the foreskin in the uncircumcised infant should not be attempted because phimosis is normal in the newborn.

TEMPERATURE

The infant is weighed once a day in most nurseries (although some physicians prefer that it be done every other day), and at this time the infant's temperature is taken. During the first few hours, many facilities take the newborn's temperature by the axillary method. The thermometer is placed in the center of the armpit, taking care to have skin on skin, with no clothing in the way. The arm and the thermometer should be held securely in place while the temperature is being taken. Electronic tympanic thermometers are often used to take the newborn's temperature after the first few hours, when the vernix caseosa has been fully absorbed. Only the initial temperature is taken rectally because of the danger of irritating or puncturing the rectal mucosa.

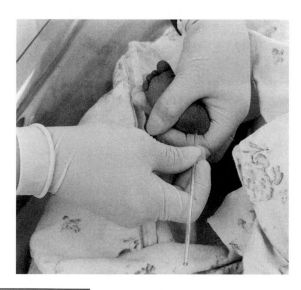

Figure 7-16
Positioning for PKU heel prick.

Newborn Screening

In the United States, each state mandates screening for specific inborn errors of metabolism so that affected neonates can be identified early and treatment started before irreversible damage occurs. Laboratory screening for phenylketonuria (PKU) is mandatory in every state for all newborns; in this simple procedure, the heel is pricked and three drops of blood are placed on filter paper (Fig. 7-16). At the same time, screening is performed for congenital hypothyroidism (T_3 and T_4), which is also required. Phenylketonuria results from the congenital lack of an enzyme necessary for the metabolism of phenylalanine, an essential amino acid, and can lead to mental retardation. Once detected, however, this disorder may be completely corrected by dietary regulation. Congenital hypothyroidism also results in mental retardation; this can be avoided by early replacement of the lacking thyroid hormone.

Additional screening tests required in some states include metabolic screening for galactosemia, homocystinuria, and maple syrup urine disease. In addition, many facilities screen all newborns for sickle cell disease and other hemoglobinopathies. See Chapter 9 for further discussion.

NEWBORN FEEDING

Feeding time is an occasion that provides stimulation and builds confidence. The infant touches and makes eye-to-eye contact with the caregiver, while the caregiver looks, touches, explores, and talks to the infant. The infant learns to trust through repeated touch, fondling, and warm physical comfort. The infant's response to her comforting care gives the mother a sense of satisfaction and confidence.

Eventually, when the infant learns that signals of need are answered promptly, the infant can wait after crying for the response. The infant should not be made to wait too long because the newly developed sense of trust is fragile if not reinforced soon.

At one time, mothers were told to put the baby on a feeding schedule and never to deviate from it. When the baby cried, they were told to check and see if anything were disturbing him or her, then to put the infant down and let him or her cry. Unfortunately, the infant did not know about being trained to conform to a schedule. The baby knew only that hunger demanded satisfaction. The infant's discomfort and sense of aloneness needed comfort and reassurance. Routine did nothing to satisfy needs, but it did potentially shake the infant's trust and belief that the world was a safe and caring place. Attitudes have changed, and infants are now fed primarily on a demand schedule. While in the healthcare facility, formula-fed newborns are basically fed on a 4-hour schedule, but this may be adjusted by the caregivers when the infant is taken home.

Both breast-fed and formula-fed infants need to suck, and sometimes this need is not satisfied by feeding. Pacifiers may be given to the infant to help satisfy this need. This decision depends on the parents' attitudes, but often the use of pacifiers is considered more desirable than having the infant suck on the fingers or a thumb. However, only commercial pacifiers should be used. Makeshift pacifiers—constructed from nipples and plastic collars from infant formula bottles—are dangerous. Deaths of infants have occurred from the aspiration of such nipples.

Family caregivers should be informed that the infant normally loses 5% to 10% of his or her body weight during the first few days of life. This loss is expected, and the weight should be regained within about 2 weeks.

Breast-Feeding

Breast-feeding is the ideal form of infant nutrition. Whether to breast-feed or to use formula, however, is the decision of the mother or the couple, unless there is a contraindication to either method. The mother often decides during pregnancy which method to use, often consulting her mate, family members, or other persons with whom she can review the advantages and possible disadvantages of breast-feeding (Table 7-4).

When breast-feeding is chosen, the infant is usually put to the breast shortly after birth in the delivery or birthing room. The infant's sucking promotes early secretion of milk, is a source of security and comfort to the infant and satisfaction to the mother, and stimulates uterine contractions. During this time, the infant is often placed skin to skin with the mother, enhancing the bonding process.

Nursing on demand seems to work best for most infants. The mother should be instructed to expect to nurse every 2 to 3 hours for the first few days. Nursing should be limited to 5 minutes on each breast. The time may be increased

TABLE 7-4. Advantages and Disadvantages of Breast-feeding

Advantages	Disadvantages
1. Nutritionally best for baby 2. Provides protection against allergies 3. Provides antibodies against illness 4. Helps to develop a special bond between mother and infant 5. Promotes involution of uterus (return of uterus to its prepregnant state) 6. Easily digested 7. Convenient, always ready, inexpensive, sterile 8. Correct temperature 9. Provides times for mother to rest while nursing 10. Mother gains a sense of accomplishment and satisfaction 11. Obesity is infrequent in breast-fed children	1. Mother may be sensitive to nursing when others are around 2. Neonatal jaundice may occur from inadequate fluid intake 3. Mother must watch what medications she takes 4. Mother must be careful about diet, limiting caffeine and other foods that may upset the infant 5. Mother cannot take oral contraceptives 6. Mother's nipples may become sore and cracked 7. Breast-feeding makes demands on mother's time

gradually until the infant nurses 10 to 15 minutes on the first breast (to empty it) and as the infant desires on the second.

The mother must wash her hands before each feeding. If this is the mother's first child, she will need help and support when she first attempts to nurse. At first, it is usually easier for the mother to nurse while lying flat with a pillow under her head and cradling the infant's head. The nurse may instruct the mother to turn to one side, place her nipple between her index and third finger, and bring it toward the infant's mouth. As she brushes her nipple near the newborn's lips, the baby will actively seek it (Fig. 7-17).

A considerable portion of the **areola** (the darkened area around the nipple) should be drawn into the infant's mouth because this stimulates the mammary glands and helps prevent sore nipples. If the mother's breasts are large and soft, the infant's nose may be obstructed by pressing against the breast while trying to nurse. The mother may be shown how to press her breast away from the infant's nose with her finger so that breathing is comfortable (Fig. 7-18).

The mother may find that she prefers sitting in bed with a pillow support for her arm or in a chair with arms at a comfortable level (many hospitals provide comfortable rocking chairs for this purpose). The infant is held in a position lying entirely on the side facing the mother, with the mother's nipple directly in front of the infant's mouth.

Nearly all mothers experience some discomfort when the infant is first put to the breast. The nurse may reassure the mother that this discomfort is normal and does not last.

For the first 2 or 3 days, the mother's breasts secrete **colostrum**, a yellowish, watery fluid with a higher protein, vitamin A, and mineral content and a lower fat and carbohydrate content than breast milk. It also contains antibodies that may play a part in the immune mechanism of the newborn. Its laxative effect helps promote evacuation of meconium from the infant's bowel.

Until lactation begins, both breasts should be used at each feeding to stimulate the secretion of milk. Later, when the breasts are full, one breast is generally sufficient at a feeding. A reminder of which breast to use each time may be needed, such as a safety pin on the bra strap of the side to be used next. One breast should be emptied at each feeding to stimulate refilling. Many physicians do not want infants to have any supplemental feedings during this initial period, so that they will be hungry and will nurse vigorously to stimulate the production of milk.

Whether breast milk or formula is used, some air is swallowed during nursing, and the infant needs burping to help expel it. After feeding, the infant may be held up on the mother's shoulder, may sit upright on her lap with the head supported, or may lie face down across her lap. With the baby in any of these positions, the mother gently rubs the infant's back. Some infants who nurse eagerly may need more than one burping during a feeding.

The mother who wishes to have support for breast-feeding after leaving the facility may appreciate a referral to the LaLeche League, a national organization dedicated to helping breast-feeding mothers have a successful experience. Most healthcare facilities have the names of local members who are happy to consult with new mothers.

Figure 7-17
When offered a nipple, the newborn responds immediately and vigorously owing to the rooting and sucking reflexes.

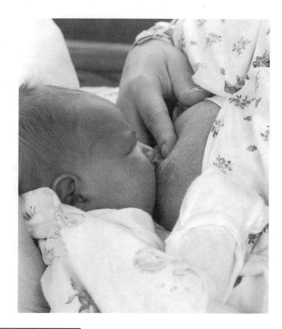

Figure 7-18
The mother presses her breast away from the infant's nose to enable more comfortable breathing while feeding.

preparation. All equipment to be used must be washed and rinsed thoroughly. Disposable bottles are available but add to the cost of infant feeding. The best plan is to prepare one bottle at a time and use it immediately.

Formula may be given to the infant at room temperature or warmed, if desired. Bottles should never be warmed in a microwave oven because they may explode or the formula may become too hot. Formula remaining in the bottle should not be saved from one feeding to the next because

Formula Feeding

If the mother does not breast-feed, for whatever reason, the caregivers may still provide all the necessary nutrients through a formula. Caregivers may also furnish the same comfort and security as they hold the infant (Fig. 7-19). However, they should be warned of the problems created by "propping" the bottle. This practice deprives the infant of the comfort and security of being held and may cause aspiration if the infant is left unattended. Infants who nurse from propped bottles become more prone to develop middle ear infections, because formula pools in the infant's mouth and pharynx, providing a medium for bacterial growth.

Formula may be purchased already prepared in individual bottles, but this can be quite expensive. More economical formulas are prepared from dry powder or cans of formula that may be mixed with water. Water used to mix the formula should be boiled. The person preparing the formula must wash his or her hands before starting the

Figure 7-19
Fed babies need the warmth and closeness of a caregiver.

Figure 7-20
The football hold is one of many methods for holding the newborn.

of the risk of bacterial growth. Open cans of formula may be covered and refrigerated until the next feeding.

Bottle-fed infants should be burped after every ½ to 1 oz they consume. The newborn takes about 2 oz at each feeding. After the feeding, the infant should be positioned on the right side to minimize regurgitation and to allow swallowed air to rise above the level of fluid and escape. The feeding should take about 15 to 20 minutes. If the bottle is tilted so that formula fills the nipple, the amount of air swallowed is reduced.

The new caregiver should be encouraged to find a comfortable position with arm support when preparing to feed the infant. The caregiver's comfort transfers to the infant and makes feeding time more pleasant for both of them. The father or other support person may need encouragement to help with feeding.

TEACHING THE NEW PARENT

Nurses have a major responsibility for patient teaching, so it is of the utmost importance that they are well informed. Most new parents are eager to learn all they can about their new roles. Many realize suddenly that they have taken on a tremendous task: raising a healthy, well-adjusted child. Although many may have attended parenting classes, the situation has changed from a theoretical study to serious business.

Some parents who have older children feel comfortable in their ability to care for a new infant. Others may want

an update on infant care. Some parents have definite ideas about how they want to care for their infants, so nurses should be objective in the way they present information. Information and instruction should be made available to all the infant's prospective caretakers, if possible.

The most effective teaching often occurs on an individual basis when the nurse and the mother and father or support person are together with the infant. In addition to determining how much the parent already knows, the nurse needs to know if the family has any anxieties and perhaps any misunderstandings and misinformation that need to be corrected. Mother–baby nursing is ideal for this, offering both parents (or the mother and a support person) a chance to care for the infant under the guidance of the nurse.

Short stays have created additional problems in finding time to teach infant care. Audiovisual materials, such as slide-and-tape programs and videocassettes, are being used in many hospitals. Often the videocassette programs are set up on an in-hospital television channel or on separate patient teaching carts (equipped with a videocassette recorder and monitor) that the patient may view in her own room with members of her support system. The nurse must take care to follow up after these programs, encouraging questions and clarifying any misunderstandings. The nurse

Family Teaching
Skin Rashes—Points to Cover

1. The infant may break out with heat rash when dressed too warmly. Dress infant with only light covering or diapers only.
2. The plastic in disposable diapers may cause some infants to develop a rash. Observe infant for rash if using disposable diapers. Switching brands may help, but if the rash persists, cloth diapers may be necessary.
3. Cloth diapers may also cause a rash. Keep infant as dry as possible. If cloth diapers are used, close the safety pins when removing them and insert them into the diaper with points outward.
4. Good laundry practices are important.
   a. Wash baby's clothing separate from the rest of your laundry. Use a mild soap and rinse well (twice if possible).
   b. Avoid using softeners or strong detergents on baby's clothes.
   c. White vinegar (⅔ cup) may be added to the final wash rinse as a fabric softener. It softens the clothes without leaving an odor.
5. If the infant develops diaper rash, keep the area dry and expose it to air, if possible. Urine irritates diaper rash. A soothing ointment (such as A&D or lanolin) may be used to protect the skin. If the rash persists, notify the physician, who may order a special ointment.
6. Dry skin may be soothed with an over-the-counter ointment.

1. One way infants get infectious diseases is through handling by other people. Be careful who handles the baby. No one with any type of infection should visit. Avoid taking the baby into crowded places for the first month or so. Newborns have low resistance to disease.
2. If you think your infant is getting sick, note symptoms. Take the temperature and call the baby's physician.
3. Check with the baby's physician before giving any medications to be certain of the type and amount of medicine to use.
4. Handwashing carried out by anyone who is going to handle the infant is one of the most important ways to avoid infections.
5. Anything that is going into the infant's mouth should be washed before being given to the child.

must be familiar with these materials to handle questions effectively.

Particularly with a first baby, the mother and support person should observe a newborn bath and bathe the infant under the supervision and guidance of the nurse (if possible, given the time constraints of short hospitalizations).

Written materials are also widely used, but the nurse must not assume that all patients can read and understand these materials. The nurse must be sensitive to possible reading problems and language differences, with the goal of making the information clear to all. See the Family Teaching displays on skin rashes, infections, stools, and bathing.

FAMILY ADJUSTMENT

The family is reshaped each time an infant is born, because every member of that family is affected by the presence of this new person. By the same token, the family shapes the child. First-time parents probably have the greatest anxieties because they have totally new roles to learn. Early research on parent–infant attachment studied the "mothering" aspect of the relationship; more recent studies of neonatal behavior indicate that the infant has a definite role in the attachment process. Fathers also have been the subject of increasing research, all of which has aided the understanding of how relationships are formed, what factors help or hinder the process, and how potential problems can be avoided. However, although early contact has been carefully studied, no definite conclusions have been reached, and parents and families should not be made to feel that all is lost if early bonding does not take place for one reason or another.

The Parents' Adjustment

Regardless of how much preparation the mother has had for her new role, it is still a totally new experience. She is prepared to love her child, but the fact remains that she has a new child who needs total care 24 hours a day. It looms as a terrific responsibility.

She perhaps has expected that a surge of motherly love instinctively will enable her to love and care for her baby without any doubt or trouble. This does not happen on the first day, or even after a week, but it does develop over time. If she has had a previous child, she may find that this child does not "measure up" in the same way that the previous child did. This reaction may contribute to feelings of guilt and self-doubt. When she feels inadequate, exhausted, and discouraged—as many people do when confronted with a new and seemingly overwhelming responsibility—she is likely to feel resentful, and then guilty for actually resenting the new baby. Although she loves the baby, no one has prepared her for the normal resentment that the responsibility of total care for a helpless, demanding infant often brings.

Rather than trying to deny her resentment and what she considers to be unworthy feelings, the mother needs help to admit them and, furthermore, to understand that resentment is a normal reaction. She needs to understand that as she grows into her task and as she and her child begin to adjust to each other, resentment and feelings of inadequacy will fade away. Those who can learn to admit that they are normal women with a right to normal emotions have come a long way toward reaching equilibrium.

Another way to help is to find some way in which the mother may be relieved of some of the burden until her strength rises to the occasion. The father or another sup-

1. Breast-fed infants average two to four stools a day, with a range of one to seven for the first few months. Occasionally, an infant may have one movement every few days and still be comfortable and normal. After breast-feeding is established, the stool will be yellow to golden with a consistency of liquid paste and an odor of sour milk.
2. Bottle-fed infants average one to four stools per day. An infant may have more or less and still be normal. The stool may range from pale yellow to light brown, and the consistency may be firmer and more solid than stools from a breast-fed baby.
3. When solid food is added, stools tend to become darker, firmer, and stronger in odor.
4. Constipation is rare. A change in the stool's consistency (hard or dry and difficult to pass) rather than the frequency of stools is the sign of constipation. Notify the physician for treatment.

Family Teaching
Newborn Bath

Purposes of the Bath

1. The bath removes waste products from the infant's skin and removes odors.
2. This is a time when the bath giver can inspect the infant's body carefully and note any changes such as rashes, discolorations, and abnormal movements of the extremities.
3. The infant has the opportunity to kick and exercise.
4. This is a time to be alone with the infant and become acquainted. It is also a time for the baby to begin to feel more secure. Talking, cooing, cuddling, and stroking are an important part of the bath procedure. The more the bath giver can relax and enjoy the infant, the happier the time will be for both of them.

Topics Most Often Covered in a Bath Demonstration

1. *Picking up and holding a young baby.* Slide an arm under the baby up toward the head; with hand under head, lift the infant up. One comfortable method of holding a baby is the *football hold,* in which the infant's head rests in the palm of the holder's hand, and the body lies along the inside of the holder's arm, with the infant resting on the holder's hip (Fig. 7-20, p. 118).
2. *Types of baths appropriate for the young baby.* Until the cord stump falls off and the navel is healed, the baby should have sponge baths only because the cord stump should be kept as dry as possible. Many parents like to give their baby a daily bath, but it is not really necessary. Every other day is adequate. On the nonbathing day, wipe the baby's face with water and a clean cloth, and cleanse the diaper area at each change.
3. *Use of baby powders and lotions.* Generally, use of baby powders and lotions is discouraged, because they can irritate the infant's skin. They should be used only after consultation with the infant's physician.
4. *Temperature taking.* During the bath the nurse can demonstrate how to take the infant's temperature and how to read the thermometer. The mother should practice reading the thermometer. The nurse should make clear that the infant's temperature needs to be taken only when the infant is ill in order to be able to report it to the physician. When the temperature is to be taken rectally, lubricate the bulb end of the rectal thermometer. With the infant in a dorsal recumbent position, grasp the ankles in one hand and raise the legs toward the head with knees bent outward. This will expose the rectum so that the end of the thermometer can slip in easily. The thermometer should not be inserted more than 0.8" (2 cm). Continue to hold the infant's legs and the thermometer for about 3 minutes if a mercury thermometer is used. Normal rectal temperature for a neonate is 98.6° to 100°F (37°–37.8°C).
5. *Use of bulb syringe.* Some hospitals provide bulb syringes for each newborn for use in clearing the nares and mouth of excess mucus. This is a good time to teach the use of the bulb syringe.
6. *Cord care and circumcision care in circumcised males.* These topics are appropriate to discuss even if the circumcision care has already been covered. New families can be quite anxious about taking care of these two "wounds" as they heal.
7. *Cradle cap.* After the infant's face is washed, the scalp should be washed. The nurse can point out the "soft spot" and reassure the family caregiver that it is not easily injured. The importance of regular shampooing to prevent cradle cap should be stressed. The hair can be combed at the end of the bath.
8. *Positioning of infant.* This is a good time to explain the importance of positioning the infant on either side or on the back but not on the abdomen. This is recommended until the infant is older than 6 months of age as a measure to prevent sudden infant death syndrome.
9. *Good hygiene measures.* People who are going to handle the infant should wash their hands and arms well before touching the baby. Anyone with any type of infection should be discouraged from visiting.

port person may be helpful by giving her some relief from care responsibilities each day and encouraging her to rest or get out of the house for a short period. If there are older children, she needs to spend time with them, perhaps while the newborn is sleeping, but she still needs time completely for herself.

Even a father who loves his new baby very much may feel left out and neglected when the mother and the baby come home and all her time and attention seem to be devoted to the baby. He may resent the fact that she seems exhausted, unless he understands just how much effort it takes to care for a helpless infant. This is especially true

Family Teaching
Sponge Bath

Assemble the necessary articles on the bathing table. Any sturdy table covered with a clean cloth can be used. Articles needed are the following:

Basin of warm water, warm to the elbow, 100° to 105°F (37.5°–40.6°C). The basin should be used for this purpose only.

Cake of mild, unscented soap to be used only if needed

Soft washcloth; towel for drying baby; large soft towel or cotton blanket on table on which to lay baby

Alcohol–70% (rubbing)

Cotton balls

Comb and/or brush

Ointment such as A&D for dry skin

Clean clothes for baby

Procedure

Have everything ready before picking up the baby. *Never* leave the baby on the table unattended. Small infants can easily roll off the table; keep one hand on the infant at all times.

Place the baby on the blanket or towel and wash the face with clear water. If eyes have been draining, sponge them with a clean piece of cotton, wiping from the inner canthus outward and using clean cotton for each eye. Wash the outer folds of the ears and behind them, but do not poke in the infant's ear because serious harm can be done. Remember, "Nothing smaller than your elbow in the ear."

If the infant has a nasal discharge, wash the edge of nostrils with cotton but do not poke in the nose. To dislodge dried mucus just inside the nostril, cleanse with a small piece of cotton dipped in water. This will usually make the infant sneeze and dislodge any mucus lodged further up in the nose.

Pick up the baby and hold like a football. Wet the head, lather well with soap and rinse well and dry. Combing the hair gently with a fine-toothed comb helps loosen and rid the scalp of debris that could cause cradle cap. *Do not* use shampoo until the infant is 1 month old.

Undress the baby. Cleanse the diaper area with a clean wet cloth if the diaper is soiled. Always clean from front to back to avoid contamination of the urinary system with fecal material. Wash hands before continuing the bath. (It is a good idea to have another small basin of water handy for handwashing.)

Wash the baby's arms, trunk, and legs. Lather the body with soap, getting into skin folds, such as in the neck and underarms. Rinse soap from the skin and dry thoroughly, making certain to dry well in the skin folds and in the groin.

Wash the genital area, getting into the creases. Gently cleanse around the labia of girls, but do not try to retract the foreskin in an uncircumcised boy unless under the specific direction of the pediatrician. Circumcision care should be performed on circumcised boys.

Dry the infant, then turn him or her on the abdomen and wash the back of the neck, the trunk, and lastly the buttocks, cleansing around the rectum.

Wet a cotton ball with alcohol, and wipe the cord stump and the skin immediately around it. This should be done until the cord falls off. The cord may take 3 to 4 weeks to dry and fall off. If a few drops of blood appear when the cord falls off, simply wipe the area with alcohol. There should not be any drainage the next day.

Remove the wet towel on which the baby had been lying, and dress the baby according to the season. Fold the undershirt up and the diaper down so that the cord is exposed to the air to promote drying.

---

of the first-time father. Like the mother, he needs to be encouraged to admit his feelings because they are normal reactions to the situation. He also needs to be encouraged to give the mother a break or to arrange for someone to come in to give her a break. If a family member or other person will relieve them for short periods regularly, the couple should take advantage of this and do something together, even if it is only taking a walk. These little breathers can do much to refresh the spirit.

The Infant's Adjustment

Each infant affects and reacts to the family environment uniquely. The infant's primary developmental task, according to Erikson, is to develop a sense of trust. After 9 months of security, the infant has been thrust into a world in which needs must be made known, with no assurance that they will be met. At birth, the infant entered a strange country where the language, customs, and rules are unknown. Now another move—to home—occurs, and the difference is noticeable. The infant is sensitive to attitudes that alter the touch or the tone of voice of the caretakers. Likewise, the caretakers are affected by the infant's reactions and characteristics. The infant needs reassurance that this is a friendly world.

Nurses must be aware of the variety of life situations into which infants are born and must adjust their teaching and nursing care appropriately.

The Sibling's Adjustment

Sibling attachment and adjustment are as important as those of other family members. Increased knowledge about sibling rivalry and the detrimental effects of separation anxiety make it important to include the other children in the events surrounding the birth of a new family member. The practice of allowing siblings to witness the actual birth is controversial, but policies generally allow siblings to visit after the birth (Fig. 7-21). Many birthing centers promote the inclusion of siblings during labor and delivery and the immediate postpartum period. Many hospitals provide prenatal sibling classes in which the prenatal instructor talks about feelings of new babies, how they look, how they behave, how to handle them, the amount of care they take, and feelings of rivalry. The classes often include a tour of the obstetric department to see where the mother will be. Studies indicate that newborns who have direct contact with their siblings have no higher incidence of infection than do those who have contact with adults. However, maternity units must monitor the siblings to prevent those with possible infections from visiting.

Anderberg says that after the birth of a baby, siblings

Figure 7-21
Shortly after birth, Dad introduces the new baby to her big sister.

are more concerned about reunion with the mother than acquaintance with the newborn.[2] However, after reassurances from the mother, the child accepts the new infant. Children who had established prenatal relationships with the fetus demonstrate a higher frequency of attachment behavior with the newborn than do siblings who had not established such a relationship.

■ KEY POINTS

■ The neonate is an intriguing, exciting being. Although helpless and vulnerable, the neonate is complex and capable of responding to and eliciting many responses from caregivers.

■ The trauma of birth and abrupt changes in environment make the first day of life a time of stabilization for the neonate. Careful observation and appropriate interventions by the nurse are necessary to prevent complications. These observations and interventions include maintaining a patent airway and stable temperature, protecting the baby from infection, and providing nutrition.

■ One of the goals of family-centered care is to create a positive atmosphere in which the family is helped to learn about, care for, appreciate, and enjoy their infant. The new family has much to learn, and the nurse has a great responsibility to aid in that process. Shortened hospital stays make this learning process intense, but it must be thorough.

■ All members of the family have adjustments to make to include the newest family member. The family will find that as they make adjustments in their lives, they can learn to live in harmony with each other.

? CRITICAL THINKING

1. Draw a simple sketch of a newborn's circulatory system, indicating the changes that occur at birth or within the first weeks of life.
2. The parent of a dark-skinned infant questions you about a large area on the infant's right buttock that appears to be a bruise. What response will you give to this parent to provide reassurance?
3. Sue Smith needs guidance with breast-feeding. Describe in detail how you will help her.
4. Jack, the father of a newborn, asks about the rash he notices on his new daughter's abdomen. What can you say to reassure him?
5. You walk by Mary Greene's room and notice that her baby is crying loudly while Mary apparently is watching a television soap opera. Identify appropriate nursing interventions to help Mary care for her baby.

6. You are teaching Rosa about infant care. She is upset by her baby's caput succedaneum. Describe the teaching you will offer Rosa and her family about this condition.

REFERENCES

1. Schuster CS, Ashburn SS. The process of human development: A holistic life-span approach, 3d ed. Philadelphia: JB Lippincott, 1992.
2. Anderberg GJ. Initial acquaintance and attachment behavior of siblings with the newborn. J Obstet Gynecol Neonatal Nurs 17:49–54, 1988.

BIBLIOGRAPHY

Davis R, Truesdale M. Creative approaches to promoting parent–infant bonding. J Pediatr Nurs 8(24):201, 1993.
DiFlorio I. Mothers' comprehension of terminology associated with the care of a newborn baby. Pediatr Nurs 17(2):193–196, 1991.
Edgehouse L, Radzuminski SG. A device for supplementing breastfeeding. MCN 15(1):34–35, 1990.
Evans CJ. Description of a home follow-up program for childbearing families. J Obstet Gynecol Neonatal Nurs 20(2):113–118, 1991.
Greenspan S, Greenspan N. First feelings. New York: Viking Press, 1986.
Hill PD. The enigma of insufficient milk supply. MCN 16(6): 313–315, 1991.
Klaus MH, Klaus PH. The amazing newborn. Reading, MA: Addison-Wesley, 1985.
Murphy SO. Siblings and the new baby: Changing perspectives. J Pediatr Nurs 8(5):277, 1993.
Olds SB, London ML, Ladewig PW. Maternal–newborn nursing, 5th ed. Menlo Park: Addison-Wesley, 1996.
Pillitteri A. Maternal and child health nursing, 2d ed. Philadelphia: Lippincott-Raven, 1996.
Reeder SJ, Martin LL, Koniak D. Maternity nursing, 18th ed. Philadelphia: Lippincott-Raven, 1997.
Schuster CS, Ashburn SS. The process of human development, 3d ed. Philadelphia: JB Lippincott, 1992.
Shrago L, Bocar D. The infant's contribution to breastfeeding. J Obstet Gynecol Neonatal Nurs 19(3):209–220, 1990.
Spadt SK, Martin KR, Thomas AM. Experiential classes for siblings-to-be. MCN 15(3):184–186, 1990.
Wong DL. Whaley and Wong's nursing care of infants and children, 5th ed. St Louis: Mosby, 1995.

The High-Risk Newborn

STUDENT OBJECTIVES

On completion of this chapter, the student will be able to:

1. State four possible causes of prematurity.
2. Differentiate between prematurity and small for gestational age.
3. Identify the characteristics of the preterm infant.
4. List eight systems and the symptoms that are most likely to cause problems in the preterm infant.
5. Discuss hydration and feeding of the preterm infant.
6. Describe phototherapy.
7. Discuss ways to comfort the parents of a preterm infant.
8. Describe the postterm infant.
9. State two problems that occur that place the postterm infant in danger.
10. List six possible problems of an infant born to a diabetic mother.
11. Describe what happens to red blood cells in hemolytic disease of an infant.
12. State which mothers are at risk for having an infant with erythroblastosis fetalis.
13. Explain how erythroblastosis fetalis may be prevented.
14. List the criteria for giving RhoGAM.
15. State the signs and symptoms of sepsis neonatorum.
16. Describe common symptoms of necrotizing enterocolitis.
17. State why newborns of HIV-positive mothers test positive for HIV antibodies.
18. Describe precautions the nurse must use when caring for the newborn of an HIV-positive mother.
19. List the handicaps to which an infant born to an alcoholic mother is prone.
20. Describe the symptoms of addiction in the newborn.
21. List three drugs used to treat the newborn affected by addiction.

KEY TERMS

amniocentesis	preterm (premature) infant
antigen	priapism
antigen–antibody response	pulse oximeter
apnea	respiratory distress
erythroblastosis fetalis	syndrome
fiberoptic blanket	retinopathy of prematurity
hemolysis	retrolental fibroplasia
hyaline membrane disease	RhoGAM
hydrops fetalis	small for gestational age
hyperbilirubinemia	surfactant
hyperthermia	swaddling
kernicterus	term infant
lecithin	thermoregulation
necrotizing enterocolitis	tissue perfusion
phototherapy	
postterm (postmature)	
infant	

Box 8-2. *Terms Used to Describe Newborns According to Size*

SGA—small for gestational age; newborns in the lowest 10th percentile of weight for gestational age

AGA—appropriate for gestational age; newborns between the 10th and 90th percentile of weight for gestational age

LGA—large for gestational age; newborns in the top 10th percentile of weight for gestational age

IUGR—intrauterine growth retardation; used to describe fetus who is small for gestational age

LBW—low birth weight; newborn weighing 1,500 to 2,500 g, regardless of reason

VLBW—very low birth weight; newborn whose birth weight was less than 1,500 g, regardless of gestational age

Preterm (premature)—an infant born before the end of the 37th week of gestation, regardless of cause

Postterm (postmature)—an infant born after the end of the 42d week of gestation

A high-risk neonate is defined as any neonate who is in danger of serious illness or death as a result of prenatal, perinatal, or neonatal conditions, regardless of birth weight or gestational age. Only technologically advanced, expert care by skilled health professionals and a controlled environment can offer such an infant hope of realizing a normal life potential. Several factors may place a fetus at risk (Box 8-1).

The largest number of high-risk newborns are small infants. About two thirds of these are preterm or premature; the rest are term infants of low birth weight, or **small for gestational age** (SGA). Classifications of newborns are shown in Box 8-2. These tiny beings and their parents often have multiple problems to deal with before they can be together as a family.

The immediate physical survival of the infant is not the only factor to be considered. Research indicates that some infants who are hospitalized for a long time at birth are later victims of neglect or abuse; several reasons are suggested for this tragic statistic. The small infant, preterm or SGA, appears unlike the fantasy baby of the parents' dreams, and they may feel guilty about this. The need for the high-risk newborn to be in the neonatal intensive care unit (NICU) means that early bonding is interrupted, and the infant has little chance to be held, cuddled, and comforted, even though the emotional needs of the high-risk newborn are probably more acute than those of a normal term infant. Unmet emotional needs may make the infant irritable, unstable, and easily stressed, an added source of great tension for the family. To try to alleviate some of these problems, visits by family members are encouraged. The family often is encouraged to bring in clothing for the infant to help them feel that he or she is an individual and to encourage parent–infant attachment. Pictures of family members may be taped to the infant's unit, and small visual toys may be placed near the infant.

Health professionals who are aware of the potential problems may contribute greatly to the prevention of child abuse. Nurses in the NICU are highly skilled in the use of complicated mechanical equipment and are especially sensitive to even the most subtle change in the infant. These specially educated nurses are also sensitive to the emotional needs of both the infant and the family. In addition, they teach the family how to care for the infant after discharge or serve as a source of support for the family if the infant dies.

Box 8-1. *Factors that Place a Fetus at Risk*

Age of mother <17 or >35 years

Unmarried mother

Low socioeconomic status of mother

Prenatal care—none or late

Poor maternal nutrition

Maternal illness—diabetes, hypertension, cardiac disease

Genetic abnormalities

Multiple births

Maternal history of complications of pregnancy—placental abnormalities, premature rupture of membranes, long period of infertility

Maternal addiction

THE PRETERM INFANT

At one time, prematurity was defined only on the basis of birth weight: any live infant weighing 2,500 g (5 lb, 8 oz) or less at birth. Time proved this definition inadequate, because some term infants weigh less than 2,500 g and some premature infants weigh more than 2,500 g. The American Academy of Pediatrics advocates the use of the term **preterm (premature) infant** to mean any infant of less than 37 weeks' gestation. A **term infant** is one born between the beginning of the 38th week and the end of the 42d week of gestation, regardless of birth weight. A **postterm (postmature) infant** is one born after completion of the 42d week of gestation, regardless of birth weight.

The Dubowitz scoring system was devised as an assessment tool based on external and neurologic development. Variations of the system are currently in use in many hospitals (Fig. 8-1). The newborn is evaluated by the criteria on the chart, and the gestational age of the infant is calculated from the score. This assessment usually is performed

ESTIMATION OF GESTATIONAL AGE BY MATURITY RATING   Side 1
Symbols: X - 1st Exam   O - 2nd Exam

NEUROMUSCULAR MATURITY

	0	1	2	3	4	5
Posture						
Square Window (Wrist)	90°	60°	45°	30°	0°	
Arm Recoil	180°		100°-180°	90°-100°	< 90°	
Popliteal Angle	180°	160°	130°	110°	90°	< 90°
Scarf Sign						
Heel to Ear						

PHYSICAL MATURITY

	0	1	2	3	4	5
SKIN	gelatinous red, transparent	smooth pink, visible veins	superficial peeling &/or rash, few veins	cracking pale area, rare veins	parchment, deep cracking, no vessels	leathery, cracked, wrinkled
LANUGO	none	abundant	thinning	bald areas	mostly bald	
PLANTAR CREASES	no crease	faint red marks	anterior transverse crease only	creases ant. 2/3	creases cover entire sole	
BREAST	barely percept.	flat areola, no bud	stippled areola, 1–2 mm bud	raised areola, 3–4 mm bud	full areola, 5–10 mm bud	
EAR	pinna flat, stays folded	sl. curved pinna, soft with slow recoil	well-curv. pinna, soft but ready recoil	formed & firm with instant recoil	thick cartilage, ear stiff	
GENITALS Male	scrotum empty, no rugae		testes descending, few rugae	testes down, good rugae	testes pendulous, deep rugae	
GENITALS Female	prominent clitoris & labia minora		majora & minora equally prominent	majora large, minora small	clitoris & minora completely covered	

Gestation by Dates _____ wks

Birth Date _____ Hour _____ am/pm

APGAR _____ 1 min _____ 5 min

MATURITY RATING

Score	Wks
5	26
10	28
15	30
20	32
25	34
30	36
35	38
40	40
45	42
50	44

SCORING SECTION

	1st Exam=X	2nd Exam=O
Estimating Gest Age by Maturity Rating	_____ Weeks	_____ Weeks
Time of Exam	Date _____ am Hour _____ pm	Date _____ am Hour _____ pm
Age at Exam	_____ Hours	_____ Hours
Signature of Examiner	M.D.	M.D.

Figure 8-1

Estimation of gestational age by maturity rating. (Scoring system: Ballard JL, Kazmaierk K, Driver M. A simplified assessment of gestational age. Pediatr Res, 11:374, 1977. Figures adapted from Sweet AY. Classification of the low-birth-weight infant. In Kalus MH, Fanaroff AA, et al. eds: Care of the High-Risk Infant. Philadelphia: WB Saunders, 1977.)

Figure 8-2
The difference between full-term and premature infants is striking. The premature infant has a relatively large head and loose skin. Sometimes loops of intestine are visible through the thin abdominal wall.

within the first 24 hours of life and at least by the time the newborn is 42 hours old.

The preterm infant's untimely departure from the uterus may mean that various organs and systems are not sufficiently mature to adjust to extrauterine life. Small

community hospitals or birthing centers are often not equipped to care adequately for the preterm infant. When premature delivery is expected, the mother often is taken to a facility with an NICU before delivery, if possible. However, unexpected problems arise, and transportation of a newborn may be necessary. Teams of specially trained personnel may come from the NICU to transport the neonate by ambulance, van, or helicopter. The newborn is transported in a self-contained, battery-powered unit that provides warmth and oxygen. Intravenous (IV) fluids, monitors, and other emergency equipment also may be used during the transport of the newborn.

Characteristics of the Preterm Infant

Compared with the term infant, the preterm infant is tiny, scrawny, and red (Fig. 8-2). The extremities are thin, with little muscle or subcutaneous fat. The head and abdomen are disproportionately large, and the skin is thin, relatively translucent, and usually wrinkled. Veins of the abdomen and scalp are more visible. Lanugo is plentiful over the extremities, back, and shoulders. The ears have soft, minimal cartilage and thus are extremely pliable. The soft bones of the skull tend to flatten on the sides, and the ribs yield with each labored breath. Testes are undescended in the male; the labia and clitoris are prominent in the female. The soles of the feet and the palms of the hands have few creases. Many of the typical newborn reflexes are weak or absent (Fig. 8-3).

Figure 8-3
The grasp reflex present in the premature newborn (**A**) is much weaker than that noted in the full-term infant (**B**).

Box 8-3. *Systems and Situations That are Most Likely to Cause Problems in the Premature Infant*

The premature infant has altered physiology due to immature and often poorly developed systems. The severity of any problem depends on the gestational age of the infant.

Respiratory System

Alveoli begin to form at 26–28 weeks' gestation; therefore, lungs are poorly developed.
Respiratory muscles are poorly developed.
Chest wall lacks stability.
Production of surfactant is reduced.
The lung has reduced compliance and low functional residual capacity.
Breathing may be labored and irregular with periods of apnea and cyanosis.
Infant is prone to atelectasis.
Gag and cough reflexes are poor; thus, aspiration may be a problem.

Digestive System

The stomach is small, and vomiting is likely because of poor muscle tone at the cardiac sphincter. It is difficult to provide caloric requirements in the early days.
Tolerance is decreased related to decreased enzymes.
Lacks bile salts that aid digestion of fats and absorption of vitamin D and other fat-soluble vitamins
Limited ability to convert glucose to glycogen and break down glycogen to glucose
Limited and immature ability to release insulin in response to glucose
Lacks coordinated sucking-swallowing reflex before 32–34 weeks gestational age; immature esophageal motility

Poor Thermal Stability

Little subcutaneous fat; thus, no heat storage or insulation; poor glycogen and lipid stores
Limited ability to shiver; poor vasomotor control of blood flow to skin capillaries
Relatively large surface area in comparison to body weight
Sweat glands are decreased; infant cannot perspire before 32 weeks gestational age.
Reduced muscle and fat deposits restrict metabolic rate and heat production. Brown fat is deposited after 28 weeks' gestation in adipose tissue around axillae, kidneys, scapula, neck, and adrenal glands.
Usually is less active
Posture flaccid, increasing surface area exposed

Renal Function

Sodium excretion is probably increased, which may lead to hyponatremia; there is difficulty in excreting potassium.
Ability to concentrate urine decreases; thus, when vomiting or diarrhea occurs, dehydration is likely to follow.
Decreased ability to conserve or excrete fluid.

Ability to acidify urine decreases.
Glomerular tubular imbalance accounts for sugar, protein, amino acids, and sodium present in urine.

Nervous System

Response to stimulation is slow.
Suck, swallow, and gag reflexes are poor; therefore, feeding and possible aspiration are problems.
Cough reflex is weak or absent.
Centers that control respirations, temperature, and other vital functions are poorly developed.

Infection

Actively formed antibodies are lacking at birth (active immunity).
No immunoglobulin M is present at birth.
Limited chemotaxis (reaction of cell to chemical stimuli)
Decreased opsonization (preparation of cells for phagocytosis)
Limited phagocytosis (digestion of bacteria by cells)
Hypofunctioning adrenal gland contributes to a decreased antiinflammatory response.

Liver Function

Lacks ability to handle and conjugate bilirubin.
Does not store or release glucose well; thus, there is a tendency toward hypoglycemia.
There is a steady decrease in hemoglobin after birth and in the production of blood; therefore, anemia may occur.
Does not make or store vitamin K; thus, infant is susceptible to hemorrhagic disease.

Eyes

Oxygen may cause retinal arteries to constrict, resulting in anoxic damage.
The retinae detach from the surface of posterior chambers and a fibrous mass forms, resulting in an inability to receive visual stimulation. This is *retrolental fibroplasia* (RLF).
The exact amount and level of oxygen needed to produce RLF is unknown. An infant weighing less than 1,000 g is at high risk for RLF. It is also related to conditions such as sepsis, transfusions, chronic disease, and hypoxia.

Skin

Sensitive because of permeability and collagen instability
Decreased cohesion between epidermis and dermis
Decreased thickness of stratum corneum (outer layer of epidermis)
Delayed skin pH recovery to acidity following washing with alkaline-based soaps, creams, and emollients
Increased risk of toxicity from topical application and percutaneous absorption of drugs and substances

Adapted from Suddarth D. Lippincott manual of nursing practice, 6th ed. Philadelphia: JB Lippincott, 1991.

Problems of the Preterm Infant

The preterm infant's physiologic immaturity causes many difficulties (Box 8-3), the most critical of which is respiratory. Typically, respirations are shallow, rapid, and irregular, with periods of **apnea** (temporary interruption of the breathing impulse). Respirations may become so labored that the chest wall, perhaps even the sternum, is retracted.

Pediatricians and nursery staff should be alerted to an impending birth of a preterm infant so that equipment for resuscitation and emergency care is ready. If the birth occurs in a facility without a NICU, plans should be made to transport the newborn immediately after birth.

RESPIRATORY DISTRESS SYNDROME

Respiratory distress syndrome (RDS), also known as **hyaline membrane disease**, occurs in about 50,000 of the 250,000 premature infants born in the United States each year. It occurs because the lungs are too immature to function properly. Normally, the lungs remain partially expanded after each breath due to a substance called **surfactant**, a biochemical compound that reduces surface tension inside the air sacs. The premature infant's lungs are deficient in surfactant and thus collapse after each breath, greatly reducing the infant's vital supply of oxygen. This damages the lung cells, and these damaged cells combine with other substances present in the lungs to form a fibrous substance called *hyaline membrane*. This membrane lines the alveoli and blocks gas exchange in the alveoli.

Surfactant replacement therapy with surfactant made synthetically, obtained from animal sources, or extracted from human amniotic fluid has proved successful in the treatment of RDS. Surfactant is administered as an inhalant through a catheter inserted into an endotracheal tube, at or soon after birth. The therapy may be used as preventive treatment ("rescue") to avoid the development of RDS in the newborn at risk. Neonates with RDS usually receive additional oxygen through continuous positive airway pressure, using intubation or a plastic hood. This helps the lungs to remain partially expanded until they begin producing surfactant, usually within the first 5 days of life. If premature delivery is expected, an attempt may be made to prevent RDS. Through amniocentesis, the amount of **lecithin**, the major component of surfactant, may be measured to determine lung maturity. If insufficient lecithin is present 24 to 48 hours before delivery, the mother may be given a glucocorticosteroid drug (betamethasone) that crosses the placenta and causes the infant's lungs to produce surfactant. The infant begins to produce surfactant about 72 hours after birth; therefore, the critical time comes within these first several days. Infants who survive the first 4 days have a much improved chance of recovery unless other problems are overwhelming.

HEAT LOSS

Cold stress is a greater threat to the preterm newborn than to the term infant. The preterm infant cannot shiver and has no integration of reflex control of peripheral blood vessels. Cold stress may result in hypoxia, metabolic acidosis, and hypoglycemia. Therefore, to prevent heat loss and to control other aspects of the premature infant's environment, an isolette or a radiant warmer is used (Fig. 8-4). The isolette has a clear Plexiglas top that allows a full view of the infant from all aspects. The isolette maintains ideal temperature, humidity, and oxygen concentrations and isolates the infant from infection. Portholes at the side afford access to the infant with minimal temperature and oxygen loss. The temperature of the isolette or the radiant warmer is controlled by a heat-sensing probe attached to the infant's skin. If oxygen is administered through an oxygen hood, it must be warmed and moisturized before it is administered.

INTRAVENTRICULAR HEMORRHAGE

Intraventricular hemorrhage (IVH) is a complication of prematurity that occurs more often in the neonate of less than 32 weeks' gestation. In addition to early gestational age, other factors commonly associated with IVH are birth asphyxia, low birth weight, respiratory distress, and hypotension. Ultrasonography, computed tomography, and magnetic resonance imaging can be used to determine if a bleed has occurred.

Signs of possible IVH include hypotonia, apnea, bradycardia, a full (or bulging) fontanelle, cyanosis, and increased head circumference. Neurologic signs such as twitching, convulsions, and stupor are also possible warning signs. However, mild bleeds can occur without these symptoms.

Figure 8-4
The preterm infant in a radiant warmer with oxihood. The parents are encouraged to participate in the care of their newborn, who is in the radiant warmer.

A Personal Glimpse

My son was born 5½ weeks before his expected due date. I was unable to hold him until twelve hours after his birth. I was discharged from the hospital with a Polaroid snapshot of him and the phone number of the hospital's neonatal intensive care unit.

For two weeks I visited him, learning new medical terms and gaining an understanding of all the obstacles he would have to overcome before being released. These days were an emotional roller-coaster filled with feelings of joy over being blessed with a son; enormous concern over his condition; and a great deal of guilt. The thing I wanted most in the world was to take him home, healthy and without the I.V.'s, equipment, monitors and the hard hospital chairs. When I left him each day, I was leaving a part of myself, and I felt as though I would not be whole until he was home with me.

Looking back, I so appreciated that the medical staff was optimistic when informing me of things, but not overly so. Unmet expectations can be devastating! There is not a moment that I am not thankful for my son and his health and not a night that I don't sleep better after I have checked on him sleeping in bed.

Kerry

Nursing interventions to avoid increasing or causing fluctuations in the cerebral blood pressure are important in trying to prevent IVH. Measures that avoid these fluctuations are keeping the head and body in alignment when moving and turning the neonate (avoiding twisting the head at the neck), reducing procedures that cause crying (as a result of pain), minimizing endotracheal suctioning, and generally avoiding unnecessary disturbance of the neonate. In addition, the danger of increased intracranial blood pressure can be lessened by administering analgesics to relieve or reduce discomfort.

OTHER PROBLEMS

The preterm infant desperately needs nourishment but has a digestive system that may be unprepared to receive and digest food. The stomach is small, with a capacity that may be less than 1 to 2 oz. The sphincters at either end of the stomach are immature, causing regurgitation or vomiting if feedings distend the stomach. The immature liver cannot manage all the bilirubin produced by **hemolysis** (destruction of red blood cells with the release of hemoglobin), making the infant prone to jaundice and high blood bilirubin levels (**hyperbilirubinemia**) that may result in brain damage.

The preterm infant does not receive enough antibodies from the mother and cannot produce them. This characteristic makes the infant particularly vulnerable to infection.

Muscle weakness in the premature infant contributes to nutritional and respiratory problems and to a posture distinct from that of the term infant (Fig. 8-5). The infant may not be able to change positions and is prone to fatigue and exhaustion, even from eating and breathing. Skilled, gentle intensive care is needed for the infant to survive and develop.

Nursing Process in the Care of the Preterm Infant

The physical condition of a preterm infant demands the skilled assessment and planning of nursing care, emphasizing maintenance of adequate oxygenation, continuous electronic cardiac and respiratory monitoring, frequent manual monitoring of vital signs, **thermoregulation** (regulation of the infant's temperature), infection control, hydration, and provision of adequate nutrition, sensory stimulation for the infant, and emotional support for the parents.

ASSESSMENT

The initial assessment focuses on the status of the respiratory, circulatory, and neurologic systems to determine the immediate needs of the infant.

NURSING DIAGNOSIS

Based on the initial assessment, some of the nursing diagnoses that may be included are:

- Ineffective Breathing Patterns related to an immature respiratory system

- Ineffective Thermoregulation related to immaturity and transition to extrauterine life

- Risk for Infection related to an immature immune system and environmental factors

- Risk for Altered Nutrition, Less than Body Requirements related to an inability to suck adequately because of weakness

- Risk for Impaired Skin Integrity related to urinary excretion of bilirubin and exposure to phototherapy light

Figure 8-5
It is easy to distinguish the premature newborn from the term infant when both are in the prone position. **(A)** The premature infant lies with pelvis flat and legs spread in a froglike position. **(B)** Term infant lies with limbs flexed, pelvis raised, and knees drawn up under abdomen.

- Activity Intolerance related to poor oxygenation and weakness

- Parental Anxiety related to an unpredictable prognosis

- Altered Parenting related to separation from the infant and difficulty accepting an impaired infant

- Altered Family Process related to the effect of prolonged hospitalization on the family

OUTCOME IDENTIFICATION AND PLANNING

The major goals for the preterm infant include improving respiratory function, maintaining body temperature, preventing infection, maintaining adequate nutrition, preserving skin integrity, and conserving energy. Goals for the family include reducing anxiety and improving parenting skills and family process. The premature infant is cared for by highly skilled nurses in an NICU. Nursing care is implemented to address each of the nursing diagnoses identified for the infant.

IMPLEMENTATION

IMPROVING RESPIRATORY FUNCTION. Not all preterm infants need extra oxygen, but many do. Isolettes are made with oxygen inlets and humidifiers for raising the oxygen concentration in the incubator from 20% to 21% (room air) to a higher percentage. Also, clear plastic hoods placed over the infant's head supply humidified oxygen at the concentration desired. Oxygen saturation of the blood may be monitored by pulse oximetry, or the oxygen and carbon dioxide levels may be measured by transcutaneous

monitoring. Both of these methods help establish the desirable oxygen concentration in the infant.

High blood concentrations of oxygen are associated with a disease of the blood vessels of the eye called **retinopathy of prematurity** (ROP). This disease begins with vasoconstriction of the eye vessels. In later stages, there is an increase in capillaries that, in some infants, results in scarring, causing retinal detachment. This final stage is called **retrolental fibroplasia** (RLF). Although the disease is associated with high oxygen levels (higher than 40% is considered dangerous), the exact reason for this mechanism is unknown. Usually, the younger the preterm infant, the higher the probability of ROP. This complex disease of prematurity has many causes and is therefore difficult to prevent. Laser treatment has been successful in stopping the progression of the abnormal vessels by photocoagulation. Laser treatment has proved more effective and less damaging to surrounding eye tissues than cryosurgery.

Observe the neonate's pulse and respiratory rates, retractions, skin color, muscle tone, alertness, and activity. In the absence of lung pathologic changes, it is safer to keep the oxygen concentration lower than 40%, unless hypoxia is documented.

Observing the preterm infant's respirations is obviously of utmost importance (Fig. 8-6). Measure the rate of respiration and identify retractions to help determine proper oxygen concentrations. One of the most hazardous characteristics of the preterm infant is the tendency to stop breathing periodically (apnea). The hypoxia caused by this apnea and general respiratory difficulty may cause mental retardation or other neurologic problems.

Score

Feature observed	0	1	2
Chest movement	Synchronized respirations	Lag on inspiration	Seesaw respirations
Intercostal retraction	None	Just visible	Marked
Xiphoid retraction	None	Just visible	Marked
Nares dilatation	None	Minimal	Marked
Expiratory grunt	None	Audible by stethoscope	Audible by unaided ear

Figure 8-6
Grading of neonatal respiratory distress based on Silverman-Anderson index (Adapted from Silverman WA, Anderson DH [1956]: A controlled clinical trial of effects of water and mist on obstructive respiratory signs, death rate, and necroscopy findings among premature infants. Pediatrics, 17, 1.)

Electronic apnea alarms are used routinely. Electrodes are placed across the infant's chest with leads to the apnea monitor, providing a continuous reading of the respiratory rate. Visual and audio alarms may be set to alert the nurse when the rate goes too high or too low or if the infant waits too long to take a breath.

It is a nursing responsibility to place, check, and replace the leads on the infant. Remove electrodes and slightly relocate electrodes at least daily to protect the infant's sensitive skin from being damaged by the electrode paste and adhesive. Cleanse the skin carefully between applications of the electrodes. Many false alarms are the result of leads that have come loose. Some of these false alarms may be prevented by using a small amount of electrode paste and being careful to keep the paste inside the circle of adhesive on the electrode.

Respiratory assistance may be used to handle apnea. Usually, gentle stimulation, such as wiggling a foot, is enough to remind the infant to breathe. However, sometimes respirations need to be assisted by a bag and mask. Every nursery nurse should know how to "bag" an infant. The principles of this form of assisted respiration are similar to those of mouth-to-mouth artificial respiration:

1. Slightly extend the neck to open the airway.
2. Cover the infant's mouth and nose with the mask. Maintain a tight seal between the mask and the infant's face.

3. Quickly squeeze the small bag, filled with oxygen or air. The quantity of air needed is relatively small, and the pressure is gentle.

MAINTAINING BODY TEMPERATURE.   The high-risk infant must be monitored closely and continuously. Monitors that record temperature, pulse, respirations, and blood pressure, transcutaneous oxygen and carbon dioxide monitors, and **pulse oximeters** (monitors used to measure oxygen saturation) are all routinely used in the NICU. However, close observation by a nurse who is regularly assigned to the same infant remains an essential part of the infant's care. Observe the monitoring and life-support equipment, making sure it is functioning properly, and systematically assess the infant. Time assessment and other procedures should be timed so that the infant is disturbed as little as possible to conserve energy.

Most isolettes have a control system for temperature regulation. Attach a temperature-sensitive electrode to the infant's abdomen and connect it to the isolette thermostat. The unit may then be set to turn the heater on and off according to the infant's skin temperature. Open units with overhead radiant warmers allow maximum access to the infant when sophisticated equipment or frequent manipulation for treatment and assessment is necessary. The temperature remains more constant than in the closed unit, which is constantly having the door or portholes opened and the atmosphere breached. The infant must not be overheated (**hyperthermia**), because this causes consumption of oxygen and calories and may jeopardize the infant. Use clothing, a head covering (such as a stockinette cap), and blankets when the infant is removed from the warm environment of the isolette or radiant warmer to be held for feeding or cuddling. It is still standard practice to take and record axillary temperatures when the infant is being warmed by either of these methods.

Although monitoring equipment provides a continual reading of the heart rate, take apical pulses periodically, listening to the heart through the chest using a stethoscope for 1 full minute so as not to miss an irregularity in rhythm. Observations should include rate, rhythm, and strength. The pulse rate is normally rapid (120–140 beats per minute [bpm]) and unstable. Premature infants are subject to dangerous periods of bradycardia (as low as 60–80 bpm) and tachycardia (as high as 160–200 bpm). The nurse's observations of the pulse rate, rhythm, and strength are essential to determining how the infant is tolerating treatments, activity, feedings, and the temperature and oxygen concentration of the isolette.

PREVENTING INFECTION.   Infection control is an urgent concern in the care of the high-risk newborn. The preterm infant cannot resist bacterial invasions, so the caretakers must provide an atmosphere that protects him or her from such attacks. The primary means of preventing infection is handwashing. All persons who come in contact with the newborn must practice good handwashing immediately before touching the infant and when moving from one infant to another. Handwashing is the most important aspect of infection control.

Other important aspects of good housekeeping include regular cleaning or changing of humidifier water, IV tubing, and suction, respiratory, and monitoring equipment. The high-risk nursery is separate from the normal newborn nursery and usually has its own staff. This separation helps eliminate sources of infection. Personnel in this area usually wear scrub suits or gowns. Personnel from other departments (radiology, respiratory therapy, or laboratory) put a cover gown over their uniforms while working with high-risk infants.

MAINTAINING ADEQUATE NUTRITION.   When born, a preterm infant may be too weak to suck or may not yet have adequate sucking and swallowing reflexes. Specifically, the preterm infant has poorly coordinated suck, swallow, and gag reflexes, leading to possible aspiration; a limited stomach capacity, contributing to distention and inadequate intake; poor muscle tone of the cardiac sphincter, leading to regurgitation and secondary apnea and bradycardia; and finally muscle weakness, which leads to exhaustion. In addition, preterm neonates do not tolerate carbohydrates and fats well.

For several hours or even 1 day, the preterm infant may be able to manage without fluids, but soon IV fluids will be necessary. In many instances, an IV "life line" is established immediately after delivery. Fluids are infused through a catheter passed into the umbilical vein in the stub of the umbilical cord if it is still fresh. Intravenous fluids may be given through other veins, particularly the peripheral veins of the hands or feet. Extremely small amounts of fluid are needed, perhaps as little as 5 to 10 mL/hr or even less. They may be measured accurately and administered at a steady rate by using an infusion pump. Keep accurate, complete records of IV fluids and frequently observe for infiltration or overhydration. Measure and record all urinary output by weighing the diapers before and after they are used. Urine volume is normally 35 to 40 mL/kg per 24 hours during the first few days, increasing to 50 to 100 mL. Also observe and record the number of urinations, the color of the urine, and edema. Edema changes the loose, wrinkled skin to tight, shiny skin.

At first, some preterm infants receive all their fluid, electrolyte, vitamin, and calorie needs by the IV route; others can start with a nipple and bottle (Fig. 8-7). Premature infants are likely to have problems with aspiration because the gag reflex does not develop until about the 32d to 34th week of gestation. Many infants need gavage feedings. The frequency and quantity of gavage feedings are determined for each infant, but usually feedings are given every 2 hours. Extending the feeding time too long may tire the infant: a feeding should be completed in less than 30 minutes, or the next feeding should be given by gavage to allow the infant to rest. If the stomach is not being emptied by

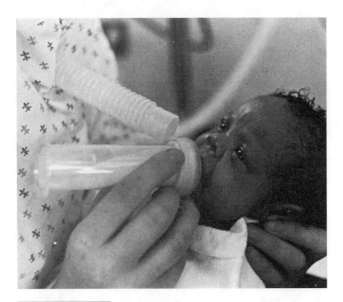

Figure 8-7
This preterm infant with chronic lung disease still requires a small amount of supplementary oxygen but is able to be out of the isolette for short periods to be held for feedings.

the next feeding, allow more time between feedings or give smaller feedings. Usually, the quantity given is just as much as the infant can tolerate and is increased milliliter by milliliter as quickly as tolerated. Starting an infant on 5 to 10 mL per feeding is not unusual. Special premature infant nursers are used that are calibrated in 1-mL markings. The feeding is too large if the infant's stomach is so distended that it causes respiratory difficulty, vomiting, or regurgitation and if there is formula left in the stomach by the next feeding.

Breast milk is the preferred source of nutrition for the preterm infant. The breast milk of mothers of preterm infants is thought to be higher in protein, sodium, chloride, and immunoglobulin A than mothers of term infants. Mothers can pump their breast milk and freeze it to use for bottle or gavage feedings until the infant is strong enough to breast-feed. The use of her own milk to nourish her newborn is a tremendous boost to the emotional satisfaction of the mother.

The most common premature infant formula has 13 cal/oz (often called half-strength formula). A formula with 20 cal/oz (the usual strength for newborns) also may be used. If the formula is too rich (too high in carbohydrates and fats), the infant may vomit and have diarrhea. If the infant does not gain weight after the initial postnatal weight loss, the formula may be too low in calories.

When an infant who is being gavage fed begins to suck vigorously on the fingers, hands, pacifier, or gavage tubing and demonstrates evidence of a gag reflex, nipple feeding should be tried. The infant who can take the same quantity of formula by nipple that was tolerated by gavage without becoming too tired is ready. Some infants need alternating gavage and nipple feedings to see them through the transition period. The nipple for a preterm infant is of softer rubber than the regular nipple. It is also smaller, but no shorter, than the regular nipple.

Burp preterm infants often during and after feedings. Sometimes simply changing the infant's position is enough assistance; at other times, it may help to rub or pat the infant's back gently. Throughout feedings, be careful to prevent aspiration. Hold the infant for the feeding, keeping oxygen available as needed. After a feeding, the best position for the infant is probably on his or her right side, with the head of the mattress slightly elevated.

Other feeding methods can be used if neither gavage nor nipple feeding is tolerated and if IV fluids are inadequate. Some babies do better if fed with a rubber-tipped medicine dropper. Other babies need gastrostomy feedings. The infant who is not receiving nipple feedings should be given nonnutritive sucking opportunities, such as a pacifier.

Weigh the infant daily. These daily weights give an indication of the infant's overall health and indicate whether enough calories are being consumed. The physicians and parents probably will want to know the infant's current weight each day. Using the same scale and the same clothing and taking the weight at the same time each day help ensure accurate, comparable data.

CARING FOR THE INFANT UNDERGOING PHOTOTHERAPY.
Jaundice is common in premature infants. The bilirubin level may be measured noninvasively with transcutaneous bilirubinometry or by a heel stick, results of which may be interpreted by the nursery nurse with specialized equipment. Babies with elevated bilirubin levels are exposed to specially designed fluorescent lights to prevent bilirubin levels from reaching the danger point of 20 mg/dL, beyond which **kernicterus** (severe brain damage from excessive bilirubin levels) is a threat.

The criteria for treatment with **phototherapy** varies with the infant's size and age. The lights are placed above and outside the isolette. The infant is nude, with the eyes shielded from the ultraviolet light. The eye patches may promote infection if they are not clean and changed frequently, or they may cause eye damage if they are not applied so that they stay in place. The light may cause the infant to have skin rashes, "sunburn" or tanning, loose, greenish stools, hyperthermia, an increased metabolic rate, increased evaporative loss of water, and **priapism** (a perpetual abnormal erection of the penis). Infants undergoing phototherapy need as much as 25% more fluids to prevent dehydration. Monitor the serum bilirubin level routinely when the infant is receiving phototherapy.

A **fiberoptic blanket** (a pad attached to a halogen light source, with plastic fibers that are illuminating, covered with a disposable protective cover) can be wrapped about the infant to disperse therapeutic light (Fig. 8-8). These blankets can be used at home, cutting hospitalization costs

Figure 8-8
Infant with fiberoptic light wrap to treat hyperbilirubin jaundice.

for the infant with hyperbilirubinemia and reducing the separation time for the infant and family. The neonate's eyes do not need to be covered. The light can stay on all the time and the neonate is available for care as needed.

PROMOTING ENERGY CONSERVATION AND SENSORY STIMULATION.

The preterm newborn uses the most energy to breathe and pump blood. Plan the infant's day to avoid exhaustion from constant handling and moving about. The infant's energy may be conserved by eliminating regular bathing and giving only "face and fanny" care as needed. Preterm infants usually are dressed in only a diaper, if anything, to conserve energy, provide more freedom of movement, and allow a better opportunity to observe the infant. However, do not be misled into ignoring or avoiding the infant or discourage the contact essential to establishing a normal relationship.

Older preterm infants have a special need for sensory stimulation. Mobiles hung over the isolette and toys placed in or on the infant unit may provide visual stimulation. A radio with the volume turned low, a music box, or a wind-up toy in the isolette may provide auditory stimulation. An excellent form of auditory stimulation comes from the voices of the infant's family, physicians, and nurses talking and singing. Being bathed, held, cuddled, and fondled provides needed tactile stimulation. Contact is essential to the infant and the family. Some NICUs have "foster grandparents" who regularly visit long-term NICU infants and provide them with sensory stimulation—cuddling, loving, crooning, and talking. These programs have proven beneficial to both the infants and the volunteer grandparents.

Position the preterm infant carefully, and change the position periodically. The infant may be positioned from side to side. If the infant is placed on the back, make sure that aspiration of vomitus does not occur. Preterm infants have a knack for wriggling into corners and cracks from which they cannot extract themselves, so close observation is necessary.

REDUCING PARENTAL ANXIETY.

The birth of a preterm infant creates a crisis for the family caregivers. Their long-awaited baby is whisked away from them, sometimes to a distant neonatal center, and hooked up to a maze of machines. Parents feel anxiety, guilt, fear, depression, and perhaps anger. They cannot share the early, sensitive attachment period. It may take weeks to establish touch and eye contact, ordinarily achieved in 10 minutes with a term infant. Parents often leave the hospital empty-handed, without the perfect, healthy infant of their dreams. How can they learn to know and love the strange, scrawny creature who now lives in that plastic box? These feelings are normal, but studies have shown that if these feelings are not expressed and resolved, they can damage the long-term relationship of parents and child, even resulting in child neglect or abuse.

The mother's condition also must be considered. If the infant was delivered by cesarean birth, or if the labor was difficult or prolonged, she may feel abandoned or too weak to become involved with the baby.

Nurses who work with high-risk infants can do much to help families cope with the crisis of prematurity and early separation. To ease some of the apprehension of the family caregivers, transport teams prepare the infant for transportation, then take the infant in the transport incubator into the mother's room so that they may see (and touch, if possible) the infant before the child is whisked away. In many cases, instant photos provide the family some concrete reminder of the infant until they can visit in person. Explain what is happening to the infant in the NICU and periodically report on the infant's condition (by phone if the NICU is not in the same hospital) to reassure the family that the child is receiving excellent care and that they are being kept informed. Listen to the family and encourage them to express their feelings and support one another. As soon as possible, the family should see, touch, and help care for the infant (Fig. 8-9). Most NICUs do not restrict visiting hours for parents or support persons, and they encourage families to visit their infants often, whenever it is convenient for the family. Many hospitals offer 24-hour phone privileges to families so that they are never out of touch with their infant's caregivers.

IMPROVING PARENTING AND FAMILY PROCESS.

Before the mother is discharged from the hospital, plans are made for both parents or other support persons to visit the infant and to participate in the care. They need to feel that the infant belongs to them, not to the hospital. To help foster this feeling and strengthen the attachment, work closely with families to help them progress toward successful parenthood (Fig. 8-10). Siblings should be included in the visits to see the infant. The monitors, warmers, ventilators, and other equipment may be frightening to siblings and family caregivers. Make the family feel wel-

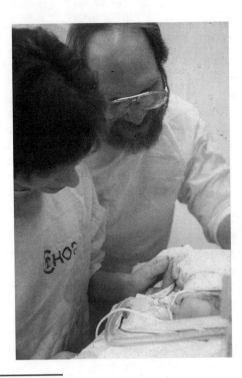

Figure 8-9
Parents should be encouraged to establish bonds with their high-risk newborn in the early postpartum period.

come and comfortable when they visit. A primary nurse assigned to care for the infant gives the family a constant person to contact, increasing their feelings of confidence in the care the infant is receiving.

Support groups of families who have experienced the crisis that a preterm infant causes are of great value to new families of high-risk infants. Members of these groups visit new high-risk families in the hospital and at home. These groups can help high-risk parents deal with their feelings and solve the problems that may arise when their infant is ready to come home or if the infant dies.

As the time for discharge of the infant nears, the family is understandably apprehensive. The NICU nurses must teach the mother and her support persons the skills they need to care for the infant. This knowledge gives them confidence that they can take care of the infant. Some hospitals allow caregivers to stay overnight before the infant's discharge so that they can participate in around-the-clock care. The knowledge that they can telephone the physician and nurse at any time after discharge to have questions answered is reassuring.

Before discharge, most preterm infants will have successfully made the transition from isolette to open crib, thriving without artificial support systems. In addition to the feeding, bathing, and general care of the infant, many families of premature infants need to learn infant cardio-

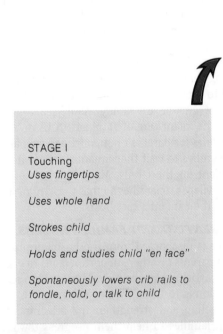

STAGE I
Touching
Uses fingertips

Uses whole hand

Strokes child

Holds and studies child "en face"

Spontaneously lowers crib rails to fondle, hold, or talk to child

STAGE II
Care-Taking
Provides clean clothing, toys, grooming aids

Performs activities of daily living (bathing, diapering, feeding, dressing)

Performs care-taking tasks with proficiency and expresses pleasure in meeting infant's needs

Able to comfort child when distressed or crying

Able to meet child's special health needs (suctioning, cleaning stoma sites, treatments)

STAGE III
Identity
Brings linens from home

Takes photographs

Brings individualized toys

Can make personalized observations about child

Offers suggestions and makes demands for personalized care

Demonstrates "advocacy" behavior

Feels he can care for child better than anyone else

Demonstrates consistent visiting and/or calling pattern

Questions focus on total child, not only physiological parameters

Figure 8-10
Stages of parenting behaviors observed in parents of high-risk infants. (Adapted from the work of Rubin R, Schaeffer Jay S, Schraeder B. *In* Schraeder BD. Attachment and parenting despite lengthy intensive care. Am J Matern Child Nurs 5:37–41,1980.)

COMMUNICATIONS BOX

A mother (Jewel) stands by her infant in the NICU. Her eyes are downcast and she appears to be near tears.

INEFFECTIVE COMMUNICATION

Nurse: (Brightly) Hi, Jewel, how're we doing this morning?
Jewel: (Quietly) OK.
Nurse: It sure is hot this morning. It feels like a heat wave.
Jewel: Oh. ..... Yes.
Nurse: Well, I need to do some things for the baby, so you can go for a break if you want to.
Jewel: (Hesitating) Uh........ OK.
Nurse: Take your time.

The nurse either did not observe the obvious downcast appearance of Jewel or deliberately chose to ignore it. By choosing to say "we" instead of "you" in the initial greeting, the nurse did not acknowledge Jewel as an individual. Also, by diverting the conversation to the weather, the nurse negated any feeling that Jewel was having. In addition, the nurse chose to suggest that Jewel go out for a break instead of staying and learning about the baby's needs for care. The nurse may think that Jewel needs a break, but she did not check with Jewel to see if she was reading her correctly.

EFFECTIVE COMMUNICATION

Nurse: (Noticing Jewel's downcast look) Hi, Jewel. You look kind of down this morning.
Jewel: (Quietly) Yes, I guess I am.
Nurse: Care to talk about what's bothering you?
Jewel: (Unsure, hesitating) Oh, I don't know. It's just silly, I guess.
Nurse: You feel it's silly that you're worried about something.
Jewel: Right.
Nurse: Can you tell me what is bothering you?
Jewel: I'm worried that I won't be able to take care of the baby when I take him home.
Nurse: You think you won't have the experience and know how to take care of him.
Jewel: Right, I feel so inadequate.
Nurse: I understand your feeling that way. Let's sit down together and do some planning to go over the care the baby will need. We'll do it in small segments so that you will feel comfortable with it and will have lots of chances to ask questions. We'll also go over the support system you will have after the baby's discharge.
Jewel: (Visibly brightening) Oh, thanks! That will help a lot.
Nurse: How about staying here with me now while I do this treatment? It will give you some idea of some of the baby's care.

The nurse observed Jewel initially and responded to her apparent downcast appearance. By responding to her and showing concern for her feelings, the nurse was able to discover what was worrying Jewel and offer some concrete help. The nurse also assured Jewel that the help would not be overwhelming but in limited amounts at a time so that Jewel could handle it and have lots of opportunity for questions. The nurse also included Jewel in the immediate care the baby was about to receive.

pulmonary resuscitation and the use of an apnea monitor before the infant is discharged. Some high-risk infants are being sent home with oxygen, gastrostomy feeding tubes, and many other kinds of sophisticated equipment. This helps place the infant in the home much earlier, but it requires intensive training and support of the family members who care for the infant.

After the baby goes home, a nurse, usually a community health nurse, visits the family to check on the health of the mother and the baby. The nurse provides additional support and teaching about the infant's care, if necessary, and answers any questions the family might have.

EVALUATION: GOALS AND OUTCOME CRITERIA

Evaluation of the preterm infant is an ongoing process that demands continual readjustment of the nursing diagnoses, planning, and implementation. Goals for the nursing diagnoses include:

■ *Goal*: Respiratory function will improve.
Criteria: Respiratory rate remains less than 60 bpm; no grunting or retractions are evidenced; breath sounds are clear; no episodes of apnea occur.

■ *Goal*: The infant's temperature will remain stable.
Criteria: Temperature is maintained at 97.7° to 100°F (36.5°–37.8°C).

■ *Goal*: The infant will remain clear of infection.
Criteria: Signs of infection are not noted as evidenced by vital signs within normal limits; breath signs are clear.

■ *Goal*: The infant's nutritional status will remain adequate.
Criteria: The infant can take increased amounts of oral nutrition and gains weight daily; skin turgor improves.

■ *Goal*: The infant will remain free from negative effects of phototherapy.
Criteria: The infant's skin is free of redness, rashes, and irritation; eyes are protected from damage if phototherapy light is used.

■ *Goal*: The infant's energy will be conserved and sensory needs will be met.
Criteria: The infant rests for long periods and responds to auditory and tactile cues.

■ *Goal*: Anxiety of family caregivers will be reduced.
Criteria: Family caregivers express feelings and anxieties concerning the infant's condition, visit and establish a relationship with the infant, and hold and help care for the infant.

■ *Goal*: Family caregivers will learn home care for the infant.
Criteria: Family caregivers demonstrate knowledge of appropriate infant care.

■ *Goal*: The family will have an adequate support system.
Criteria: The family uses available support systems and contacts a support group for families of high-risk infants.

OTHER HIGH-RISK CONDITIONS

The Postterm Infant

When pregnancy lasts longer than 42 weeks, the infant is considered to be postterm (postmature), regardless of birth weight. About 12% of all infants are postterm. The causes of delayed birth are unknown. However, some predisposing factors are first pregnancies between the ages of 15 and 19, the woman over 35 years of age with multiple pregnancies, and certain fetal anomalies, such as anencephaly.

Some postterm neonates have an appearance similar to term infants, but others look like infants 1 to 3 weeks old. Little lanugo or vernix remains, scalp hair is abundant, and fingernails are long. The skin is dry, cracked, wrinkled, peeling, and whiter than that of the normal newborn. These infants have little subcutaneous fat and appear long and thin. This lack of subcutaneous fat may lead to cold stress. These infants are threatened by failing placental function and are at risk for intrauterine *hypoxia* (deficient level of oxygen) during labor and delivery. It is customary, therefore, for the physician or nurse midwife to induce labor or perform a cesarean delivery when the baby is markedly overdue. Many physicians believe that pregnancy should be terminated by the end of 42 weeks.

Often, the postterm infant has expelled meconium in utero. At birth, the meconium may be aspirated into the lungs, obstructing the respiratory passages and irritating the lungs, and this may lead to pneumonia. Whenever meconium-stained amniotic fluid is detected in any delivery, oral and nasopharyngeal suctioning often is performed as soon as the head is born. After delivery, gastric lavage also may be performed to remove any meconium swallowed and to prevent aspiration of vomitus.

In the last weeks of gestation, the infant relies on glycogen for nutrition. This depletes the liver glycogen stores and may result in hypoglycemia. Another complication of the postterm infant may be *polycythemia* (excess red blood cells) in response to intrauterine hypoxia. This puts the infant at risk for cerebral ischemia, hypoglycemia, thrombus formation, and respiratory distress as a result of hyperviscosity of polycythemia.

The Infant of a Diabetic Mother

The severity of the mother's diabetes has a direct relation to the risk for the infant. The diabetic woman who can closely control her blood glucose level before conception

Figure 8-11
Infant of diabetic mother.

and throughout pregnancy, particularly in the early months, can avoid having an infant with the congenital anomalies commonly associated with diabetes. Infants of mothers with poorly controlled diabetes have a distinctive appearance (Fig. 8-11). They are large for gestational age, plump and full-faced, and coated with vernix caseosa. Both the placenta and the umbilical cord are oversized. In contrast infants of mothers with poorly controlled, long-term, or severe diabetes actually may suffer from intrauterine growth retardation.

Infants of diabetic mothers often are at risk for hypoglycemia in the first few hours after birth (Box 8-4). The mother's high blood glucose levels increase the blood glucose level of the fetus before birth and cause the fetal pancreas to secrete increased amounts of insulin. This process leads to the increased intrauterine growth of the fetus. After birth, however, the high levels of glucose are suddenly cut off, and the infant's pancreas cannot readjust quickly enough—thus, hypoglycemia (or hyperinsulinism) occurs.

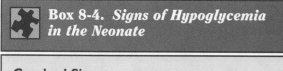

Box 8-4. *Signs of Hypoglycemia in the Neonate*

Cerebral Signs
Jitteriness
Tremors
Twitching
Limpness
Lethargy
Weak or high-pitched cry
Apathy
Convulsions
Coma

Other Signs
Cyanosis
Apnea
Irregular, rapid respirations
Poor feeding
Sweating

This may be fatal if not detected quickly and treated with oral or IV glucose to raise the level of the infant's blood glucose. Hypoglycemia, if untreated, may cause severe, irreversible damage to the central nervous system.

The usual range of blood glucose levels for newborns is 45 to 90 mg/dL. If the newborn's blood glucose level is 25 mg/dL or lower, the infant is treated with IV fluids, early feedings, and IV or oral glucose. The newborn's blood glucose level is checked by heel stick on a frequent schedule for the first 24 hours of life.

These infants are subject to many other hazards, including congenital anomalies, hypocalcemia, hyperbilirubinemia, and hyaline membrane disease. Infants of diabetic mothers require especially careful observation.

The Infant With Hemolytic Disease of the Newborn

Hemolytic disease of the newborn is another name for **erythroblastosis fetalis**, a condition in which the infant's red blood cells are broken down (hemolyzed) and destroyed, producing severe anemia and hyperbilirubinemia. This rapid destruction of red blood cells may produce heart failure, brain damage, and death.

Before the mid-1960s, hemolytic disease was largely the result of Rh incompatibility between the blood of the mother and the blood of the fetus. The introduction of Rho immune globulin, or **RhoGAM**, in the mid-1960s has markedly reduced the incidence of this disorder. Hemolytic disease occurring today is principally the result of ABO incompatibility and is generally much less severe than the Rh-induced disorder.

RH INCOMPATIBILITY

Rh factor is a protein substance that is called an **antigen** and is found on the surface of red blood cells. It is called Rh because it was first identified in the blood of rhesus monkeys. Persons who have the factor are Rh positive (D); those lacking it are Rh negative (d). A person's blood type is inherited, following the same hereditary rules regarding dominant and recessive traits. Rh positive is dominant. If both members of a couple are Rh negative, there will be no hemolytic disorder with their children. However, if the mother is Rh negative, the father is Rh positive, and the child inherits Rh-positive blood, the disorder may occur.

If the father is homozygous positive, then both of his genes carry the D (dominant) trait, but if he is heterozygous positive, one of the genes is a D and the other a d. Thus, if the father is heterozygous positive and the mother Rh negative, there is a 50% probability of their having a baby who is Rh negative (without hemolytic disease). Because of the mechanism by which the mother is sensitized to the Rh factor, there is little chance of the first baby being affected.

Pathophysiology   The mechanism is based on the principles of the **antigen–antibody response**. Although fetal and maternal circulations are completely separate, a break in the placental barrier may allow some fetal red blood cells to escape into the maternal circulation. The break often occurs when the placenta separates during delivery, or it may take place after an abortion. The Rh-positive fetal cells entering the maternal circulation act as a "mini-transfusion," causing the mother to form protective antibodies. It may take some time, however, for the antibodies to form; thus, the first baby is rarely affected.

With the next pregnancy, if any of the baby's red blood cells enter the maternal circulation, antibodies form rapidly. Consequently, the maternal antibodies enter the fetal circulation and begin to hemolyze the baby's red blood cells (Fig. 8-12). The rapid destruction of red blood cells causes excretion of bilirubin into the amniotic fluid. The fetus makes a valiant attempt to replace the red blood cells being destroyed by sending out large amounts of immature red blood cells (erythroblasts) into the bloodstream (hence the name *erythroblastosis fetalis*). As the process of rapid destruction of red blood cells continues, anemia develops. If the anemia is severe enough, heart failure and death of the fetus in utero may result.

Treatment   All expectant mothers should have their blood tested for blood group and Rh type at the initial prenatal visit. If the woman is found to be Rh negative, she should then be followed closely throughout her pregnancy. (The father's blood also should be typed; if he is Rh positive, a genotype may be done to determine if he is homozygous or heterozygous.) The woman should have blood titers performed periodically as a screening method to detect the presence of antibodies. This allows the physician to evaluate the health of the fetus and plan for the infant's delivery and care.

When titers show the presence of antibodies, the physician then tries to determine to what degree the fetus is affected. Because there is no direct way to sample fetal blood to determine the degree of anemia, indirect means must be used. Diagnosis may be made through the use of **amniocentesis**. Through a needle inserted into the amniotic sac, 10 to 15 mL of amniotic fluid is removed. The fluid is sent to the laboratory for spectrophotometric analysis, which shows the amount of bile pigments (bilirubin) in the amniotic fluid. Thus, it can be determined if the fetus is mildly, moderately, or severely affected.

If analysis of the amniotic fluid shows that the fetus is severely affected, the obstetrician will either perform an intrauterine transfusion of Rh-negative blood or, if the fetus is beyond 32 weeks' gestation, induce labor or perform a cesarean delivery. After delivery, the baby is turned over to a pediatrician, who will arrange for exchange transfusions.

Prevention   The dramatic reduction in the incidence of erythroblastosis fetalis is due largely to the introduction of RhoGAM. It is effective only in mothers who do not have Rh antibodies, and it must be injected into the mother within 72 hours after delivery of an Rh-positive infant or after abortion of an Rh-positive fetus. Most obstetricians also give the mother an injection of RhoGAM in the 28th week of pregnancy to prevent any sensitization occurring during the pregnancy. RhoGAM essentially neutralizes any Rh-positive cells that may have escaped into the mother's system, preventing isoimmunization. As mentioned earlier, RhoGAM also must be given to the Rh-negative mother after an abortion. It is *never* given to an infant or to a father. The use of RhoGAM on all patients who are candidates for it offers the hope of eliminating hemolytic disease caused by Rh incompatibility. The criteria for giving RhoGAM are:

- The mother must be Rh negative.
- The mother must not be sensitized by an earlier pregnancy.
- The infant must be Rh positive.
- The direct Coombs' test (a test for antibodies performed on cord blood at delivery) is weakly reactive or negative.

ERYTHROBLASTOSIS FETALIS

Infants with known incompatibility to the mother's blood are examined carefully at birth for pallor, edema, jaundice, and an enlarged spleen and liver. If prenatal care was inadequate or absent, a severely affected infant may be stillborn or have **hydrops fetalis**, a condition marked by extensive edema, marked anemia and jaundice, and enlargement of

Figure 8-12
In Rh incompatibility, antibodies from the mother enter the child and begin destroying its blood cells.

the liver and spleen. These babies are in critical condition and need exchange transfusions at the earliest possible moment. If untreated, severely affected infants are at risk for severe brain damage or kernicterus from excess bilirubin levels. Death occurs in about 75% of infants with kernicterus; those who survive may be mentally retarded or develop spastic paralysis or nerve deafness. Exchange transfusions are given at once to infants who have signs of neurologic damage when first seen, although there is no proof that the damage is reversible. Fortunately, our current ability to detect and treat hemolytic disease has reduced the number of infants who become permanently damaged to just a few.

A severely affected newborn usually is transfused without waiting for laboratory confirmation. All other suspected infants have a sample of cord blood sent to the laboratory for a Coombs' test for the presence of damaging antibodies, Rh and ABO typing, hemoglobin and red blood cell levels, and measurement of plasma bilirubin. A positive direct Coombs' test indicates the presence of antibodies on the surface of the infant's red blood cells. A negative direct Coombs' test indicates that there are no antibodies on the infant's red blood cells.

Treatment A positive Coombs' test indicates the presence of the disease but not the degree of severity. If bilirubin and hemoglobin levels are within normal limits, the infant is watched carefully and frequent laboratory blood tests are performed. The nurse may perform a microbilirubin screening doing a heel stick and using specialized equipment in the nursery. Phototherapy also may be ordered (see earlier section). Exchange transfusions are performed at the discretion of the physician. The infant is cared for in the NICU.

Any infant admitted to the newborn nursery should be examined for jaundice during the first 36 hours or more. Early development of jaundice (within the first 24–48 hours) is a probable indication of hemolytic disease.

Infants whose bilirubin has been restored to normal levels may be discharged to routine home care like any well newborn. The nurse should be sensitive to the parents' feelings of guilt and anxiety. They may feel that they caused the condition and need to ventilate their feelings. They must never be made to feel that they are responsible for the condition.

ABO INCOMPATIBILITY

The major blood groups are A, B, AB, and O, and each has antigens that may be incompatible with those of another group. The most common incompatibility in the newborn occurs between an infant with type O blood and a mother with type A or B. Although the reactions are usually less severe than in Rh incompatibility, the clinical manifestations are similar, including jaundice and an enlarged liver and spleen, but usually without severe anemia. Treatment is also similar, but no preventive measures exist.

The Infant With Neonatal Sepsis

Newborns are at increased risk for infections because their immune systems are immature and they cannot localize infections. High-risk infants are even more susceptible than normal newborns. A primary responsibility of the nursing staff is to prevent infection in these high-risk infants. Infections may be acquired prenatally from the mother (through the placenta), during the intrapartum period (during labor and delivery) from maternal vaginal infection or inhalation of contaminated amniotic fluid, and after birth from cross-contamination with other infants, health care personnel, or contaminated equipment.

The newborn often does not have any specific signs of illness. The clue that alerts the nurse to a possible problem may be signs such as cyanosis, pallor, thermal instability (difficulty keeping temperature within normal range), convulsions, lethargy, apnea, jaundice, or just "not looking right." Diagnosis is made through blood, urine, and cerebrospinal fluid cultures and other laboratory and radiographic tests necessary to isolate the specific organism. Treatment consists of intensive antibiotic therapy, IV fluids, respiratory therapy, and other supportive measures.

The Infant With Necrotizing Enterocolitis

Necrotizing enterocolitis, an acute inflammatory disease of the intestine, occurs most often in small preterm infants, but it may occur in full-term neonates. The cause is not clearly defined. Precipitating factors are hypoxia, causing poor **tissue perfusion** (filling with blood) to the bowel; bacterial invasion of the bowel; and feedings of formula, which provide material on which bacterial enzymes can work. Clinical manifestations are distention of the abdomen, return of more than 2 mL of undigested formula when the gastric contents are aspirated before a feeding, and occult blood in the stool. This disorder usually occurs within the first 10 days of life. Diagnosis is confirmed by abdominal radiographs. The infant with necrotizing enterocolitis is gravely ill and must be cared for in the NICU.

Treatment begins with the discontinuation of oral feedings and nasogastric suction, IV fluids and antibiotics. There is a danger that a necrotic area will rupture, causing peritonitis. A temporary colostomy may be needed to relieve the obstruction, and surgical removal of the necrotic bowel may be necessary.

The Infant of a Human Immunodeficiency Virus-Positive Mother

The newborn of a human immunodeficiency virus (HIV)-positive mother may not show any signs of infection at birth and appears much the same as any other newborn.

Human immunodeficiency virus may be transmitted to the fetus across the placenta, from the mother's body fluids during birth, or through breast milk. If the mother is known to be positive for HIV, she should not breast-feed her newborn. The infant's test results are positive for HIV antibodies for as long as 15 months because he or she has passively acquired antibodies from the mother. Only 20% to 40% of infants born to known HIV-infected mothers are infected themselves.[1] Signs of HIV infection usually are not seen in infants younger than 4 to 6 months of age. By 1 year of age, about half of those who are infected are symptomatic, and by 2 years of age, most HIV-infected infants become symptomatic. The prognosis is poor for infants who have symptoms before 1 year of age and those who develop *Pneumocystis carinii* pneumonia. Bacterial infections, such as pneumonia, meningitis, and bacteremia, are common in infected newborns. These infants also commonly have thrush, mouth sores, and severe diaper rash. Gloves must be worn by personnel when they are performing the first bath on every newborn. Gloves also must be worn by the nurse when performing any procedure in which the nurse could be exposed to blood or body fluids that may contain blood (see Chap. 19 for further discussion of HIV-infected children).

The Infant of an Addicted Mother

As mentioned in Chapter 6, alcohol is one of the many teratogenic substances that crosses the placenta to the infant. No amount of alcohol is believed to be safe, and women should stop drinking at least 3 months before they plan to become pregnant. Fetal alcohol syndrome is often apparent in infants of mothers with chronic alcoholism and sometimes appears in infants whose mothers are low to moderate consumers of alcohol. The ability of the mother's liver to detoxify the alcohol is apparently of greater importance than the actual amount consumed. Fetal alcohol syndrome is characterized by low birth weight, smaller height and head circumference, short palpebral fissures (eyelid folds), reduced ocular growth, and a flattened nasal bridge. These infants are prone to respiratory difficulties, hypoglycemia, hypocalcemia, and hyperbilirubinemia. Their growth continues to be slow and their mental development is retarded despite expert care and nutrition.

Infants of mothers addicted to cocaine, heroin, methadone, or other narcotics are born addicted, and many of these infants suffer withdrawal symptoms during the early neonatal period. These symptoms include tremors, restlessness, hyperactivity, disorganized reflexes, increased muscle tone, sneezing, tachypnea, and a shrill cry. Ineffective sucking and swallowing reflexes create feeding problems, and regurgitation and vomiting occur often after feeding. Typical treatment is the administration of chlorpromazine, diazepam, paregoric, or phenobarbital intra-

muscularly, orally, or both. Many of these babies respond favorably to movement and close body contact with their caregivers; therefore, some nurseries place the infants in special carriers that hold them close to the nurse's chest while moving about the nursery. **Swaddling** the infant (wrapping securely in a small blanket) with arms across the chest also is recommended as a method of quieting the agitated infant.

Unfortunately, identifying the pregnant woman who abuses alcohol or drugs may be difficult. Many of these women have no prenatal care or only infrequent care. They may not keep appointments because of apathy or simply because they are not awake during the day. As a result, many of these infants have suffered prenatal insults that result in intrauterine growth retardation, congenital abnormalities, and premature birth. (For further discussion of the problems of drug abuse, see Chaps. 20 and 21.)

THE DEATH OF A FETUS OR NEWBORN

When a child dies, either before birth or in the first weeks after birth, parents are faced with the crisis of mourning someone they never had a chance to know. They had expected a joyous event; instead, they experienced a devastating loss. Nurses who work with these families need to understand the grieving process and their own feelings about death to help parents cope with this crisis.

Mothers sometimes are aware that the fetus is dead long before any signs of labor appear, but many mothers deny that something is wrong until they are informed by the physician. Parents, particularly the mothers of a stillborn infant or one who dies immediately after birth, may need to see and touch the infant to accept the reality of the infant's death. This is an issue that should be decided by each parent individually, after discussing it with the nurse, physician, social worker, or pastoral counselor. Before seeing the infant, parents need to be prepared for the infant's appearance—the temperature, color, size, and any deformities or bruises. The mother must be able to mourn this baby as a real person. Well-meaning comments such as "You can have another baby" deny this baby as an individual.

Many maternity units have set procedures in which photos are taken of the infant. Parents are given the opportunity to hold the infant in private. Memory books with footprints, bracelets, locks of hair, and photos are given to the parents. If the parents do not want these mementos at the time of delivery, they are kept for a period (sometimes 5 years) and are available for the parents whenever they choose. Parents are encouraged to name the child to add to the reality of the life. Both parents need to feel that the nurse has the time and interest to listen and that it is important for them to express their feelings. Attempts to cheer them up do not aid in the grieving process but strike a note of insincerity and insensitivity. Nurses need to know that it is all right for them to grieve with the parents, to touch or hold them, and to cry with them.

The crisis of stillbirth or neonatal death is another instance in which parent support groups may be effective. No one can better understand the feelings and problems of this tragic situation than parents who have lived through it and managed to rebuild their lives. They are proof that life can go on, even though it seems impossible at the time of the crisis. Compassionate Friends and SHARE are two support groups with chapters throughout the United States and Canada. Most maternity units have information about local support groups and may make referrals to them. In addition, parents who have previously experienced such a loss sometimes volunteer to contact these families to provide personal support. These people often provide the maternity nurses with their phone number so that they may be contacted when their support is desired.

The mother whose infant dies often asks, "Why me?" and "What did I do wrong?" and feels that the death is "not fair." The family may be upset and confused. One of the most important aspects of caring for the parent whose newborn has died is to give him or her an opportunity to talk about the death. Friends and relatives may try to talk about everything else to distract the parents, but often their need to talk is great. The nurse may say, "Do you want to talk about your baby?" Use active listening techniques and avoid using clichés or false assurances. It does hurt; it is devastating; it is overwhelming. The parents must be allowed to express these feelings in a nonjudgmental atmosphere, and the nurse can encourage this outpouring.

KEY POINTS

■ The high-risk infant starts extrauterine life with many problems, regardless of the cause for the high-risk classification. Several factors may have contributed to the infant's compromised condition, including prematurity, substance abuse or addiction, postmaturity, maternal conditions such as diabetes or HIV infection, and neonatal sepsis.

■ Breathing, feeding, and regulating temperature are difficult, if not impossible, for the preterm infant without skilled medical and nursing intervention.

■ The high-risk infant may need to be transported to a distant facility with a NICU. The separation of the infant

and the family and the concern for the infant's condition cause added stress for the family.

■ In addition to the urgent need for skilled physical care, the infant has emotional needs that the nurse must respond to with sensitivity.

■ The infant's family must be counseled and supported to deal with this crisis. The family may need long-term support and assistance in caring for the infant after discharge.

■ If the infant dies, the family needs care, understanding, guidance, and support in mourning their loss.

CRITICAL THINKING

1. Describe the characteristics commonly seen in the preterm infant.
2. What is missing in the lungs of the newborn who has RDS? What treatment is helpful in RDS?
3. Baby James is receiving gavage feedings. You are planning his care. Identify the criteria you will use to evaluate whether he is ready to begin nipple feedings.
4. Discuss nursing measures you would implement to conserve energy of the premature infant.
5. Your friend Kati, a diabetic, tells you that she has decided that she is ready to start a family and is planning to get pregnant. What advice will you give her that will help ensure a healthy baby?
6. Teenager Carla admits to drinking at parties. She is pregnant now. What can you tell her that will help her understand the impact of drinking on her unborn child?

REFERENCE

1. Lambert J. Maternal issues regarding HIV infection. Pediatr Ann 19(7):468, 1991.

BIBLIOGRAPHY

Barron DF, Sivulich KA. Laser therapy as a treatment for retinopathy of prematurity. Pediatr Nurs 20(1):90–92, 1994.
Bell EH, Geyer J, Jones L. A structured intervention improves breastfeeding success for ill or preterm infants. MCN 20(6):309–314, 1995.
Brown CE, Kozick P. Impressioning: A way to preserve memories. MCN 19(5):285–287, 1994.
Jacques JT, Snyder N. Newborn victims of addiction. RN 54(4):47–52, 1991.
Kelley SJ, Walsh JH, Thompson K. Birth outcomes, health problems, and neglect with prenatal exposure to cocaine. Pediatr Nurs 17(2):130–135, 1991.
Lindberg CE. Perinatal transmission of HIV: How to counsel women. MCN 20(4):207–212, 1995.

Olds SB, London ML, Ladewig PW. Maternal-newborn nursing, 5th ed. Menlo Park, CA: Addison-Wesley, 1996.

Pillitteri A. Maternal and child health nursing, 2d ed. Philadelphia: JB Lippincott, 1995.

Reeder SJ, Martin LL, Koniak D. Maternity nursing, 18th ed. Philadelphia: Lippincott-Raven, 1997.

Ross T, Dickason EJ. Vertical transmission of HIV and HBV. MCN 17(4):193–195, 1992.

Van Cleve L, Andrews S. Pain responses of hospitalized neonates to venipuncture activities. MCN 20(3):148–152, 1995.

Wong DL. Whaley and Wong's nursing care of infants and children, 5th ed. St. Louis: Mosby, 1995.

The Newborn With Special Needs

STUDENT OBJECTIVES

On completion of this chapter, the student will be able to:

1. Differentiate between cleft lip and cleft palate.
2. Identify the early signs that indicate the presence of an esophageal fistula.
3. Name the greatest preoperative danger for infants with tracheoesophageal atresia.
4. List and describe the five types of hernias that infants may have.
5. Differentiate the three types of spina bifida that may occur.
6. Name the type of spina bifida that is most difficult to treat, and state why this is so.
7. Describe the two types of hydrocephalus that may occur.
8. State the most obvious symptoms of hydrocephalus.
9. Describe two types of shunting performed for hydrocephalus.
10. State the signs and symptoms of congestive heart failure in the child with congenital heart disease.
11. List five common types of congenital heart defects, and trace the blood flow of each defect, indicating if blood is oxygen-poor or oxygen-rich.
12. State the two most common skeletal deformities in the newborn.
13. Discuss the importance of early treatment for clubfoot.
14. List three signs and symptoms of congenital dislocation of the hip.
15. Describe the treatment for congenital dislocation of the hip.
16. Describe congenital rubella, and discuss its prevention.
17. State the cause of gonorrheal ophthalmia neonatorum.
18. State the effect of herpes simplex virus on the newborn.
19. Identify the test to detect phenylketonuria in the newborn.
20. Describe the treatment for phenylketonuria.
21. Name the tests performed on newborns to detect congenital hypothyroidism.
22. State the one serious outcome that is common to untreated phenylketonuria, congenital hypothyroidism, and galactosemia.

KEY TERMS

atresia	overriding aorta
bilateral	phenylketonuria
chordee	pulmonary stenosis
congestive heart failure	right ventricular
cyanotic heart disease	hypertrophy
ductus arteriosus	spina bifida
ductus venosus	supernumerary
foramen ovale	talipes equinovarus
galactosemia	unilateral
hernia	ventricular septal defect
hip dysplasia	ventriculoatrial shunting
hypothermia	ventriculoperitoneal
imperforate anus	shunting
interstitial keratitis	

As with other high-risk infants, the birth of an infant with a congenital defect or birth injury is a crisis for parents and caregivers. Depending on the defect, immediate or early surgery may be necessary. Early, continuous skilled observation and highly skilled nursing care are required. Rehabilitation of the infant and education of the family caregivers in the care of the infant are essential. The emotional needs of the infant and the family must be integrated into the plans for nursing care. Many of these infants have a brighter future today as a result of increased diagnostic and medical knowledge and advances in surgical techniques.

Family caregivers experience a grief response whether the infant's defect is a result of injury at birth or of abnormal intrauterine development. They mourn the loss of the perfect child of their dreams, question why it happened, and possibly wonder how they will show the infant to family and friends without shame or embarrassment. This grief may interfere with the process of parent–infant attachment. Parents need to understand that their response is normal and that they are entitled to honest answers to their questions about the infant's condition. Other children in the family should be informed gently but honestly about the infant and should be allowed to visit the infant accompanied by adult family members. Sufficient time and attention must be devoted to the older siblings to avoid jealousy toward the infant.

CONGENITAL ANOMALIES

Congenital anomalies may be caused by genetic or environmental factors. These anomalies include facial deformities, such as cleft lip and palate, and defects of the gastrointestinal, central nervous, cardiovascular, skeletal, and genitourinary systems. Defects such as the facial deformities and severe neural tube defects are apparent at birth, but others may be discovered only after a complete physical examination. Congenital anomalies account for a large percentage of the health problems seen in infants and children.

Facial Deformities

The birth of an infant with a facial deformity may change the atmosphere of the delivery from one of joyous anticipation to one of awkward tension. The most common facial malformations, cleft lip and cleft palate, occur either alone or in combination. Cleft lip occurs in about one in 1,000 live births and is more common in males. Cleft palate occurs in one in 25,000, more often in females. Its cause is not entirely clear; it appears to be genetically influenced but sometimes occurs in isolated instances with no genetic history.

CLEFT LIP AND PALATE

Parents and family are naturally eager to see and hold their newborn infant and must be prepared for the shock of seeing the disfigurement of a cleft lip. Their emotional reaction to such an obvious malformation is usually much greater than to a "hidden" defect such as congenital heart disease. They need encouragement and support, as well as considerable instruction about the feeding and care of this infant. The child born with a cleft palate (but with an intact lip) does not have the external disfigurement that may be so distressing to the new parent, but the problems are more serious.

Although a cleft lip and a cleft palate often appear together, either defect may appear alone. In embryonic development, the palate closes later than the lip, and the failure to close occurs for different reasons.

The cleft lip and palate defects result from failure of the maxillary and premaxillary processes to fuse during the fifth to eighth week of intrauterine life. The cleft may be a simple notch in the vermilion line, or it may extend up into the floor of the nose (Fig. 9-1). It may be either **unilateral** (one side of the lip) or **bilateral** (both sides). Cleft palate occurs with a cleft lip about 50% of the time, most often with bilateral cleft lip. Cleft palate, which develops sometime between the seventh and 12th weeks of gestation, often is accompanied by nasal deformity and dental disorders such as deformed, missing, or **supernumerary** (excessive in number) teeth.

When the embryo is about 8 weeks old, there is still no roof to the mouth: the tissues that are to become the palate are two shelves running from the front to the back of the mouth and projecting vertically downward on either side of the tongue. The shelves move from a vertical position to a horizontal position, their free edges meeting and fusing in midline. Later, bone forms within this tissue to form the hard palate.

Normally, the palate is intact by the 10th week of fetal life. Exactly what happens to prevent this closure is not

Figure 9-1
(A) A 2-week-old infant with unilateral cleft lip. (B) Same at age 14 months, showing surgical repair.

known for sure. It is more common in close relatives of people with the defect than in the general population, and some evidence indicates that environmental and hereditary factors play a part in this defect.

Clinical Manifestations and Diagnosis The physical appearance of the infant confirms the diagnosis of cleft lip. Diagnosis of cleft palate is made at birth with the close inspection of the newborn's palate. To be certain that a cleft palate is not missed, the examiner must insert a gloved finger into the newborn's mouth to feel the palate to determine that it is intact. If a cleft is found, consultation is set up with a clinic specializing in cleft palate repair.

Treatment Surgery, usually performed by a plastic surgeon, is a major part of the treatment of a child with a cleft lip, palate, or both. Total care involves many other specialists, including pediatricians, nurses, orthodontists, prosthodontists, otolaryngologists, speech therapists, and occasionally psychiatrists. Long-term, intensive, multidisciplinary care is needed for infants with major defects.

Plastic surgeons' opinions differ as to the best time for repair of the cleft lip. Some surgeons favor early repair, before the infant is discharged from the hospital, believing they can alleviate some of the family's feelings of rejection of the infant. Other surgeons prefer to wait until the infant is 1 or 2 months old, weighs about 10 lb, and is gaining weight steadily. Infants who are not born in large medical centers with specialists on the staff are discharged from the birth hospital and referred to a center or physician specializing in cleft lip and palate repair.

If early surgery is contemplated, the infant should be healthy and of average or above-average weight. The infant must be observed constantly, because a newborn has greater difficulty dealing with excess mucus than does an older infant. These infants must be cared for by competent plastic surgeons and experienced nurses.

The goal in repairing the cleft palate is to give the child a union of the cleft parts to allow intelligible and pleasant speech and to avoid injury to the maxillary growth. The timing of cleft palate repair is individualized, according to the size, placement, and degree of deformity. The surgery may need to be done in stages over several years to achieve the best results. The optimal time for surgical repair of the cleft palate is considered to be between 6 months and 5 years of age. Because the child cannot make certain sounds when starting to talk, undesirable speech habits are formed that are difficult to correct. If surgery must be delayed beyond the third year, a dental speech appliance may help the child develop intelligible speech.

⬛ Nursing Process for the Infant With Cleft Lip and Palate

ASSESSMENT

One of the primary concerns in the nursing care of the infant with a cleft lip, with or without a cleft palate, is the emotional care of the infant's family. Assessment of the infant must include exploration of the family's acceptance of the infant. Practice active listening with reflective responses, accept the family's emotional responses, and demonstrate complete acceptance of the infant.

The family caregivers who return to the hospital with the young infant for the beginning repair of a cleft palate already have been faced with the challenges of feeding their infant. Conduct a thorough interview with the caregivers, including the methods they found to be most effective in feeding the infant.

Physical assessment of the infant includes temperature, apical pulse, and respirations. Listen to breath sounds to detect any pulmonary congestion. Evaluate skin turgor and color, noting any deviations from normal. Also, perform a neurologic assessment, noting alertness and responsiveness. Document assessment and description of the cleft.

NURSING DIAGNOSES

Formulation of nursing diagnoses depends partly on the timing of the initial cleft lip surgery. If the infant is to be discharged from the hospital before surgery, the nursing diagnoses are directed to the emotional care of the family and the feeding and nutrition of the infant. If the newborn is to have lip repair surgery before discharge, nursing diagnoses also include the preoperative aspects. The nursing diagnosis is based in part on the operative plans.

Nursing diagnoses for the newborn infant may include:

- Altered Nutrition: Less than Body Requirements related to inability to suck secondary to cleft lip

- Risk for Altered Parent/Infant Attachment related to visible physical defect

- Anxiety of family caregivers related to lack of knowledge about surgery

Some preoperative and postoperative nursing diagnoses applicable to the infant admitted for surgical repair are:

- Risk for Aspiration related to a reduced level of consciousness postoperatively

- Ineffective Breathing Pattern related to anatomic changes

- Risk for Fluid Volume Deficit related to NPO status postoperatively

- Altered Nutrition: Less than Body Requirements related to difficulty in feeding postoperatively

- Risk of Injury to the operative site related to infant's desire to suck thumb or fingers and anatomic changes

- Risk for Altered Oral Mucous Membranes related to surgical incision

- Risk for Infection related to postoperative period

- Pain related to surgical procedure

- Risk for Altered Growth and Development related to hospitalizations and surgery

- Health Seeking Behaviors of family caregivers related to long-term aspects of cleft palate

OUTCOME IDENTIFICATION AND PLANNING: PREOPERATIVE CARE

Goal setting and planning must be modified to adapt to the surgical plans. If the infant is to be discharged from the birth hospital to have surgery a month or two later,

the nurse may focus on preparing the family to care for the infant at home and helping them cope with their emotions. The major goals include maintaining adequate nutrition, improving parent–infant attachment, reducing parental guilt and anxiety regarding the infant's physical defect, and preparing for the future repair of the cleft lip and palate.

IMPLEMENTATION

MAINTAINING ADEQUATE NUTRITION

The infant's nutritional condition is important to the planning of surgery because the infant must be in good condition before surgery can be scheduled. Feeding the infant with a cleft lip before repair is a challenge. The procedure may be time-consuming and tedious. The infant's ability to suck is inadequate, making feeding difficult. Breast-feeding may be successful because the breast tissue may mold to close the gap. If the infant cannot breast-feed, the mother's breast milk may be expressed and used instead of formula until after the surgical repair is healed. Use of various nipples may be tried to find the method that works best. A soft nipple with a crosscut made to promote easy flow of milk or formula may work well. Lamb's nipples (extra-long nipples) have been used with success, as well as special cleft palate nipples that are molded to fit into the open palate area to close the gap. One of the simplest and most effective methods may be the use of an eyedropper or an Asepto syringe with a short piece of rubber tubing on the tip (Breck feeder). The dropper or syringe is used carefully to drip formula into the infant's mouth at a rate slow enough to allow the infant to swallow. As the infant learns to eat, much coughing, sputtering, and choking may occur. The nurse or family caregiver feeding the infant must be alert for signs of aspiration.

Whatever feeding method is used, the experience may be frustrating for both the feeder and the infant. Have family caregivers practice the feeding techniques under supervision. During the teaching process, give them ample opportunity to ask questions so they feel able to care for the infant (see Family Teaching Tips for Cleft Palate).

PROMOTING FAMILY COPING. Encourage the family to verbalize their feelings regarding the defect and their disappointment. Convey to the family that their feelings are acceptable and normal. While caring for the infant, demonstrate behavior that clearly displays acceptance of the infant. Serve as a model for the family caregivers' attitudes toward the child.

REDUCING FAMILY ANXIETY. Give the family caregivers information about cleft repairs. Pamphlets are available that present photographs of before-and-after corrections that will answer some of their questions. Encourage them to ask questions and reassure them that any question is valid. By the time the infant is actually admitted for the repair, the family will have received a lot of information,

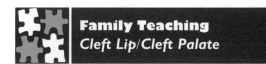

Family Teaching
Cleft Lip/Cleft Palate

1. Sucking is important to speech development.
2. Holding the baby upright while feeding helps avoid choking.
3. Burp the baby frequently, because a lot of air is swallowed during feeding.
4. Don't tire the baby. Limit feeding times to 20 to 30 minutes maximum. If necessary, feed the baby more often.
5. Feed strained foods from the side of the spoon in small amounts, slowly.
6. Don't be alarmed if food seeps through cleft and out nose.
7. Have baby's ears checked any time he or she has a cold or upper respiratory infection.
8. Talk normally to baby (no "baby talk"). Talk a lot; repeat baby's babbling and cooing. This helps in speech development.
9. Try to understand early talking without trying to correct baby.
10. Good mouth care is a must.
11. Early dental care is essential to observe teething and prevent caries.

but all families need additional support throughout the procedure. Explain the usual routine of preoperative, intraoperative, and postoperative care. Written information is helpful, but be certain the parents understand the information. Simple things are important: show them where they may wait during surgery, inform them how long the surgery should last, tell them about the postanesthesia care unit procedure, and let them know where the surgeon will expect to find them to report on the surgery.

OUTCOME IDENTIFICATION AND PLANNING: POSTOPERATIVE CARE

Major goals for the postoperative care of the infant who is hospitalized for surgical repair of cleft lip or palate include preventing infection, preventing aspiration, improving respiration, preventing injury to the surgical site, relieving pain, and increasing the family caregivers' knowledge about the long-term care of the child.

IMPLEMENTATION

PREVENTING ASPIRATION. To facilitate drainage of mucus and secretions, position the infant on the side after a cleft lip repair and on the side or abdomen after a cleft palate repair. Watch the infant closely in the immediate postoperative period. Do not put anything in the infant's mouth to clear mucus because of the danger of damaging the surgical site, particularly with a palate repair.

CHANGING BREATHING PATTERN. Immediately after a palate repair, the infant must change from a mouth-

breathing pattern to nasal breathing. This change may frustrate the infant, but if positioned to ease breathing and given encouragement, the infant should be able to adjust quickly.

MONITORING FLUID VOLUME. In the immediate postoperative period, the infant needs parenteral fluids. Follow all the usual precautions; check placement, discoloration of the site, swelling, and flow rate every 2 hours. Document intake and output levels and use of restraints. Parenteral fluids are continued until the infant can take oral fluids without vomiting.

MAINTAINING ADEQUATE NUTRITION. As soon as the infant is no longer nauseated (vomiting should be avoided if possible), the surgeon usually permits clear liquids.

Sucking is important to the development of speech muscles, so it should be encouraged. If the infant does not have a cleft lip, or if the lip has had an early repair, sucking may be learned more easily even though the suction generated is not as good as in the infant with an intact palate. A large nipple, with holes that allow the milk to drip freely, makes sucking easier. If the cleft is unilateral, the nipple should be aimed at the unaffected side.

For an infant who has had a palate repair, no nipples, spoons, or straws are permitted, just a drinking glass or cup. A favorite cup from home may be reassuring to the infant. Offer clear liquids such as flavored gelatin water, apple juice, and synthetic fruit-flavored drinks. Red juices should not be given because they may conceal bleeding. Usually, infants do not like broth. The diet is increased to full liquid, and the infant usually is discharged on a soft diet. When permitted, foods such as cooked infant cereals, ice cream, and flavored gelatin are often favorites. The surgeon determines the progression of the diet. Nothing hard or sharp should be placed in the infant's mouth.

PREVENTING POSTOPERATIVE INJURY. Continuous, skilled observation is essential. Swollen mouth tissues cause excessive secretion of mucus that is poorly handled by a small infant. For the first few postoperative hours, never leave the infant alone, because aspiration of mucus occurs quickly and easily. Because nothing is permitted in the infant's mouth, particularly that beloved thumb or finger, elbow restraints are necessary. The thumb, although comforting, may quickly undo the repair or cause scarring along the suture line, which is undesirable. On this occasion, the infant's ultimate happiness and well-being must take precedence over immediate satisfaction. It helps to accustom the infant to elbow restraints gradually before admission.

Elbow restraints must be applied properly and checked frequently (see Fig. 4-12 in Chap. 4). Tie these restraints firmly around the arm and pin them to the infant's shirt or gown to prevent them from sliding down below the elbow. The infant's arms can move freely but cannot bend at the elbows to reach the face. Apply the restraint snugly but do not allow the circulation to be hindered. The older infant may need to be placed in a jacket restraint. Make every effort to prevent the infant with a lip repair from crying to prevent excessive tension on the suture line.

Remove restraints at least every 4 hours, but remove them only one at a time and control the released arm so that the thumb or fingers do not pop into the mouth. Comfort the infant and explore other means of comforting. Talk to the infant continuously while providing care. Playing "Peek-a-Boo" and other baby games may be helpful; however, "Patty Cake" does not work well with an infant in elbow restraints! Inspect and massage the skin, apply lotion, and perform range-of-motion exercises. Replace restraints when they become soiled.

PROMOTING HEALING. Gentle mouth care with tepid water or clear liquid may be recommended to follow feeding. This care helps clean the suture area of any food or liquids to promote a cleaner incision for optimal healing.

Care of Lip Suture Line. The lip suture line is left uncovered after surgery and must be kept meticulously clean and dry to prevent infection and subsequent scarring. A wire bow called a Logan bar or a butterfly closure is applied across the upper lip and attached to the cheeks with adhesive tape to prevent tension on the sutures caused by crying or other facial movement (Fig. 9-2). Carefully clean the sutures after feeding and as often as necessary to prevent collection of dried formula or serum. Frequent cleaning is essential as long as the sutures are in place. Clean the

Figure 9-3
This child may need a revision of the vermilion line.

sutures gently with sterile cotton swabs and saline or the solution of the surgeon's choice. Application of an ointment such as bacitracin also may be ordered. Care of the suture line is of utmost importance because it has a direct effect on the cosmetic appearance of the repair. Teach the family how to care for the suture line, because the infant will probably be discharged before the sutures are removed. The sutures are removed 7 to 10 days after surgery. The infant probably will be allowed to suck on a soft nipple at this time.

After effective surgery and skilled, careful nursing care, the appearance of the baby's face should be greatly improved. The scar fades in time. Family caregivers need to know that the baby will probably need a slight adjustment of the vermilion line in later childhood, but they can expect a repair that is barely—if at all—noticeable (Fig. 9-3).

PREVENTING INFECTION. Aseptic technique is important while caring for the infant undergoing lip or palate repair. Good handwashing technique is essential. Instruct the family caregivers about the importance of preventing anyone with an upper respiratory infection from visiting the infant. Observe for signs of otitis media that may occur from drainage into the eustachian tube.

RELIEVING PAIN. Observe the infant for signs of pain or discomfort from the surgery. Administer ordered analge-

Figure 9-2
Logan bar for easing strain on sutures.

sics as needed. Relieving pain not only comforts the infant, but it may also prevent crying, which is important because of the danger of disrupting the suture line.

PROMOTING SENSORY STIMULATION. The infant needs stimulating, safe toys in the crib. The nurse and family caregivers must use every opportunity to provide sensory stimulation. Talking to the infant, cuddling and holding him or her, and responding to cries are all important interventions. Provide freedom from restraints within the limitations of safety as much as possible. One caregiver should be assigned to provide stability and consistency of care. Family caregivers and health care personnel must encourage the older child to use speech and help enhance the child's self-esteem. The baby suffers emotional frustration because of the restraints, so satisfaction must be provided in other ways. Rocking, cuddling, and other soothing techniques are an important part of nursing care. Family members and other caregivers are the best people to supply this loving care.

PROVIDING FAMILY TEACHING. Cleft lip and cleft palate centers have teams of specialists who can provide the services that these children and their families need through infancy, preschool, and school years. Explain to the caregivers the services offered by the pediatrician, plastic surgeon, orthodontist, speech therapist, nutritionist, and public health nurse. These professionals can give explanations and counseling about the child's diet, speech training, immunizations, and general health. Encourage family caregivers to ask these people any questions they may have. Be alert for any evidence that the caregivers need additional information, and arrange appropriate meetings.

Dental care for the deciduous teeth is even more important than usual. The incidence of dental caries is high in children with a cleft palate, but preservation of the deciduous teeth is important for the best results in speech and appearance.

EVALUATION: GOALS AND OUTCOME CRITERIA

PREOPERATIVE

- *Goal*: The infant will show appropriate weight gain.
  Criteria: The infant's weight increases at a predetermined goal of 1 oz or more per day.

- *Goal*: The family will demonstrate acceptance of the infant.
  Criteria: Family caregivers vocalize their feelings about the infant and cuddle and talk to the infant.

- *Goal*: Family caregiver anxiety will be reduced.
  Criteria: Family caregivers ask appropriate questions about surgery, openly discuss their concerns, and voice reasonable expectations.

POSTOPERATIVE

- *Goal*: The infant will not aspirate mucus or secretions.
  Criteria: No episodes of aspiration occur.

- *Goal*: The infant will adjust his or her breathing pattern.
  Criteria: The infant breathes nasally with little stress.

- *Goal*: Signs of adequate hydration will be evident during NPO period.
  Criteria: Skin turgor is good and mucous membranes are moist; there is no evidence of parenteral fluid infiltration in the urine.

- *Goal*: The infant will retain and tolerate oral nutrition.
  Criteria: The infant doesn't experience nausea or vomiting and gains 0.75 to 1 oz (22–30 g) per day if under 6 months of age or 0.5 to 0.75 oz (13–22 g) per day if over 6 months of age.

- *Goal*: The surgical site will remain intact.
  Criteria: The infant is content most of the time and responds appropriately to the caregiver and parents. The infant puts nothing into the mouth, such as straws, sharp objects, thumb, or fingers.

- *Goal*: The infant will remain infection-free.
  Criteria: Caregivers and family members practice good handwashing and aseptic technique. Infant shows no evidence of respiratory or other infection.

- *Goal*: The infant will remain pain-free.
  Criteria: The infant rests quietly, does not cry, and is not fretful.

- *Goal*: The infant will engage in diversional activities.
  Criteria: The infant engages in age- and development-appropriate activities within the limits of restraints.

- *Goal*: The family will learn how to care for the infant.
  Criteria: Family caregivers ask appropriate questions and demonstrate an understanding of the infant's long-term treatment when responding to queries by the staff.

Digestive Tract Defects

Most digestive tract anomalies are apparent at birth or shortly thereafter. The anomalies are often the result of embryonic growth that was interrupted at a crucial stage. Many of these anomalies interfere with the normal nutrition and digestion that are essential to the normal growth and development of the infant. Many anomalies require immediate surgical intervention.

ESOPHAGEAL ATRESIA

Atresia is the absence of a normal body opening or the abnormal closure of a body passage. Esophageal atresia, with or without fistula into the trachea, is a serious congenital anomaly and is among the most common anomalies causing respiratory distress. This condition occurs in about one in 2,500 live births. There are several types of esophageal atresia, but in more than 90% of affected infants the upper, or proximal, end of the esophagus ends in a blind pouch and the lower, or distal, segment from the stomach is connected to the trachea by a fistulous tract (Fig. 9-4).

Blind pouch
of esophagus

Trachea

Distal portion
of esophagus

A

Figure 9-4
(A) The most common form of
esophageal atresia. (B) Both
segments of the esophagus are
blind pouches. (C) Esophagus is
continuous but with narrowed
segment. (D) Upper segment of
esophagus opens into trachea.

Clinical Manifestations and Diagnosis   Any mucus
or fluid that an infant swallows goes into the blind pouch of
the esophagus. This pouch soon fills and overflows, usually
resulting in aspiration into the trachea. Few other conditions depend so greatly on careful nursing observation for
early diagnosis and, therefore, improved chances of survival. The infant with this disorder has frothing and excessive drooling and periods of respiratory distress with chok-

ing and cyanosis. Many newborns have difficulty with
mucus, but the nurse should be alert to the possibility of
an anomaly and report such difficulties immediately. No
feeding should be given until the infant has been examined.

If early signs are overlooked and feeding is attempted,
the infant chokes, coughs, and regurgitates as the food
enters the blind pouch. The newborn becomes deeply cyanotic and appears to be in severe respiratory distress. Dur-

Figure 9-5
Repair of tracheal esophageal atresia and fistula showing chest incision and drainage tube. Gastrostomy tube is also in place.

ing this process, some of the formula may be aspirated, resulting in pneumonitis and increasing the risk of surgery. In a sense, this infant's life may depend on the careful observations of the nurse. If there is a fistula of the distal portion of the esophagus into the trachea, the gastric contents may reflux into the lungs, causing a chemical pneumonitis.

Treatment   Surgical intervention is necessary to correct the defect. Timing of the surgery depends on the surgeon's preference, the anomaly, and the infant's condition. Aspiration of mucus must be prevented, and continuous, gentle suction may be used. The infant needs intravenous fluids to maintain optimal hydration. The first stage of surgery may involve a gastrostomy and a method of draining

the proximal esophageal pouch. A chest tube is inserted to drain chest fluids. An end-to-end anastomosis is sometimes possible. If the repair is complex, surgery may need to be done in stages.

Often these defects occur in premature infants; thus, additional factors may complicate the surgical repair and prognosis (Fig. 9-5). If there are no other major problems, the long-term outcome should be good. Regular follow-up is necessary to observe for and dilate esophageal strictures that may be caused by scar tissue.

IMPERFORATE ANUS

Early in intrauterine life, the membrane between the rectum and the anus should be absorbed, and a clear passage from the rectum to the anus should exist. If the membrane remains, blocking the union between the rectum and the anus, an **imperforate anus** results. In an infant with imperforate anus, the rectal pouch ends blindly at a distance above the anus, and there is no anal orifice. There may be a fistula between the rectum and the vagina in females or between the rectum and the urinary tract in males.

Diagnosis   In some newborns, only a dimple indicates the site of the anus (Fig. 9-6**A**). When the initial rectal temperature is attempted, it is apparent that there is no anal opening. However, there may be a shallow opening in the anus, with the rectum ending in a blind pouch some distance higher (see Fig. 9-6**B**). Thus, being able to pass a thermometer into the rectum does not guarantee that the rectoanal canal is normal. More reliable presumptive evidence is obtained by watching carefully for the first meconium stool. If the infant does not pass a stool within the first 24 hours, the physician should be notified. Abdominal

Figure 9-6
Imperforate anus (anal atresia). (**A**) Membrane between anus and rectum. (**B**) Rectum ending in a blind pouch at a distance above the perineum.

distention also occurs. Definitive diagnosis is made by radiographic studies.

Surgical Treatment If the rectal pouch is separated from the anus by only a thin membrane, the surgeon may repair the defect from below. For a high defect, abdominoperineal resection is indicated. In these infants, a colostomy is performed, and extensive abdominoperineal resection is delayed until the age of 3 to 5 months or later.

Home Care When the infant goes home with a colostomy, the family must learn how to give colostomy care. Teach caregivers to keep the area around the colostomy clean with soap and water and to diaper the baby in the usual way. A protective ointment is useful to protect the skin around the colostomy.

HERNIAS

A **hernia** is the abnormal protrusion of a part of an organ through a weak spot or other abnormal opening in a body wall. Complications occur depending on the amount of circulatory impairment involved and how much the herniated organ impairs the functioning of another organ. Most hernias can be repaired surgically.

Diaphragmatic Hernia In a congenital hernia of the diaphragm, some of the abdominal organs are displaced into the left chest through an opening in the diaphragm. The heart is pushed toward the right, and the left lung is compressed. Rapid, labored respirations and cyanosis are present on the first day of life, and breathing becomes increasingly difficult. Surgery is essential and may be performed as an emergency procedure. During surgery, the abdominal viscera are withdrawn from the chest and the diaphragmatic defect is closed.

This defect may be minimal and easily repaired or so extensive that pulmonary tissue has failed to develop normally. The outcome of surgical repair depends on the degree of pulmonary development. The prognosis in severe cases is guarded.

Hiatal Hernia More common in adults than in newborns, hiatal hernia is caused when the cardiac portion of the stomach slides through the normal esophageal hiatus into the area above the diaphragm. This action causes reflux of gastric contents into the esophagus and subsequent regurgitation. If upright posture and modified feeding techniques do not correct the problem, surgery is necessary to repair the defect.

Omphalocele Omphalocele is a relatively rare congenital anomaly. Some of the abdominal contents protrude through into the root of the umbilical cord and form a sac

Figure 9-7
Omphalocele.

lying on the abdomen (Fig. 9-7). This sac may be small, with only a loop of bowel, or large, containing much of the intestine and the liver. The sac is covered with peritoneal membrane instead of skin. These defects may be detected during prenatal ultrasonography so that prompt repair may be anticipated. At birth, the defect should be covered immediately with gauze moistened in sterile saline, which then may be covered with plastic wrap to prevent heat loss. Surgical replacement of the organs into the abdomen may be difficult with a large omphalocele because there may not be enough space in the abdominal cavity. Other congenital defects are often present.

With large omphaloceles, surgery may be postponed and the surgeon will suture skin over the defect, creating a large hernia. The abdomen may enlarge enough as the child grows to allow replacement.

Umbilical Hernia Normally, the ring that encircled the fetal end of the umbilical cord closes gradually and spontaneously after birth. When this closure is incomplete, portions of omentum and intestine protrude through the opening. More common in preterm and African-American infants, umbilical hernia is largely a cosmetic problem (Fig. 9-8). It is upsetting to parents but is associated with little or no morbidity. In rare instances, the bowel may strangulate in the sac, requiring immediate surgery. Almost all these hernias close spontaneously by the age of 3 years; hernias that do not should be surgically corrected before the child enters school.

Inguinal Hernia Primarily common in males, inguinal hernias occur when the small sac of peritoneum surrounding the testes fails to close off after the testes descend from the abdominal sac into the scrotum. This failure allows the intestine to slip into the inguinal canal, with resultant swelling. If the intestine becomes trapped (incarcerated) and the circulation to the trapped intestine is impaired (strangulated), surgery is necessary to prevent

Figure 9-8
Unusually large umbilical hernia in infant.

intestinal obstruction and gangrene of the bowel. As a preventive measure, inguinal hernias normally are repaired as soon as they are diagnosed.

Central Nervous System Defects

Central nervous system defects include disorders caused by an imbalance of cerebrospinal fluid (as in hydrocephalus) and a range of disorders (often called neural tube defects) resulting from malformations of the neural tube during embryonic development. These defects vary from mild to severely disabling.

SPINA BIFIDA

Caused by a defect in the neural arch, generally in the lumbosacral region, **spina bifida** is a failure of the posterior laminae of the vertebrae to close, leaving an opening through which the spinal meninges and spinal cord may protrude (Fig. 9-9).

Clinical Manifestations A bony defect that occurs without soft-tissue involvement is called *spina bifida occulta*. In most instances, it is asymptomatic and presents no problems. A dimple in the skin or a tuft of hair over the site may cause one to suspect its presence, or it may be entirely overlooked.

When part of the spinal meninges protrudes through the bony defect and forms a cystic sac, the condition is termed *spina bifida with meningocele*. No nerve roots are involved; therefore, no paralysis or sensory loss below the lesion appears. The sac may, however, rupture or perforate, thus introducing infection into the spinal fluid and causing meningitis. For this reason, as well as for cosmetic purposes, surgical removal of the sac, with closure of the skin, is indicated.

In *spina bifida with myelomeningocele*, there is a protrusion of the spinal cord and the meninges, with nerve roots embedded in the wall of the cyst (Fig. 9-10). The effects of this defect vary in severity from sensory loss or partial paralysis below the lesion to complete flaccid paralysis of all muscles below the lesion. Complete paralysis involves the lower trunk and legs as well as bowel and bladder sphincters.

It is not always possible to make a clear-cut differentiation in diagnosis between a meningocele and a myelomen-

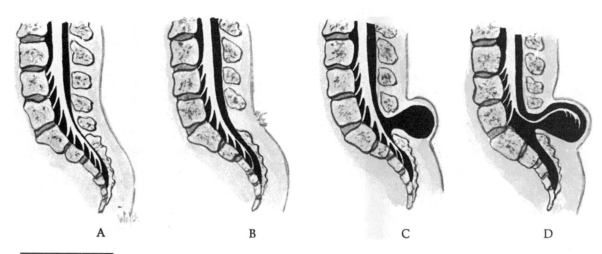

Figure 9-9
Degrees of spinal cord anomalies. **(A)** The normal spinal closure. **(B)** Occulta defect. **(C)** Meningocele defect. **(D)** Myelomeningocele defect to clearly show the spinal cord involvement.

Figure 9-10
A myelomeningocele showing an additional defect of clubfeet.

A Personal Glimpse

A child with "special needs." I never thought I would have to understand just what that really means. Courtney was our second child. A perfect pregnancy. Absolutely no problems. I didn't drink, never smoked, so I planned on a perfectly healthy baby. Until the AFP test. I will never forget that test now. I was 4 months pregnant and went in for the routine test. A few days later the results were in. A neurotube defect . . . . what in the world was that?

I have been asked many times if I was glad I knew before I had Courtney that she would have problems. I've thought a lot about it and even though it made the last several months of the pregnancy a little (well, maybe more than a little) worrisome, yes, I'm very glad we knew. Courtney was born C-section at a regional medical center that is about 60 miles from home. She was in surgery just a few hours after she was born.

Words like spina bifida, hydrocephalus, v. p. shunt, catheterizations, glasses, walkers, braces, kidney infections, all became everyday words at our home. We have learned a lot in the last 5 years. Courtney has frequent doctor visits to all her specialists. She is the only 5-year-old concerned if her urine is cloudy and making sure her mom gives her medication on time.

A little over 5 years ago a "special" child was born and we feel very blessed she was given to us!!

Rhonda

ingocele on the basis of symptoms alone. Myelomeningo-cele also may be termed *meningomyelocele*; the associated "spina bifida" is always implied but not necessarily named. *Spina bifida cystica* is the term used to designate either of these protrusions.

Diagnosis   Elevated maternal alphafetoprotein (AFP) levels, followed by ultrasonographic examination of the fetus, may show an incomplete neural tube. An elevated AFP level in the maternal serum or amniotic fluid indicates the probability of central nervous system abnormalities. Further examination may confirm this and allow the pregnant woman to terminate the pregnancy, because the best time to perform these tests is between 13 to 15 weeks' gestation, when peak levels are reached. Most obstetricians perform AFP testing.

Diagnosis of the newborn with spina bifida is made from clinical observation and examination. Further evaluation of the defect may include magnetic resonance imaging (MRI), ultrasonography, computed tomography (CT) scanning, and myelography. The newborn needs to be examined carefully for other associated defects, particularly hydrocephalus, genitourinary defects, and orthopedic anomalies.

Treatment   Many specialists are involved in the treatment of these infants, especially in the case of myelomenin-

gocele.[1] These specialists may include neurologists, neurosurgeons, orthopedic specialists, pediatricians, urologists, and physical therapists. After a thorough evaluation of the infant, a plan of surgical repair and treatment is developed.

Highly skilled nursing care is necessary in all aspects of the infant's care. The child requires years of ongoing follow-up and therapy. Surgery is required to close the open defect but may not be performed immediately, depending on the surgeon's decision. Waiting several days does not seem to cause additional problems, and this period gives the family an opportunity to adjust to the initial shock and become involved in making the necessary decisions.

📖🗹 Nursing Process for the Infant With 🖎 🔾 Myelomeningocele

ASSESSMENT

A routine newborn assessment is conducted, with emphasis on the neurologic impairment. During the assessment, observe the movement and response to stimuli of the lower extremities. Carefully measure the head circumference and examine the fontanelles. Thoroughly document the assessment. When the infant is handled, take great care to prevent injury to the sac.

The family needs support and understanding during the initial care of the infant as well as for the many years of care during the child's life. Assess the family's knowledge and understanding of the defect, as well as their attitude concerning the birth of an infant with such serious problems.

NURSING DIAGNOSES

The nursing diagnoses suggested here are appropriate for the newborn infant, but because this child will be hospitalized periodically throughout his or her life, suitable diagnoses will vary and need to be made at each admission after careful assessment. Possible nursing diagnoses are:

- Risk for Infection related to vulnerability of the myelomeningocele sac

- Risk for Impaired Skin Integrity related to exposure to urine and feces

- Risk for Injury related to neuromuscular impairment

- Grieving, Anticipatory, by the family related to the perceived loss of the perfect newborn

- Anxiety by the family related to the complexities of caring for an infant with serious neurologic and musculoskeletal defects

OUTCOME IDENTIFICATION AND PLANNING: PREOPERATIVE CARE

The preoperative goals for care of the infant with myelomeningocele include preventing infection, maintaining skin integrity, preventing trauma related to disuse, reducing family anxiety, and increasing family support and education about the condition.

IMPLEMENTATION

PREVENTING INFECTION. Monitor the infant's vital signs, neurologic signs, and behavior frequently to observe for any deviations from normal that may indicate an infec-

tion. Prophylactic antibiotics may be ordered. Carry out routine aseptic technique with conscientious handwashing, gloving, and gowning as appropriate. Until surgery is performed, the sac must be covered with a sterile dressing moistened in a warm sterile solution (often sterile saline). Change this dressing every 2 hours; do not allow it to dry to avoid damage to the covering of the sac. The dressings may be covered with a plastic protective covering. Maintain the infant in a prone position so that no pressure is placed on the sac. After surgery, continue this positioning until the surgical site is well healed.

Diapering is not advisable with a low defect, but the sac must be protected from contamination with fecal material. This contamination may be prevented by placing a protective barrier between the anus and the sac. If the anal sphincter muscles are involved, the infant may have continual loose stools, adding to the challenge of keeping the sac free from infection.

PROMOTING SKIN INTEGRITY. The nursing interventions discussed in the previous section on infection also are necessary to promote skin integrity around the area of the defect as well as the diaper area. As mentioned earlier, there may be continual leakage of stool as well as urine. This leakage causes skin irritation and breakdown if the infant is not kept clean and the diaper area is not free of stool and urine. Scrupulous perineal care is necessary.

PREVENTING CONTRACTURES OF LOWER EXTREMITIES. Infants with spina bifida often have talipes equinovarus (clubfoot) and congenital hip dysplasia (dislocation of the hips), both of which are discussed later in this chapter. If there is loss of motion in the lower limbs due to the defect, conduct range-of-motion exercises to prevent contractures. Position the infant so that the hips are abducted and the feet are in a neutral position. Massage the knees and other bony prominences with lotion regularly, then pad them, and protect them from irritation. When handling the infant, avoid putting pressure on the sac.

PROMOTING FAMILY COPING. The family of an infant with such a major anomaly is in a state of shock on first learning of the problems. Be especially sensitive to their needs and emotions. Encourage the family to express their emotions as openly as possible. Recognize that some families express their emotions much more freely than others, and adjust your responses to the family with this in mind. Provide privacy as needed for the family to mourn together over their loss, but do not avoid the family, because this only exaggerates their feelings of loss and depression. If possible, encourage the family members to cuddle or touch the infant, with proper precautions for the safety of the defect. With the permission of the physician, the infant may be held chest to chest to provide closer contact.

PROVIDING FAMILY TEACHING. Give the family information about the defect and encourage them to discuss their concerns and ask questions. Provide information about the infant's present state, the proposed surgery, and follow-up care. Remember that anxiety may block the understanding and processing of knowledge, so information may need to be repeated. Information should be broken down into small segments to facilitate comprehension.

After surgery, the family needs to be prepared to care for the infant at home. Teach the family to hold the infant's head, neck, and chest slightly raised in one hand during feeding. Also teach them that stroking the infant's cheek helps stimulate sucking. Teaching the family how to care for the infant, allowing them to participate in the care, and guiding them in performing return demonstrations are all methods to use.

For long-term care and support, refer the family to the Spina Bifida Association. Give them materials concerning spina bifida. These children need long-term care involving many aspects of medicine and surgery as well as education and vocational training. Although children with spina bifida have many long-term problems, their intelligence is not affected, and many of these children grow into productive young adults who may live independently (Fig. 9-11).

Figure 9-11
Learning to use new braces, this boy underwent successful surgery for repair of a myelomeningocele during infancy.

EVALUATION: GOALS AND OUTCOME CRITERIA

■ *Goal*: Infection will be prevented.
Criteria: Vital signs and neurologic signs are within normal limits; there are no signs of irritability or lethargy.

■ *Goal*: The infant's skin will remain clean, dry, and intact.
Criteria: There are no areas of reddening or other signs of irritation on the skin; bony prominences are protected from irritation and show no redness or irritation.

■ *Goal*: Trauma to the lower limbs will be prevented.
Criteria: The lower limbs show no evidence of contracture, and skin integrity is maintained.

■ *Goal*: The family will show positive signs of beginning coping.
Criteria: Family members verbalize their anxieties and needs and hold, cuddle, and soothe the infant as appropriate.

■ *Goal*: The family will learn to care for the infant.
Criteria: The family demonstrates competence in performing care for the infant, verbalizes understanding of the signs and symptoms that should be reported, and has information about support agencies.

HYDROCEPHALUS

Hydrocephalus is a condition characterized by an excess of cerebrospinal fluid (CSF) within the ventricular and subarachnoid spaces of the cranial cavity. Normally, there is a delicate balance between the rate of formation and absorption of CSF: the entire volume is absorbed and replaced every 12 to 24 hours. In hydrocephalus, this balance is disturbed.

Cerebrospinal fluid is formed by the choroid plexus, mainly in the lateral ventricles. It is absorbed into the venous system through the arachnoid villi. Cerebrospinal fluid circulates within the ventricles and the subarachnoid space. It is a colorless fluid, consisting of water with traces of protein, glucose, and lymphocytes.

In the *noncommunicating* type of congenital hydrocephalus, there is an obstruction in the free circulation of CSF. This blockage causes increased pressure on the brain or spinal cord. The site of obstruction may be at the foramen of Monro, the aqueduct of Sylvius, the foramen of Lushka, or the foramen of Magendie (Fig. 9-12). In the *communicating* type of hydrocephalus, there is no obstruction of the free flow of CSF between the ventricles and the spinal theca; rather, the condition is caused by defective absorption of CSF, thus causing increased pressure on the brain or spinal cord. Congenital hydrocephalus is most often the obstructive or noncommunicating type.

Hydrocephalus may be recognized at birth, or it may not be evident until after a few weeks or months of life. The condition may not be congenital but may instead occur

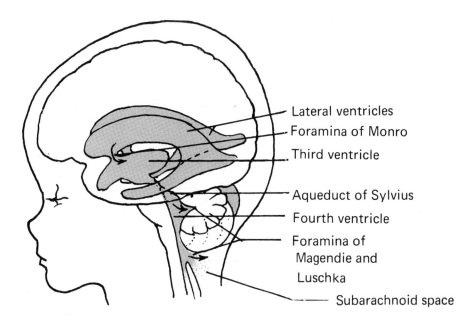

Figure 9-12
Ventricles of the brain and channels for the normal flow of cerebrospinal fluid.

during later infancy or during childhood as the result of a neoplasm, a head injury, or an infection such as meningitis.

When hydrocephalus occurs early in life, before the skull sutures close, the soft, pliable bones separate to allow head expansion. This condition is manifested by a rapid increase in head circumference. The fact that the soft bones can yield to pressure in this manner may partially explain why many of these infants fail to show the usual symptoms of brain pressure and may exhibit little or no damage in mental function until later in life. Other infants show severe brain damage, often occurring before birth.

Clinical Manifestations An excessively large head at birth is suggestive of hydrocephalus. Rapid head growth with widening cranial sutures is also strongly suggestive. A rapidly enlarging head may be the first manifestation of this condition. An apparently large head in itself is not necessarily significant. Normally, every infant's head is measured at birth, and the rate of growth is checked at subsequent examinations. If an infant's head appears to be abnormally large at birth or appears to be enlarging, it should be measured frequently.

As the head enlarges, the suture lines separate and the spaces may be felt through the scalp. The anterior fontanelle becomes tense and bulging, the skull enlarges in all diameters, and the scalp becomes shiny and its veins dilate. If pressure continues to increase without intervention, the eyes appear to be pushed downward slightly, with the sclera visible above the iris—the so-called "setting sun" sign (Fig. 9-13).

If the condition progresses without adequate drainage of excessive fluid, the head becomes increasingly heavy, the neck muscles fail to develop sufficiently, and the infant has difficulty raising or turning the head. Unless hydrocephalus is arrested, the infant becomes increasingly help-

less and symptoms of increased intracranial pressure (ICP) develop. These symptoms may include irritability, restlessness, personality change, high-pitched cry, ataxia, projectile vomiting, failure to thrive, seizures, severe headache, changes in level of consciousness, and papilledema.

Diagnosis Clinical manifestations, particularly an excessive increase in the head circumference, are indications

Figure 9-13
A child with hydrocephalus. Note the pull on the eyes giving the "setting sun" appearance. Note also the site of incision for a shunt.

of hydrocephalus. Positive diagnosis is made with CT and MRI. Echoencephalography and ventriculography also may be performed for further definition of the condition.

Treatment   Surgical intervention is the only effective means of relieving brain pressure and preventing further damage to the brain tissue. If minimal brain damage has occurred, the child may be able to function within a normal mental range. Motor function is usually retarded. In some instances, surgical intervention may remove the cause of the obstruction, such as a neoplasm, a cyst, or a hematoma, but most children require placement of a shunting device that bypasses the point of obstruction, draining the excess CSF into a body cavity. This procedure arrests excessive head growth and prevents further brain damage.

Shunting Procedures.   All shunt procedures use a silicone rubber catheter that is radiopaque so that its position may be checked by radiographic examination. The silicone rubber catheter reduces the problem of tissue reaction. A valve or regulator is an essential part of each catheter that prevents excessive build-up of fluid or too-rapid decompression of the ventricle.

The most common procedure, particularly for infants and small children, is **ventriculoperitoneal shunting**. In this procedure, the CSF is drained from a lateral ventricle in the brain, running subcutaneously and emptying into the peritoneal cavity. This procedure allows the insertion of some excess tubing to accommodate growth. As the child grows, the catheter needs to be revised and lengthened (Fig. 9-14).

In **ventriculoatrial shunting**, CSF drains into the right atrium of the heart. This procedure cannot be used in children with pathologic changes in the heart. The CSF drained from the ventricle is absorbed into the bloodstream.

Other pathways of drainage have been used with varying degrees of success. All types of shunts may have problems with kinking, blocking, moving, or shifting of tubing. The danger of infection in the tubing is a constant concern. Children with shunts must be constantly observed for signs of malfunction or infection.

The long-term outcome for a child with hydrocephalus depends on several factors. If untreated, the outcome is very poor, often leading to death. With shunting, the outcome depends on the initial cause of the increased fluid, the treatment of the cause, the brain damage sustained before shunting, complications with the shunting system, and continued long-term follow-up. Some of these children can lead relatively normal lives, with follow-up and revisions as they grow.

✺ ✎ Nursing Process for the Postoperative ✎ ✺ Infant With Hydrocephalus

ASSESSMENT

Complete assessment of vital and neurologic signs is necessary preoperatively and postoperatively. Measurement of the infant's head is essential. If the fontanelles are not closed, carefully observe them for any signs of bulging. Observe, report, and document all signs of ICP. If this is a child who has returned for revision of an existing shunt, obtain a complete history preoperatively from the family to provide a baseline of the child's behavior.

Assess the level of knowledge family members have about the condition. For the family of the newborn or young infant, the diagnosis will probably come as an emotional shock. Conduct the assessment with sensitivity and understanding.

NURSING DIAGNOSES

The nursing diagnoses vary with the results of the assessment, the child's age, and the procedure to be performed (first placement of a shunt or a revision). Possible nursing diagnoses may be:

- Risk for Injury related to increased ICP

- Risk for Impaired Skin Integrity related to pressure from physical immobility

Figure 9-14
Ventriculoperitoneal shunt.

Ventriculostomy catheter

Incision

Incision

Coiled peritoneal catheter

- Risk for Infection related to the presence of a shunt
- Risk for Altered Growth and Development related to impaired ability to achieve developmental tasks
- Family Anxiety related to fear of surgical outcome
- Risk for Altered Health Maintenance related to the family's insufficient knowledge about the child's condition and home care

OUTCOME IDENTIFICATION AND PLANNING

The goals for the postoperative care of the infant with shunt placement for hydrocephalus include preventing injury, maintaining skin integrity, preventing infection, maintaining growth and development, and reducing family anxiety. Family goals include increasing knowledge about the condition and providing loving, supportive care to the infant.

IMPLEMENTATION

PREVENTING INJURY. Every 2 to 4 hours, assess the infant's level of consciousness, check the pupils for equality and reaction, assess the neurologic signs, and observe for a shrill cry, lethargy, or irritability. Measure and record the occipitofrontal circumference daily. Carry out appropriate procedures to care for the shunt as directed. To prevent a rapid decrease in ICP, keep the infant flat. Observe for signs of seizure, and initiate seizure precautions. Keep suction and oxygen equipment convenient at the bedside.

PROMOTING SKIN INTEGRITY. After a shunting procedure, keep the infant's head turned away from the operative site until the physician allows a change in position. If the infant's head is enlarged, prevent pressure sores from forming on the side on which the child rests. Support the head when the child is moved or picked up. Egg-crate pads, lamb's wool, or a special mattress may be used, if necessary, to prevent pressure breakdown of the scalp. Reposition the infant at least every 2 hours as permitted. Immediately after surgery, frequently inspect the dressings over the shunt site; later, inspect them every 4 hours.

PREVENTING INFECTION. Infection is the primary threat after surgery. Closely observe for and promptly report any signs of infection: redness, heat, or swelling along the surgical site, fever, and signs of lethargy. Perform wound care meticulously as ordered. Administer antibiotics as prescribed.

PROMOTING GROWTH AND DEVELOPMENT. Every infant has the need and the right to be picked up and held, cuddled, and comforted. An uncomfortable or painful experience increases the need for emotional support. An infant perceives such support principally through physical contact made in a soothing, loving manner.

The infant needs social interaction and needs to be talked to, played with, and given the opportunity for activity. Provide toys appropriate for his or her physical and mental capacity. If the child has difficulty moving about

the crib, place toys within easy reach and vision, such as a cradle gym tied close enough for the infant to maneuver its parts.

Unless the infant's nervous system is so impaired that all activity increases irritability, the infant needs stimulation just like any child does. If repositioning from side to side means turning the infant away from the sight of activity, the crib may be turned around so that vision is not obstructed.

An infant who is given the contact and support that all infants require develops a pleasing personality because he or she is nourished by emotional stimulation. Use the time spent on physical care as a time for social interaction. Talking, laughing, and playing with the infant are all important aspects of the infant's care. Make frequent contacts, and do not limit them to the times when physical care is being performed.

REDUCING FAMILY ANXIETY. In terms they can understand, explain to the family the condition and the anatomy of the surgical procedure. Discuss the overall prognosis for the child. Encourage the family to express their anxieties and ask questions. Giving accurate, nontechnical answers is extremely helpful. Give the family information about support groups such as the National Hydrocephalus Foundation, and encourage them to contact the group.

PROVIDING FAMILY TEACHING. Demonstrate care of the shunt to the family, and have them perform a return demonstration. Give the family a list of signs and symptoms that should be reported. Review these with the family and make sure they understand them. Discuss appropriate growth and developmental expectations for the child, stressing realistic goals.

EVALUATION: GOALS AND OUTCOME CRITERIA

- *Goal*: The infant will not experience increased ICP.
  Criteria: There are no signs of ICP, as evidenced by an absence of lethargy, irritability, and seizure activity, and the presence of a stable level of consciousness.

- *Goal*: The infant's skin will remain intact.
  Criteria: The infant's skin shows no evidence of pressure sores, redness, or other signs of breakdown.

- *Goal*: The infant will remain free of infection.
  Criteria: There are no signs of infection, vital signs are stable, and there is no redness or swelling at the surgical site.

- *Goal*: The infant's social and developmental needs will be met.
  Criteria: The infant responds to social interaction and plays appropriately with toys and surroundings.

- *Goal*: The family's anxiety will be reduced.
  Criteria: The family expresses its fears and interacts appropriately with the infant.

■ *Goal*: The family will learn care of the child.
Criteria: The family participates in the care of the infant and demonstrates an understanding of the equipment and signs and symptoms to report.

Cardiovascular System Defects

Cardiovascular system defects range from mild to severe. They may be detected immediately at birth or may not be detected for several months.

CONGENITAL HEART DISEASE

When a newborn is suspected of having a heart abnormality, the family is understandably upset. The heart is *the* vital organ; one can live without a number of other organs and appendages, but life itself depends on the heart. The family will have many questions, some of which may be answered by the nurse and others that must be answered by the physician. Many answers will not be available until after various evaluation procedures have been conducted.

Technologic advances have progressed rapidly in this field, making earlier detection and successful repair much more likely. However, heart defects are the leading cause of death from congenital anomalies in the first year of life.

A brief discussion of the development and function of the embryonic heart is useful to understanding the malformations that occur.

Pathophysiology   The heart begins beating early in the third to eighth week of intrauterine life. When first formed, the heart is a simple tube receiving blood from the placenta and pumping it out into its developing body. During this period, it rapidly develops into the normal, but complex, four-chambered heart.

Adjustments in circulation must be made at birth. During fetal life, the lungs are inactive, requiring only a small amount of blood to nourish their tissues. Blood is circulated through the umbilical arteries to the placenta, where waste products and carbon dioxide are exchanged for oxygen and nutrients. The blood is then returned to the fetus through the umbilical vein.

At birth, the umbilical cord is cut, and the infant's own independent system is established. Certain circulatory bypasses, such as the **ductus arteriosus**, the **foramen ovale**, and the **ductus venosus**, are no longer necessary. They close and atrophy during the first several weeks after birth. In addition, the pressure in the heart, which has been higher on the right side during fetal life, now changes so that the left side of the heart has the higher pressure (Fig. 9-15; see also Fig. 7-2 in Chapter 7).

During this period of complex development, any error in formation may cause serious circulatory difficulty. The incidence of cardiovascular malformations is about eight in 1,000 live births.

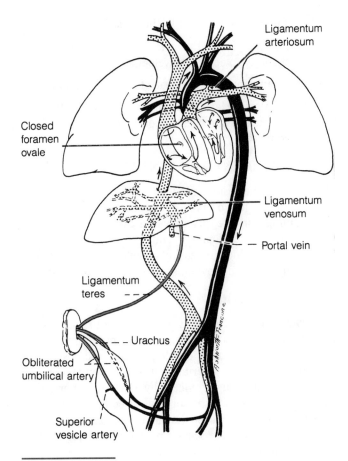

Figure 9-15
Normal blood circulation. Highlighted ligaments indicate pathways which should close at or soon after birth. Arrows indicate normal flow of blood.

Etiology   Rubella in the expectant mother during the first trimester is a common cause of cardiac malformation. Maternal alcoholism, maternal irradiation, ingestion of certain drugs during pregnancy, maternal diabetes, and advanced maternal age (older than 40 years) also increase the incidence. Maternal malnutrition and heredity are also contributing factors. Recent studies have shown that the offspring of mothers who had congenital heart anomalies have a much higher risk. If one child in the family has a congenital heart abnormality, later siblings have a very high risk for such a defect.

The newborn with a severe abnormality, such as a transposition of the great vessels, is cyanotic from birth, requiring oxygen and special treatment. A less seriously affected child, whose heart can compensate to some degree for the impaired circulation, may not have symptoms severe enough to call attention to the difficulty until he or she is a few months older and more active. Others may live a fairly normal life and not be aware of any heart trouble until a murmur or an enlarged heart is discovered on physical examination in later childhood. Some abnormalities are slight and allow the person to lead a normal life without correction. Others cause little apparent difficulty but need correction to improve the chance for a longer life and for optimal health. Some severe anomalies are incompatible with life for more than a short time, and others may be helped but not cured by surgery.

Clinical Manifestations A cardiac murmur discovered early in life necessitates frequent physical examinations. This murmur may be a functional, "innocent" murmur that may disappear as the child grows older, or it may be the chief manifestation of an abnormal heart or an abnormal circulatory system. The most common parental complaint is that of feeding difficulties. Infants with cardiac anomalies severe enough to cause circulatory difficulties have a history of being poor eaters, tiring easily from the effort to suck, and fail to grow or thrive normally.

Manifestations of **congestive heart failure** (CHF) may appear during the first year of life in infants with conditions such as large ventricular septal defects, coarctation of the aorta, and other defects that place an increased workload on the ventricles. One indication of CHF in infancy is easy fatigability, manifested by feeding problems. The infant tires, breathes hard, and refuses a bottle after 1 or 2 oz but soon becomes hungry again. Lying flat causes stress, and the infant appears to be more comfortable if held upright over an adult's shoulder.

Other signs are failure to gain weight, a pale, mottled, or cyanotic color, a hoarse or weak cry, and tachycardia. Rapid respiration (with an expiratory grunt), flaring of the nares, and the use of accessory respiratory muscles with retractions at the diaphragmatic and suprasternal levels are other clinical manifestations of CHF. Edema is a factor, and the heart generally shows enlargement. Anoxic attacks (fainting spells) are common.

Diagnosis The clinical symptoms of CHF are the primary basis for diagnosis. Chest radiographs that reveal an enlarged heart and electrocardiography indicate ventricular hypertrophy.

Treatment Treatment of CHF includes digitalization to improve the contractility of the heart, angiotensin-converting enzyme inhibitors to reduce the afterload on the heart, diuretics to reduce any edema, administration of oxygen, and the use of small doses of morphine for relaxation, if necessary. The infant should be placed with the head elevated. Energy requirements should be minimized to ease the workload of the heart. Small, frequent feedings improve nutrition with minimal energy output.

Advances in medical technology have enabled heart repairs to be performed in infants as young as less than 1 day old. Miniaturization of instruments, earlier diagnosis through the use of improved diagnostic techniques, pediatric intensive care facilities staffed with highly skilled nurse specialists, and more sophisticated monitoring techniques all have contributed to these advances.

Most physicians now think it is important to operate as early as possible to repair defective hearts. Inadequate circulation may prevent adequate growth and development and cause permanent, irreparable physical, mental, and emotional damage. If the child is diagnosed early, before CHF occurs, correction may occur and CHF is avoided if effective repair is possible.

Care at Home Before Surgery A child with congenital heart disease may show easy fatigability and retarded growth. If the child has a cyanotic type of heart disease with clubbing of the fingers or toes, periods of cyanosis and reduced exercise tolerance are evident. This young child may assume a squatting position, which reduces the return flow to the heart, thus temporarily reducing the workload of the heart.

Such a child should be allowed to lead as normal a life as possible. Families are naturally apprehensive and find it difficult not to overprotect the child. They often increase the child's anxiety and cause fear in the child about participating in normal activities. Children are rather sensible about finding their own limitations and usually limit their activities to their capacity if they are not made unduly apprehensive.

Some families can adjust well and provide guidance and security for the sick child. Others may become confused and frightened and show hostility, disinterest, or neglect; these families need guidance and counseling. The nurse has a great responsibility to support the family. The nurse's primary goal is to reduce anxiety in the child and family. This goal may be accomplished through open communication and ongoing contact.

Routine visits to a clinic or a physician's office become a way of life, and the child may come to feel different from other people. Physicians and nurses have a responsibility both to the family caregivers and the child to give clear explanations of the defect, using readily understandable terms and diagrams, pictures, or models. A child who knows what is happening can accept a great deal and can continue with the business of living.

Cardiac Catheterization Cardiac catheterization may be performed before heart surgery to obtain more accurate information about the child's condition. The child or infant is sedated or anesthetized for this process, and a radiopaque tube is inserted through a vein into the right atrium. In the infant or young child, the femoral vein often is used. Close observation of the child after the procedure is essential. Carefully monitor the site used, and check the extremity for pulses, edema, skin temperature and color, and any other signs of poor circulation or infection.

Preoperative Preparation When a child enters the hospital for cardiac surgery, it is seldom a first admission; generally, it has been preceded by cardiac catheterization or perhaps other hospitalizations. The child may be admitted a few days before surgery to allow time for adequate preparation. However, with the current emphasis on cost containment, many preoperative procedures are done on an outpatient basis. Preoperative teaching should be intensive for the family and the child as appropriate to the age level. They should understand that blood may be obtained for typing and cross-matching and for other determinations as ordered. Additional roentgenograms may be made.

The apparatus to be used after surgery should be described with drawings and pictures. If possible, the family caregivers and the child should be taken to a cardiac recovery room and should be shown chest tubes and an oxygen tent. They should meet the nursing personnel and see the general appearance of the unit. Of course, nurses should use good judgment about the timing and the extent of such preparation: nothing is gained by arousing additional anxiety with premature or excessively graphic descriptions. A young child may become familiar with the surgical clothing worn by personnel and with the oxygen tent, and can perhaps listen to a heart beat. The child should be taught how to cough and should practice coughing. He or she should understand that coughing is important after surgery and must be done regularly, even though it may hurt.

Cardiac Surgery Open-heart surgery, using the heart-lung machine, has made extensive heart correction possible for many children who otherwise would have been disabled throughout their limited lives. Machines have been refined for use with infants and small children. Heart transplants may be performed when no other treatment is possible.

Hypothermia—reducing the body temperature to 68° to 78.8°F (20°–26°C)—is a useful technique that helps make early surgery possible. A reduced body temperature increases the time that the circulation may be stopped without causing brain damage. The blood temperature is reduced by the use of cooling agents in the heart-lung machine. This also provides a dry, bloodless, motionless field for the surgeon.

Postoperative Care At the end of surgery, the child is taken to the pediatric intensive care unit for skillful nursing by specially trained personnel for as long as necessary. Children who have had closed-chest surgery need the same careful nursing as those who have had open-heart surgery.

By the time the child returns to the regular pediatric unit, chest drainage tubes usually have been removed and the child has started taking oral fluids and is ready to sit up in bed or in a chair. The child probably feels weak and helpless after such an experience and needs encouragement and reassurance. With recovery, however, a child is usually ready for activity. Improving health provides the incentive. Family caregivers usually need to reorient themselves and to accept their child's new status, an attitude that is not easy to acquire after what seemed like a long period of anxious watching. The surgeon and the surgical staff evaluate the results of the surgery and make any necessary recommendations regarding resumption of the child's activities. Plans should be made for follow-up and supervision as well as counseling and guidance.

COMMON TYPES OF CONGENITAL HEART DEFECTS

Traditionally, congenital heart defects have been described as cyanotic or acyanotic conditions. **Cyanotic heart disease** implies an oxygen saturation of the peripheral arterial blood of 85% or less. This condition occurs when a heart defect allows any appreciable amount of oxygen-poor blood in the right side of the heart to mix with the oxygenated blood in the left side of the heart. Defects that permit right-to-left shunting may occur at the atrial, ventricular, or aortic level. However, since defects are often complex, occurring in various combinations, this is an inadequate means of classification. A more clear-cut classification system is based on blood flow characteristics. These are: 1) increased pulmonary blood flow, 2) decreased pulmonary blood flow, 3) obstruction of blood flow out of the heart, and 4) mixed blood flow, where saturated and desaturated blood mix in the heart, aorta, and pulmonary vessels.

Since defects often occur in combination, they give rise to complex situations. Many of the complex defects and most of the rare, isolated defects may never be seen by most nurses. The conditions discussed here are common enough that the pediatric nurse needs to be familiar with their diagnosis and treatment.

Ventricular Septal Defect This is the most common intracardiac defect. It consists of an abnormal opening in the septum between the two ventricles that allows blood to pass directly from the left to the right ventricle. There is no leakage of unoxygenated blood into the left ventricle and thus no cyanosis (Fig. 9-16).

Small, isolated defects are usually asymptomatic and often are discovered during a routine physical examination. A characteristic loud, harsh murmur, associated with a systolic thrill, occasionally is heard on examination. There may be a history of frequent respiratory infections during infancy, but growth and development are unaffected. The child leads a normal life.

Corrective surgery may be postponed until the age of 18 months to 2 years, when the surgical risk is less than that for infants. However, surgical techniques have improved to the degree that the repair may be made in the first year of life with high rates of success. The child is observed closely and may be placed on prophylactic antibiotics to prevent frequent respiratory infections. If pulmonary involvement becomes a problem, the repair is done without further delay. Clinical trials are underway to study the use of cardiac catheterization for repair in children at high risk.

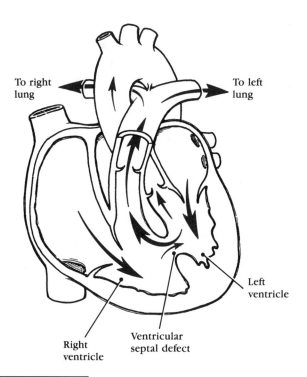

Figure 9-16
A ventricular septal defect is an abnormal opening between the right and left ventricle. Ventricular septal defects vary in size and may occur in the membranous or muscular portion of the ventricular septum. Owing to higher pressure in the left ventricle, a shunting of blood from the left to the right ventricle occurs during systole. If pulmonary vascular resistance produces pulmonary hypertension, the shunt of blood is then reversed from the right to the left ventricle, with cyanosis resulting.

Atrial Septal Defects   In general, left-to-right shunting occurs in all true atrial septal defects. However, many healthy people have a patent foramen ovale, which is situated in the atrial septum, and it normally causes no problems. This is because the valve of the foramen ovale is anatomically structured to withstand left chamber pressure, making the patent foramen ovale functionally closed (Fig. 9-17).

True atrial septal defects are common heart anomalies and may occur as isolated defects or in combination with other heart anomalies.

Atrial septal defects are amenable to surgery, with a low surgical mortality risk. Since the advent of the heart–lung bypass machine, this repair may be performed in a dry field, replacing the older "blind" technique. The opening is closed with sutures or a nylon patch.

Patent Ductus Arteriosus   The ductus arteriosus is a vascular channel between the left main pulmonary artery and the descending aorta. In fetal life, this allows blood to bypass the nonfunctioning lungs and go directly into the systemic circuit. After birth, the duct normally closes,

eventually becoming obliterated and forming the ligamentum arteriosum. If the ductus arteriosus remains patent, however, blood continues to be shunted from the aorta into the pulmonary artery. This situation floods the lungs and overloads the left heart chambers (Fig. 9-18).

Normally, the ductus arteriosus is nonpatent after the first or second week of life and should be obliterated by the fourth month. Why it fails to close is unknown. Patent ductus arteriosus is common in infants who exhibit the rubella syndrome, but most of the infants with this anomaly have no history of exposure to rubella during fetal life. It is also common in preterm infants weighing less than 1,200 g and infants with Down syndrome.

Symptoms of patent ductus arteriosus are often absent during childhood. Growth and development may be retarded in some children, with an easy fatigability and dyspnea on exertion. The diagnosis may be based on a characteristic machinery-like murmur over the pulmonary area, a wide pulse pressure, and a bounding pulse. Cardiac catheterization is diagnostic but is not required in the presence of classic clinical features.

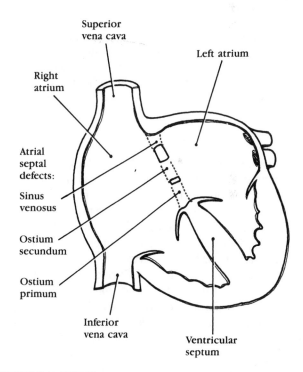

Figure 9-17
An atrial septal defect is an abnormal opening between the right and left atria. Basically, three types of abnormalities result from incorrect development of the atrial septum. An incompetent foramen ovale is the most common defect. The high ostium secundum defect results from abnormal development of the septum secundum. Improper development of the septum primum produces a basal opening known as an ostium primum defect, frequently involving the atrioventricular valves. In general, left to right shunting of blood occurs in all atrial septal defects.

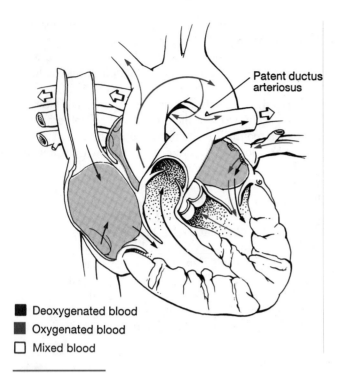

■ Deoxygenated blood
■ Oxygenated blood
☐ Mixed blood

Figure 9-18
The patent ductus arteriosus is a vascular connection that, during fetal life, short-circuits the pulmonary vascular bed and directs blood from the pulmonary artery to the aorta. Functional closure of the ductus normally occurs soon after birth. If the ductus remains patent after birth, the direction of blood flow in the ductus is reversed by the higher pressure in the aorta.

Surgery is indicated in all diagnosed cases, even if they are asymptomatic. Some persons live a normal life span without correction, but the risks involved far outweigh the surgical ones. Indomethacin (Indocin), a prostaglandin inhibitor, may be administered to premature infants with respiratory distress syndrome to promote closure of the ductus arteriosus with some success. If this fails to close the ductus, surgery is performed. Surgical correction consists of closure of the defect by ligation or by division of the ductus. Division is the method of choice if the child's condition permits because the ductus occasionally reopens after ligation. The optimal age for surgery is before the age of 2 years, with earlier surgery for severely affected infants. Prognosis is excellent after a successful repair.

Coarctation of the Aorta   This congenital cardiovascular anomaly consists of a constriction or narrowing of the aortic arch or the descending aorta, usually adjacent to the ligamentum arteriosum (Fig. 9-19).

Most children with this condition are asymptomatic until later childhood or young adulthood. A few infants have severe symptoms in their first year of life, showing dyspnea, tachycardia, and cyanosis, all signs of developing CHF.

In older children, the condition is easily diagnosed based on hypertension in the upper extremities and hypotension in the lower extremities. The radial pulse is readily palpable, but the femoral pulses are weak or even impalpable. Blood pressure is normal or elevated in the arms and is low or undetectable in the legs. A high-pitched systolic murmur is usually present, heard over the base of the heart and over the interscapular area of the back. The diagnosis may be confirmed by aortography.

Obstruction to blood flow caused by the constricted portion of the aorta does not cause early difficulty in an average child because the blood bypasses the obstruction by way of collateral circulation. The bypass is chiefly from the branches of the subclavian and carotid arteries, which arise from the arch of the aorta. Eventually, the enlarged collateral arteries erode the rib margins, and the rib notching may be visualized by radiographic examination.

Uncorrected coarctation may cause hypertension and cardiac failure later in life. The optimal age for elective surgery is before the age of 2 years. Early surgery may be necessary for a gravely ill infant who may present with severe CHF. In early infancy, the mortality rate depends on the presence of other congenital heart problems.

Surgery consists of resection of the coarcted area with an end-to-end anastomosis of the proximal and distal ends of the aorta. Occasionally, a long defect may necessitate an

Normally closed ductus arteriosus

Coarctation of aorta

Figure 9-19
Coarctation of the aorta is characterized by a narrowed aortic lumen. It exists as a preductal or postductal obstruction, depending on the position of the obstruction in relation to the ductus arteriosus. Coarctations exist with great variation in anatomic features. The lesion produces an obstruction to the flow of blood through the aorta, causing an increased left ventricular pressure and work load.

end-to-end graft using tubes of Dacron or similar material. Prognosis is excellent for the restoration of normal function after surgery.

Tetralogy of Fallot   This is a fairly common congenital heart defect, involving 50% to 70% of all cyanotic congenital heart diseases. It consists of a grouping of heart defects (*tetralogy* denotes four abnormal conditions): 1) **pulmonary stenosis**, 2) **ventricular septal defect**, 3) **overriding aorta**, and 4) **right ventricular hypertrophy**. The pulmonary stenosis is usually of the infundibular type, in which there is a narrowing of the upper portion of the right ventricle; however, it may include stenosis of the valve cusps. Pulmonary stenosis results, in turn, in right ventricular hypertrophy. The aorta appears to straddle the ventricular septum, overriding the ventricular septal defect. This defect allows a shunt of unsaturated blood from the right ventricle into the aorta or into the left ventricle (Fig. 9-20).

The child with tetralogy of Fallot may be precyanotic in early infancy, with the cyanotic phase starting at 4 to 6 months of age. Some severely affected infants, however, may show cyanosis earlier. As long as the ductus arteriosus remains open, enough blood apparently passes through the lungs to prevent cyanosis.

The infant presents with feeding difficulties and poor weight gain, resulting in retarded growth and development. Dyspnea and easy fatigability become evident. Exercise tolerance depends in part on the severity of the disease, some children becoming fatigued after little exertion. In the past, on experiencing fatigue, breathlessness, and increased cyanosis, the child was described as assuming a squatting posture for relief. Squatting apparently increased the systemic oxygen saturation. However, squatting rarely is seen today because these infants' defects usually are repaired by the time they are 2 years old.

Attacks of paroxysmal dyspnea are common during infancy and early childhood. An anoxic spell is heralded by sudden restlessness, gasping respiration, and increased cyanosis, leading to a loss of consciousness and possibly convulsions. These attacks, called "tet spells," last from a few minutes to several hours and appear to be unpredictable, although stress does seem to trigger some episodes.

The history and clinical manifestations are usually sufficient to make a diagnosis. However, cardiac catheterization, electrocardiography, chest radiography, and laboratory tests to determine polycythemia and arterial oxygen saturation may be performed for further definition.

The preferred repair of these defects is total surgical correction. This procedure may be carried out only in a dry field, necessitating the use of a cardiopulmonary bypass machine. The heart is opened and extensive resection is done. The septal defect is closed by use of a patch, and the valvular stenosis and infundibular chamber are resected.

Successful total correction transforms a grossly abnormal heart into a functionally normal one. Most of these children are left without a pulmonary valve, however.

In infants who cannot withstand the total surgical correction until they are older, the Blalock-Taussig procedure is performed. This procedure is an end-to-end anastomosis of a vessel arising from the aorta, usually the subclavian artery, to the corresponding right or left pulmonary artery. These shunts are used less commonly than before because total surgical repair is meeting with much greater success and lower mortality rates.

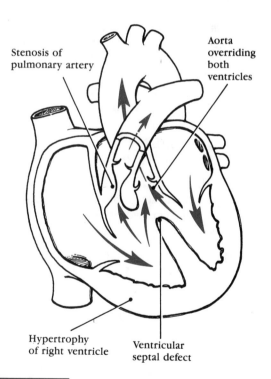

Figure 9-20
Tetralogy of Fallot is characterized by the combination of four defects: (1) pulmonary stenosis, (2) ventricular septal defect, (3) overriding aorta, and (4) hypertrophy of the right ventricle. It is the most common defect causing cyanosis in patients surviving beyond 2 years of age. The severity of symptoms depends on the degree of pulmonary stenosis, the size of the ventricular septal defect, and the degree to which the aorta overrides the septal defect.

*Labels in figure:*
Stenosis of pulmonary artery
Aorta overriding both ventricles
Hypertrophy of right ventricle
Ventricular septal defect

▶ � ◀ Nursing Process for the Infant With Congestive Heart Failure

ASSESSMENT

The interview of the family caregiver of an infant with CHF must include the gathering of information about the present illness and any previous episodes. Ask about any problems the infant may have during feeding, episodes of rapid or difficult respirations, episodes of turning blue, and difficulty with lying flat. Determine if the infant has been gaining weight. Avoid causing any feelings of guilt in the caregiver.

The physical assessment of the infant includes a complete assessment of vital signs. Note the quality and rhythm of the apical pulse. Assess respirations, including any use of accessory muscles, retractions, breath sounds, rate, and type of cry. Examine the skin and extremities for color, skin temperature, and evidence of edema. Observe the infant closely for signs of easy fatigability or an increase in symptoms on exertion.

NURSING DIAGNOSES

Some infants are so acutely ill on admission that they are admitted immediately to the pediatric intensive care unit, if one is available. The nursing diagnoses depend on the severity of the symptoms that determine the priority of care. Some diagnoses that may be useful include:

- Decreased Cardiac Output related to structural defects of the heart
- Ineffective Breathing Pattern related to pulmonary congestion and anxiety
- Activity Intolerance related to insufficient oxygenation secondary to heart defects
- Risk for Altered Nutrition: Less than Body Requirements related to fatigue and dyspnea
- Knowledge Deficit related to the infant's life-threatening illness

OUTCOME IDENTIFICATION AND PLANNING

The major goals include improving cardiac output and oxygenation, relieving inadequate respirations, and maintaining adequate nutritional intake. The family's goals include relieving the infant's symptoms of distress and increasing understanding of the condition and its prognosis.

IMPLEMENTATION

MONITORING VITAL SIGNS. Monitor vital signs regularly. If digoxin is ordered, count the apical pulse for a full minute before it is administered. Withhold digoxin and notify the physician if the apical rate is lower than the established norms for the child's age and baseline information (90–110 beats per minute for infants, 70–85 beats per minute for older children). Always check the dosage of digoxin with another nurse before administering it. Regularly evaluate the child for evidence of periorbital or peripheral edema. Weigh the child daily early in the morning, before the first feeding of the day, using the same scale with the infant undressed. Maintain careful intake and output measurements. If diuretics are administered, monitor serum electrolyte levels, especially potassium levels.

IMPROVING RESPIRATORY FUNCTION. Elevate the head of the crib mattress so that it is at a 30° to 45° angle.

Do not allow the infant to shift down in the crib and become "scrunched up," causing decreased expansion room for the chest. Avoid constricting clothing. Administer oxygen as ordered. Monitor respirations at least every 4 hours, paying close attention to breath sounds, dyspnea, tachypnea, retractions, and inspection of the nail beds for cyanosis. Monitor oxygen saturation levels with pulse oximetry.

PROMOTING ENERGY CONSERVATION. Plan nursing care so that the infant has long periods of uninterrupted rest. While nursing procedures are being carried out, talk to the infant softly and soothingly and handle him or her gently, giving loving care. Respond to the infant's cries quickly to avoid tiring.

MAINTAINING ADEQUATE NUTRITION. Give frequent feedings in small amounts to avoid overtiring the infant. Use a soft nipple with a large opening to ease the workload of the infant. If adequate nutrition cannot be taken during feedings, gavage feedings may be needed.

PROVIDING FAMILY TEACHING. The family of this infant has reason to be apprehensive and anxious. Be understanding, empathetic, and nonjudgmental when communicating with them. Give them information about CHF in such a way that they can understand it. Repeat information about signs and symptoms and offer explanations as many times as necessary. Include teaching about medication, feeding, and care techniques, growth and development expectations, and future plans for correction of the defect, if known. Involve the family in the care of the infant as much as possible within the limitations of the infant's condition.

EVALUATION: GOALS AND OUTCOME CRITERIA

- *Goal*: The child's cardiac output will improve.
  Criteria: The heart rate is within the normal limits for age; no arrhythmia or evidence of edema exists. Peripheral perfusion is adequate.

- *Goal*: The child's respiratory function will improve.
  Criteria: The child's respirations are regular, with no retractions; breath sounds are clear.

- *Goal*: The child will exhibit no cardiac or respiratory stress.
  Criteria: The child rests quietly.

- *Goal*: The child's nutrition will remain adequate.
  Criteria: The child feeds with minimal tiring and consumes most of the feeding each time.

- *Goal*: The family will be prepared for home care of the child.
  Criteria: The family verbalizes anxieties, asks appropriate questions, and demonstrates understanding of and participates in the care of the child.

Figure 9-21
Unilateral clubfoot. (A) Front view. (B) Back view.

Skeletal System Defects

Infants or children with congenital skeletal defects usually receive primary treatment on the general nursery or pediatric unit; thus, nurses need to understand the nature and treatment of these anomalies. Children with these conditions and their parents often face long periods of exhausting, costly treatment and therefore need continuing support, encouragement, and education.

The two most common and important skeletal defects are congenital **talipes equinovarus** (clubfoot) and congenital **hip dysplasia** (dislocation of the hip).

CONGENITAL TALIPES EQUINOVARUS

Congenital clubfoot is a deformity in which the entire foot is inverted, the heel is drawn up, and the forefoot is adducted. The Latin *talus*, meaning ankle, and *pes*, meaning foot, make up the word *talipes*, which is used in connection with many foot deformities. Equinus, or plantar flexion, and varus, or inversion, denote the kind of foot deformity present in this condition. The equinovarus foot has a club-like appearance—hence the term clubfoot (Fig. 9-21).

Congenital talipes equinovarus is the most common congenital foot deformity, occurring in about seven in 1,000 births. It appears as a single anomaly or in connection with other defects, such as myelomeningocele. It may be bilateral (both feet) or unilateral (one foot). The cause is unclear; a hereditary factor occasionally is observed. A hypothesis that has received some acceptance proposes an arrested embronic growth of the foot during the first trimester of pregnancy.

Diagnosis   Talipes equinovarus is easily detected in a newborn infant but must be differentiated from a persisting "position of comfort" assumed in utero. The positional de-

formity may be easily corrected by the use of passive exercise, but the true clubfoot deformity is fixed. The positional deformity should be explained to the parents at once to prevent anxiety.

Nonsurgical Treatment   If treatment is started during the neonatal period, correction usually may be accomplished by manipulation and bandaging or by application of a cast. The cast often is applied while the infant is still in the neonatal nursery. While the cast is being applied, the foot is first gently moved into as nearly normal a position as possible. Force should not be used. If the family caregiver can be present to help hold the infant while the cast is being applied, the caregiver will have the opportunity to understand what is being done. The very young infant gets satisfaction from sucking; therefore, a pacifier helps prevent squirming while the cast is being applied.

The cast is applied over the foot and ankle (and usually to mid-thigh) to hold the knee in right-angle flexion (Fig. 9-22). Casts are changed frequently to provide gradual, atraumatic correction—every few days for the first several weeks, then every week or two. Treatment is continued until complete correction is confirmed by radiograph and clinical observation, usually in a matter of months.

Any cast applied to a child's body should have some type of waterproof material protecting the skin from the sharp plaster edges of the cast. One method is to apply strips of adhesive vertically around the edges of the cast in a manner called petaling. This is done by cutting strips of adhesive 2″ or 3″ long and 1″ wide. One end is notched and the other end is cut pointed to aid in smooth application. Family caregivers must be taught cast care.

After correction with a cast, a Denis Browne splint with shoes attached is used to maintain the correction for another 6 months or longer (Fig. 9-23). After overcorrection

Figure 9-22
Casting for clubfoot in typical overcorrected position showing petaling of cast.

has been attained, a special clubfoot shoe should be worn, a laced shoe with a turning out of the shoe and the outer wedge of the sole that looks like the shoe is being worn on the wrong foot. The Denis Browne splint still may be worn at night, and passive exercises of the foot should be carried out by the caregivers. The older infant may resist wearing the splint, so family caregivers must be taught the importance of gentle, but firm, insistence that the splint be worn.

Surgical Treatment   Children who do not respond to nonsurgical measures, especially older children, need surgical correction. This approach involves several procedures, depending on the age of the child and the degree of the deformity. It may involve lengthening of the Achilles tendon, capsulotomy of the ankle joint, release of medial strictures, and, for the child older than 10 years of age, an operation on the bony structure. Prolonged observation after correction by either means should be carried out at least until adolescence; any recurrence is treated promptly.

Figure 9-23
A Denis Browne splint with shoes attached.

CONGENITAL HIP DYSPLASIA

Congenital hip dysplasia results from defective development of the acetabulum with or without dislocation. The malformed acetabulum permits dislocation, the head of the femur becoming displaced upward and backward. The condition is difficult to recognize during early infancy. When there is a family history of the defect, increased observation of the young infant is indicated. The condition is about seven times more common in girls than in boys and is often bilateral.

Diagnosis   Early recognition and treatment, before an infant starts to stand or walk, are extremely important for successful correction. The first examination should be part of the newborn examination. Experienced examiners may detect an audible click when examining the newborn using the Bartow and Ortolani tests. These tests, used together on one hip at a time, involve dislocating and relocating the acetabulum in adduction and abduction and should be conducted only by an experienced practitioner. They are effective only for the first month, after which they disappear. Signs that are useful after this include:

1. Asymmetry of the gluteal skin folds (higher on the affected side) (Fig. 9-24).
2. Limited abduction of the affected hip. This is tested by placing the infant in a dorsal recumbent position with the knees flexed and then abducting both knees passively until they reach the examination table without resistance. If dislocation is present, the affected side cannot be abducted more than 45°.
3. Apparent shortening of the femur.

Later signs, after the child has started walking, include lordosis, swayback, protruding abdomen, shortened extremity, duck-waddle gait, and a positive Trendelenburg sign. To elicit this sign, the child stands on the affected leg and raises the normal leg. The pelvis tilts down rather than up toward the unaffected side.

Roentgen studies usually are made to confirm the diagnosis in the older infant. Uncorrected dislocation causes limping, easy fatigue, hip and low back discomfort, and postural deformities.

Treatment   When the dislocation is discovered during the first few months, treatment consists of manipulation of the femur into position and application of a brace. The most common type of brace used is the Pavlik harness (Fig. 9-25). The physician assesses the infant weekly while the infant is in the harness and adjusts it to align the femur gradually. Sometimes no further treatment is needed.

If treatment is delayed until after the child has started to walk, or if earlier treatment is ineffective, open reduction followed by a spica cast is usually needed. After the cast is removed, a metal or plastic brace is applied to keep the legs in wide abduction.

Figure 9-24
Congenital hip disclocation. (A) Limitation of abduction in the affected leg. (B) Asymmetry of the gluteal folds of the thighs. (C) Apparent shortening of the femur.

Figure 9-25
Proper positioning of an infant in Pavlik harness. The harness is composed of shoulder straps, stirrups, and a chest strap. It is placed on both legs, even if only one hip is dislocated.

🔖 *Nursing Process for the Infant in an Orthopedic Device or Cast*

ASSESSMENT

Although the actual hospitalization of the infant is relatively short (if no other abnormalities require hospitalization), the nurse must teach the family cast care or care of the infant in an orthopedic device, such as a Pavlik harness. Assess the family's ability to understand and cooperate in the care of the infant. Emotional support of the family is important.

The assessment of the infant varies with the orthopedic device or cast used. Immediately after the application of a cast, observe for signs that the cast is drying evenly. Check the toes for circulation and movement. Check the skin at the edges of the cast for signs of pressure or irritation. If an open reduction has been performed, assess the child for signs of shock and bleeding in the immediate postoperative period.

NURSING DIAGNOSES

The nursing diagnoses depend on the defect and the type of treatment. Some diagnoses that may be used are:

- Altered Comfort related to orthopedic device or cast (Although this diagnosis does not appear on the NANDA list, it has been included for clarity.)
- Risk for Impaired Skin Integrity related to pressure of the cast on the skin surface
- Risk for Altered Growth and Development related to restricted mobility secondary to orthopedic device or cast
- Health Seeking Behaviors by the family related to home care of the infant in the orthopedic device or cast

OUTCOME IDENTIFICATION AND PLANNING

Goals include relieving discomfort, maintaining skin integrity, promoting growth and development, and increasing family knowledge about home care of the infant. The goals for the family focus on the desire for correction of the defect with minimal disruption to the infant's growth and development and care of the infant at home.

IMPLEMENTATION

PROVIDING COMFORT MEASURES. The infant may be irritable and fussy because of the restricted movement caused by the device or cast. Useful methods of soothing the infant include nonnutritive sucking, stroking, cuddling, and talking or crooning. If irritability seems excessive, check the infant for signs of irritation from the device or cast. The infant in a cast may be held after the cast is completely dry. Do not remove the harness unless specific permission for bathing is granted by the physician. Teach the family caretakers how to reapply the harness correctly. The infant in a Pavlik harness is not difficult to handle.

PROMOTING SKIN INTEGRITY. For the first 24 to 48 hours after application of a cast, place the infant on a firm mattress, and support position changes with firm pillows. When handling the cast, use the palms of the hands to avoid excessive pressure on the cast. Carefully inspect the skin around the cast edges for signs of irritation, redness, or edema. Petal the edges of the cast around the waist and toes and protect the cast with plastic covering around the perineal area. Take great care to protect the diaper area from becoming soiled and moist. If the covering becomes soiled, remove it, wash, dry thoroughly, and reapply or replace it. With the Pavlik harness, assess the skin under the straps frequently and massage them gently to promote circulation. Place extra padding under the shoulder straps to relieve pressure in that area.

Avoid using powders and lotions, as caking and pilling of the powder or lotion cause areas of irritation. Daily sponge baths are important and must include close attention to the skin under the straps of the device or around the edge of the cast.

Observe the infant in a cast carefully to prevent any restrictions of breathing caused by tightness over the abdomen and lower chest area. Vomiting after a feeding may be an indication that the cast is too tight over the stomach.

Prevent any small particles of food or toys from being pushed down into the cast by the older infant or child.

Diapering can be a challenge for the infant in a cast. Despite environmental concerns, disposable diapers may be the most effective way to provide good protection of the cast and prevent leakage.

PROVIDING SENSORY STIMULATION. Since the infant will be in the device or cast for an extended period during which much growth and development occur, provide him or her with stimulation of a tactile nature. Provide mobiles, musical toys, and stuffed toys. Do not permit the infant to cry for long periods. Keep feeding times relaxed. Hold the infant if possible and encourage interaction. Provide a pacifier if the infant desires it. Encourage activities that use the infant's free hands. The older infant may enjoy looking at picture books and interacting with siblings.

Diversionary activities should include transporting the infant to other areas in the home or in the car. Strollers and car seats may be adapted to allow safe transportation. For toddlers, a dolly (a low solid frame on wheels) may provide a movable base to explore the environment and encourage independence.

PROVIDING FAMILY TEACHING. Assess the family's knowledge and design a thorough teaching plan, since the infant will be cared for at home for most of the time. Use complete explanations, written guidelines, demonstrations, and return demonstrations. Provide the family with a resource person who may be called when a question arises, and encourage them to feel free to call that person. Make definite plans for return visits to have the device or cast checked. The family needs to understand the importance of keeping these appointments. Provide a public health nurse referral when appropriate. (See Nursing Care Plan for the Infant With an Orthopedic Device or Cast.)

EVALUATION: GOALS AND OUTCOME CRITERIA

- *Goal:* The infant's comfort will increase.
  Criteria: The infant is alert and content with no long periods of fussiness. The infant interacts with caregivers with cooing, smiling, and eye contact.

- *Goal:* The infant's skin will remain intact.
  Criteria: The skin around the edges of the cast shows no signs of redness or irritation. The diaper area is protected from soiling.

- *Goal:* The infant will demonstrate evidence of accomplishing appropriate developmental milestones.

Nursing Care Plan
for the Infant With an Orthopedic Cast

Six-month-old Malinda has right congenital hip dysplasia. After a trial with a Pavlik harness, she has been placed in a hip spica cast. The cast has just been applied. This is a new experience to her and to her caregiver.

NURSING DIAGNOSIS

Altered Comfort related to orthopedic device*

GOAL: *The infant will experience increased comfort.*

OUTCOME CRITERIA

- Malinda is alert and contented
- Malinda has no long periods of fussiness

Nursing Intervention	Rationale
Soothe by stroking, cuddling, talking, and crooning to her.	These comfort measures help the infant feel safe and loved. Provides distraction from discomfort and restriction of cast.
Provide Malinda with a pacifier.	Nonnutritive sucking is a means of self comforting.

NURSING DIAGNOSIS

Risk for Skin Impairment related to pressure of the cast on the skin surface

GOAL: *Skin integrity will be maintained around the cast*

OUTCOME CRITERIA

- Malinda's skin around the cast shows no signs of redness or irritation
- The perineal covering remains dry and clean and Malinda has no signs of perineal redness or irritation

Nursing Interventions	Rationale
Place Malinda on firm mattress for 24 to 48 hours until cast is dry.	The cast is still. pliable until dry. Undue pressure on any point must be avoided.
Use palms when handling damp cast.	Using palms instead of fingers prevents excessive pressure in any one area.
Petal all edges of cast.	Provides a smooth edge along cast to avoid irritation.
Inspect Malinda's skin around the cast edges for redness and irritation each shift.	Early signs of irritation indicate areas which may need added protection.
Protect perineal area of cast with waterproof covering.	Urine and feces can easily cause irritation, skin breakdown or a softened and malodorous cast.
Remove, wash, and thoroughly dry perineal covering if wet or soiled.	A clean, dry perineal cast protective covering decreases the danger of breakdown.

(continued)

Nursing Care Plan (Continued)
for the Infant With an Orthopedic Cast

NURSING DIAGNOSIS

Risk for Altered Growth and Development related to restricted mobility secondary to cast

GOAL: *Malinda will show evidence of accomplishing appropriate developmental milestones*

OUTCOME CRITERIA

• Malinda responds positively and appropriately to audio, visual, and diversional activities.

Nursing Interventions	*Rationale*
Provide mobiles, musical toys, stuffed toys, and toys Malinda can manipulate.	Visual, tactile and auditory stimulation is important for infant development.
Encourage caregiver to interact with Malinda during feeding.	Interacting (babbling, cooing) with others in her environment encourages development.
Plan activities which include changes of environment.	Environmental variety provides increased visual, auditory, and tactile stimulation.

NURSING DIAGNOSIS

Family Health-Seeking Behaviors related to the home care of the infant in a cast

GOAL: *The family caregivers will learn home care*

OUTCOME CRITERIA

• Malinda's family caregivers demonstrate understanding of her home care and ask relevant questions

Nursing Interventions	*Rationale*
Assess the family caregivers' knowledge level and design a teaching plan.	An effective teaching plan is tailored to begin with the knowledge base of the family.
Choose teaching methods most suited to identified needs and learning style of the family caregivers.	The ability of the family to read, understand and follow directions, and their cognitive abilities affect the results.
Before discharge schedule follow-up appointment for return visit to have the cast checked.	Scheduling the follow-up appointment emphasizes to family caregivers the importance of close follow-up

* This diagnosis does not appear on the NANDA list.

Criteria: The infant responds positively to audio, visual, and diversionary activities.

■ *Goal:* The family will learn home care of the infant. *Criteria:* The family demonstrates understanding of the infant's care and asks pertinent questions.

Genitourinary Tract Defects

Most congenital anomalies of the genitourinary tract are not life-threatening but may present social problems with lifelong implications for the child and family. Thus, early

recognition and supportive, understanding care are essential.

HYPOSPADIAS AND EPISPADIAS

Hypospadias is a congenital condition in which the urethra terminates on the ventral (underside) surface of the penis instead of at the tip. A cordlike anomaly (a **chordee**) extends from the scrotum to the penis, pulling the penis downward in an arc. Urination is not affected, but the boy cannot void while standing in the normal male fashion. Surgical repair is desirable between the ages of 6 and 18 months, before body image and castration anxiety become problems. Microscopic surgery makes early repair possible.

Surgical repair is often accomplished in one stage and is often done as outpatient surgery. These infants should not be circumcised, because the foreskin is used in the repair. Severe hypospadias may require additional surgical procedures.

In epispadias, the opening is on the dorsal (top) surface of the penis. This condition often occurs with exstrophy of the bladder. Surgical repair is indicated.

EXSTROPHY OF THE BLADDER

This urinary tract malformation occurs in one in 30,000 live births in the United States and is usually accompanied by other anomalies, such as epispadias, cleft scrotum, cryptorchidism (undescended testes), a shortened penis, and cleft clitoris. It is also associated with malformed pelvic musculature, resulting in a prolapsed rectum and inguinal hernias. Children with this defect have a widely split symphysis pubis and posterolaterally rotated hip sockets, causing a waddling gait.

In this condition, the anterior surface of the urinary bladder lies open on the lower abdomen (Fig. 9-26). The exposed mucosa is red and sensitive to touch and allows direct passage of urine to the outside. This condition makes the area vulnerable to infection and trauma. Surgical closure of the bladder is preferred within the first 48 hours of life. Final surgical correction is completed before the

Figure 9-26
Exstrophy of the bladder.

child goes to school. If repair of the bladder is not done early in the child's life, the family caregivers must be taught how to care for this condition and how to deal with their feelings toward this less-than-perfect child. Their emotional reaction may be further complicated if the malformation is so severe that the sex of the child may be determined only by a chromosome test (see the following section on sexual ambiguity).

Nursing care of the infant with exstrophy of the bladder should be directed toward preventing infection, preventing skin irritation around the seeping mucosa, meeting the infant's need for touch and cuddling, and educating and supporting the parents during this crisis.

SEXUAL AMBIGUITY

Although rare, the birth of an infant with ambiguous genitalia presents a highly charged emotional climate and has possible long-range social implications. Regardless of the cause, it is important to establish the genetic sex and the sex of rearing as early as possible, so that surgical correction of anomalies may occur before the child begins to function in a sex-related social role. Authorities believe that the infant's anatomic structure, rather than the genetic sex, should determine the sex of rearing. It is possible to construct a functional vagina surgically and to administer hormones to offer an anatomically incomplete female a somewhat normal life. Currently, it is impossible to offer comparable surgical reconstruction to males with an inadequate penis. Parents may feel guilt, anxiety, and confusion about their child's condition and need empathic understanding and support to help them cope with this emergency.

OTHER CONGENITAL DISORDERS

Infections

There are numerous maternally derived infectious diseases, some of which are congenital rubella, syphilis, gonorrhea, and herpes simplex virus. Nursing care for these infants focuses on prompt diagnosis, strict adherence to infection control guidelines, and routine care as for any newborn. Anxious caregivers often require support, education regarding treatment and prevention, and preparation for long-term care.

CONGENITAL RUBELLA

The rubella virus infection acquired by the fetus in utero generally persists throughout fetal life and for as long as 18 months after delivery. Persons coming into intimate contact with these babies may develop the disease; therefore, all women of childbearing age who are not immune to rubella should avoid contact with an infected infant.

The congenital rubella syndrome comprises a large variety of malformations, including cataracts and other eye defects, such as glaucoma. Other complications include deafness, cardiac anomalies (especially patent ductus arteriosus) and septal defects, intrauterine growth retardation, subnormal head circumference, and retarded functional development.

It is unreliable to assume that a person has been immunized by presumed attacks of rubella during childhood, because many rashes resemble that of rubella, and symptoms of childhood rubella are mild. Children now receive rubella vaccine as part of their immunizations at 15 months of age. Testing for the presence of rubella serum antibody is routine in all pregnant women. A positive reaction shows the person to be immune either as a result of the disease itself or from immunization. As a result of these concentrated efforts, neonates are protected from this devastating disease.

Maternal immunization for rubella is discussed in Chapter 6 in the section on maternal infections.

CONGENITAL SYPHILIS

Syphilis, whether congenital or acquired, is caused by the spirochete *Treponema pallidum*. Fetal infection does not occur much before the fourth month of fetal life, after the fetal organs are formed; therefore, anomalies rarely occur. The infection is contracted through the mother by placental transfer. About one fourth of infected infants are stillborn. Infants born live may not show any clinical symptoms for months or years.

Clinical Manifestations   In early congenital syphilis, symptoms may appear before the sixth week of life. Rhinitis, with a profuse, mucopurulent nasal discharge, is usually the first symptom. A maculopapular skin rash appears next, heaviest over the back, buttocks, and backs of the thighs. Bleeding ulcerations and mucous membrane lesions appear around the mouth, the anus, and the genital areas (Fig. 9-27). Anemia is present; pseudoparalysis and pathologic fractures may occur. These symptoms usually subside without treatment while the infectious organism lies latent in the child's tissues.

Late symptoms, appearing after infancy, involve the skeletal framework, the eyes, and the central nervous system. The child may acquire a flat bridge of the nose, known as "saddle nose." The permanent teeth are affected in that the incisors are peg-shaped (Hutchinson's teeth). A condition of the eyes called **interstitial keratitis** often occurs later in the disease with lacrimation, photophobia, and opacity of the lens that may lead to blindness.

Diagnosis   A VDRL (Venereal Disease Research Laboratory) or Wassermann test on cord blood at delivery is

Figure 9-27
Some of the skin manifestations of congenital syphilis.

done when congenital syphilis is suspected. Passively acquired antibodies may give false-positive results; therefore, other serologic tests are conducted subsequently. If results are doubtful, treatment usually is instituted to avoid a full-blown infection.

Treatment   Ideally, treatment is preventive, consisting of penicillin therapy for the affected mother early in pregnancy. The physician may order the test to be repeated later in pregnancy, if infection is suspected, with penicillin therapy instituted at this point if the test is positive. Treatment for the affected infant consists of a course of penicillin therapy. Strict isolation of the infant is required.

Early congenital syphilis usually responds to vigorous treatment, and growth and development are not affected. Late congenital syphilis responds well to treatment, but pathologic changes in the bones, eyes, and nervous system are permanent.

GONORRHEAL OPHTHALMIA NEONATORUM

Gonorrheal eye infection in the newborn is a serious condition, usually resulting in blindness if prophylactic treatment at birth is omitted. The infectious agent is the gonococcus *Neisseria gonorrhoeae*. The infant becomes infected while passing through the birth canal of an infected mother.

Clinical Manifestations and Diagnosis Symptoms are acute redness and swelling of the conjunctiva with a purulent discharge from the eyes, occurring within 36 to 48 hours after birth. These symptoms usually indicate gonorrheal eye infection; however, inspection of the eye should be followed by a culture and smear to determine the causative organism. The condition is communicable for 24 hours after specific therapy is instituted or, when no therapy is used, until discharge from the eyes has ceased.

Prevention and Treatment In the United States, all states have laws requiring the use of specific preparations instilled into the eyes at birth. All states require instillation of 1% silver nitrate or antibiotic drops or ophthalmic ointments, such as tetracycline and erythromycin. Penicillin is the drug of choice for the treatment of gonorrheal infections, including gonorrheal ophthalmia (see Chap. 7).

HERPES SIMPLEX VIRUS

Herpes simplex virus, most frequently caused by herpesvirus hominis type 2, is transmitted to the neonate during vaginal delivery by a mother who has an active genital lesion. Cesarean delivery before rupture of membranes is considered a preventive measure, although a small possibility remains that the fetus could have been infected before delivery. The infant usually has no apparent signs of the disease until 6 to 9 days after delivery. In the newborn nursery, infants who have had possible exposure should be segregated or cared for in the mother's private room.

The infection may be generalized, resembling sepsis. The infant may or may not have lesions, which are highly contagious. The mortality rate is high. Infants who survive have a high probability for ocular and neurologic damage.

Inborn Errors of Metabolism

Inborn errors of metabolism include phenylketonuria, galactosemia, congenital hypothyroidism, maple syrup urine disease, and homocystinuria. Nursing care for the infant involves prompt diagnosis and initiation of treatment. Family teaching might include dietary guidelines, information about the disorder, and genetic counseling. The family also needs support and information to prepare for the long-term care of a chronically ill child (see Chap. 21).

PHENYLKETONURIA

Phenylketonuria (PKU) is a recessive hereditary defect of metabolism that, if untreated, causes severe mental retardation in most, but not all, affected children. It is uncommon, appearing in about one in 10,000 births. Children with this condition lack the enzyme that normally changes the essential amino acid phenylalanine into tyrosine.

As soon as the newborn with this defect begins to take milk (either breast or cow's milk), phenylalanine is absorbed in the normal manner. However, because the affected infant cannot metabolize this amino acid, phenylalanine builds up in the blood serum to as much as 20 times the normal level. This build-up occurs so quickly that increased levels of phenylalanine appear in the blood after only 1 or 2 days of ingestion of milk. Phenylpyruvic acid appears in the urine of these infants between the second and the sixth week of life.

Most untreated children with this condition develop severe and progressive mental deficiency, apparently because of the high serum phenylalanine level. The infant appears normal at birth but begins to show signs of mental arrest within a few weeks. Therefore, this disorder must be diagnosed as early as possible and the child must be placed immediately on a low-phenylalanine formula.

Clinical Manifestations Untreated infants may experience frequent vomiting and have aggressive and hyperactive traits. Severe, progressive retardation is characteristic. Convulsions may occur, and eczema, particularly in the perineal area, is common. There is a characteristic musty smell to the urine.

Diagnosis Most states require newborns to undergo a blood test to detect the phenylalanine level. This screening procedure, called the Guthrie inhibition assay test, uses blood from a simple heel prick. The test is most reliable after the infant has ingested some form of protein. Because most infants are discharged early, the accepted practice is to perform the test before the infant is discharged and to repeat it in the third week of life if the first test was done before the infant was 24 hours old. Health practitioners caring for infants not born in a hospital are responsible for screening these infants. When screening indicates an increased level of phenylalanine, additional testing is done to make a firm diagnosis.

Treatment Dietary treatment is required. A formula low in phenylalanine should be started as soon as the condition is detected (Lofenalac and Phenyl-free are low-phenylalanine formulas produced by Mead Johnson; Ross Laboratories produces Phenex-1 and Phenex-2). Best results are obtained if the special formula is started before the infant is 3 weeks of age. A low-phenylalanine diet is a very restricted one. Foods to be omitted are breads, meat, fish, dairy products, nuts, and legumes. The diet should be carefully supervised by a nutritionist and should be continued well into the school years. Routine blood testing is done to maintain the serum phenylalanine level at 2 to 8 mg/dL.

Maintaining the infant on the restricted diet is relatively simple compared with the problems that arise as the child grows and becomes more independent. As the child ventures into the world beyond home, more and more dietary temptations are available, and dietary compliance is difficult. The family and child need support and counseling throughout the child's developmental years. The length of time that the restrictions are necessary remains unclear. Although difficult, it seems best to follow the diet into adolescence.

GALACTOSEMIA

Galactosemia is a recessive hereditary metabolic disorder in which the enzyme necessary for converting galactose into glucose is missing. The infants generally appear normal at birth but experience difficulties after ingesting milk (breast, cow's, or goat's milk) because one of the component monosaccharides of milk lactose is galactose.

Clinical Manifestations and Diagnosis   Early feeding difficulties, with vomiting and diarrhea severe enough to produce dehydration and weight loss, and jaundice are primary manifestations. Unless milk is withheld early, other difficulties include cataracts, liver and spleen damage, and mental retardation, with a high mortality rate early in life. A blood test using the Guthrie inhibition assay method has proved a reliable diagnostic test and is now required by many states as part of routine newborn screening. It may be performed in conjunction with a test for PKU.

Treatment   Galactose must be omitted from the diet, which in the young infant means a substitution for milk. Nutramigen and Pregestimil are formulas that provide galactose-free nutrition for the infant. The diet must continue to be free of lactose when the child moves on to table foods, but the diet allows more variety than the phenylalanine-free diet.

CONGENITAL HYPOTHYROIDISM

At one time referred to by the now unacceptable term cretinism, congenital hypothyroidism is associated with either the congenital absence of a thyroid gland or the inability of the thyroid gland to secrete thyroid hormone. The incidence is about one in 5,000 births, or about twice as common as PKU.

Diagnosis   Most states require a routine test for triiodothyronine (T_3) and thyroxine (T_4) levels to determine thyroid function in all newborns before discharge to diagnose congenital hypothyroidism early. This test is done as part of the heel stick screening, which includes the Guthrie screening test for PKU.

Clinical Manifestations   The infant appears normal at birth, but at about 6 weeks of life, clinical signs and symptoms begin to be noticeable. The facial features are typical, with a short forehead, depressed nasal bridge, large tongue, and puffy eyes. The voice (cry) is hoarse, the skin is dry, and there is slow bone development. Two common features are obstinate constipation and umbilical hernia.

The infant is a poor feeder and is often characterized as a "good" baby by the parent or caretaker because he or she cries very little and sleeps for long periods.

Treatment   The thyroid hormone must be replaced as soon as the diagnosis is made. Levothyroxine sodium, a synthetic thyroid replacement, is the drug most commonly used. Blood levels of T_3 and T_4 are monitored to prevent overdosage. Unless therapy is started in early infancy, mental retardation and slow growth occur. The later the therapy is started, the more severe the mental retardation. Therapy must be continued lifelong.

MAPLE SYRUP URINE DISEASE

Maple syrup urine disease (MSUD) is an inborn error of metabolism of the branched chain amino acids. It is autosomal recessive in inheritance. It is rapidly progressive and often fatal.

Clinical Manifestations and Diagnosis   The onset of MSUD occurs very early in infancy. These infants often have feeding problems and neurologic signs such as seizures, spasticity, and opisthotonos in the first week of life. The urine has a distinctive odor of maple syrup. Diagnosis is made through a blood test for the amino acids leucine, isoleucine, and valine. This is easily done at the same time as the heel stick for PKU is performed.

Treatment   Treatment of MSUD is dietary and must be initiated within 12 days of birth to be successful. The special formula is low in the branched chain amino acids. The special diet must be continued indefinitely.

HOMOCYSTINURIA

In homocystinuria, a relatively rare inborn error of metabolism, there is a deficiency of the enzyme cystathionine B synthase. This enzyme blocks the conversion of methionine to cystine. Mental retardation, early-onset thrombosis, seizures, and behavioral disorders result from high levels of serum methionine.

Clinical Manifestations and Diagnosis   The newborn with this deficiency may have skeletal abnormalities, mental retardation, dislocation of ocular lenses, or intravascular thromboses as the result of methionine and homocystine in the blood. Diagnosis can be made through screening at the time newborn screening is performed.

Treatment   Homocystinuria is treated with a special diet low in methionine, supplemented with cystine and pyridoxine (vitamin B_6). With prompt, early diagnosis and treatment, the long-term prognosis for the prevention of mental retardation is good.

■ KEY POINTS

■ Many infants injured during birth or born with a congenital anomaly have long-term effects from their conditions.

■ Advances in medical technology have improved the outlook for many infants who have sustained damage during intrauterine development or birth, giving them a better chance for an improved quality of life, but many conditions still inflict overwhelming consequences, causing lifelong disabilities.

■ Care of the newborn with special needs is a challenging aspect of nursing.

■ All available resources must be used to deliver quality nursing care to infants with congenital anomalies or birth injuries and to the families of these infants.

■ Nursing care must stimulate the infant's optimal growth and development as well as meeting his or her immediate physical needs.

■ The nurse must prepare the family for home care of the infant and guide the family to support services that will enable them to manage the care for their child for many years.

? CRITICAL THINKING

1. Diane's baby was born with a bilateral cleft lip and cleft palate. When you bring the baby in to her for feeding, she breaks down and sobs uncontrollably. Describe your immediate response. Identify the nursing diagnosis this suggests and the nursing implementation you believe is appropriate.

2. After you talk with her for a while, Diane gets herself under control enough to tell you that she was planning to breast-feed but cannot because of the cleft lip and palate. What is your response? Detail the teaching you will plan for her.

3. Identify the reason infection control is of utmost importance in the care of the infant with myelomeningocele.

4. Tell what happens as fluid builds up in hydrocephalus a) before the suture lines close and b) after the sutures line close. Identify the symptoms an infant would display if fluid build-up in the brain is not relieved.

5. Identify an appropriate nursing diagnosis for the infant in an orthopedic cast for whom you plan to provide comfort and developmental stimulation.

6. Explain some of the maternal risk factors that may cause congenital heart defects.

REFERENCE

1. Alexander MA, Steg NL. Myelomeningocele: Comprehensive treatment. Arch Phys Med Rehabil 70:637–641, 1989.

BIBLIOGRAPHY

Carpenito LJ. Handbook of nursing diagnosis, 6th ed. Philadelphia: JB Lippincott, 1995.

Combs VL, Marino BL. A comparison of growth patterns in breast- and bottle-fed infants with congenital heart disease. Pediatr Nurs 19(2):175–179, 1993.

Evans-Berro EA. How to defeat a "tet spell." Am J Nurs 91(7): 46–48, 1991.

Peterson PM. Spina bifida: Nursing challenge. RN 55(3):40–46, 1992.

Pillitteri A. Maternal and child health nursing, 2d ed. Philadelphia: JB Lippincott, 1995.

Powell ML, Costanzo JM. Tricuspid atresia: Surgical treatment, pediatric nursing care. AORN J 52(3):567–570, 1990.

Richard ME. Weight comparisons of infants with complete cleft lip and palate. Pediatr Nurs 20(2):191–196, 1994.

Schaming D, Gorry M, Soroka K, et al. When babies are born with orthopedic problems. RN 53(4):62–67, 1990.

Shaw N. Common surgical problems in the newborn. J Perinat Neonat Nurs 3(3):50–56, 1990.

Turley KM, Higgens SS. When parents participate in critical pathway management following pediatric cardiovascular surgery. MCN 21(5):229–234, 1996.

Wong DL. Whaley and Wong's nursing care of infants and children, 5th ed. St. Louis: Mosby, 1995.

Unit **III**

A Child Grows

Chapter 10

Growth and Development of the Infant: 28 Days to 1 Year

PHYSICAL DEVELOPMENT
Head and Skull
Skeletal Growth and Maturation
Eruption of Deciduous Teeth
Circulatory System
Body Temperature and Respiratory Rate
Neuromuscular Development
PSYCHOSOCIAL DEVELOPMENT

NUTRITION
Addition of Solid Foods
Weaning the Infant
Women, Infants, Children Food Program
HEALTH PROMOTION AND MAINTENANCE
Routine Checkups
Immunizations
Family Teaching
Accident Prevention
THE INFANT IN THE HEALTH CARE FACILITY
Parent–Nurse Relationship

STUDENT OBJECTIVES

On completion of this chapter, the student will be able to:

1. State the ages at which the a) anterior fontanelle and b) posterior fontanelle normally close.
2. State the ages at which the infant's birth weight a) doubles and b) triples.
3. Discuss the eruption of deciduous teeth: a) approximate age of the first tooth, b) first teeth to erupt, c) factors that may interfere with eruption, and d) role of fluoride in dental health.
4. Discuss the appropriate use of developmental tables.
5. State the age at which the child becomes aware of himself or herself as a person.
6. Name the age when the fear of strangers usually appears.
7. State one useful purpose of the game "Peek-a-Boo."
8. State why a baby tends to push food out of the mouth with the tongue.
9. State the rationale for introducing new foods one at a time.
10. Discuss weaning: a) the usual age when the baby becomes interested in a cup and b) criteria to determine the appropriate time.
11. State the cause and prevention of "bottle mouth" caries.
12. List three foods to offer the infant who does not drink enough milk from the cup.
13. List seven communicable diseases against which children are immunized.
14. State at what age immunizations usually begin and which are given in the first year.
15. Identify caregiver teaching the nurse should present during routine health maintenance visits.
16. Describe early dental care for the infant.
17. Discuss the family caregivers' role in the infant's hospital care.

The infant who has lived through the first month of life has a busy year ahead. During this year, the infant grows and develops skills more rapidly than will ever be experienced again. In the brief span of a single year, this tiny, helpless bit of humanity becomes a person with strong emotions of love, fear, jealousy, and anger and gains the ability to rise from a supine to an upright position and move about purposefully.

In the first year, both weight and height increase rapidly. During the first 6 months, the infant's birth weight doubles and height increases about 6". Growth slows slightly during the second 6 months but is still rapid. By 1 year of age, the infant has tripled his or her birth weight and has grown 10" to 12".

Thinking in terms of the "average" child is misleading. To determine whether an infant is reaching acceptable levels of development, birth weight and height must be the standard with which later measurements are compared. A baby weighing 6 lb at birth cannot be expected to weigh as much at 5 or 6 months of age as the baby who weighed 9 lb at birth, but each is expected to double his or her birth weight at about this time. A growth graph is helpful to the nurse, pediatrician, or caregiver for charting a child's progress (Fig. 10-1).

PHYSICAL DEVELOPMENT

Despite the many factors, such as genetic background, environment, health, gender, and race, that affect growth in the first year of life, the healthy infant progresses in a predictable pattern. By the end of the year, the dependent infant who at 1 month of age had no teeth and could not roll over, sit, or stand blossoms into an emerging toddler with teeth who can sit alone, stand, and begin to walk alone. The miracle of growth, seen in the prenatal development of the fetus, continues.

Head and Skull

At birth, an infant's head circumference averages about 13.75" (35 cm) and is usually slightly larger than the chest circumference. The chest measures about the same as the abdomen at birth. At about 1 year of age, the head circumference has grown to about 18" (47 cm). The chest also grows rapidly, catching up to the head circumference at

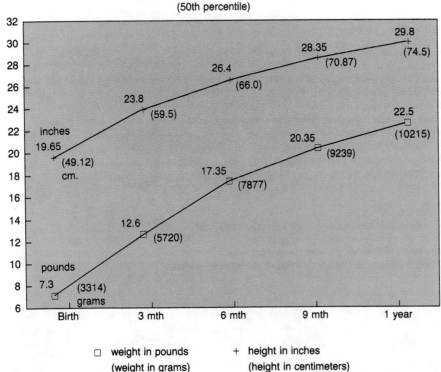

Height and Weight First Year
(50th percentile)

□ weight in pounds
(weight in grams)

+ height in inches
(height in centimeters)

Figure 10-1
Chart of infant growth representing an infant in the mid-range–birthweight 7.3 lb (3314 g) and birth length 19.65 inches (49.12 cm). Infants of different races vary in average size. Asian infants tend to be smaller, African American infants larger.

about 5 to 7 months of age. From then on, the chest can be expected to exceed the head in circumference.

FONTANELLES AND CRANIAL SUTURES

The posterior fontanelle is usually closed by the second or third month of life. The anterior fontanelle may increase slightly in size during the first few months of life. After the sixth month it begins to decrease in size, closing between the 12th and the 18th months. The sutures between the cranial bones do not ossify until later childhood.

Skeletal Growth and Maturation

During fetal life, the skeletal system is completely formed in cartilage at the end of 3 months' gestation. Ossification and growth of bones occur during the remainder of fetal life and throughout childhood. The pattern of maturation is so regular that the "bone age" can be determined by radiologic examination. When the bone age matches the child's chronologic age, the skeletal structure is maturing at a normal rate. To avoid unnecessary exposure to radiation, radiologic examination is performed *only* if a problem is suspected.

Eruption of Deciduous Teeth

Calcification of the primary or **deciduous teeth** starts early in fetal life. Shortly before birth, calcification begins in the permanent teeth that are the first to erupt in later childhood. The first deciduous teeth usually erupt between 6 and 8 months of age. The first teeth to erupt are usually the lower central incisors (Fig. 10-2).

Time of eruption of deciduous teeth

Upper

Lower

		(Upper)	(Lower)
1	Central incisor	8–12 mos.	5–9 mos.
2	Lateral incisor	8–12 mos.	12–18 mos.
3	Cuspid	18–24 mos.	
4	First molar	12–18 mos.	
5	Second molar	24–30 mos.	

Figure 10-2
Approximate ages for the eruption of deciduous teeth.

Babies in good health who show normal development may differ in the timing of tooth eruption. Some families show a tendency toward very early or very late eruption, without other signs of early or late development. Some infants may become restless or fussy from swollen, inflamed gums during teething. A cold teething ring may be helpful in soothing the baby's discomfort. Teething is a normal process of development and does not cause high fever or upper respiratory conditions.

Nutritional deficiency or prolonged illness in infancy may interfere with calcification of both the deciduous and the permanent teeth. The role of fluoride in strengthening calcification of teeth has been well documented. The American Dental Association recommends administration of fluoride to infants and children in areas where the fluoride content of drinking water is inadequate or absent.

Circulatory System

In the first year of life, the circulatory system undergoes several changes. During fetal life, high levels of hemoglobin and red blood cells are necessary for adequate oxygenation. After birth, when oxygen is supplied through the respiratory system, hemoglobin decreases in volume, and red blood cells gradually decrease in number until the third month of life. Thereafter, the count gradually increases until adult levels are reached.

It is difficult to obtain an accurate blood-pressure measurement in an infant. The flush method is sometimes used to determine the systolic pressure (see Chap. 3). Electronic or ultrasonographic monitoring equipment is often used. The average blood pressure during the first year of life is 85/60 mmHg. However, variability is expected among children of the same age and body build.

An accurate determination of the infant's heart beat requires an apical pulse count. A pediatric stethoscope with a small-diameter diaphragm is placed over the left side of the chest in a position where the heart beat can be clearly heard. A count is then taken for 1 full minute. During the first year of life, the average apical rate ranges from 70 (asleep) to 150 (awake) beats per minute and as high as 180 beats per minute while the infant is crying.

Body Temperature and Respiratory Rate

Body temperature follows the average normal range after the initial adjustment to postnatal living. Respirations average 30 breaths per minute, with a wide range (20–50 breaths per minute) according to the infant's activity.

Neuromuscular Development

As the infant grows, nerve cells mature and fine muscles begin to learn to coordinate in an orderly pattern of development. Naturally, the family caregivers are full of pride

TABLE 10-1. Growth and Development Chart: Birth to 1 Year

Age	Physical	Psychosocial	Fine Motor	Gross Motor	Language	Cognition
Birth–4wk	Weight gain of 5–7 oz (150–270 g) per wk. Height gain of 1″ per mo first 6 mo. Head circumference increases ½″ per mo. Moro, Babinski, rooting, and tonic neck reflexes present	Some smiling. Begins Erikson's stage of "trust vs. mistrust"	Grasp reflex very strong. Hands flexed	Catches and holds objects in sight that cross visual field. Can turn head from side to side when lying in a prone position (see Fig. 10-3A). When prone, body in a flexed position. When prone, moves extremities in a crawling fashion	Cries when upset. Makes enjoyment sounds during mealtimes	At 1 mo, sucking activity associated with pleasurable sensations
6 wk	Tears appear	Smiling in response to familiar stimuli	Hands open. Less flexion noted	Tries to raise shoulders and arms when stimulated. Holds head up when prone. Less flexion of entire body when prone	Cooing predominant. Smiles to familiar voices. Babbling	**Primary Circular Reactions** Begins to repeat actions
10–12 wk	Posterior fontanelle closes	Aware of new environment. Less crying. Smiles at significant others	No longer has grasp reflex. Pulls on clothes, blanket, but does not reach for them	No longer has Moro reflex. Symmetric body positioning. Pumps arms, shoulders, and head from prone position (see Fig. 10-3B)	Makes noises when spoken to	Beginning of coordinated responses to different kinds of stimuli
16 wk	Moro, rooting, and tonic neck reflexes disappear; drooling begins	Responds to stimulus. Sees bottle, squeals, laughs. Aware of new environment and shows interest	Grasps objects with two hands. Grasps objects in crib voluntarily and brings them to mouth. Eye–hand coordination beginning	Plays with hands. Brings objects to mouth. Balances head and body for short periods in sitting position	Laughs aloud. Sounds "n," "k," "g," and "b"	Likes social situations. Defiant, bored if unattended
20 wk	May show signs of teething	Smiles at self in mirror. Cries when limits are set or when objects are taken away	Holds one object while looking for another one. Grasps objects wanted	Able to sit up (see Fig. 10-3C). Can roll over. Can bear weight on legs when held in a standing position. Able to control head movements	Cooing noises. Squeals with delight	Visually looks for an object that has fallen
24 wk	Birth weight doubles; weight gain slows to 3–5 oz (90–150 g) per wk. Height slows to ½″ per mo. Teething begins with lower central incisors	Likes to be picked up. Knows family from strangers. Plays "Peek-a-Boo". Knows likes and dislikes. Fear of strangers	Holds a bottle fairly well. Tries to retrieve a dropped article	Tonic neck reflex disappears. Sits alone in high chair, back erect. Rolls over and back to abdomen	Makes sounds "guh," "bah". Sounds "p," "m," "b," and "t" are pronounced. Bubbling sounds	**Secondary Circular Reactions** Repeats actions that affect an object. Beginning of object permanence
28 wk	Lower lateral incisors are followed in the next month by upper central incisors	Imitates simple acts. Responds to "no". Shows preferences and dislikes for food	Holds cup. Transfers objects from one hand to the other	Reaches without visual guidance. Can lift head up when in a supine position	Babbling decreases. Duplicates "ma-ma" and "pa-pa" sounds	

(continued)

Age	Physical	Psychosocial	Fine Motor	Gross Motor	Language	Cognition
TABLE 10-1. Growth and Development Chart: Birth to 1 Year *(Continued)*						
32wk	Teething continues	Dislikes diaper and clothing change Afraid of strangers Fear of separating from mother	Adusts body position to be able to reach for an object May stand up while holding on	Craws around (see Fig. 10-3D) Pulls toy toward self	Combines syllables but has trouble attributing meaning to them	
40 wk–1 yr	Birth weight tripled; has six teeth; Babinski reflex disappears Anterior fontanelle closes between now and 18 mo	Does things to attract attention Tries to follow when being read to Imitates parents Looks for objects not in sight	Holds tool with one hand and works on it with another Puts toy in box after demonstration Stacks blocks Holds crayon to scribble on paper	Stands alone; begins to walk alone Can change self from prone to sitting to standing position	Words emerge Says 'da-da' and "ma-ma" with meaning	Coordination of secondary schemes; masters barrier to reach goal, symbolic meanings

in the infant who learns to sit or stand before the neighbor's baby does, but accomplishing such milestones early means little. Each child follows a unique rhythm of progress, within reasonable limits.

Average rates of growth and development are useful for purposes of evaluation. There are a few landmarks that call for special attention, even though their absence may indicate the need for additional environmental stimulation. Do not emphasize routine developmental tables with family caregivers; a mild time lag may be insignificant. A large lag may require greater stimulation from the environment or a watchful attitude to discover how overall development is proceeding.

Table 10-1 summarizes the accepted norms in physical, psychosocial, motor, language, and cognitive growth and development in the first year of life (Fig. 10-3).

PSYCHOSOCIAL DEVELOPMENT

The give-and-take of life is experienced by the infant who actively seeks food to fulfill feelings of hunger. The infant begins to develop a sense of trust when fed on demand. However, the infant eventually learns that every need is not always met immediately when demanded. Slowly, the infant becomes aware that one's needs are fulfilled by something or someone separate from oneself. Gradually, as a result of the loving care of family caregivers, the infant learns that the environment responds to desires expressed through one's own efforts and signals. The infant is now aware that the environment is separate from self.

Caregivers who expect too much too soon from the infant are not encouraging optimal development. Rather than teaching the rules of life before the infant has learned to trust the environment, the caregivers are actually teach-

Family Teaching
Tips for Infants from Birth to 1 Year

First 6 weeks: Frequent holding of infant gives infant feeling of being loved and cared for. Rocking and soothing baby are important.

6 weeks to 3½ months: Continue to give infant feeling of being loved and cared for; respond to cries; provide visual stimulation with toys, pictures, and mobiles and auditory stimulation by talking and singing to baby; repeat sounds infant makes to encourage vocal stimulation.

3½ to 5 months: Play regularly with baby; give child variety of things to look at; talk to baby; offer a variety of items to touch—soft, fuzzy, smooth, and rough—to provide tactile stimulation; continue to respond to infant's cries; move baby around home to provide additional visual and auditory stimulation; begin placing infant on floor to provide freedom of movement.

5 to 8 months: Continue to give infant feeling of being loved and cared for by holding, cuddling, and responding to needs; talk to infant; put infant on floor more to roll and move about; fear of strangers is common at this age.

8 to 12 months: Accident-proof the house; give the infant maximum access to living area: supply infant with toys; stay close by to support infant in difficult situations; continue to talk to infant to provide language stimulation. The baby at this age loves surprise toys like jack-in-the-box and separation games like "Peek-a-Boo"; loves putting-in and taking-out activities. The child is developing independence, and temper tantrums may begin.

Figure 10-3
Growth and development of the infant.
(A) At 4 weeks, this infant turns her head when lying in a prone position.
(B) At 12 weeks, this infant pushes up from a prone position to look at his toy.
(C) At 21 weeks, this infant sits up but tilts forward for balance.
(D) At 30 weeks, this infant is crawling around and on the go.
(E) At 43 weeks, this infant is getting ready to walk.

TABLE 10-2.	Criteria of Positive Caregiver–Infant Interactions
Area of Interaction	*Positive Caregiver Response*
Feeding	Offers infant adequate amounts and proper types of food and prepares food appropriately
	Holds infant in comfortable, secure position during feeding
	Burps infant during or after feeding
	Offers food at a comfortable pace for infant
Stimulation	Provides appropriate nonaggressive verbal stimulation to infant
	Provides a variety of tactile experiences and touches infant in caring ways other than during feeding times or when moving infant away from danger
	Provides appropriate toys and interacts with infant in a way satisfying to infant
Rest and sleep	Provides a quiet, relaxed environment and a regular, scheduled sleep time for infant
	Makes certain infant is adequately fed and warm and dry before putting down to sleep
Understanding of infant	Has realistic expectations of infant and recognizes infant's developing skills and behavior
	Has realistic view of own parenting skills
	View of infant's health condition similar to the view of medical or nursing diagnosis
Problem-solving initiative	Motivated to manage infant's problems; diligently seeks information about infant; follows through on plans involving infant
Interaction with other children	Demonstrates positive interaction with other children in home without aggression or hostility
Caregiver's recreation	Seeks positive outlets for own recreation and relaxation
Parenting role	Expresses satisfaction with parenting role; positive attitudes expressed

ing that nothing is gained by one's own activity and that the world does not respond to one's needs.

Conversely, caregivers who rush to anticipate every need give the infant no opportunity to test the environment. The opportunity to discover that through one's own actions the environment may be manipulated to suit one's own desires is withheld from the infant by these "smothering" caregivers. The box on Family Teaching Tips for infants in the first year of life suggests healthy childrearing patterns during infancy.

No one is perfect, and every family caregiver misinterprets the infant's signals at times. The caregiver may be tired, preoccupied, and responding momentarily to his or her own needs. The caregiver may not be able to ease the infant's pain or soothe the restlessness, but this also is a learning experience for the baby.

As mentioned earlier, the infant's development depends on a mutual relationship, with give and take, between the infant and the environment, of which the family caregivers play the most important role. Table 10-2 summarizes significant caregiver–infant interactions indicating positive behaviors.

During the first few weeks of life, actions such as kicking and sucking are simple reflex activities. In the next sequential stage, reflexes are coordinated and elaborated. For example, the eyes follow random hand movements (Fig. 10-4A). The infant finds that repetition of chance movements brings interesting changes, and in the latter part of the first year these acts become clearly intentional (see Fig. 10-4B). The infant expects that certain results follow certain actions.

The smiling face looking down is soon connected by the infant with the pleasure of being picked up, fed, or bathed. Anyone who smiles and talks softly to the infant may make that small face light up and cause squirming of anticipation. In only a few weeks, however, the infant learns that one particular person is the main source of comfort and pleasure.

An infant cannot apply abstract reasoning but understands only through the five senses. As the infant matures enough to recognize the mother or primary caregiver, the infant becomes fearful when this person disappears. Out of sight has always meant, to the infant, out of existence, and the infant cannot tolerate this. Thus, to the infant, self-assurance is necessary to confirm that objects and people do not cease to exist when out of sight. This is a learning experience on which the infant's entire attitude toward life depends.

The ancient game of "Peek-a-Boo" is a universal example of this learning technique. It is also one of the joys of infancy, as the child affirms the ability to control the disappearance and reappearance of self. In the same manner by which the infant affirms self-existence, the existence of others is confirmed even when temporarily out of sight.

NUTRITION

During the first year of life, the infant's rapid growth creates a need for nutrients greater than at any other time of life. The Academy of Pediatrics Committee on Nutrition

Figure 10-4
(A) In the early stages of infancy, hand movements are random.
(B) Later in infancy, hand movements are coordinated and intentional. The child follows her hands with her eyes as she brings an object to her mouth.

has endorsed breast-feeding as the best method of feeding infants.

Most of the infant's requirements for the first 4 to 6 months of life are supplied by either breast milk or commercial infant formulas. Nutrients that may need to be supplemented are vitamins C and D, iron, and fluoride. Breast-fed infants need supplements of iron as well as vitamin D, which can be supplied as vitamin drops. Most commercial infant formulas are enriched with vitamins C and D. Some infant formulas are fortified with iron. Infants who are fed home-prepared formulas (based on evaporated milk) need supplemental vitamin C and iron; however, evaporated milk has adequate amounts of vitamin D, which is unaffected by heating in the preparation of formula. Vitamin C can be supplied in orange juice or juices fortified with vitamin C.

Fluoride is needed in small amounts (0.25 mg/day) for strengthening calcification of the teeth and preventing tooth decay. A supplement is recommended for breast-fed and commercial formula-fed babies and for those whose home-prepared formulas are made with water that is deficient in fluoride. Vitamin preparations are available combined with fluoride.

Addition of Solid Foods

There is no exact time or order requirement for starting foods. However, at about 4 to 6 months of age the infant's iron supply becomes low and supplements of iron-rich foods are needed. Guidelines for introducing new foods into an infant's diet are provided in Table 10-3.

INFANT FEEDING

The infant knows only one way to take food: namely, to thrust the tongue forward as if to suck. This is called the **extrusion** (protrusion) **reflex** (Fig. 10-5) and has the effect

Figure 10-5
A baby tends to push his or her first solids out of the mouth with the tongue.

of pushing the solid food right out of the infant's mouth. The process of transferring food from the front of the mouth to the throat for swallowing is a complicated skill that must be learned. The eager, hungry baby is puzzled over this new turn of events and is apt to become frustrated and annoyed, protesting loudly and clearly. It is best to take the edge off the very hungry infant's appetite by giving part of the formula before proceeding with this new experience. If the family caregivers understand that pushing food out with the tongue does not mean rejection, their patience will be rewarded.

The baby's clothing (and the caregiver's as well) needs

TABLE 10-3.   **Suggested Feeding Schedule for the First Year of Life**

Age	Food Item	Amount*	Rationale
Birth–6 mo	Human milk or iron-fortified formula	Daily totals 0–1 mo 18–24 oz 1–2 mo 22–28 oz 2–3 mo 25–32 oz 3–4 mo 28–32 oz 4–5 mo 27–39 oz 5–6 mo 27–45 oz	Infants' well-developed sucking and rooting reflexes allow them to take in milk and formula. Infants do not accept semisolid food because their tongues protrude when a spoon is put in their mouths. They cannot transfer food to the back of the mouth. Human milk needs supplementation.
	Water	Not routinely recommended	Small amounts may be offered under special circumstances (eg, hot weather, elevated bilirubin level, or diarrhea).
4–6 mo	*Iron-fortified infant cereal;† begin with rice cereal (delay adding barley, oats, and wheat until 6th mo)	4–8 tbsp after mixing	At this age, there is a decrease of the extrusion reflex, the infant can depress the tongue and transfer semisolid food from a spoon to the back of the pharynx to swallow it.
	*Unsweetened fruit juices;†‡ plain, vitamin C–fortified	2–4 oz	Cereal adds a source of iron and B vitamins; fruit juices introduce a source of vitamin C.
	Dilute juices with equal parts of water		Delay orange, pineapple, grapefruit, or tomato juice until 6th mo.
	Human milk or iron-fortified formula	Daily totals 4–5 mo 27–39 oz 5–6 mo 27–45 oz	Do not offer water as a substitute for formula or breast milk, but rather as a source of additional fluids.
	Water	As desired	
7–8 mo	*Fruits, plain strained; avoid fruit desserts *Yogurt†	1–2 tbsp	Teething is beginning; thus, there is an increased ability to bite and chew.
	*Vegetables,† plain strained; avoid combination meat and vegetable dinners	5–7 tbsp	Vegetables introduce new flavors and textures.
	*Meats,† plain strained; avoid combination or high-protein, dinners	1–2 tbsp	Meat provides additional iron, protein, and B vitamins.
	*Crackers, toast, zwieback†	1 small serving	
	Iron-fortified infant cereal or enriched cream of wheat	4–6 tbsp	
	Fruit juices‡	4 oz	
	Human milk or iron-fortified formula	24–32 oz	Iron-fortified formula or iron supplementation with human milk is still needed because the infant is not consuming significant amounts of meat.
	Water	As desired	May introduce a cup to the infant.

(continued)

TABLE 10-3. Suggested Feeding Schedule for the First Year of Life (Continued)

Age	Food Item	Amount*	Rationale
9–10 mo	*Finger foods†—well-cooked, mashed, soft, bite-sized pieces of meat and vegetables	In small servings	Rhythmic biting movements begin; enhance this development with foods that require chewing.
	Iron-fortified infant cereal or enriched cream of wheat	4–6 tbsp	Decrease amounts of mashed foods as amounts of finger foods increase.
	Fruit juices‡	4 oz	
	Fruits	6–8 tbsp	
	Vegetables	6–8 tbsp	
	Meat, fish, poultry, yogurt, cottage cheese	4–6 tbsp	Formula or breast milk consumption may begin to decrease; thus, begin other sources of calcium, riboflavin, and protein (eg, cheese, yogurt, and cottage cheese).
	Human milk or iron-fortified formula	24–32 oz	
	Water	As desired	
11–12 mo	Soft table foods† as follows:		Motor skills are developing; enhance this development with more finger foods.
	Cereal; iron-fortified infant cereal; may introduce dry, unsweetened cereal as a finger food	4–6 tbsp	
	Breads; crackers, toast, zwieback	1 or 2 small servings	Rotary chewing motion develops; thus, child can handle whole foods, which require more chewing.
	Fruit juice‡	4 oz	
	Fruit: soft, canned fruits or ripe banana, cut up, peeled raw fruit as the infant approaches 12 mo	½ cup	Infant is relying less on breast milk or formula for nutrients; a proper selection of a variety of solid foods (fruits, vegetables, starches, protein sources, and dairy products) will continue to meet the young child's needs.
	Vegetables: soft cooked, cut into bite-sized pieces	½ cup	
	Meats and other protein sources: strips of tender, lean meat, cheese strips, peanut butter	2 oz or ½ cup chopped	Delay peanut butter until 12th month.
	Mashed potatoes, noodles		
	Human milk or iron-fortified infant formula	24–30 oz	
	Water	As desired	

* Amounts listed are daily totals and goals to be achieved gradually. Intake varies depending on the infant's appetite.
† New food items for age group.
(Adapted from Twin Cities District Dietetic Association. *Manual of clinical nutrition,* with permission from its publisher, Chronimed Publishing, 13911 Ridgedale Dr, Minneapolis, MN 55343, 1994 54–56.)
‡ The Committee on Nutrition of the American Academy of Pediatrics recommends that fruit juices be introduced when infant can drink from a cup.

protection when the baby is being held for a feeding. A small spoon fits the infant's mouth better than a large one and makes it easier to put food further back on the tongue—but not far enough to make the baby gag. If the food is pushed out, the caregiver must catch it and offer it again. The baby soon learns to manipulate the tongue and comes to enjoy this novel way of eating. To avoid the danger of aspiration, the caregiver must quiet an upset or crying baby before proceeding with feeding.

Foods are started in small amounts, 1 or 2 tsp daily.

Babies like their food smooth, thin, lukewarm, and bland. The choice of mealtime does not matter. It works best, at first, to offer one new food at a time, allowing 4 or 5 days before introducing another so that the baby becomes accustomed to it. This method also helps determine which food is the culprit if the baby has a reaction to a new food.

When teeth start erupting, anytime between 4 and 7 months of age, the infant appreciates a piece of zwieback or hard toast to practice chewing on. At about 9 or 10 months of age, after a few teeth have erupted, chopped foods can be substituted for puréed foods. Breast milk or formula gradually is replaced with whole milk as the infant learns to drink from a cup. This change takes some time because the infant doubtless continues to derive comfort from sucking at the breast or bottle. Infants need fat and should not be given reduced-fat milk (skim, 1%, or 2%).

PREPARATION OF FOODS

Various puréed baby foods, chopped junior foods, and prepared milk formulas are available on the market. These products save caregivers much preparation time, but many families cannot afford them. No matter which type of food is used, it is important for family caregivers to read food labels carefully to avoid foods that have undesirable additives, especially sugar and salt.

The nurse can point out that vegetables and fruits can be cooked and strained or puréed in a blender and are just as acceptable to the baby. Baby foods prepared at home should be made from freshly prepared foods, not canned, to avoid commercial additives. Labels of frozen foods that are used should be checked for added sugar, salt, or other unnecessary ingredients. Excess blended food can be stored in the freezer in ice cube trays for future use. Cereals may be cooked and formulas may be prepared at home as well. Instead of purchasing junior foods, the caregiver can substitute well-cooked, unseasoned table foods that have been mashed or ground.

Preparation and storage of baby food at home require careful sanitary practices. All equipment used in the preparation of the infant's food must be carefully cleaned with hot, soapy water and rinsed thoroughly.

Some families prefer to spend more money for convenience and economize elsewhere, but no one should be made to feel that a baby's health or well-being depends on commercially prepared foods.

The well baby's appetite is the best index of the proper amount of food. Healthy babies enjoy eating and accept most foods, but they do not like strongly flavored or bitter foods. If the baby shows a definite dislike for any particular food, there is no reason to force it because this may develop into a battle of wills. A dislike for a certain food is not always permanent, and the rejected food may be offered again later. The important point is to avoid making an issue of likes or dislikes. The caregiver also should avoid introducing any personal attitudes about food preferences.

SELF-FEEDING

The infant has an overpowering urge to investigate and to learn. At around 7 or 8 months of age, the baby may grab the spoon from the caregiver, examine it, and mouth it. The baby also sticks fingers in the food to feel the texture and to bring it to the mouth for tasting (Fig. 10-6). All this is an essential, although messy, part of the learning experience.

After preliminary testing, the infant's next task is to try self-feeding. The baby soon finds that the motions involved in getting a spoon right side up into the mouth are too complex; thus, fingers become favored over the spoon. However, the infant returns to the spoon again until he or she eventually succeeds in getting some food from spoon to mouth, at least part of the time. The nurse can help family caregivers understand that all this is not deliberate messing, to be forbidden, but rather a necessary part of the infant's learning.

Weaning the Infant

Weaning, either from the breast or bottle, must be attempted gradually, without fuss or strain. The infant is still testing the environment. The abrupt removal of a main source of satisfaction—sucking—before basic distrust of the environment has been conquered may prove detrimental to normal development. The speed with which weaning is accomplished must be suited to each infant's readiness

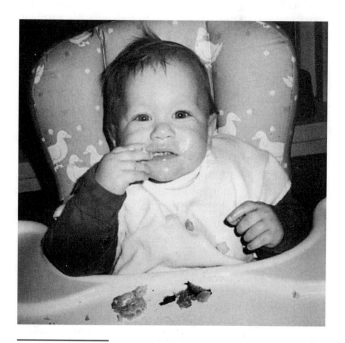

Figure 10-6
Eating by yourself is a messy business but so much fun!

to give up this form of pleasure for a more mature way of life.

At the age of 5 or 6 months, the infant who has watched others drink from a cup usually is ready to try a sip when it is offered. The infant seldom is ready at this point, however, to give up the pleasures of sucking altogether. Forcing the child to give up sucking creates resistance and suspicion. It is better to let the infant set the pace.

An infant who takes food from a dish and milk from a cup during the day may still be reluctant to give up a bedtime bottle. However, the infant must never be permitted to take a bottle of formula, milk, or juice along to bed. **Pedodontists** (dentists who specialize in the care and treatment of children's teeth) discourage the bedtime bottle because the sugar from formula or sweetened juice coats the infant's teeth for long periods and causes erosion of the enamel on the deciduous teeth, resulting in a condition known as "**bottle mouth**" or "**nursing bottle**" **caries**. This condition can also occur in infants who sleep with their mother and nurse intermittently throughout the night. In addition to the caries, liquid from milk, formula, or juice can pool in the mouth and flow into the eustachian tube, causing otitis media, if the infant falls asleep with the bottle. A bottle of plain water or a pacifier can be used if the infant needs the comfort of sucking at bedtime.

A few babies resist drinking from a cup. Milk needs (calcium, vitamin D) may be met by offering yogurt, custard, cottage cheese, and other milk products until the infant becomes accustomed to the cup. The caregiver should be cautioned not to use honey or corn syrup to sweeten milk because of the danger of botulism in these products, which the infant's system is not strong enough to combat.

During the second half of the first year, the infant's milk consumption alone is not likely to be sufficient to meet caloric, protein, mineral, and vitamin needs.

Women, Infants, Children Food Program

Women, Infants, Children (WIC) is a special supplemental food program for pregnant, breast-feeding, or postpartum women and infants and children as old as 5 years of age. This federal program provides nutritious supplemental foods, nutrition information, and health care referrals. It is available free of charge to persons who are eligible, based on financial and nutritional needs, and who live in a WIC service area. The family's food stamp benefits or schoolchildren's breakfast and lunch program benefits are unaffected. The foods prescribed by the program include iron-fortified infant formula and cereal, infant juices, milk, dry beans or peas, peanut butter, cheese, cereal, juice, and eggs. These foods may be purchased with vouchers or distributed through clinics. To encourage the use of WIC services, many health care facilities give WIC information to eligible mothers during prenatal visits or at the time of delivery.

HEALTH PROMOTION AND MAINTENANCE

Routine checkups, immunizations, family teaching, and education about accident prevention are important aspects of health promotion and maintenance. Immunizations and frequent well-baby visits help ensure good health. Family teaching and accident prevention help caregivers provide the best care for their rapidly growing child.

Routine Checkups

During the first year of life, at least six visits to the health care facility are recommended. These are essentially considered well-baby visits and usually occur at 2 weeks, 2 months, 4 months, 6 months, 9 months, and 12 months. During these visits, the nurse assesses the infant's growth

A Personal Glimpse

Prepped as we were by those "over-the-counter" baby books, our first out-of-the-hospital visit to the pediatrician seemed daunting beforehand. We had many questions. The staff answered all our questions in a respectful and unhurried way and we felt more at ease. For our second visit, we were less apprehensive. Natty received his immunization shots and all went well. But that night he was unusually fussy and he had a slight fever. We were alarmed. Was this a bad reaction to the immunization? Could he develop a seizure disorder (our neighbor had once told us that her niece developed a seizure disorder after her immunizations)? We knew that we were probably overreacting, but still we worried all night. In the morning, Natty was still sick. We immediately called the doctor's office. The nurse understood our concern and assured us that it is not uncommon for babies to have a slight fever and become irritable after an immunization. We appreciated her support but wished we had known ahead of time. That's one sleepless night we could have done without.

John and Coco

and development, nutrition, and sleep, the caregiver–infant relationship, and any potential problems. The infant's weight, height, and head circumference are documented and the infant receives immunizations to guard against disease. Family teaching, particularly for first-time caregivers, is an integral part of health promotion and maintenance.

Immunizations

Every infant is entitled to the best possible protection against disease. Obviously, infants cannot take proper precautions, so family caregivers and health professionals must be responsible for them. This care extends beyond the daily needs for food, sleep, cleanliness, love, and security to a concern for the infant's future health and well-being. Protection is available against a number of serious or disabling diseases, such as diphtheria, smallpox, tetanus, hepatitis, polio, mumps, measles, German measles (rubella), and *Haemophilus influenzae* meningitis, making it unnecessary to take chances with a child's health due to inadequate immunization.

IMMUNIZATION SCHEDULE

The Academy of Pediatrics, through its committee on the control of infectious diseases, has recommended a schedule of immunizations for healthy children living in normal conditions (Table 10-4). Immunizations should be given within the prescribed timetable, unless the child's physical condition makes this impossible. An immunization need not be postponed if the child has a cold but should be postponed if the child has an acute febrile condition or a condition causing immunosuppression, or if he or she is receiving corticosteroids, radiation, or antimetabolites.

Side effects vary with the type of immunization. The most common side effect is a fever within the first 24 to 48 hours and possibly a local reaction at the site of injection. These reactions are treated symptomatically with acetaminophen for the fever and warm compresses to the injection site.

Many children do not get their initial immunizations in infancy and may not get them until they reach school age, when immunizations are required for school entrance. Health care personnel should make every effort to encourage parents to have their children immunized in infancy to avoid the danger of possible epidemic outbreaks. For instance, measles outbreaks, resulting in the deaths of children, have been increasing at an alarming rate because of inadequate immunization. Serious illnesses, permanent disability, and deaths from inadequate immunizations are senseless and tragic. Answer any questions the caregiver may have about immunizations. Remember, however, that the caregiver has a right to refuse immunization if he or she has been fully informed about immunizations and any possible reactions. Maintain a nonjudgmental viewpoint throughout the episode.

TABLE 10-4. Recommended Childhood Immunization Schedule

Age → Vaccine ↓	Birth	1 mo.	2 mos.	4 mos.	6 mos.	12 mos.	15 mos.	18 mos.	4–6 yrs.	11–12 yrs.	14–16 yrs.
Hepatitis B	Hep B-1		Hep B-2		Hep B-3					Hep B	
Diphtheria, Tetanus, Pertussis			DTP	DTP	DTP	DTP[3] (DTap at 15 + m)			DTP or DTaP	Td	
H. influenzae type b			Hib	Hib	Hib	Hib[4]					
Polio			OPV	OPV	OPV				OPV		
Measles, Mumps, Rubella						MMR			MMR or MMR		
Varicella Zoster Virus Vaccine							Var			Var	

Approved by the Advisory Committee on Immunization Practices, the American Academy of Pediatrics, and the American Academy of Family Physicians.
Note: At 11 to 12 years of age, hepatitis B vaccine should be administered to children not previously vaccinated, and varicella zoster virus vaccine should be administered to children not previously vaccinated who lack a reliable history of chickenpox.

Family Teaching

Since mothers are discharged so early after giving birth, it is important to use every opportunity to perform teaching and promote healthy baby care. Well-baby visits provide an opportunity to ask the caregiver about concerns and to provide teaching. During well visits, offer guidance to help caregivers prepare for the many changes that occur with each developmental level. Discuss normal growth and development milestones, but emphasize that these milestones vary from infant to infant. The infant's overall progress is the most important concern, not when he or she accomplishes a given task as compared to another infant or a developmental table. Discuss any infant sleep and activity concerns that the caregiver has. Encourage the caregiver to seek information about any other problems, worries, or anxieties he or she has. Provide ample time and opportunity for the caregivers to ask questions and gain information. A perceptive nurse not only asks if the caregiver has concerns, but also suggests possible topics that may need to be reinforced. Some of those topics are discussed here.

BATHING THE INFANT

A daily bath is unnecessary but is desirable and soothing in very hot weather. Placing the baby into a small tub for a bath rather than giving a sponge bath may have a soothing and comforting effect, as long as the baby is healthy and has no open skin areas (Fig. 10-7). The small tub or large basin bath is described in the Family Teaching display.

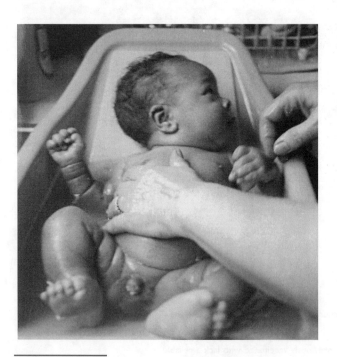

Figure 10-7
Bath time can be an enjoyable experience for the infant.

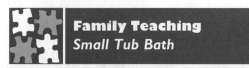

Family Teaching
Small Tub Bath

Make sure room is warm and draft-free. Wash hands, put on protective covering, and assemble the following equipment:

- Large basin or small tub
- Mild soap
- Nonsterile protective gloves
- Clean cotton balls
- Soft washcloth
- Large soft towel or small cotton blanket
- Clean diaper and clothes for infant

Fill tub with several inches of warm water (95°–100°F [35°–37°C]). This is comfortably warm to the elbow. Place basin or tub in crib or other protected surface.

Never turn from the baby during bathing. *Always* keep at least one hand holding the infant.

Procedure
Wash the infant's head and face at the beginning of the bath, following the procedure for a sponge bath (see Chap. 7). A mild shampoo may be used for the infant over 1 month old, but soap is adequate.

After drying the head, undress the infant and examine for skin rashes or excoriations. Wearing protective gloves, remove diaper and wipe any feces from diaper area.

Place infant in tub and soap the body, supporting head and shoulders on your arm. If infant's skin is dry, soap may be eliminated or a prescribed soap substitute used.

If the baby is enjoying the experience, make it a leisurely one, engaging the infant in talk, paddling in the water, and playing for a few extra minutes. When finished, lift infant from tub, place on dry towel and pat dry, with careful attention to folds and creases (underarms, neck, perineal area).

After the bath, gently separate the female infant's labia and cleanse with moistened cotton balls and clean water, wiping from *front to back* to avoid bacterial contamination from the anal region. Circumcised male infants need only be inspected for cleanliness. Uncircumcised males may have the foreskin gently retracted to remove smegma and accumulated debris. The foreskin is gently replaced. Do not force foreskin if not easily retracted, but document and report this occurrence.

The bathing procedure is essentially the same for the older infant. When old enough to sit and move about freely, the infant may enjoy the regular bathtub, but often this is frightening to him or her. Splashing about in a small tub may be more fun, especially with a floating toy. An infant in a tub should always be held securely. If possible, time should be scheduled so that this is a leisurely process, a time for the caregiver and baby to enjoy. The procedure for sponge baths is discussed in Chapter 7. As noted in Chapter 7, regular shampooing is important to prevent seborrheic dermatitis (cradle cap), which is caused by a collection of **seborrhea**, yellow crusty patches of lesions on the scalp.

Scented or talcum powder should not be used after the bath; powder tends to cake in the creases, causing irritation, and it also may be inhaled by the infant, causing respiratory problems. Scented powders and lotions cause allergic reactions in some babies. In any case, a clean baby has a sweet smell without the use of additional fragrances. Excessively dry skin may benefit from the application of lanolin or A and D Ointment, but oils are believed to block pores and cause infection. Various medicated ointments are available for excoriated skin areas.

After the bath, the baby's fingernails need to be inspected and cut if long. Otherwise, the baby may scratch his or her face during random arm movements. The nails should be cut straight across with great care, holding the arm securely and the hand firmly while cutting.

CARING FOR THE DIAPER AREA

To prevent diaper rash, soiled diapers should be changed frequently. Check every 2 to 4 hours while the infant is awake to see if the diaper is soiled. It is unnecessary to wake the baby to change the diaper. Cleanse the diaper area with water and a mild soap if needed (see Parent Teaching Tips to Prevent Diaper Rash in Chap. 11). Commercial diaper wipes also may be used, but they are an added expense (Fig. 10-8).

Diapers come in various sizes and shapes. The choice of cloth versus disposable diapers is controversial: disposable diapers have an environmental impact, but cloth diapers are inconvenient and associated with a higher risk of infection. Whatever the type, size, and folding method used,

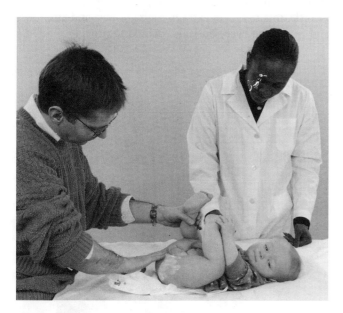

Figure 10-8
Noting that the dad has used an overly generous amount of Desitin cream, the nurse takes this opportunity to provide teaching on care of the diaper area.

there should be no bunched material between the thighs. Two popular cloth diaper styles are the oblong strip pinned at the sides or the square diaper folded kite-fashion. The latter has the advantage of being useful for different ages and sizes. When folding a cloth diaper for a boy, the excess material is folded in the front; for a girl, it is folded to the back. Safety pins must *always* be closed when they are used to fasten the diaper. When removed, they must be closed and placed out of the infant's reach.

For the older infant, the diaper must be fastened snugly at the hips and legs to prevent feces from running out the open spaces. Cleaning a soiled crib and a smeared baby once or twice serves as an effective reminder!

DRESSING THE INFANT

Dressing an infant can sometimes create a dilemma, especially for the first-time caregiver. Sometimes it is difficult just to get the clothes on the baby. For instance, babies tend to spread their little hands when the caregiver is trying to put on a top with long sleeves. The easiest way to put an infant's arm into a sleeve is to work the sleeve so that the armhole and the opening are held together, then to reach through the armhole and pull the arm through the opening. Clothing should not bind; it should allow freedom of movement and should be appropriate for the weather.

One rule of thumb is to dress the infant with the same amount of clothing that the adult is comfortable in. Overdressing in hot weather can cause overheating and prickly heat (miliaria rubra; see Chap. 11). In very hot weather, a diaper may be sufficient. When the infant begins to crawl, long pants help protect the knees from becoming chafed from the rug or flooring. When dressing the infant to go outdoors in cold weather, a head covering is important, since infants loose a great amount of heat through their heads. In hot, sunny weather, the infant should not spend much time in the direct sun, since the infant's skin is tender and burns easily.

Choosing shoes for the infant can be a problem to the new caregiver. Infants do not need hard-soled shoes; in fact, health care providers often recommend that infants be allowed to go barefoot and wear shoes only to protect them from harsh surfaces. Shoes with stiff soles actually hamper the development of the infant's foot. Sneakers made with a smooth lining with no rough surfaces to irritate the infant's foot are a good choice. They should be durable and flexible and have ample room in the toe. Properly made moccasins also are a good choice. High-topped shoes are unnecessary. Socks should provide plenty of toe room. Shoes should be replaced frequently as the infant's feet grow.

DENTAL CARE

When teething begins in the second half of the first year, the caregiver can start practicing good dental hygiene with the infant. Initially, the caregiver can rub the gums and newly erupting teeth with a clean, damp cloth while

Family Teaching
Tips for Infant Safety

1. The infant should always be placed in an approved infant car carrier when in the car.
2. Crib and playpen bars should be spaced less than 2½" apart.
3. Never leave infant unattended on a high surface.
4. Always close safety pins and keep out of infant's reach.
5. Choose toys carefully:
   a. Watch for loose or sharp parts.
   b. Avoid small buttons or parts that can come off and choke infant.
   c. Check for nontoxic material.
5. Never leave infant unattended in a car.
6. Babyproof your home:
   a. Cover unused plugs with plastic covers.
   b. Keep electrical cords out of sight.
   c. Move all toxic substances (cleaning fluids, detergents, insecticides) out of reach and keep them locked up.
   d. Keep small articles (such as buttons and marbles) off the floor and out of infant's reach.
   e. Remove tablecloths or dresser scarves that infant might grasp and pull.
   f. Remove any house plants that may be poisonous.
   g. Pad sharp corners of low furniture or remove them from infant's living area.
7. Never leave infant alone in the bath.
8. Turn household hot water to a safe temperature—120°F (48.8°C)—to avoid burns.
9. Protect infant from inhaling lead paint dust (from remodeling) or chewing on surfaces painted with lead paint.
10. Place medicines in locked cupboards; remind family and friends (especially those with grown children or no children) to do the same.
11. Be one step ahead of baby's development, prepared for the next stage.

holding the infant in the lap. This time can be made pleasant by talking or singing to the infant. Brushing the teeth, using a small, soft brush, is usually not started until several teeth have erupted. Gentle cleansing with plain water is adequate. Toothpaste is not recommended at this stage because the infant will swallow too much of it.

Accident Prevention

It is important to discuss safety issues with caregivers. Provide information about car safety and childproofing and preventing aspiration, falls, burns, poisoning, and bathing accidents. Remind caregivers that the infant is rapidly developing and safety precautions should stay one step ahead of the infant's developmental abilities. Older children in the family should be taught to be watchful for possible dangers to the infant, and caregivers must be alert to poten-

tial dangers that may be introduced by the sibling, such as unsafe toys, rough play, or jealous harmful behavior. (See Family Teaching Tips for Infant Safety.)

THE INFANT IN THE HEALTH CARE FACILITY

Hospitalization, however brief, hampers the infant's normal pattern of living. Disruption occurs even if a family caregiver can stay with the infant during hospitalization. All or most of the sick infant's energies may be needed to cope with the illness. However, if given sufficient affection and loving care and if promptly restored to the family, the infant is not likely to suffer any serious psychological problems. Long-term hospitalization, however, may present serious problems, even with the best of care.

Illness in itself is frustrating, causing pain and discomfort and limiting normal activity, none of which the infant can understand. If the hospital atmosphere is emotionally unresponsive, offering little if any cuddling or rocking, the infant may fail to respond to treatment, despite cleanliness and proper hygiene. Touching, rocking, and cuddling a child are essential elements of nursing care (Fig. 10-9).

Hospitalization may have other adverse effects. The small infant matures largely as a result of physical development. If hindered from reaching out and responding to the environment, the infant becomes apathetic and ceases to learn. This situation is particularly apparent when restraints are necessary to keep the child from undoing surgical procedures or dressings or to prevent injury. The child in restraints needs an extra measure of love and attention and the use of every possible method to provide comfort.

Figure 10-9
Holding and cuddling can ease the discomfort and fear of the hospital experience.

Parent–Nurse Relationship

The nurse's relationship with family caregivers is extremely important. The hospitalized infant needs continued stimulation, empathetic care, and loving attention from family caregivers. Encourage caregivers to feed, hold, diaper, and participate in the care of their infant as much as they can. Through conscientious use of the nursing process, evaluate the needs of the caregivers and the infant and plan care with these needs in mind. Identify and acknowledge the caregivers' apprehensions and develop plans to resolve or eliminate them. Make arrangements for rooming-in for the family caregiver, if possible. Family caregivers often are sensitive to changes in their infant that may help to identify discomfort, pain, or fear. Caregivers may sometimes assist during treatments and other procedures by stroking, talking to, and looking directly at the infant, thus helping to provide comfort during a time of stress. After the procedure, the infant may benefit from rocking, cuddling, singing, stroking, and other comfort measures that the family caregivers may provide. If the family caregivers are unavailable or can spend only limited time with the infant, the nursing staff must meet these emotional needs.

■ KEY POINTS

- During the first year of life, the infant grows and develops skills more quickly than at any other time of life.

- During the first year of life, the infant progresses from a totally dependent being to one who is ready to "take off and cruise solo."

- The infant whose world is secure develops the basic sense of trust that will enable progression to the next stage of development.

- The infant's development depends on a mutual relationship, with give and take, between the infant and the environment. Family caregivers play the most significant role in this interaction.

- The infant's nutrition needs are met during the first 4 to 6 months of life by breast milk or formula. Additional vitamins A and C, iron, and fluoride may be needed.

- During the second 6 months of life, the infant is introduced to solid foods and learns to drink from a cup.

- Routine immunizations scheduled in the first year of life include those for hepatitis B virus, diphtheria, pertussis, tetanus, *Haemophilus influenzae* type b, and polio. Measles, mumps and rubella, and varicella (chickenpox) vaccines are scheduled between 12 and 18 months of age.

- The nurse has a primary responsibility to provide infant care health teaching during every contact with the caregiver.

- Safety, important in all stages of life, becomes critical as the infant becomes more independent.

 CRITICAL THINKING

1. Tony Ricardo brings 6-month-old Essie for a routine checkup. Formulate a plan for the visit. Identify the characteristics to observe during the physical examination, immunizations she will need at this visit (assuming she is up to date), nutritional factors to cover, and other age-appropriate teaching.

2. As you review nutrition with Mr. Ricardo, he states that Essie loves her bedtime bottle. Explain to him your concerns about this practice, and propose a plan to avoid the problems that often result from bedtime bottles.

3. Katya Lawrence brings 9-month-old Bart to the clinic. During the visit, she seems worried that Bart has only two teeth. Describe your response to her. Identify the physical trait you referred to when constructing your answer.

4. Katya and Bart live in an apartment that has a living room, kitchen, bathroom, bedroom, and nursery (baby's bedroom). Going room to room, list all the safety precautions that Katya should take to protect Bart as he becomes more mobile and independent.

5. Tammy Jackson is an unmarried 17-year-old with a 4-month-old daughter, Shari. Her income is very limited. Describe the guidance you will give her to help her get nutritious formula and baby food for Shari. Detail information specific for your area.

6. At Shari's 6-month checkup, Tammy tells you that Shari doesn't like baby food because she spits it out. What will you tell Tammy to help her understand what is happening? What other information about feeding infants will you provide for Tammy?

BIBLIOGRAPHY

Brazelton TB. To listen to a child. Reading, MA: Addison-Wesley, 1985.

Brazelton TB. What every baby knows. New York: Ballantine Books, 1987.

Castiglia PT, Harbin RE. Child health care: Process and practice. Philadelphia: JB Lippincott, 1992.

Coryell J, Provost B. Stability of Bayley Motor Scale scores in the first year of life [abstr]. Phys Ther 69(10):834–841, 1989.

Eschleman MM. Introductory nutrition and diet therapy, 3d ed. Philadelphia: Lippincott-Raven, 1996.

Pillitteri A. Maternal and child health nursing, 2d ed. Philadelphia: JB Lippincott, 1995.

Premomo J, Bruck AM, Greenstreet PK, et al. The high environmental cost of disposable diapers. MCN 15(5):279, 1990.

Schuster CS, Ashburn SS. The process of human development, 3d ed. Philadelphia: JB Lippincott, 1992.

Spock B, Rothenberg MB. Dr. Spock's baby and child care. New York: Pocket Books, 1992.

Wong DL. Whaley and Wong's nursing care of infants and children, 5th ed. St. Louis: Mosby, 1995.

Chapter II

Health Problems of the Infant

SPECIAL NURSING CONSIDERATIONS

PSYCHOLOGICAL PROBLEMS
  Nonorganic Failure to Thrive
  Nursing Process for the Infant With Nonorganic Failure to Thrive

GASTROINTESTINAL DISORDERS
  Malnutrition
  Food Allergies
  Nursing Process for the Nutritionally Deprived Infant
  Diarrhea and Gastroenteritis
  Nursing Process for the Infant With Diarrhea and Gastroenteritis
  Colic
  Pyloric Stenosis
  Nursing Process for the Infant With Pyloric Stenosis
  Congenital Aganglionic Megacolon
  Nursing Process for the Infant Undergoing Surgery for Congenital Megacolon
  Intussusception

CIRCULATORY SYSTEM DISORDERS
  Iron Deficiency Anemia
  Sickle Cell Disease
  Nursing Process for the Child With Sickle Cell Crisis

RESPIRATORY SYSTEM DISORDERS
  Acute Nasopharyngitis (Common Cold)
  Otitis Media
  Acute Bronchiolitis
  Bacterial Pneumonia
  Nursing Process for the Infant With a Respiratory Disorder
  Sudden Infant Death Syndrome

GENITOURINARY DISORDERS
  Hydrocele
  Cryptorchidism
  Urinary Tract Infections
  Nursing Process for the Child With a Urinary Tract Infection
  Wilms' Tumor (Nephroblastoma)

NERVOUS SYSTEM DISORDERS
  Acute or Nonrecurrent Seizures
  Nursing Process for the Child at Risk for Seizures
  Haemophilus influenzae Meningitis
  Nursing Process for the Children With Meningitis

SKIN AND MUCOUS MEMBRANE DISORDERS
  Miliaria Rubra
  Diaper Rash
  Candidiasis
  Seborrheic Dermatitis
  Impetigo
  Acute Infantile Eczema
  Nursing Process for the Child With Infantile Eczema

STUDENT OBJECTIVES

On completion of this chapter, the student will be able to:

1. Identify seven ways the infant's respiratory system differs from the adult's.
2. Describe the characteristics of the child with nonorganic failure to thrive.
3. Differentiate between mild diarrhea and severe diarrhea.
4. Identify the symptoms of pyloric stenosis.
5. State another name for congenital megacolon, and list the common symptoms.
6. Describe the diagnosis and treatment of intussusception.
7. Identify the common causes of iron deficiency anemia.
8. Explain how a) sickle cell trait and b) sickle cell anemia are inherited.
9. Describe the behavior of the infant with acute otitis media.
10. Describe the effect sudden infant death syndrome has on the infant's family.
11. Describe the nursing care specific to a child at high risk for seizures.
12. List four complications of *Haemophilus influenzae* meningitis.
13. Identify the causative organism of thrush.

KEY TERMS

colic	myringotomy
craniotabes	nuchal rigidity
currant jelly stools	opisthotonos
febrile seizure	orchiopexy
gastroenteritis	pruritus
invagination	purpuric rash
kwashiorkor	rumination
lactose	teratogenicity
lactose intolerance	urticaria
marasmus	

Infancy is a period of continuing adjustment for the child and the family. The infant is adjusting to physical life outside the uterus and social life within the family. Family members are adjusting to their new roles as parents or siblings and to the presence of this new person in their midst. Although the adjustment is more gradual than the abrupt transition required at birth, it can still involve sufficient physiologic and psychosocial stresses to create health problems during the first year of life.

Three factors that help determine how health problems are manifested in the infant are:

1. The pathogenic agent—how virulent the organism or how great the stress
2. The environment—how favorable or unfavorable external conditions are, including nutrition and hygiene
3. The infant—his or her resistance to stress and ability to adapt to it, and body responses to biologic, chemical, and physical injuries.

All three factors need to be considered when planning nursing care for the infant and family. Remember that even a minor health problem can create great anxiety for concerned caregivers.

Infants can rapidly become very ill, often with a high fever (102°–104°F [38.9°–40°C] or more). Fortunately, with prompt intervention, they usually recover just as quickly. Diagnosis of an infant's health problem is no simple matter, partly because the infant cannot say where it hurts and partly because the clinical manifestations are similar for many different disorders, some minor, some serious.

Most acute health problems result from a respiratory or gastrointestinal (GI) infection or from an uncorrected, or perhaps even undetected, congenital deviation. Respiratory problems occur more often and with greater severity in infants because of their immature body defenses and small and undeveloped anatomic structures (Fig. 11-1). Sometimes these problems require hospitalization, interrupting development of the infant–family relationship and the infant's patterns of sleeping, eating, and stimulation. Although the illness may be acute, if recovery is rapid and

the hospitalization brief, the infant probably will experience few if any long-term effects. If, however, the condition is chronic or so serious that it requires long-term care, both infant and family may suffer serious consequences.

SPECIAL NURSING CONSIDERATIONS

Some special nursing considerations are evident in most nursing plans of care for the ill infant. They include infection control, the promotion of normal growth and development, and safety precautions. General nursing diagnoses and interventions are discussed below.

A common nursing diagnosis for the infant with a health problem is *Risk for Infection*. The infant may be especially susceptible to infectious diseases because the immature immune system can easily become weakened. Malnutrition, dehydration, and surgery are typical conditions that place the infant at risk. To protect the infant, the guidelines shown in Box 11-1 should be carefully followed.

"Altered Growth and Development related to inadequate environmental stimulation or a chronic condition" is another common nursing diagnosis for the ill infant. In the first weeks and months of life, the infant is developing quickly. Illness can slow the developmental process.

Provide age-appropriate sensory stimulation, within the constraints of the infant's condition. Coo to and cuddle the infant, talk to him or her in warm, soft tones, and provide opportunities to fulfill sucking needs. Engage the infant in play. Singing songs, looking at picture books, reading stories, reciting rhymes, playing "Peek-a-Boo," and other activities are strongly recommended. Toys should be introduced that are safe and age-appropriate and stimulate interest and responsiveness. Balloons are not safe if kept within the infant's reach. Provide family caregivers with information about normal developmental activities appropriate for the infant and encourage them to provide sensory and cognitive stimulation. This approach helps the infant

Box 11-1. *Guidelines to Prevent Infection*

- Follow good handwashing procedures.
- Follow aseptic technique and transmission precautions.
- Teach good handwashing and aseptic techniques to family and all who come in contact with the infant.
- Keep anyone with viral or respiratory infections from contact with the infant.
- Report any signs of systemic infection—for example, fever, pulse or respiratory changes, pain, swelling, tenderness, lethargy, elevated white cell count
- Observe neurologic signs—for example, nuchal rigidity, irritability, behavior changes

The infant's respiratory system differs from the adult's in that the infant's:

Soft palate is much greater

Larynx is 2–3 cervical vertebrae higher, which makes him more vulnerable to aspiration

Tongue is larger in proportion to mouth, so potential for airway obstruction is greater

Lungs have fewer true alveoli at birth, but continue to gain new alveoli and existing ones increase in size

Airway has larger proportion of soft tissue, so potential for edema is greater

Cricoid cartilage encircles airway, so support is less; cartilaginous support increases in late school-age

Mucous membranes lining the airway are more loosely attached, so potential for airway edema is greater

Figure 11-1
The infant or young child is at greater risk than the adult for airway obstruction due to anatomic differences in the respiratory tract. Alveolar damage in infancy is often not permanent, but airway damage remains throughout life.

build trust in the caregiver, which is a major developmental task according to Erikson. It also helps caregivers feel needed and useful.

Risk for Injury related to the infant's developmental age is a nursing diagnosis relevant to the nursing process for all illnesses. Follow safety practices conscientiously. Keep side rails completely up, except when directly attending the infant. Infant seats are recommended instead of high chairs. Never leave equipment within the reach of an infant. Restraints should be used with extreme caution, only if necessary to keep the infant or child from interfering with treatments. Teach the family caregivers safety practices and reinforce good safety rules at every opportunity. Always consider these nursing diagnoses when developing a nursing careplan.

PSYCHOLOGICAL PROBLEMS

Nonorganic Failure to Thrive

Four principal factors are necessary for human growth: food, rest and activity, adequate secretions of hormones, and a satisfactory relationship with a caregiver or nurturing person who provides consistent, loving human contact and stimulation. When one of these four factors is missing, or when the infant has a major birth defect, such as congenital heart disease or a metabolic disorder, growth is disturbed and development can be delayed.

Infants who fail to gain weight and who show signs of delayed development are classified as failure-to-thrive infants. Failure to thrive can be divided into two classifications: organic failure to thrive, which is a result of a disease condition, and nonorganic failure to thrive (NFTT), which has no apparent physical cause. The section below discusses NFTT, as organic failure to thrive is covered under specific diseases.

CLINICAL MANIFESTATIONS

Infants with NFTT are often listless, seriously below average weight and height, and immobile for long periods. They may be unresponsive to (or actually try to avoid) cuddling and vocalization. Examination of the infant is likely to reveal no organic cause for this condition. Examination of the family relationship, particularly the mother–infant relationship, however, often provides important insights into the problem.

The family relationships of these infants are often so disrupted that there is no warm, close relationship with a family caregiver. For some reason, proper attachment has not occurred. Often the father is absent or emotionally unavailable, adding to the mother's feelings of isolation and inadequacy and leading to an atmosphere of additional stress and conflict.

The problem is not with the caregiver alone, nor with the infant, but instead with their interaction and mutual lack of responsiveness. They are not in harmony. The caregiver does not stimulate the infant; therefore, the infant has no one to respond to and fails to do the "cute baby" things that would gain attention and stimulation. The infant cannot accomplish the developmental task of establishing basic trust.

Infants with NFTT often fall into the classification of "difficult" or irritable babies, but others may be listless and passive and do not seem to care about feedings. A common characteristic is **rumination** (voluntary regurgitation), perhaps as a means of self-satisfaction when the desired response is not received from the caregiver. When rumination occurs, a chain of events is activated that further strains the caregiver–infant relationship. The infant loses weight, sometimes becoming severely emaciated, grows increasingly listless and irritable, and because of frequent vomiting smells "sour." None of this makes for an attractive baby to love, cuddle, and show off.

DIAGNOSIS

The infant must be thoroughly evaluated by the physician to rule out a systemic or congenital disorder. Signs of deprivation are important elements in the diagnosis. When the infant begins to improve in a nurturing atmosphere, the diagnosis is confirmed.

TREATMENT

Treatment initially depends almost entirely on good nursing care. By teaching child care skills, acting as a role model, and supporting caregiver–infant interactions, the nurse can help reverse the infant's growth failure and begin an improved caregiver–infant relationship.

Prognosis is uncertain. Much depends on the support and counseling the family receives. Long-term care is almost certainly necessary and may require several members of the health care team, such as a family therapist, clergy, social worker, and public health nurse. Avoid judgmental, stereotyped feelings when dealing with the family of such an infant. A positive, nonjudgmental attitude on the part of the nurse can have a direct and lasting effect on the family's interaction with their infant.

🔊🏷 *Nursing Process for the Infant With*
📣🏷 *Nonorganic Failure to Thrive*

ASSESSMENT

Conduct a careful physical assessment of the infant, including skin turgor, assessment of the anterior fontanelle, signs of emaciation, weight, temperature, apical pulse, respira-

tions, responsiveness, listlessness, and irritability. Observe for rumination or odor of vomitus.

When interviewing the family caregiver, carefully observe the interaction between the caregiver and the infant and note the caregiver's responsiveness to the infant's needs and the infant's response to the caregiver. Listen carefully for underlying problems while talking with the family caregivers. Note if other supportive, involved people are present or if the caregiver is a single parent with no support system. Take a careful history of feeding and sleeping patterns or problems. Assess the caregiver's confidence in handling the infant and note any apparent indication of feelings of stress or inadequacy.

NURSING DIAGNOSES

The nursing diagnoses for the infant with NFTT must include as much interaction with the family caregiver as possible. Careful assessment, diagnosis, and planning provide for sensory stimulation, adequate food intake (140 cal/kg) for weight gain, and tender loving care. As the infant becomes less fretful and more responsive and gains weight, the caregiver will find the infant much more appealing. In addition to the nursing diagnoses identified under special considerations, some nursing diagnoses might include:

- Sensory/Perceptual Alteration related to deficient nurturing

- Altered Nutrition: Less than Body Requirements and Fluid Volume Deficit related to inadequate intake

- Constipation and Altered Urinary Elimination related to dehydration

- Altered Parenting related to lack of knowledge and confidence in parenting skills

- Risk for Impaired Skin Integrity related to malnourishment

OUTCOME IDENTIFICATION AND PLANNING

The major goals for the NFTT infant focus on improving alertness and responsiveness and increasing oral intake. Other goals for the infant and family include improving parenting skills, building parental confidence, and maintaining skin integrity. The caregiver's participation in the infant's care is essential. Plan individualized nursing according to these goals.

IMPLEMENTATION

PROVIDING SENSORY STIMULATION. The nurse plays a critical role in reversing the infant's growth failure and improving the caregiver–infant relationship. Providing sensory stimulation is vital in the care of the NFTT infant. Therefore, it is especially important to follow the guidelines detailed in the beginning of this chapter.

MAINTAINING ADEQUATE NUTRITION AND FLUID INTAKE. Feed the infant slowly and carefully in a quiet environment. During feeding, the infant might be closely snuggled and gently rocked. It may be necessary to feed the infant every 2 or 3 hours initially. Burp the infant frequently during and at the end of each feeding, then place him or her on the side with the head slightly elevated or held in a chest-to-chest position. Feed the infant until good eating habits are established. Extra fluids of unsweetened juices are encouraged. If a family caregiver is present, encourage him or her to become involved in the infant's feedings. Demonstrate the importance of talking encouragingly as the baby eats. An older child can sit at a low table facing the feeder while eating. Make the feeding time pleasant and comforting. Carefully document food intake with caloric intake and strict intake and output records.

MONITORING ELIMINATION PATTERNS. As food and fluids are gradually increased and the infant becomes hydrated, bowel activity and urine production return to normal. Daily stools are of a soft consistency, and the hourly urinary output is 2 to 3 mL/kg.

PROVIDING FAMILY TEACHING. While caring for the infant, point out to the caregiver the infant's development and responsiveness, noting and praising any positive parenting behaviors the caregiver displays. The caregiver who has not had a close, warm childhood relationship may not understand the infant's needs for cuddling and stimulation. Teaching about these needs must be done carefully, so as not to damage the caregiver's self-esteem still further. Many of these family caregivers are overly concerned about spoiling the infant. It is important to dispel these fears. Explain the need for the infant to develop trust, and teach the caregiver about the developmental tasks appropriate for infants. Involve other health care team members as needed.

PROMOTING SKIN INTEGRITY. Protect the infant's skin to prevent irritation. Lanolin or A and D Ointment can be used to lubricate dry skin. Apply the ointment at least once each shift and turn the infant at least every 2 hours.

EVALUATION: GOALS AND OUTCOME CRITERIA

- *Goal*: The infant will be more alert and responsive.
  Criteria: The infant visually follows the caregiver around the room.

- *Goal*: Oral intake will be appropriately increased.
  Criteria: The infant's weight increases at a predetermined goal of 1 oz or more per day.

- *Goal*: The family caregivers will demonstrate positive signs of good parenting.
  Criteria: The family caregivers feed the infant successfully and exhibit an appropriate response to the child.

- *Goal*: Skin integrity will be maintained.
  Criteria: The infant's skin shows no signs of redness or irritation.

GASTROINTESTINAL DISORDERS

The GI system is responsible for taking in and processing nutrients that nourish all parts of the body. As a result, any problem of the GI system, whether it is a lack of nutrients, an infectious disease, or a congenital disorder, can quickly affect other parts of the body and can ultimately affect general health and growth and development.

Malnutrition

The World Health Organization has widely publicized the malnutrition and hunger that affect more than half the world's population. In the United States, malnutrition contributes to the high death rate of the children of migrant workers and Native Americans. Malnourished children grow at a slower rate, have a higher rate of illness and infection, and have more difficulty concentrating and achieving in school. Appendix E lists foods that are good sources of the nutrients a child needs for healthy growth.

PROTEIN MALNUTRITION

Protein malnutrition results from an insufficient intake of high-quality protein or from conditions in which protein absorption is impaired or there is an increased loss of protein. Clinical evidence of protein malnutrition may not be apparent until the condition is well advanced.

Kwashiorkor results from severe deficiency of protein with an adequate caloric intake. It accounts for most of the malnutrition in the world's children today. The highest incidence is in children 4 months to 5 years of age. The affected child develops a swollen abdomen, edema, and GI changes; the hair is thin and dry, with patchy alopecia; and the child becomes apathetic and irritable and has retarded growth with muscle wasting. In untreated patients, mortality rates are 30% or higher. Although strenuous efforts are being made around the world to prevent this condition, its causes are complex.

Traditionally, these babies have been breast-fed until the age of 2 or 3 years. The child is weaned abruptly when the next child is born. In fact, the term *kwashiorkor* in African dialect means "the sickness the older baby gets when the new baby comes" (Fig. 11-2). The older child is then given the regular family diet, which consists mostly of starchy foods with little meat or vegetable protein. Cow's milk generally is unavailable, and in many places where goats are

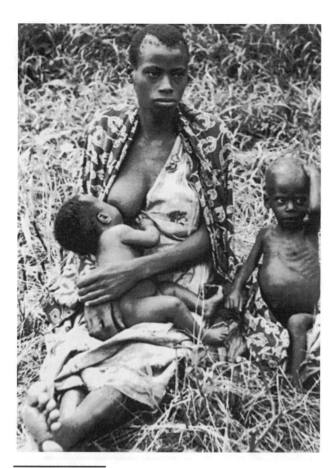

Figure 11-2
The older child in this picture shows the protein-calorie deprivation and the malnutrition that occurred when he was dispossessed or replaced at his mother's breast by the new baby.

kept, their milk is not considered fit for human consumption.

Marasmus is a deficiency in calories as well as protein. The child with marasmus is seriously ill. The condition is common in children in Third World countries because of severe drought conditions. There is not enough food to supply everyone in these countries, and the children are not fed until adults are fed. The child is severely malnourished and highly susceptible to disease. This syndrome may be seen in the child with NFTT.

VITAMIN DEFICIENCY DISEASES

Rickets, a disease affecting the growth and calcification of bones, is caused by a lack of vitamin D. The absorption of calcium and phosphorus is diminished due to the lack of vitamin D, which is needed to regulate the use of these minerals. Early manifestations include **craniotabes** (softening of the occipital bones) and delayed closure of the fontanelles. There is delayed dentition, with defects in tooth enamel and a tendency to develop caries. As the dis-

ease advances, thoracic deformities, softening of the shafts of long bones, and spinal and pelvic bone deformities develop. The muscles are poorly developed and lacking in tone, thus delaying standing and walking. Deformities occur during periods of rapid growth, and although rickets itself is not a fatal disease, complications such as tetany, pneumonia, and enteritis are more likely to cause death in rachitic children (children with rickets) than in healthy children.

Infants and children require an estimated 400 U of vitamin D daily to prevent rickets. Because a small child living in a temperate climate may not receive sufficient exposure to ultraviolet light, vitamin D is administered orally in the form of fish liver oil or synthetic vitamin. Whole milk and evaporated milk, fortified with 400 U of vitamin D per quart, are available throughout the United States. Breast-fed infants should receive vitamin D supplements, especially if the mother's intake of vitamin D is poor.

Scurvy is caused by inadequate dietary intake of vitamin C (ascorbic acid). Early inclusion of vitamin C in the diet, in the form of orange or tomato juice or a vitamin preparation, prevents the development of this disease. Febrile diseases seem to increase the need for vitamin C. A variety of fresh vegetables and fruits supply vitamin C for the older infant and child. Because much of the vitamin C content is destroyed by boiling or by exposure to air for long periods, the family caregivers should be taught to cook vegetables with minimal water in a covered pot and to store juices in a tightly covered opaque container. Vegetables cooked in a microwave oven retain more vitamin C because little water is added in the cooking process.

Early clinical manifestations of scurvy are irritability, loss of appetite, and digestive disturbances. A general tenderness in the legs severe enough to cause a pseudoparalysis develops. The infant is apprehensive about being handled and assumes a frog position, with the hips and knees semiflexed and the feet rotated outward. The gums become red and swollen, and hemorrhage occurs in various tissues. Characteristic hemorrhages in the long bones are subperiosteal, especially at the ends of the femur and tibia.

Recovery is rapid with adequate treatment, but death may occur from malnutrition or exhaustion in untreated cases. Treatment consists of therapeutic daily doses of ascorbic acid.

Thiamine is one of the major components of the vitamin B complex. Children whose diets are deficient in thiamine exhibit irritability, listlessness, loss of appetite, and vomiting. A severe lack of thiamine in the diet causes *beriberi*, a disease characterized by cardiac and neurologic symptoms. Beriberi does not occur when balanced diets that include whole grains are eaten.

Riboflavin deficiency usually occurs in association with thiamine and niacin deficiencies. It is manifested mainly by skin lesions. The primary source of riboflavin is milk. Riboflavin is destroyed by ultraviolet light; thus, opaque milk cartons are best for storage. Whole grains are also a good source of riboflavin.

Niacin insufficiency in the diet causes a disease known as *pellagra*, which presents with GI and neurologic symptoms. Pellagra does not occur in children who ingest adequate whole milk or who eat a well-balanced diet.

MINERAL INSUFFICIENCY

Iron deficiency results in anemia. This condition is the most common cause of nutritional deficiency in children older than 4 to 6 months of age whose diets lack iron-rich foods. Anemia is often found in poor children younger than 6 years of age in the United States. Iron deficiency anemia is discussed more fully later in this chapter in the section on circulatory system disorders.

Calcium is necessary for bone and tooth formation and is also needed for proper nerve and muscle function. *Hypocalcemia* (insufficient calcium) causes neurologic damage, including mental retardation. Rich sources of calcium include milk and milk products. Children with milk allergies are at an increased risk for hypocalcemia.

Food Allergies

The symptoms of food allergies vary from one child to another. Common symptoms are **urticaria** (hives), **pruritus** (itching), stomach pains, and respiratory symptoms. Some of the symptoms may appear quickly after the child has eaten the offending food, but other foods may cause a delayed reaction. Thus, the investigation needed to find the cause can be frustrating.

MILK

Milk allergy is the most common food allergy in the young child. Symptoms that may indicate an allergy to milk are diarrhea, vomiting, colic, irritability, respiratory symptoms, or eczema. Infants who are breast-fed for the first 6 months or more may avoid developing milk allergies entirely unless there is a strong family history of allergies. Infants with severe allergic reactions to milk are given commercial formulas that are soybean- or meat-based and formulated to be similar in nutrients to other infant formulas. If the infant has a severe milk allergy, the caregiver must learn to read the labels on prepared foods carefully to avoid lactose or lactic acid ingredients.

OTHER FOOD ALLERGIES

Foods should be introduced to the infant one at a time, with an interval of 4 or 5 days between each new food. If any GI or respiratory reaction occurs, the food should be eliminated. Among the foods most likely to cause allergic reactions are eggs, wheat, corn, legumes (including peanuts and soybeans), oranges, strawberries, and chocolate (Table 11-1). Suspected foods are eliminated and reintro-

TABLE 11-1. Some Foods That May Cause Allergies and Possible Sources

Food	Sources
Milk	Yogurt, cheese, ice cream, puddings, hot dogs, foods made with nonfat dry milk, lunch meat, chocolate candies
Eggs	Baked goods, ice cream, puddings, meringues, candies, mayonnaise, salad dressings, custards
Wheat	Breads, baked goods, hot dogs, lunch meats, cereals, cream soups. Oat, rye, and cornmeal products may have wheat added.
Corn	Products made with cornstarch, corn syrup, or vegetable starch; many children's juices, popcorn, cornbreads or muffins, tortillas
Legumes	Soybean products, peanut butter and peanut products
Citrus fruits	Oranges, lemons, limes, grapefruit, gelatins, children's juices, some pediatric suspensions
Strawberries	Gelatins, some pediatric suspensions
Chocolate	Cocoa, candies, chocolate drinks or desserts, colas

duced one at a time in small amounts to test for reaction. This testing should be done in a carefully controlled manner to avoid serious or life-threatening reactions. Many allergies disappear as the child's GI tract matures.

LACTOSE INTOLERANCE

Congenital lactose intolerance is seen in some infants of African-American, Native American, Eskimo, Asian, and Mediterranean heritage. Infants with **lactose intolerance** cannot digest **lactose**, the primary carbohydrate in milk, because of an inborn deficiency of the enzyme lactase. Symptoms include cramping, abdominal distention, flatus, and diarrhea after ingesting milk. Commercially available formulas such as Isomil, Nursoy, Nutramigen, and Prosobee are made from soybean, meat-based, or protein mixtures and contain no lactose. The infant needs supplemental vitamin D. Yogurt is tolerated by these infants.

Nursing Process for the Nutritionally Deprived Infant

ASSESSMENT

Carefully interview the family caregiver to determine the underlying cause. If the difficulty lies in the caregiver's inability to give proper care, try to determine if this can be attributed to lack of information, financial problems, indifference, or other reasons. Do not make assumptions until the interview is completed. Several cases of malnutrition have been reported in infants of families who believed it was better for their infants to eat vegetables only; this severely limits fat intake, which the infant needs. If food allergies are suspected as the cause of malnourishment, include a careful history of food intake. Obtain a history of stools and voiding from the caregiver.

The physical assessment of the infant includes an evaluation of skin turgor and skin condition, assessment of the anterior fontanelle, signs of emaciation, weight, temperature, apical pulse, respirations, responsiveness, listlessness, and irritability.

NURSING DIAGNOSES

The malnourished infant is often seriously ill. The nursing diagnoses depend on the physical as well as the sociocultural causes of the condition. Some specific nursing diagnoses that may be used include:

- Altered Nutrition: Less than Body Requirements related to inadequate intake of nutrients secondary to poor sucking ability, lack of interest in food, lack of adequate food sources, or caregiver knowledge deficit

- Knowledge Deficit related to the caregivers' lack of knowledge regarding infant nutritional requirements

- Fluid Volume Deficit and Constipation related to insufficient fluid intake

- Impaired Skin Integrity related to malnourishment

OUTCOME IDENTIFICATION AND PLANNING

The major goals for the nutritionally deprived infant focus on increasing nutritional intake, improving hydration, and maintaining skin integrity. Other goals concentrate on improving caregiver knowledge and understanding of nutrition and facilitating the infant's ability to suck. Even with focused and individualized goals, developing a plan of care for the malnourished infant may be challenging. It may be necessary to try a variety of tactics to feed the child successfully. Include the family caregiver in the plan of care, as this is in the best interest of both the infant and the caregiver.

IMPLEMENTATION

MAINTAINING ADEQUATE NUTRITION

One of the primary nursing care problems may be persuading the infant to take more nourishment than he or she wants. Inexperienced nurses may find it difficult to persuade an uninterested infant to take formula, and this can become frustrating. Perhaps the nurse's insecurity and uncertainty communicate themselves to the infant in the way he or she handles the child. An experienced nurse may

succeed in feeding an infant 3 or 4 oz in a short period, whereas the inexperienced nurse who seems to be going through the same motions persuades the infant to take only 1 oz or less. As the nurse and the infant become accustomed to each other, however, they both relax, and feeding becomes easier.

The baby who is held snugly, wrapped closely, and rocked gently finds it easier to relax and take in a little more feeding. An impatient, hurried attitude nearly always communicates tension to the child. Ask for help if the need to attend to other feedings causes tension. Never prop the bottle in the crib.

Gavage feedings or intravenous (IV) fluids may be needed to improve the infant's nutritional status, but it is important for the infant to develop an interest in food and in the process of sucking. A hard or small-holed nipple may completely discourage the infant. The nipple should be soft, with holes large enough to allow the formula to drip without pressure. However, it should not be so soft that it offers no resistance and collapses when sucked on. The holes should not be so large that milk pours out, causing the infant to choke. This situation can frustrate a weak infant, who then no longer attempts to nurse.

Scheduling feedings every 2 or 3 hours is best because most weak babies can handle frequent, small feedings better than every-4-hour feedings. With more frequent feedings, promptness is important. Feedings should be limited to 20 to 30 minutes so that the infant does not tire. Demand schedules are not wise because the infant has probably lost the power to regulate the supply and demand schedule.

PROVIDING FAMILY TEACHING. If malnutrition is related to economic factors or inadequate caregiver knowledge of the infant's needs, teach the family caregivers the essential facts of infant and child nutrition and make referrals for social services. Be alert to the possibility that the caregiver cannot read or understand English, and be certain that the teaching materials used are understood. Simply asking the family caregivers if they have questions is not sufficient to determine whether the material has been understood.

Family caregivers may need information regarding assistance in obtaining nutritious food for the infant. Infant formulas and baby food can be expensive, and economic factors may be the actual cause of the infant's malnutrition. A referral to social services or the Women, Infant, Children (WIC) program may be appropriate (see Chap. 10).

IMPROVING FLUID INTAKE. In addition to having a lack of interest, the infant often is weak and debilitated, with little strength to suck. Intravenous fluids may be needed initially to build up the infant's energy so that he or she can take more oral nourishment and correct the fluid and electrolyte imbalance. During IV therapy, restraints should be adequate but kept to a minimum. Accurately document intake and output. Check the fontanelles each shift and weigh the infant daily in the early morning

Box 11-2. *Weighing the Infant*

1. Prepare the scale by covering it with paper, cloth diaper, or sheet and by balancing it.
2. Place the naked infant on the scale and weigh the infant. *Always* hold your hand within an inch or so of the infant to be ready to take hold if necessary.
3. Pick up the infant and discard the scale cover.
4. Read the weight and record it on the worksheet or scrap paper.
5. Clean the scale according to the facility's policy.

If the baby's weight varies significantly from the previous weight, have another person check it with you. Document and report the weight as appropriate. The ill infant often needs to be weighed daily to assess growth or fluid balance. Weights should be taken every day at the same time, with the same scale.

(Box 11-2). Every 2 hours, monitor the IV infusion placement, its patency, and the site for redness and induration. Report any unusual signs immediately.

MONITORING ELIMINATION PATTERNS. Improved nutritional status is evidenced by improved hydration, which is assessed by monitoring skin turgor, fontanelle tension, and intake and output. Carefully document intake and output, as well as the character, frequency, and amount of stools. Report any unusual characteristics of the stools or urine at once.

PROMOTING SKIN INTEGRITY. Closely observe the skin condition, with careful attention to the mucous membranes. Use A and D Ointment or lanolin for dry or reddened skin, and promptly change soiled diapers to prevent skin breakdown in weakened infants.

EVALUATION: GOALS AND OUTCOME CRITERIA

- *Goal*: Nutritional intake will improve.
  Criteria: The infant gains 0.75 to 1 oz (22–30 g) per day if under 6 months of age and 0.5 to 0.75 oz (13–22 g) per day if over 6 months of age.

- *Goal*: The infant will show interest in feedings.
  Criteria: The infant shows evidence of adequate sucking and the ability to extend the amount of time nursing without showing signs of tiring.

- *Goal*: The family caregivers will demonstrate a beginning knowledge of appropriate nutrition for a growing infant.
  Criteria: Family caregivers verbalize five essential facts about infant nutrition.

- *Goal*: Fluid intake will improve.
  Criteria: The infant's fontanelles are of normal tension, skin turgor is good, and weight gain is as above.

- *Goal*: If parenteral fluids are administered, the site will remain intact.
  Criteria: The skin shows no signs of redness or induration.

- *Goal*: Urine and bowel output will improve.
  Criteria: Hourly urine output is 2 to 3 mL/kg; stool is soft and of normal character.

- *Goal*: Skin and mucous membranes will show evidence of improved hydration.
  Criteria: Mucous membranes are moist and pink, skin turgor is good, and skin shows no signs of breakdown.

Diarrhea and Gastroenteritis

Diarrhea in infants is a fairly common symptom of a variety of conditions. It may be mild, with a small amount of dehydration, or it may be extremely severe, requiring prompt and effective treatment. Simple diarrhea that does not respond to treatment can quickly turn into severe, life-threatening diarrhea.

Chronically malnourished infants with diarrheal symptoms are a common problem in many areas of the world. This condition is prevalent in areas where adequate clean water and sanitary facilities are lacking. Certain metabolic diseases, such as cystic fibrosis, have diarrhea as a symptom. Diarrhea also may be caused by antibiotic therapy.

Some conditions that cause diarrhea require readjustment of the infant's diet. Allergic reactions to food are not uncommon and can be controlled by avoiding the offending food. Overfeeding as well as underfeeding or an unbalanced diet may also be the cause of diarrhea in an infant. Adjusting the infant's diet, adding less sugar to formula, or reducing bulk or fat in the diet may be necessary.

Many diarrheal disturbances in infants are caused by contaminated food or from human or animal fecal waste through the oral–fecal route. Infectious diarrhea is commonly referred to as **gastroenteritis**. The infectious organisms may be salmonella, *Escherichia coli*, dysentery bacilli, and various viruses, most notably rotaviruses. It is difficult to determine the causative factor in many instances. Because of the seriousness of infectious diarrhea in infants and the danger of spreading diarrhea, the child with moderate or severe diarrhea is often isolated until the causative factor has been proved to be noninfectious.

CLINICAL MANIFESTATIONS

Mild diarrhea may present as little more than loose stools; the frequency of defecation may be two to 12 per day. The infant may be irritable and have a loss of appetite. Vomiting and gastric distention are not significant factors, and dehydration is minimal.

Mild or moderate diarrhea can rather quickly become severe diarrhea in an infant. Vomiting usually accompanies the diarrhea; together, they cause large losses of body water and electrolytes. The infant becomes severely dehydrated and is gravely ill. The skin becomes extremely dry and loses its turgor. The fontanelle becomes sunken, and the pulse is weak and rapid. The stools become greenish liquid and may be blood-tinged.

DIAGNOSIS

Stool specimens may be collected for culture and sensitivity testing to determine the causative infectious organism, if there is one; subsequently, effective antibiotics can be prescribed as indicated.

TREATMENT

Treatment to stop the diarrhea must be initiated immediately. Establishing normal fluid and electrolyte balance is the primary concern in treating gastroenteritis. The infant with acute dehydration may be given oral feedings of commercial electrolyte solutions, such as Pedialyte, Rehydralyte, and Infalyte unless there is shock or severe dehydration. This treatment is called *oral rehydration therapy*. As the diarrhea clears, food may be offered. Once commonly used, the BRAT diet (ripe *b*anana, *r*ice cereal, *a*pplesauce, and *t*oast) has become somewhat controversial because it is high in calories and low in energy and protein and does not provide adequate nutrition. Salty broths should be avoided. Infants can return to breast-feeding, if they have been NPO, and formula-fed infants are given their formula. Foods can be added as the infant's condition improves, returning to a regular diet. Early return to the usual diet has been shown to reduce the number of stools and to decrease weight loss and the length of the illness.

In severe diarrhea with shock and severe dehydration, oral feedings are discontinued completely. Fluids to be given IV must be carefully calculated to replace the lost electrolytes. Frequent laboratory determinations of the infant's blood chemistries are necessary to guide the physician in this replacement therapy. For the infant who has had a serious bout of diarrhea, the physician may prescribe soybean formula for a few weeks to avoid a possible reaction to milk proteins.

🏃🏿 *Nursing Process for the Infant With* *Diarrhea and Gastroenteritis*

ASSESSMENT

In addition to basic information about the infant, the interview with the family caregiver must include specific information about the history of bowel patterns and the onset of diarrheal stools, with details on number and type of stools per day. Suggest terms to describe the color and odor of stools to assist the caregiver with descriptions. In-

quire about recent feeding patterns, nausea, and vomiting. Ask the caregiver about fever and other signs of illness in the infant and signs of illness in any other family members.

The physical assessment of the infant involves evaluation of skin turgor and condition, including excoriated diaper area, temperature, anterior fontanelle (depressed, normal, or bulging), apical pulse rate (observing for weak pulse), stools (character, amount, and color and presence of blood), irritability, lethargy, vomiting, urine (amount and concentration), lips and mucous membranes of the mouth (dry, cracked), eyes (bright, glassy, sunken, dark circles), and any other notable physical signs.

NURSING DIAGNOSES

A primary nursing diagnosis is "Diarrhea related to (whatever the cause is)." Other nursing diagnoses vary with the intensity of the diarrhea (mild or severe) as determined by the physical assessment and caregiver interview. In addition to the nursing diagnoses suggested earlier in this chapter, some appropriate nursing diagnoses are:

- Altered Skin Integrity related to the constant presence of diarrheal stools

- Fluid Volume Deficit related to dehydration

- Ineffective Family Coping: Compromised related to the seriousness of the infant's illness

- Altered Nutrition: Less than Body Requirements related to malabsorption of nutrients

- Hyperthermia related to dehydration

- Parental Health Seeking Behaviors related to therapy for diarrhea

- Risk for Infection related to inadequate secondary defenses or insufficient knowledge to avoid exposure to pathogens.

OUTCOME IDENTIFICATION AND PLANNING

The major goal for the family with an infant who has diarrhea or gastroenteritis is eliminating the risk of infection transmission. Other important goals for the ill infant include improving hydration, maintaining good skin condition, increasing comfort levels, improving nutritional intake, and satisfying sucking needs. Plan individualized nursing care according to these goals. Remember that stopping the diarrhea is a vital aspect of nursing care.

IMPLEMENTATION

PREVENTING INFECTION. To prevent the spread of possibly infectious organisms to other pediatric patients, follow standard precautions issued by the Centers for Disease Control. All caregivers must wear gowns and gloves when handling articles contaminated with feces, but masks are unnecessary. Place contaminated linens and clothing in specially marked containers to be processed according to the policy of the health care facility. Place disposable diapers and other disposable items in specially marked bags and dispose of them according to policy. Visitors are limited to family only.

Teach the family caregivers the principles of aseptic technique and observe them to ensure understanding and compliance. Good handwashing must be carried out and also taught to the family caregivers. Stress that gloves are needed for added protection, but careful handwashing is also necessary.

PROMOTING SKIN INTEGRITY. To reduce irritation and excoriation of the buttocks and genital area, cleanse those areas frequently and apply a soothing protective preparation such as lanolin or A and D Ointment. Change diapers as quickly as possible after soiling. Some infants may be sensitive to cloth diapers, and others may be sensitive to disposable diapers, so it may be necessary to try both types. It is often helpful to leave the diaper off, exposing the buttocks and genital area to the air. Placing disposable pads under the infant can facilitate easy and frequent changing. Teach caregivers that waterproof diaper covers hold moisture in and do not allow circulation of air, increasing irritation and excoriation of the diaper area.

PREVENTING DEHYDRATION. An infant can dehydrate quickly and can get into serious trouble after only 3 days or less of diarrhea. Carefully count diapers and weigh them to determine the infant's output more accurately, if necessary. Carefully observe all stools. Document the number and character of the stools, as well as the amount and character of any vomitus.

SUPPORTING FAMILY COPING. Being the family caregiver of an infant who has become so ill in such a short time is frightening. Meeting the infant's emotional needs is difficult but very important. Suggest to the caregiver ways that the infant might be consoled without interfering with care. Soothing, gentle stroking of the head, and speaking softly help the infant bear the frustrations of the illness and its treatment. The infant can be picked up and rocked, as long as this can be done without jeopardizing the IV infusion site. If the IV infusion is in a position that may be displaced, this is not permitted. Threading a needle into the small veins of a dehydrated infant is difficult, and replacement may be nearly impossible, but the infant's life may depend on receiving the proper parenteral fluids. Help fulfill the infant's emotional needs, and encourage the family caregiver to have some time away from the infant's room without feeling guilty about leaving.

MAINTAINING ADEQUATE NUTRITION. Weight the infant daily on the same scale. Take measurements in the early morning before the morning feeding, if infant is on oral feedings. Maintain precautions to prevent contamination of equipment while the infant is weighed. Monitor intake and output strictly.

In severe dehydration, IV fluids are given to rest the GI tract and restore hydration. Monitor the placement, patency, and site of the IV infusion at least every 2 hours. The use of restraints, with relevant nursing interventions, may be necessary. Good mouth care is essential while the infant is NPO.

When oral fluids are started, the infant is given oral replacement solutions such as those listed earlier. After the infant tolerates these solutions, half-strength formula may be introduced, then several days later full-strength formula (possibly lactose-free or soy formula to avoid disaccharide intolerance or reaction to milk proteins). The breast-fed infant can continue breast-feeding. Give the mother of a breast-fed infant access to a breast pump if her infant is NPO. Breast milk may be frozen for later use, if desired. The infant who is NPO needs to have his or her sucking needs fulfilled. To accomplish this, offer the infant a pacifier.

MAINTAINING BODY TEMPERATURE. Monitor vital signs at least every 2 hours if there is fever. Do *not* take the temperature rectally, as insertion of a thermometer into the rectum can cause stimulation of stools as well as trauma and tissue injury to sensitive mucosa. Follow the appropriate procedures for fever reduction, and administer antipyretics and antibiotics as prescribed. Take the temperature with a thermometer that is used only for that infant.

PROMOTING FAMILY TEACHING. Explain to the family caregivers the importance of GI rest for the infant. The family caregivers (especially if young or poorly educated) may not understand the necessity for NPO status. Cooperation of the caregiver is improved with increased understanding. See the Family Teaching Tips on Diarrhea and Vomiting.

EVALUATION: GOALS AND OUTCOME CRITERIA

- *Goal*: Infection control will be maintained.
  Criteria: Family caregivers verbalize standard precautions for infection control.

- *Goal*: Skin integrity will be maintained.
  Criteria: The infant's diaper area shows no evidence of redness or excoriation.

- *Goal*: Dehydration will be prevented.
  Criteria: Intake is sufficient to produce hourly urine output of 2 to 3 mL/kg; skin turgor is good; mucous membranes are moist and pink; and fontanelles exhibit normal tension.

- *Goal*: Caregiver anxiety will be reduced.
  Criteria: Caregivers participate in the care and soothing of the infant.

- *Goal*: The infant will be comforted.
  Criteria: The infant rests quietly and is effectively consoled by caregivers or health care personnel.

Family Teaching
Tips on Diarrhea

The danger in diarrhea is dehydration (drying out). If the child becomes dehydrated, he or she can become very sick. Increasing the amount of liquid the child drinks is helpful. Solid foods may need to be decreased so the child will drink more.

Suggestions
1. Give liquids in small amounts (3 or 4 tbsp) about every half hour. If this goes well, increase the amount a little each half hour. Don't force the child to drink, because he or she may vomit.
2. Give solid foods in small amounts. Do not give milk for a day or two, because this can make diarrhea worse.
3. Give only nonsalty soups or broths.
4. Liquids recommended for vomiting may be given for diarrhea also.
5. Soft foods to give (small amounts): applesauce, fine chopped or scraped apple without peel, bananas, toast, rice cereal, plain unsalted crackers or cookies, any meats.

Call the Physician if:
1. Child develops sudden high fever.
2. Stomach pain becomes severe.
3. Diarrhea becomes bloody (more than a streak of blood).
4. Diarrhea becomes more frequent or severe.
5. Child becomes dehydrated (dried out).

Signs of Dehydration
1. Child has not urinated for 6 hours or more.
2. Child has no tears when crying.
3. Child's mouth is dry or sticky to touch.
4. Child's eyes are sunken.
5. Child is less active than usual.
6. Child has dark circles under eyes.

Warning
Do not use medicines to stop diarrhea for children younger than 6 years of age unless specifically directed by the physician. These medicines can be dangerous if not used properly.

Diaper Area Skin Care
1. Change diaper as soon as it is soiled.
2. Wash area with mild soap, rinse, and dry well.
3. Use soothing, protective lotion recommended by your physician or hospital.
4. Do not use waterproof diaper covers—they increase diaper area irritation.
5. Wash hands with soap and water after changing diapers or wiping the child.

■ *Goal*: The infant will be well hydrated.
Criteria: The infant consumes an age-appropriate amount of full-strength formula or breast milk 3 days after therapy with oral replacement solution.

■ *Goal*: The infant will satisfy nonnutritive sucking needs.
Criteria: The infant uses a pacifier to satisfy sucking needs.

Family Teaching
Tips on Vomiting

Vomiting will usually stop in a couple of days and can be treated at home as long as the child is getting some fluids.

Warning
Some medications used to stop vomiting in older children or adults are dangerous in infants or young children. DO NOT use any medicine unless your physician has told you to use it for *this child*.

Give child clear liquids to drink in small amounts.

Suggestions
1. Flat soda (no fizz). Use caffeine-free type; do not use diet soda.
2. Jello water—double the amount of water, let stand to room temperature.
3. Ice popsicles
4. Gatorade
5. Pedialyte, Lytren, Rehydralyte, Infalyte
6. Tea
7. Solid Jell-O
8. Broth (not salty)

How to Give
Give small amounts often. One tbsp every 20 minutes for the first few hours is a good rule of thumb. If this is kept down without vomiting, increase to 2 tbsp every 20 minutes for the next couple of hours. If there is no vomiting, increase the amount the child may have. If the child vomits, wait for 1 hour before offering more liquids.

■ *Goal*: Hyperthermia does not occur.
Criteria: The infant's temperature is 98.6° to 100°F (37°–37.8°C).

■ *Goal*: The family will demonstrate an understanding of the infant's treatment.
Criteria: Family caregivers verbalize three suggestions to increase hydration and the warning signs of dehydration.

Colic

Colic consists of recurrent paroxysmal bouts of abdominal pain and is fairly common in young infants. It often disappears around the age of 3 months, but this is small comfort to the caregiver vainly trying to soothe a colicky infant. Although many theories have been proposed, none has been accepted as the causative factor.

CLINICAL MANIFESTATIONS AND DIAGNOSIS

Attacks occur suddenly, usually late in the day or evening. The infant cries loudly and continuously. The infant appears to be in considerable pain but otherwise seems

COMMUNICATIONS BOX

Conversation with first-time mother of 10-week-old infant with colic:

INEFFECTIVE COMMUNICATION

Mother: I can't stand it! Joey cries for hours every evening.

Nurse: Can't you figure out what's making him cry?

Mother: Well, not really; he pulls up his legs and just screams.

Nurse: He must have colic. Don't let that upset you. A lot of babies have that.

Mother: It makes me feel helpless.

Nurse: Don't worry. It will only last a few months and then he'll outgrow it.

Mother: I'm not sure I can take it.

Nurse: Oh, it won't last forever; just keep hanging in there.

During this conversation, the nurse just continues to offer answers without acknowledging the mother's feelings. At the end of the conversation, the mother still feels helpless and perhaps out of control.

EFFECTIVE COMMUNICATION

Mother: I can't stand it! Joey cries for hours every evening.

Nurse: You are really frustrated by Joey's crying.

Mother: Yeah. I feel like screaming.

Nurse: It makes you feel like you are losing control, and this is upsetting to you.

Mother: I just feel like shaking him.

Nurse: You want to make him stop, but you really don't know what to do. You know that shaking him is dangerous and won't really do any good.

Mother: That's right. I feel so helpless. What can I do?

Nurse: Having a baby crying from colic is very upsetting to a parent. I have a handout on tips on caring for a baby with colic. Let me go over it with you. Some of these suggestions may help you cope with Joey's crying.

From the beginning of this conversation, the nurse recognizes the mother's feelings and validates them. The nurse concludes the conversation by telling the mother this is a common problem and provides support by offering her some concrete solutions.

---

healthy, nurses or takes formula well, and gains weight as expected. The baby may be momentarily soothed only by rocking or holding but eventually falls asleep, exhausted from crying. The infant with colic is often considered a "difficult" baby.

Differential diagnosis should be made to rule out an allergic reaction to milk or certain foods. Changing to a nonallergenic formula helps determine if there is an allergic factor or if the infant has lactose intolerance. If the baby is breast-fed, the mother's diet should be studied to determine if anything she is eating may be affecting the baby. Intestinal obstruction or infection also must be ruled out.

TREATMENT AND NURSING CARE

No single treatment is consistently successful. A number of measures may be employed, one or more of which might work. Medications such as sedatives, antispasmodics, and antiflatulents are sometimes prescribed, but their effectiveness is inconsistent. The family must remember that the condition will pass, even though at the time it seems it will last forever. Family caregivers need to be reassured that their parenting skills are not inadequate. The nurse can support the family and promote coping skills by providing family teaching. See Family Teaching Tips for Colic.

Pyloric Stenosis

Pyloric stenosis is rarely symptomatic during the first days of life. It has occasionally been recognized shortly after birth, but the average affected infant does not show symptoms until about the third week of life. Symptoms rarely appear after the second month. Although symptoms appear late, pyloric stenosis is classified as a congenital defect. Its cause is unknown, but it occurs more frequently in white males and has a familial tendency.

The pylorus is the muscle that controls the flow of food from the stomach to the duodenum. Pyloric stenosis is characterized by hypertrophy of the circular muscle fibers of the pylorus, with a severe narrowing of its lumen. The pylorus is thickened to as much as twice its size, is elongated, and has a consistency resembling cartilage. As a result of this obstruction at the distal end of the stomach, the stomach becomes dilated (Fig. 11-3).

CLINICAL MANIFESTATIONS

During the first weeks of life, the infant with pyloric stenosis often eats well and gains weight, but then starts vomiting occasionally after meals. Within a few days, the vomiting increases in frequency and force, becoming projectile. The vomited material is sour, undigested food; it may con-

Figure 11-3
Pyloric stenoiss. (narrowed lumen of the pylorus).

tain mucus but never bile, because it has not progressed beyond the stomach.

Because the obstruction is a mechanical one, the baby does not feel ill, is ravenously hungry, and is eager to try again and again, but the food invariably comes back. As the condition progresses, the baby becomes irritable, loses weight rapidly, and becomes dehydrated. Alkalosis develops from the loss of potassium and hydrochloric acid, and the baby becomes seriously ill.

Constipation becomes progressive because little food gets into the intestine, and the urine is scanty. Gastric peristaltic waves passing from left to right across the abdomen usually can be seen during or after feedings.

DIAGNOSIS

Diagnosis is usually made on the clinical evidence. The nature, type, and times of vomiting, observation of gastric peristaltic waves, and a history of weight loss with hunger and irritability point in this direction. The olive-sized pyloric tumor often can be felt through deep palpation by an experienced physician. Ultrasonographic or radiographic studies with barium swallow show an abnormal retention of barium in the stomach and increased peristalsis.

TREATMENT

A surgical procedure called a pyloromyotomy (also known as Fredet-Ramstedt operation) is the treatment of choice. This procedure simply splits the hypertrophic pyloric muscle down to the submucosa, allowing the pylorus to expand so that food may pass. Prognosis is excellent if surgery is performed before the infant is severely dehydrated.

Nursing Process for the Infant With Pyloric Stenosis

ASSESSMENT

When the infant of 1 or 2 months of age has a history of projectile vomiting, pyloric stenosis is suspected. Carefully interview the family caregivers. Ask when the vomiting started and determine the character of the vomiting (undigested formula with no bile, vomitus progressively more projectile). The caregiver will relate a story of a baby who is an eager eater but cannot retain food. Ask the caregiver about constipation and scanty urine.

Physical assessment reveals an infant who may show signs of dehydration. Assess the infant's weight, skin turgor and skin condition (including excoriated diaper area), anterior fontanelle (depressed, normal, or bulging), temperature, apical pulse rate (observing for weak pulse and tachycardia), irritability, lethargy, urine (amount and concentration), lips and mucous membranes of the mouth (dry, cracked), and eyes (bright, glassy, sunken, dark circles). Observe for visible gastric peristalsis when the infant is eating. Document and report signs of severe dehydration to help determine the need for fluid and electrolyte replacement.

NURSING DIAGNOSES

The severity of dehydration and malnutrition determines to some extent the appropriate nursing diagnoses for this infant. Some diagnoses that may be used are:

Preoperative:

- Altered Nutrition: Less than Body Requirements related to inability to retain food

- Fluid Volume Deficit related to frequent vomiting

- Ineffective Family Coping: Compromised related to seriousness of illness and impending surgery

- Altered Oral Mucous Membranes and Increased Sucking Needs related to NPO status

- Risk for Impaired Skin Integrity related to dehydration

Postoperative:

- Risk for Aspiration related to postoperative condition

- Altered Nutrition: Less than Body Requirements related to postoperative condition

- Ineffective Family Coping: Compromised related to postoperative condition

- Risk for Impaired Skin Integrity related to surgery

- Pain related to surgical trauma

OUTCOME IDENTIFICATION AND PLANNING: PREOPERATIVE

Preoperatively, the major goals for the infant with pyloric stenosis include improving nutrition and hydration, relieving family anxiety, and maintaining mouth and skin integrity. Plan individualized nursing care according to these goals, including interventions to prepare the infant for surgery.

IMPLEMENTATION: PREOPERATIVE

MAINTAINING ADEQUATE NUTRITION AND FLUID INTAKE. The pylorus is hypertrophied, and food (breast milk or formula) cannot pass through because of the narrow passage from the stomach into the duodenum. As a result, the infant loses weight and becomes dehydrated. If the infant is severely dehydrated and malnourished, IV fluids and electrolytes are necessary for rehydration to prepare for surgery and to correct hypokalemia and alkalosis. Carefully monitor the IV site for redness and induration. Improved nutrition and hydration is evidenced by improved skin turgor, weight gain, correction of hypokalemia and alkalosis, adequate intake of fluids, and no evidence of gastric distention.

Feedings of formula thickened with infant cereal and fed through a large-holed nipple may be given to improve nutrition before surgery. A smooth muscle relaxant may be ordered before feedings. Feed the infant slowly while he or she is sitting in an infant seat or being held upright. During the feeding, burp the infant frequently to avoid gastric distention. Document the feeding given and the approximate amount retained. Also record the frequency and type of emesis.

The infant must be prepared for surgery. Oral fluids are omitted for a specified time before the procedure, and the infant is placed on an IV infusion. Fluid and electrolyte balance must be restored and the stomach emptied. The physician may order placement of a nasogastric (NG) tube with saline lavage to empty the stomach after the barium swallow. The NG tube is left in place when the infant goes to surgery.

PROMOTING FAMILY COPING. The family caregivers are anxious because their infant is obviously seriously ill, and when they learn that the infant is to undergo surgery, their apprehensions increase. Include the caregivers in the preparation for surgery and explain:

- The importance of added IV fluids preoperatively to improve electrolyte balance and rehydrate the infant

- The reason for ultrasonographic or barium swallow examination

- The function of the NG tube and saline lavage.

Explain the location of the pylorus (at the distal end of the stomach) and what happens when the circular muscle fibers hypertrophy. You can liken it to a doughnut that thickens, so that the opening closes and very little food gets through. Describe the surgical procedure to be performed. During the procedure, the muscle is simply split down to, but not through, the submucosa, allowing it to balloon and let food pass through.

Direct the family caregivers to the appropriate waiting area during surgery so that the surgeon can find them immediately after surgery. Explain to the caregivers what to expect and about how long the operation will last. Describe the procedure for the postanesthesia care unit so that the caregivers know the infant will be under close observation postoperatively until fully recovered.

PROVIDING MOUTH CARE AND NONNUTRITIVE SUCKING. The infant needs good mouth care because the mucous membranes of the mouth may be dry because of dehydration, and oral fluids are omitted before surgery. A pacifier can satisfy the baby's need for sucking due to the interruption in normal feeding and sucking habits.

PROMOTING SKIN INTEGRITY. Depending on the severity of dehydration, the skin may easily break down and become irritated. The infant is repositioned, the diaper is changed, and lanolin or A and D Ointment is applied to dry skin areas. Intravenous therapy may also affect skin integrity. Closely observe and document the infant's skin condition.

OUTCOME IDENTIFICATION AND PLANNING: POSTOPERATIVE

Postoperatively, the major goals for the infant include maintaining airway clearance, improving nutrition and fluid balance, reducing family anxiety, maintaining comfort, and preserving skin integrity. Individualize the nursing plan of care according these goals.

IMPLEMENTATION: POSTOPERATIVE

PREVENTING ASPIRATION.   Postoperatively, position the infant on the side and prevent aspiration of mucus or vomitus, particularly during the anesthesia recovery period. After fully waking from surgery, the infant may be held by a family caregiver. Help the caregiver find a position that does not interfere with IV infusions and that is comforting to both caregiver and child.

PROVIDING NUTRITION.   The first feeding, given 4 to 6 hours postoperatively, is usually an electrolyte replacement, such as Lytren or Pedialyte. Give feedings in small amounts, slowly, with frequent burping. Intravenous fluid is necessary until the infant is taking sufficient oral feedings. Continue to use all nursing measures for IV care that were followed preoperatively. Accurate intake and output and daily weight determinations are required.

PROMOTING FAMILY COPING.   The family caregivers will be anxious if the infant vomits after surgery, but reassure them that this is not uncommon in the first 24 hours after surgery. The caregivers should be involved in postoperative care. Reassure them that the care they gave at home did not cause the condition. Offer them support and understanding and encourage them in feeding and providing for the infant's needs. They can be told that the likelihood of a satisfactory recovery in a few weeks, with steady progression to complete recovery, is excellent. The operative fatality rate under these conditions has become less than 1%.

PROMOTING SKIN INTEGRITY.   Closely observe the surgical site for blood, drainage, and secretions. Make observations at least every 4 hours. Record and report any odor. Care for the incision and dressings as ordered by the physician.

RELIEVING PAIN.   The infant's behavior is observed to evaluate discomfort and pain. Excessive crying, restlessness, listlessness, resistance to being held and cuddled, rigidity, and increased pulse and respiratory rates can indicate pain. Administer analgesics as ordered. Nursing interventions that may provide comfort include rocking, holding, cuddling, and offering a pacifier. Include the family caregivers in helping to comfort the infant.

EVALUATION: GOALS AND OUTCOME CRITERIA

Preoperative:

- *Goal*: Nutrition and fluid intake will improve.
  Criteria: The infant's skin turgor improves, mucous membranes are moist and pink, and the hourly urine output is 2 to 3 mL/kg.

- *Goal*: The IV infusion site will remain intact.
  Criteria: No signs of redness or induration are evident.

- *Goal*: Family caregiver anxiety will be reduced.
  Criteria: Family caregivers verbalize an understanding of the procedures and treatments, cooperate with the nursing staff, ask appropriate questions, and express confidence in the treatment plan.

- *Goal*: Mucous membranes of the mouth will remain intact.
  Criteria: The mucous membranes of the mouth are moist and pink and saliva is sufficient, as evidenced by typical drooling.

- *Goal*: Sucking needs will be satisfied.
  Criteria: The infant uses a pacifier sufficiently to meet sucking needs.

- *Goal*: Skin integrity will be maintained.
  Criteria: No signs of skin irritation or breakdown are evident.

Postoperatively:

- *Goal*: The infant will not aspirate vomitus or mucus.
  Criteria: The infant rests quietly in a side-lying position without choking or coughing.

- *Goal*: Nutrition and fluid intake will improve.
  Criteria: The infant retains oral fluids with minimal vomiting. Hourly urine output is 2 to 3 mL/kg; daily weight gain is 0.75 to 1 oz (22–30 g).

- *Goal*: Family caregiver anxiety will be reduced.
  Criteria: The family caregivers are involved in the postoperative feeding of the infant and demonstrate an understanding of feeding technique.

- *Goal*: Skin integrity will remain intact.
  Criteria: The surgical site shows no signs of infection, as evidenced by absence of redness, foul odor, or drainage.

- *Goal*: The infant will show limited signs of discomfort.
  Criteria: The infant sleeps and rests in a relaxed manner, cuddles with caregivers and nurses, and does not cry excessively.

Congenital Aganglionic Megacolon

Congenital aganglionic megacolon, also called Hirschsprung disease, is characterized by obstinate constipation resulting from partial or complete intestinal obstruction of mechanical origin. The condition may be severe enough to be recognized during the neonatal period, but in others it may not be diagnosed until later infancy or early childhood.

Parasympathetic nerve cells regulate peristalsis in the intestine. The name *aganglionic megacolon* actually describes the condition because there is an absence of parasympathetic ganglion cells within the muscular wall of the distal colon and the rectum. As a result, the affected portion of the lower bowel has no peristaltic action. Thus, it narrows, and the portion directly proximal to (above) the affected area becomes greatly dilated and filled with feces and gas (Fig. 11-4).

CLINICAL MANIFESTATIONS

Accurate reporting of the first meconium stool in the newborn is vital. Failure of the newborn to have a stool in the first 24 hours may indicate a number of conditions, one of which is megacolon. Other neonatal symptoms are suggestive of complete or partial intestinal obstruction, such as bile-stained emesis and generalized abdominal distention. Gastroenteritis with diarrheal stools may be present, and ulceration of the colon may occur.

The affected older infant or young child has obstinate, severe constipation dating back to early infancy. Stools are ribbonlike or consist of hard pellets. Formed bowel movements do not occur except with the use of enemas, and soiling does not occur. The rectum is usually empty because the impaction occurs above the aganglionic segment.

As the child grows older, the abdomen becomes progressively enlarged and hard (Fig. 11-5). General debilitation and chronic anemia are usually present. Differentiation must be made between this condition and psychogenic megacolon due to coercive toileting or other emotional problems. The child with aganglionic megacolon does not withhold stools or defecate in inappropriate places, and there is no soiling.

Figure 11-5
A baby with Hirschsprung disease.

DIAGNOSIS

In the newborn, the absence of a meconium stool within the first 24 hours, and in the older infant or young child, a history of obstinate, severe constipation may indicate the need for further evaluation. Definitive diagnosis is made through barium studies and must be confirmed by rectal biopsy.

TREATMENT

Treatment involves surgery, with the ultimate resection of the aganglionic portion of the bowel. A colostomy is often performed to relieve the obstruction. This allows the infant to regain any weight lost and also gives the bowel a period of rest to return to a more normal state. Resection is deferred until later in infancy.

⬔ ⬔ Nursing Process for the Infant ⬔ ⬔ Undergoing Surgery for Congenital Megacolon

ASSESSMENT

Carefully gather a history from the family caregivers, noting especially the history of stooling. If the child is not a young infant, ask about the onset of constipation, the character and odor of stools, the frequency of bowel movements, and the presence of poor feeding habits, anorexia, and irritability.

During the physical assessment, observe for a distended abdomen and signs of poor nutrition (see the earlier sec-

Figure 11-4
Dilated colon in Hirschsprung disease.

tion on the malnourished infant). Record weight and vital signs. Assess for developmental milestones.

NURSING DIAGNOSES

Many of the nursing diagnoses for pyloric stenosis also may be appropriate for congenital megacolon, with some adjustment. The following are some specific diagnoses that may apply:

Preoperative:

- Risk for Injury related to decreased bowel motility

- Fluid Volume Deficit and Altered Nutrition: Less than Body Requirements related to anorexia

- Fear (in the older child) related to impending surgery

- Ineffective Family Coping: Compromised related to the serious condition of the infant and lack of knowledge about impending surgery

Postoperative:

- Risk for Impaired Skin Integrity related to irritation from the colostomy

- Pain related to the surgical procedure

- Fluid Volume Deficit related to postoperative condition

- Altered Oral and Nasal Mucous Membranes related to NPO status and irritation from NG tube

- Parental Health Seeking Behaviors related to postoperative care of the colostomy

OUTCOME IDENTIFICATION AND PLANNING: PREOPERATIVE CARE

The preoperative goals for the infant undergoing surgery for congenital megacolon include preventing injury, maintaining fluid balance, and relieving fear (in the older child). The major goal for the family is reducing anxiety. Base the preoperative nursing plan of care on these goals. Plan interventions that prepare the infant for surgery.

IMPLEMENTATION: PREOPERATIVE CARE

PREVENTING INJURY. Decreased bowel motility may lead to constipation, which in turn may result in injury. Therefore, empty the colon of fecal material before diagnostic and surgical procedures are performed. Administer colonic irrigations with isotonic saline solution and neomycin or other antibiotics to cleanse the bowel and prepare the GI tract. Never administer soapsuds or tap water enemas, because the lack of peristaltic action causes the enemas to be retained and absorbed into the tissues, causing water intoxication. This could cause syncope, shock, or even death after only one or two irrigations.

MAINTAINING ADEQUATE NUTRITION AND FLUID INTAKE. Parenteral fluids may be needed to improve hydration because the constipation and distended abdomen cause loss of appetite; thus, the child is in a poor nutritional state. All the precautions used with parenteral fluid administration are appropriate.

REDUCING FEAR. Children who are preschool-age and older are more aware of the approaching surgery and have a number of fears as a result of their developmental stage. Preschoolers are still in the age of magical thinking. They may overhear a word or two that they misinterpret and exaggerate, imagining pain and danger. Careful explanations must be provided for the preschooler to reduce any fears about mutilation. Talk about the surgery, reassuring the child that the "insides won't come out," and answer questions seriously and sincerely. Encourage family caregivers to stay with the young child if possible to increase the child's feelings of security.

The older school-age child may have a more realistic view of what is going to happen but may still fear the impending surgery. Peer contact may help comfort the school-age child. For more information on reducing preoperative fears and anxiety, see Chapters 4 and 17.

PROMOTING FAMILY COPING. Family caregivers are apprehensive about the preliminary procedures as well as the impending surgery. Explain all aspects of the preoperative care, including examinations, colonic irrigations, and IV fluid therapy. As with other surgical procedures, inform the caregivers about the waiting area, the postanesthesia care unit, and the approximate length of the operation, and answer any questions. Building good rapport preoperatively is an essential aspect of good nursing care. Answer the family caregivers' questions about the later resection of the aganglionic portion. With successful surgery, these children grow and develop normally.

OUTCOME IDENTIFICATION AND PLANNING: POSTOPERATIVE CARE

The major postoperative goals for the infant include maintaining skin integrity, preventing intense pain, maintaining fluid balance and nutrition, and maintaining moist, clean nasal mucous membrane. Goals for the family include reducing caregiver anxiety and preparing for home care of the infant. Develop the individualized nursing plan of care according to these goals.

IMPLEMENTATION: POSTOPERATIVE CARE

PROMOTING SKIN INTEGRITY. Skin integrity of the surgical site, especially around the colostomy stoma, is very important. When routine colostomy care is performed, give careful attention to the area around the colostomy. Record and report redness, irritation, and rashy appearances of the skin around the stoma. Prepare the skin with skin-toughening preparations that strengthen the skin and provide better adhesion of the appliance.

RELIEVING PAIN.   The child may have abdominal pain postoperatively. Assess for signs of pain, such as crying, pulse and respiration rate increase, restlessness, and guarding of the abdomen or drawing up the legs. Administer analgesics promptly as ordered. Additional nursing measures that can be used are changing the child's position, holding the child when possible, stroking, cuddling, and engaging in age-appropriate activities. Observe for abdominal distention, which must be documented and reported promptly.

MAINTAINING FLUID INTAKE.   The NG tube is left in place after surgery, and IV feedings are given until bowel function is established. Accurate intake and output determinations and reporting of the character, amount, and consistency of stools help determine when the child may have oral feedings. Record and report the drainage from the NG tube every 8 hours. Immediately report any unusual drainage, such as bright-red bleeding.

PROVIDING ORAL AND NASAL CARE.   Perform good mouth care at least every 4 hours. At the same time, gently clean the nares to relieve any irritation from the NG tube. If the infant is young, sucking needs can be satisfied with a pacifier.

PROVIDING FAMILY TEACHING.   Show the family caregiver how to care for the colostomy at home. If available, an ostomy nurse may be consulted to help teach the family caregivers. Discuss topics such as devices and their use, daily irrigation, and skin care. The caregivers should demonstrate their understanding by caring for the colostomy under the supervision of nursing personnel several days before discharge. Family caregivers also need referrals to support personnel.

EVALUATION: GOALS AND OUTCOME CRITERIA

Preoperative:

- *Goal*: Injury related to constipation will be avoided.
  Criteria: The colon is clean and well prepared for surgery.

- *Goal*: The child will be well hydrated preoperatively.
  Criteria: Hourly urine output measures 2 to 3 mL/kg. No signs of dehydration are evident: skin turgor is good, mucous membranes are moist and pink, and fontanelles have normal tension.

- *Goal*: Family caregivers will demonstrate an understanding of preoperative procedures.
  Criteria: Family caregivers cooperate with care, ask relevant questions, and accurately explain procedures when asked to repeat information.

- *Goal*: The older child will display minimal fear of bodily injury.

Criteria: The older child realistically describes what will happen in surgery and interacts with family, peers, and nursing staff in a positive manner.

Postoperative:

- *Goal*: Skin integrity will be maintained.
  Criteria: No skin irritation is noted at the colostomy site; no redness, foul odor, or purulent drainage is noted at the surgical site.

- *Goal*: The child will have minimal pain.
  Criteria: The child rests quietly without signs of restlessness; he or she verbalizes comfort if old enough to communicate.

- *Goal*: Adequate fluid intake will be maintained.
  Criteria: Hourly urine output is 2 to 3 mL/kg, indicating adequate hydration.

- *Goal*: Oral and mucous membranes will remain intact.
  Criteria: Oral and mucous membranes are moist and pink; the infant uses a pacifier to meet sucking needs.

- *Goal*: Family caregivers will demonstrate skill and knowledge in caring for the colostomy.
  Criteria: The family caregivers irrigate the colostomy and clean the surrounding skin under the supervision of nursing personnel.

Intussusception

Intussusception is the **invagination**, or telescoping, of one portion of the bowel into a distal portion. It occurs most commonly at the juncture of the ileum and the colon, although it can appear elsewhere in the intestinal tract. The invagination is from above downward, the upper portion slipping over the lower portion and pulling the mesentery along with it (Fig. 11-6).

This condition occurs more often in boys than in girls and is the most common cause of intestinal obstruction

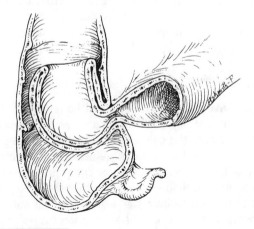

Figure 11-6
In this drawing of intussusception, note the telescoping of a portion of the bowel into the distal portion.

in childhood. The highest incidence occurs in infants between the ages of 4 and 10 months. The condition usually appears in healthy babies without any demonstrable cause. Possible contributing factors may be the hyperperistalsis and unusual mobility of the cecum and ileum normally present in early life. Occasionally, a lesion such as Meckel's diverticulum or a polyp is present.

CLINICAL MANIFESTATIONS

The infant who previously appeared healthy and happy suddenly becomes pale, cries out sharply, and draws up the legs in a severe colicky spasm of pain. This spasm may last for several minutes, after which the infant relaxes and appears well until the next episode, which may occur 5, 10, or 20 minutes later.

Most of these infants start vomiting early. Vomiting becomes progressively more severe and eventually is bile-stained. The infant strains with each paroxysm, emptying the bowels of fecal contents. The stools consist of blood and mucus, thereby earning the name **currant jelly stools**.

Signs of shock appear quickly and characteristically include a rapid, weak pulse, increased temperature, shallow, grunting respirations, pallor, and marked sweating. Shock, vomiting, and currant jelly stools are the cardinal symptoms of this condition. Because these signs, coupled with the paroxysmal pain, are quite severe, professional health care is often initiated early.

The nurse, who is often consulted by neighbors, friends, and relatives when things go wrong, needs to be informed and alert; therefore a word of caution is needed. The nurse needs to be aware that on rare occasions a more chronic form of the condition appears, particularly during an episode of severe diarrheal disturbance. The onset is more gradual and the infant may not show all the classic symptoms, but the danger of sudden, complete strangulation is present. Such an infant should already be in the care of a physician because of the diarrhea.

DIAGNOSIS

Diagnosis usually can be made by the physician from the clinical symptoms, rectal examination, and palpation of the abdomen during a calm interval when it is soft. A baby is often unwilling to tolerate this palpation, and sedation may be ordered. A sausage-shaped mass can often be felt through the abdominal wall.

TREATMENT AND NURSING CARE

Unlike pyloric stenosis, this condition is an emergency in the sense that prolonged delay is dangerous. The telescoped bowel rapidly becomes gangrenous, thus markedly reducing the possibility of a simple reduction. Adequate treatment during the first 12 to 24 hours should have a good outcome, with complete recovery. The outcome becomes more uncertain as the bowel deteriorates, making resection necessary.

Immediate treatment consists of IV fluids, NPO status, and a diagnostic barium enema. The barium enema can often reduce the invagination simply by the pressure of the barium fluid pushing against the telescoped portion. The barium enema should not be done if signs of bowel perforation or peritonitis are evident. Abdominal surgery is performed if the barium enema does not correct the problem. Surgery may consist of manual reduction of the invagination or resection with anastomosis, or possible colostomy if the intestine is gangrenous.

If the invagination was reduced, the infant is returned to normal feedings within 24 hours and discharged in about 48 hours. Carefully observe for recurrence during this period. If surgery is necessary, many of the same preoperative and postoperative nursing diagnoses can be used as for congenital aganglionic megacolon.

CIRCULATORY SYSTEM DISORDERS

Anemia is a common childhood blood disorder. It may result from inadequate production or excessive loss of red blood cells or hemoglobin. The following are examples of the more common types of anemia found in childhood; there are many others:

- Inadequate production of erythrocytes or of hemoglobin, as in iron deficiency anemia and in anemia of chronic infection
- Excessive loss of red cells, as in hemorrhage
- Hemolytic anemia associated with congenital abnormalities of erythrocytes or hemoglobin, as in thalassemia or sickle cell disease
- Hemolytic anemia associated with acquired abnormalities of erythrocytes or hemoglobin, from drugs, chemicals, or bacterial reaction.

Iron Deficiency Anemia

Iron deficiency anemia is a common nutritional deficiency in young children. It is a hypochromic, microcytic anemia—in other words, the blood cells are deficient in hemoglobin and smaller than normal—and is common between the ages of 9 and 24 months. The full-term newborn has a high hemoglobin level (needed during fetal life to provide adequate oxygenation) that decreases during the first 2 or 3 months of life. However, considerable iron is reclaimed and stored, usually in sufficient quantity to last for 4 to 9 months of life.

A child needs to absorb 0.8 to 1.5 mg of iron per day. Because only 10% of dietary iron is absorbed, a diet containing 8 to 10 mg of iron is needed for good health. During the first years of life, it is often difficult for a child to obtain this quantity of iron from food. If the diet is inadequate, anemia quickly results. (In addition, adolescent girls may have iron deficiency anemia because of improper dieting to lose weight.)

Babies with an inordinate fondness for milk can take in an astonishing amount and, with their appetites satisfied, show little interest in solid foods. These babies are prime candidates for iron deficiency anemia. They may have a history of consuming 2 or 3 quarts of milk daily while not accepting any other foods, or at best only foods with a high carbohydrate content. Many caregivers believe, incorrectly, that milk is a perfect food, so why not let the baby have all the milk desired? These infants are commonly known as milk babies. They have pale, almost translucent (porcelain-like) skin and are chubby and susceptible to infections.

Many children with iron deficiency anemia, however, are undernourished because of the family's economic problems. Along with the economic factor, a caregiver knowledge deficit about nutrition is often present. The WIC program, discussed in Chapter 10, does much to alleviate this problem.

CLINICAL MANIFESTATIONS

The signs of iron deficiency anemia include below-average body weight, pale mucous membranes, anorexia, growth retardation, and listlessness, in addition to the characteristics of milk babies described earlier.

DIAGNOSIS

In blood tests that measure hemoglobin, a level lower than 11 g/dL or a hematocrit lower than 33% is highly suspect. Stool is tested for occult blood to rule out low GI bleeding as a cause for the depleted hemoglobin and hematocrit.

TREATMENT AND NURSING CARE

Treatment consists of improved nutrition, with ferrous sulfate administered between meals with juice (preferably orange juice, since vitamin C aids in iron absorption). For best results, iron should not be given with meals. Teach the family caregivers to brush the child's teeth after administering ferrous sulfate to prevent staining. Tell the caregivers that ferrous sulfate can cause constipation or turn the child's stools black.

A few children have a hemoglobin level so low or anorexia so acute that they need additional therapy. An iron/dextran mixture for intramuscular use (Imferon) is administered. This medication should be administered in the vastus lateralis by the Z-track method to avoid leakage into the subcutaneous tissues because of its irritating nature. For infants who are seriously ill, refer to the nursing process for the nutritionally deprived infant.

For most infants with iron deficiency anemia, teaching for home care is needed. When teaching caregivers, remember that attitudes and food choices are often influ-

Family Teaching
Tips for Iron Deficiency Anemia

Foods High in Iron

1. One of the most important things you can do for your baby and family is to learn about the foods that will help them stay healthy.
2. Milk is good for your baby, but no more than a quart a day (four 8-oz bottles).
3. Shop for baby cereals fortified with iron.
4. Some baby formulas are iron-fortified.
5. Egg yolks are rich in iron. Avoid egg white for young babies because of allergies.
6. Green vegetables such as peas, green beans, lettuce, and spinach are good sources of iron.
7. Dried beans, dried peas, canned refried beans, and peanut butter provide good sources for toddlers and older children.
8. Fruits that are iron-rich include peaches, prune juice, and raisins (don't give to child younger than 3 years of age because of danger of choking).
9. For older children, fortified instant oatmeal and cream of wheat are good sources of iron.
10. Read labels to check for iron content of processed foods.
11. Organ meat, poultry, and fish are good iron sources.
12. Orange juice helps the body absorb iron.
13. Liquid iron preparations should be taken through a straw to prevent staining of teeth.

enced by cultural differences. See Family Teaching Tips for Iron Deficiency Anemia.

Sickle Cell Disease

Sickle cell disease is a hereditary trait occurring most commonly in blacks. It is characterized by the production of an abnormal hemoglobin that causes the red blood cells to assume a sickle shape. It appears as an asymptomatic trait when the sickling trait is inherited from one parent alone (heterozygous state). There is a 50% probability that each child born to one parent carrying the sickle cell trait will inherit the trait from that parent. When inherited from both parents (homozygous state), the child has sickle cell disease, and anemia develops (Fig. 11-7). A rapid breakdown of red blood cells carrying hemoglobin S, the abnormal hemoglobin, causes a severe hemolytic anemia. Those who inherit the gene for the sickle cell trait from only one parent are asymptomatic, with normal hemoglobin levels and red blood cell counts.

The sickling trait occurs in about 10% of African-Americans; there is a much higher incidence in parts of Africa. In African-Americans, the disease itself, sickle cell anemia, has an incidence of 0.3% to 1.3%. The tendency to sickle can be demonstrated by a laboratory test.

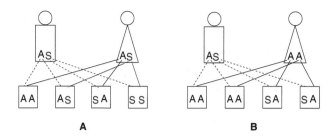

Figure 11-7
Inheritance patterns. **(A)** Heterozygous type. One parent
carries a hemoglobin S gene, and one does not. Two children
will be free of the gene (AA), and two will be carriers (AS). **(B)**
Homozygous type. Each parent is carrying one hemoglobin A
gene and one hemoglobin S gene. One child is free of the gene
(AA), two are carriers (AS), and one has sickle cell disease (SS).

CLINICAL MANIFESTATIONS

Clinical symptoms of the disease itself do not usually appear before the latter half of the first year of life because sufficient fetal hemoglobin is still present to prevent sickling. Sickle cell disease causes a chronic anemia with a hemoglobin level of 6 to 9 g/dL (the normal level in an infant is 11 to 15 g/dL). The chronic anemia causes the child to be tired and have a poor appetite and pale mucous membranes.

Sickle cell crisis is the most severe manifestation of the condition. Normal red blood cells, which carry oxygen to the tissues, are disc-shaped and normally move through the blood vessels, bending and flexing to flow through smoothly. The smooth, uniform shape of the red blood cells and the low viscosity (thickness) of the blood is such that these cells split relatively easily at Y-intersections and go single file through the capillaries with little or no clustering. The affected red blood cells (hemoglobin S) do much the same thing until there is an episode that causes sickling. These episodes (sickle cell crises) can be precipitated by low oxygen levels (which can be caused by a respiratory infection or extremely strenuous exercise), dehydration, acidosis, or stress. When sickling occurs, the affected red blood cells become crescent-shaped and therefore do not slip through as easily as do the disc-shaped cells. The viscosity of the blood increases (becomes thicker), causing slowdown and sludging of the red blood cells. The impaired circulation results in tissue damage and infarction.

A sickle cell crisis may be the first clinical manifestation of the disease and may recur frequently during early childhood. This disturbance presents a variety of symptoms. The most common symptom is severe, acute abdominal pain (caused by sludging, which leads to enlargement of the spleen), together with muscle spasm, fever, and severe leg pain that may be muscular, osseous (bony), or localized in the joints, which become hot and swollen. The abdomen becomes boardlike, with an absence of bowel sounds. This makes it extremely difficult to distinguish the condition

from an abdominal condition requiring surgery. Several days after a crisis, the child will be jaundiced, evidenced by yellow sclera, as a result of the hemolysis that has occurred. The crisis may have a fatal outcome caused by cerebral, cardiac, or hemolytic complications.

DIAGNOSIS

Screening for the presence of hemoglobin S may be done with a test called Sickledex, a finger stick screening test that gives results in 3 minutes. Definite diagnosis is made through hemoglobin electrophoresis ("fingerprinting"). This can be done if the Sickledex screening results are positive to determine if the child is carrying the trait or has sickle cell disease.

TREATMENT

Prevention of crises is the goal between episodes. Adequate hydration is vital; fluid intake of 1,500 to 2,000 mL daily is desirable for a child weighing 20 kg, and this should be increased to 3,000 mL during the crisis. Extremely strenuous activities that may cause oxygen depletion are to be avoided. These children should also avoid visiting areas of high altitude. Small blood transfusions help bring the hemoglobin to a near-normal level temporarily. Iron preparations have no effect in sickle cell disease.

Treatment for a crisis is supportive for each presenting symptom, and bed rest is indicated. Oxygen may be administered. Analgesics are given for pain. Dehydration and acidosis are vigorously treated. Prognosis is guarded, depending on the severity of the disease.

Nursing Process for the Child With Sickle Cell Crisis

ASSESSMENT

The parents who have a child with sickle cell disease may suffer a great deal of guilt for having passed the disease to their child. Take care not to increase this guilt, but help them cope with it. During the interview with the family caregivers, ask about activities or events that led to this crisis, obtain a history of the child's health and any previous episodes, and evaluate the caregivers' knowledge about the condition.

Assessment of the child varies somewhat with his or her age. Record vital signs, particularly noting fever, abdominal pain, presence of bowel sounds, pain or swelling and warmth in the joints, and muscle spasms. Observe the young child for dactylitis (hand–foot syndrome), which results from soft-tissue swelling caused by interference with circulation. This swelling further impairs circulation.

NURSING DIAGNOSES

Nursing diagnoses vary somewhat with the child's age and the stage of advancement of the disease. Some diagnoses that may be used, in addition to those suggested early in this chapter, are:

- Activity Intolerance related to oxygen depletion and pain

- Ineffective Family Coping: Compromised related to child's condition

- Fluid Volume Deficit related to low fluid intake, impaired renal function, or both

- Parental Health Seeking Behaviors related to the disorder and appropriate care measures

- Impaired Physical Mobility related to muscle and joint involvement

- Pain related to disease condition affecting abdominal organs or joints and muscles

- Risk for Impaired Skin Integrity related to altered circulation

OUTCOME IDENTIFICATION AND PLANNING

Conserving energy, improving gas exchange, and increasing fluid intake are major goals for the child with sickle cell disease. Other goals include maintaining comfort, improving physical mobility, maintaining skin integrity, and reducing the caregivers' anxiety. Another important goal is decreasing the number of future episodes by improving knowledge about the causes of crisis episodes. Plan individualized nursing care according to these goals.

IMPLEMENTATION

PROMOTING ENERGY CONSERVATION. The child may become dyspneic on any kind of activity. Plan nursing activities so that the child is disturbed as little as possible and can rest. Bed rest is necessary to decrease the demands on oxygen supply. Oxygen may be administered by mask or nasal cannula to improve tissue perfusion.

MAINTAINING FLUID INTAKE. The child is prone to dehydration because of the inability of the kidneys to concentrate urine. Observe for signs of dehydration such as dry mucous membranes, weight loss, or, in the case of infants, sunken fontanelles. Strict intake and output measurements and daily weights are necessary. In sickle cell crisis, urine specific gravity is not a good indicator of dehydration. Teach the family caregivers that fluid intake is important, and intake should be maintained at 1,500 to 2,000 mL when the child is not in crisis. Offer the child appealing fluids, such as juices, popsicles, noncaffeinated soda, and favorite flavored gelatins. Teach family caregivers that increased fluid intake will help to avoid a crisis during activities in which the child may be involved, such as hik-

ing, swimming, or sports. The child also needs increased fluids during episodes of infections.

PROMOTING FAMILY COPING. Guilt plays an important part in the anxiety that the family caregivers experience. Explain procedures, planned treatments, and care to help the caregivers feel that they are being included in the care. Caregivers need to feel that they have some control over the disease. Teach measures that may help alleviate pain or encourage fluid intake. Also emphasize the importance of protecting the child from situations that may cause overexhaustion or that may otherwise deplete the child's oxygen supplies or lead to dehydration. This knowledge may give the family caregivers a feeling of control. In addition, caregivers may need more information concerning the disorder. If the child has been previously diagnosed, the caregivers should already have had information presented to them. In this instance, assess their knowledge level and supplement and reinforce that information.

IMPROVING PHYSICAL MOBILITY. Sickling that affects the muscles and joints causes a great deal of pain for the child. The child needs careful handling and should be moved slowly and gently. Joints can be supported with pillows. Warm soaks and massages may help relieve some of the discomfort. Administer analgesics before exercise and as needed. Passive exercises help prevent contractures and wasting of muscles.

RELIEVING PAIN. The child in sickle cell crisis often has severe pain. Enlargement of the spleen (splenomegaly) causes severe abdominal pain. Joint and muscle pain are also common due to poor perfusion of the tissues. Assessment of pain, nursing measures to relieve pain, and prompt administration of analgesics are essential. The family caregivers can be involved, if they wish, in helping administer comfort measures to the child. Sometimes diversional activities can help alleviate perceived pain, but be assured that these children are in pain and need analgesics promptly.

PROMOTING SKIN INTEGRITY. Increased fluid intake and improved nutrition are important. Observe the child's skin regularly each shift, and provide good skin care, consisting of lotion, massage, and skin-toughening agents, especially over bony prominences. Additional padding in the form of foam protectors and egg-crate pads or mattresses may be helpful where there is irritation from bedding.

EVALUATION: GOALS AND OUTCOME CRITERIA

- *Goal*: The child's energy will be conserved.
  Criteria: The child's activities are restricted to conserve energy. The oxygen saturation is greater than 90%.

- *Goal*: The child's fluid intake will improve.
  Criteria: The child has an intake of at least 3,000 mL/day.

- *Goal*: The family caregivers' anxiety will be reduced.
  Criteria: Family caregivers are more self-confident, cooperate with nursing personnel, and verbalize an understanding of the disease process.

- *Goal*: The child's muscles and joints will remain flexible.
  Criteria: The child cooperates with daily passive exercises.

- *Goal*: Pain will be reduced or eliminated.
  Criteria: The child rests quietly and, if possible, reports his or her comfort.

- *Goal*: Skin integrity will be maintained.
  Criteria: The child's skin shows no signs of redness, irritation, or breakdown.

RESPIRATORY SYSTEM DISORDERS

Acute Nasopharyngitis (Common Cold)

The common cold is one of the most common infectious conditions of childhood. The young infant is as susceptible as the older child but is generally not as frequently exposed.

The illness is of viral origin, such as rhinoviruses, respiratory syncytial virus (RSV), influenza virus, parainfluenza virus, or adenovirus. Bacterial invasion of the tissues may cause complications such as ear, mastoid, and lung infections. The young child appears to be more susceptible to complications than an adult. The infant should be protected from people who have colds because complications in the infant can be serious.

CLINICAL MANIFESTATIONS

The infant older than the age of 3 months usually develops fever early in the course of the infection, often as high as 102° to 104°F (38.9°–40°C). Younger infants usually are afebrile. The infant sneezes and becomes irritable and restless. The congested nasal passages interfere with nursing, increasing the infant's irritability. The infant may have vomiting or diarrhea, which may be caused by mucous drainage into the digestive system.

DIAGNOSIS

This nasopharyngeal condition may appear as the first symptom of many childhood contagious diseases, such as measles, and must be observed carefully. The common cold also needs to be differentiated from allergic rhinitis.

TREATMENT

The child with an uncomplicated cold may not need any treatment in addition to rest, increased fluids and nutrition, normal saline nose drops, suction with a bulb syringe,

and a humidified environment. In the older child, acetaminophen can be administered as an analgesic and antipyretic. Aspirin is best avoided. If the nares or upper lip become irritated, cold cream or petrolatum (Vaseline) can be used. The infant needs to be comforted by holding, rocking, and soothing. If the symptoms persist for several days, the child must be seen by a physician to rule out complications such as otitis media.

Otitis Media

Otitis media is one of the most common infectious diseases of childhood. Two out of three children have at least one episode of otitis media by the time they are 1 year old.[1] The eustachian tube in an infant is shorter and wider than in the older child or adult (Fig. 11-8). The tube is also straighter, thereby allowing nasopharyngeal secretions to enter the middle ear more easily. *Haemophilus influenzae* is an important causative agent of otitis media in infants.

Figure 11-8
Comparison of the eustachian tube in the adult (**A**) and the infant (**B**).

CLINICAL MANIFESTATIONS

A restless infant who repeatedly shakes the head and rubs or pulls at one ear should be checked for an ear infection. Symptoms include fever and irritability. There may be vomiting or diarrhea.

DIAGNOSIS

Examination of the ear with an otoscope reveals a bright-red, bulging eardrum. Spontaneous rupture of the eardrum may occur, in which case there will be purulent drainage, and the pain caused by the pressure build-up in the ear will be relieved. If present, purulent drainage is cultured to determine the causative organism and appropriate antibiotic.

TREATMENT

Antibiotics are used during the period of infection and for several days following to prevent mastoiditis or chronic infection. A 10-day course of amoxicillin is a common treatment. Most infants respond well to antibiotics.

Some infants and young children have repeated episodes of otitis media. Children with chronic otitis media may be put on a prophylactic course of an oral penicillin or sulfonamide drug. **Myringotomy** (incision of the eardrum) may be performed to establish drainage and to insert tiny tubes into the tympanic membrane to facilitate drainage. In most cases, the tubes eventually fall out spontaneously. Attention to chronic otitis media is essential because permanent hearing loss can result from frequent occurrences.

Mastoiditis (infection of the mastoid sinus) is a possible complication of untreated acute otitis media. Mastoiditis was much more common before the advent of antibiotics. Currently, it is seen only in children who have an untreated ruptured eardrum or inadequate treatment (through non-compliance of caregivers or improper care) of an acute episode.

Most infants and young children with otitis media are cared for at home; therefore, a primary responsibility of the nurse is to teach the family caregivers about prevention and the care of the child (see Family Teaching Tips for Otitis Media).

Acute Bronchiolitis

Acute bronchiolitis (acute interstitial pneumonia) is most common during the first 6 months of life and is rarely seen after the age of 2 years. Most cases occur in infants who have been in contact with older children or adults with upper respiratory viral infections. It usually occurs in the winter and early spring.

Acute bronchiolitis is caused by a viral infection. The causative agent in more than 50% of cases has been shown to be RSV. Other viruses associated with the disease are parainfluenza virus, adenoviruses, and other viruses not always identified.

Family Teaching
Tips for Otitis Media

The eustachian tube is a connection between the nasal passages and the middle ear. The eustachian tube is wider, shorter, and straighter in the infant, allowing organisms from respiratory infections to travel into the middle ear to cause infection (otitis media).

Prevention
1. Hold infant in an upright position or with head slightly elevated while feeding to prevent formula from draining into the middle ear through the wide eustachian tube.
2. Never prop a bottle.
3. Do not give infant a bottle in bed. This allows fluid to pool in the middle ear, encouraging organisms to grow.
4. Protect infant from exposure to others with upper respiratory infections.
5. Protect infant from passive smoke; don't permit smoking in baby's presence.
6. Remove sources of allergies from home.
7. Observe for clues to ear infection: shaking head, rubbing or pulling at ears, fever, combined with restlessness or screaming and crying.
8. Be alert to signs of hearing difficulty in toddlers and preschoolers. This may be the first sign of an ear infection.
9. Teach toddler or preschooler gentle nose blowing.

Care of Child with Otitis Media
1. Have child with upper respiratory infection who shows symptoms of ear discomfort checked by a health care professional.
2. Complete the entire amount of antibiotic prescribed, even though the child seems better.
3. Heat (such as a heating pad on low setting) may provide comfort, but an adult must stay with the child.
4. Soothe, rock, and comfort child to help relieve discomfort. The child is more comfortable sleeping on side of infected ear.
5. Give pain medications (such as acetaminophen) as directed. Never give aspirin.
6. Provide liquid or soft foods; chewing causes pain.
7. Hearing loss may last up to 6 months after infection.
8. Follow-up with hearing test should be scheduled as advised.

The bronchi and bronchioles become plugged with a thick, viscid mucus, causing air to be trapped in the lungs. The infant can breathe air in but has difficulty expelling it. This hinders the exchange of gases, and cyanosis appears.

CLINICAL MANIFESTATIONS

The onset of dyspnea is abrupt, sometimes preceded by a cough or nasal discharge. There is a dry, persistent cough, extremely shallow respirations, air hunger, and cyanosis, which is often marked. Suprasternal and subcostal retractions are present. The chest becomes barrel-shaped from the trapped air. Respirations are 60 to 80 breaths per minute.

Fever is not extreme, seldom higher than 101° to 102°F (38.3°–38.9°C). Dehydration may become a serious factor if competent care is not given. The infant appears apprehensive, irritable, and restless.

DIAGNOSIS

Diagnosis is made from clinical findings and can be confirmed by laboratory testing (enzyme-linked immunosorbent assay) of the mucus obtained by direct nasal aspiration or nasopharyngeal washing.

TREATMENT

The infant is usually hospitalized and treated with high humidity by mist tent, rest, and increased fluids (Fig. 11-9). Oxygen may be administered in addition to the mist tent. Monitoring of oxygenation may be done by means of capillary gases or pulse oximetry. Antibiotics are not prescribed because the causative organism is a virus. Intravenous fluids often are administered to ensure an adequate intake and to permit the infant to rest. The hospitalized infant is placed on contact transmission precautions to prevent the spread of infection.

Ribavirin (Virazole) is an antiviral drug that may be used to treat certain infants with RSV. It is administered as an inhalant by hood, mask, or tent. The American Academy of Pediatrics states that the use of ribavirin must be limited to infants at high risk for severe or complicated RSV, such as infants with chronic lung disease, premature infants,

transplant recipients, and infants receiving chemotherapy. Ribavirin is classified as a category X drug, signifying a high risk for **teratogenicity** (causing damage to a fetus). Health care personnel and others may inhale the mist that escapes into the room, so women who might be pregnant should stay out of the room where ribavirin is being administered.

Bacterial Pneumonia

Pneumococcal pneumonia is the most common form of bacterial pneumonia in infants and children. Its incidence has decreased during the last several years. This disease occurs mainly during the late winter and early spring, principally in children younger than 4 years of age.

In the infant, pneumococcal pneumonia is generally of the bronchial type rather than the lobar type seen in older children. It is usually secondary to an upper respiratory viral infection. The most common finding in infants is a patchy infiltration of one or several lobes of the lung. Pleural effusion is often present.

H influenzae pneumonia also occurs in infants and young children. Its clinical manifestations are similar to those of pneumococcal pneumonia, but its onset is more insidious, its clinical course is longer and less acute, and it is usually lobar in distribution. Complications in the young infant are common—usually bacteremia, pericarditis, and empyema (pus in the lungs). The treatment is the same. Immunization with *H influenzae* type B conjugate vaccine (HbCV) is currently recommended beginning at 2 months of age.

Figure 11-9
The infant in the mist tent. The mom continues to hold and feed the child. (Side rails are down for purpose of photography.)

CLINICAL MANIFESTATIONS

The onset of the pneumonic process is usually abrupt, following a mild upper respiratory illness. Temperature increases rapidly to 103° to 105°F (39.4°–40.6°C). Respiratory distress is marked, with obvious air hunger, flaring of the nostrils, circumoral cyanosis, and chest retractions. Tachycardia and tachypnea are present, with a pulse rate frequently as high as 140 to 180 beats per minute and respirations as high as 80 breaths per minute.

Generalized convulsions may occur during the period of high fever. Cough may not be noticeable at the onset but may appear later. Abdominal distention due to swallowed air or paralytic ileus commonly occurs.

DIAGNOSIS

Diagnosis is made based on clinical symptoms, chest radiograph, and culture of the organism from secretions. The white blood cell count may be elevated. The antistreptolysin titer (ASO titer) is usually elevated in children with staphylococcal pneumonia.

TREATMENT

The use of antibiotics early in the disease gives a prompt and favorable response. Penicillin or ampicillin has proved to be the most effective treatment and is generally used unless the infant has a penicillin allergy. Oxygen started early in the disease process is important. Infants are sometimes placed in a croupette or mist tent. There is some controversy concerning the safety of mist tents unless constant observation can be provided. Children have become cyanotic in mist tents, with subsequent arrest, due to the difficulty in seeing the child; therefore, a mask or hood is thought to be the better choice. Intravenous fluids are often necessary to supply the needed amount of fluids. Prognosis for recovery is excellent.

A Personal Glimpse

The first time I put Bobbie in the hospital it was very scary. I knew the nurses, but still I was afraid for him. I felt like someone was punishing me. I couldn't leave him for a minute. I was afraid he wouldn't be alive when I came back. I was also afraid he would be frightened. He was so small he needed me to protect him, but I couldn't help him. We were in the hospital every couple of weeks. He would get better then have another attack. It got to the point where I would call the doctor and say that Bobbie was having another attack and they would just send us to admitting. After a few times, I got used to caring for him in the hospital. The nurses taught me how to keep his tent humidified and I could just take care of it myself. Finally I was able to go back to work during the day and care for him on my breaks and time off. It was very difficult each and every time, but we adjusted to hospital life. Although I was afraid for him, I knew he was a fighter and I had to be too I feel this experience made him a stronger person. He is now 8-years-old and has had no severe attacks since he was about 2-years-old. He has had a few mild attacks but it doesn't affect him or myself.

Tracee

Nursing Process for the Infant With a Respiratory Disorder

ASSESSMENT

Conduct a thorough interview with the caregiver, including the standard information as well as specific information such as when the caregiver first noticed the symptoms; the course of the fever thus far; the caregiver's description of respiratory difficulties; how well the infant was taking nourishment and fluids; nausea; vomiting; urinary and bowel output; and history of exposure to other family members with respiratory infections.

Conduct a physical assessment of temperature, apical pulse, respirations (rate, respiratory effort, retractions [costal, intercostal, sternal, suprasternal, substernal], and flaring of nares), breath sounds (crackles, wheezing), cough (dry, productive, hacking), irritability, restlessness, skin color (pallor, cyanosis), circumoral (around the mouth) cyanosis, skin turgor, anterior fontanelle (depressed or bulging), nasal passage congestion (color, consistency), mucous membranes (mouth dry, lips dry or cracked), and eyes (bright, glassy, sunken, moist, crusted).

NURSING DIAGNOSES

Nursing diagnoses are based on the interview with the family caregivers and the physical findings and should be reasonable and realistic. Some nursing diagnoses that may be used for the infant with a respiratory condition are:

- Impaired Gas Exchange related to inflammatory process

- Ineffective Airway Clearance related to nasal and chest congestion and obstructed airway

- Altered Nutrition: Less than Body Requirements related to inability to nurse, suck, or swallow adequately with congested nasal passages

- Risk for Hyperthermia related to infection process

- Risk for Infection related to location and anatomic structure of the eustachian tubes

- Ineffective Family Coping: Compromised related to child's illness

- Activity Intolerance related to inadequate gas exchange

OUTCOME IDENTIFICATION AND PLANNING

The major goals for the infant with a respiratory disorder include maintaining respiratory function, maintaining adequate nutrition and fluid intake, maintaining body temperature, preventing otitis media, preventing injury, reducing family anxiety, and conserving energy. Plan nursing plan care according to these goals and the infant's status.

The infant may need to be placed on respiratory precautions according to the policy of the health care facility to prevent nosocomial spread of infection. Many infants with a respiratory condition need to be placed in a croupette or mist tent. Plan additional nursing interventions for the infant in a mist tent. If IV fluids are ordered, interventions that promote tissue and skin integrity are needed. To ensure that the infant does not interfere with the IV infusion site, it may be necessary to prepare restraints. Intravenous administration and the use of restraints are discussed in Chapter 3.

IMPLEMENTATION

MONITORING RESPIRATORY FUNCTION. Monitor respirations by observing for tachypnea and retractions and assessing breath sounds at least every 4 hours. If deep retractions are noted, make observations more frequently. Oxygen saturation may be monitored by pulse oximeter. Oxygen can be administered by hood or mist tent if the physician desires, especially in cases of pneumococcal pneumonia.

MAINTAINING AIRWAY CLEARANCE. A moisturized atmosphere is provided with an ice-cooled mist tent or cool vaporizer. The moisturized air helps thin the mucus in the respiratory tract to ease respirations. Suction or clear secretions as needed to keep the airway open. Position the child to provide maximum ventilation. Use pillows and padding to maintain the infant's position. Observe frequently for slumping, which causes crowding of the infant's diaphragm. Avoid the use of constricting clothes and bedding. Stuffed toys are not recommended in mist tents, as they become saturated and provide an environment in which organisms flourish.

MAINTAINING ADEQUATE NUTRITION AND FLUID INTAKE. Clear the infant's nasal passages with a bulb syringe. Be certain to clear the passages immediately before feeding. Administer normal saline nose drops to thin secretions about 10 to 15 minutes before feedings and at bedtime. Feed the infant slowly, allowing frequent stops, with suctioning during feeding as needed. Avoid overtiring the infant during feeding. Offer juices and water appropriate for the infant's age between meals. Use a relatively small-holed nipple so that the infant does not choke, but be careful not to make the infant work too hard. Maintain accurate intake and output measurements. Observe the infant for dehydration: skin turgor, anterior fontanelle, and urine output are good indicators. Maintain diaper counts, and if necessary weigh diapers to determine the amount of urine output (1 mL urine weighs 1 g).

The infant may be so exhausted by respiratory effort that IV fluids are necessary. Observe patency, placement, site integrity, and flow rate at least hourly.

MAINTAINING BODY TEMPERATURE. Monitor the infant's temperature frequently, at least every 2 hours if it is higher than 101.3°F (38.5°C). If the infant has a fever, remove excess clothing and covering. Antipyretic medications may be ordered. A tepid sponge bath may be administered in accordance with the policy of the health care facility. Use tepid water to sponge the infant for about 20 minutes, then redress the infant lightly. Obtain, record, and report the temperature 30 minutes after completing the sponge bath.

PREVENTING OTITIS MEDIA. Turn the infant from side to side every hour so that mucus is less likely to drain into the eustachian tubes. An infant seat may help facilitate breathing and prevent the complication of otitis media. Observe the infant for irritability, shaking of the head, or pulling at the ears. Do not give the infant a bottle while he or she is lying in bed. The best position for feeding is upright to avoid excessive drainage into the eustachian tubes.

PROMOTING FAMILY COPING. Family caregivers need teaching and reassurance. Talk to the caregivers while working with the infant, explaining what is happening and why. Explain equipment and treatments to caregivers so that their questions (both spoken and unspoken) are answered. Actively listen to caregivers and use communication skills to respond to their worries. Teach the family caregivers:

- To clear the nasal passage with a bulb syringe

- To feed the infant slowly. Allow the infant to nurse without tiring, burping frequently to expel swallowed air.

- The importance of a croup tent and the need to leave the infant in it except for feedings and bathing (unless otherwise indicated)

- How to soothe the infant in the tent

- The need for respiratory precautions and good handwashing technique

- The importance of extra fluids for the infant

- The desirability of using a humidifier at home after discharge

- How to clean a humidifier properly

- The importance of preventing people who have infections from visiting the infant.

PROMOTING ENERGY CONSERVATION. During an acute stage, allow the infant to rest as much as possible. Plan work so that rest and sleep are interrupted no more than necessary. See Nursing Care Plan for an Infant With Respiratory Dysfunction.

EVALUATION: GOALS AND OUTCOME CRITERIA

- *Goal*: Respiratory function will be normal.
  Criteria: Respiratory rate is 25 to 35/min, regular, with breath sounds clear, and the infant no longer uses respiratory accessory muscles to aid in breathing.

- *Goal*: Airway will remain patent.
  Criteria: Mucous secretions are thin and scant; airway remains clear.

- *Goal*: The infant will have an adequate intake.
  Criteria: The infant consumes an amount of oral nutrition appropriate for age with no signs of tiring; skin turgor is good, fontanelles are of normal tension, and hourly urine output is 2 to 3 mL/kg.

- *Goal*: Fever will be controlled.
  Criteria: The temperature is 98.6° to 100°F (37°–37.8°C).

- *Goal*: The child will be free from complications of otitis media.
  Criteria: The infant shows no signs of ear pain such as irritability, shaking of the head, and pulling on the ears.

- *Goal*: The family caregivers' anxiety will be reduced.
  Criteria: Family caregivers verbalize methods to care for the infant with a respiratory disorder.

- *Goal*: The infant's energy will be conserved.
  Criteria: The infant has extended periods of uninterrupted rest and tolerates increased activity.

Sudden Infant Death Syndrome

Sudden infant death syndrome (SIDS) has caused much grief and anxiety among many families for centuries. One of the leading causes of infant mortality worldwide, SIDS claims an estimated 7,000 to 8,000 lives annually in the United States alone. It is the leading cause of death in infants older than 1 month of age.[2]

Throughout history, this syndrome has presented a most exasperating problem. Commonly called "crib death," it is the sudden, unexpected death of an apparently healthy infant in whom the postmortem fails to reveal an adequate cause. The term *SIDS* is not a diagnosis, but rather a description of a syndrome.

Varying theories have been suggested about the cause of SIDS. In ancient writings, it was attributed to "overlaying" by the infant's mother or nurse. The adult supposedly rolled over onto the infant during sleep. This cause was eventually ruled out, particularly because many affected infants were alone in their cribs when they ceased breathing. Over the years, much research has been done, but no single cause has been identified, and physicians can neither prevent nor predict the event.

Infants who die of SIDS are usually 2 to 3 months of age, although some deaths have occurred during the first and second weeks of life. Few infants older than 6 months of age die of SIDS. It is a greater threat to low-birth weight infants than to term infants. It occurs more often in winter and affects more male infants than female infants, as well as more infants from minority and lower socioeconomic groups. Babies born to mothers younger than 20 years of age, infants who are not firstborn, and infants whose mothers smoked during pregnancy also have been found to be at greater risk. Research has revealed that a greater number of infants with SIDS have been sleeping in a prone position than in a supine position. As a result of these studies, the American Academy of Pediatrics recommends that infants must *not* be placed in a prone position to sleep. Infants must be placed only in a supine or side-lying position until they are 6 months old.

Sudden infant death syndrome is rapid and silent. Previous studies had suggested that nighttime was the peak time of death, but recent studies reveal that about half the attacks occur during the day. The history reveals that no cry has been heard, nor is there any evidence of a struggle. People who have been sleeping nearby claim to have heard nothing unusual before the death was discovered. It is not uncommon for the infant to have been recently examined by a physician and found to be in excellent health. The autopsy often reveals a mild respiratory disorder, but nothing considered serious enough to have caused the death.

Emergency personnel must be observant for clues that may indicate child abuse, but they must be careful not to cast any suspicion on the family caregivers. The guilt feelings of the caregivers are overwhelming, and any suggestion from medical personnel that the cause of death is questionable is inexcusable and may be more than the caregivers can handle.

A closely related syndrome is apparent life-threatening events (ALTE). These are episodes in which the infant is found in distress but, when quickly stimulated, recovers with no lasting problems. These were formerly called "near-miss SIDS." These infants are placed on home apnea monitors. The apnea monitor is set to sound an alarm if the infant has not taken a breath within a given number of seconds. Family caregivers are taught infant cardiopulmonary resuscitation so that they can respond quickly if the alarm sounds. Infants who have had an episode of ALTE

Nursing Care Plan
for an Infant with Respiratory Infection

Chad, a 6-month-old infant with a respiratory infection, has been brought to the hospital from the doctor's office by his mother. He has a copious amount of thick nasal discharge end has rapid, shallow respirations with substernal and intercostal retractions. His temperature is 101.5°F (39.1°C). His young mother appears very anxious.

NURSING DIAGNOSIS

Ineffective Airway Clearance related to infectious process

GOAL: *Respiratory function will improve*

OUTCOME CRITERIA

- The infant no longer uses respiratory accessory muscles to aid in breathing.
- The infant's breath sounds are clear and respirations are regular.
- Mucous secretions become thin and scant.

Nursing Interventions	*Rationale*
Provide moist atmosphere by placing him in ice-cooled mist	Moisture helps liquefy and thin secretions for easier respirations.
Monitor respiratory function by assessing retractions, respiratory rate, and breath sounds at least every 4 hours. Monitor more frequently if tachypnea or deep retractions are noted.	Changes in the infant's breathing may be early indicators of respiratory distress.
Monitor infant's bedding and clothing every 4 hours	Clothing and bedding can become very wet from mist. Dry clothing and bedding helps prevent chilling.

NURSING DIAGNOSIS

Altered Nutrition: Less than Body Requirements related to inability to suck or swallow with congested nasal passages or fatigue from difficulty breathing

GOAL: *Adequate food and fluid intake is maintained*

OUTCOME CRITERIA

- The infant has an adequate intake as evidenced by weight.
- Skin turgor returns to normal.
- Nasal passages are clear.

Nursing Interventions	*Rationale*
Keep nasal passages clear, using bulb syringe. Clear nasal passages immediately before feeding. Teach family caregiver to use bulb syringe.	Infants are obligatory nasal breathers. Clearing eases infant's breathing to permit adequate feeding. Family caregiver can use this technique at home as needed.
Administer normal saline nose drops before feedings and at bedtime.	Normal saline nose drops help thin mucous secretions.
Weigh infant daily in morning before first feeding.	Infant will maintain weight with gain of 1 to 2 oz in a week.

(continued)

Nursing Care Plan *(Continued)*
for an Infant with Respiratory Infection

NURSING DIAGNOSIS

Risk for Otitis Media related to current respiratory infection and the size and location of infant's eustachian tube

GOAL: *Otitis media will be prevented*

OUTCOME CRITERIA

- The child is free of the complication of otitis media.

Nursing Interventions	Rationale
Change infant's position, turning from side to side every hour.	Turning infant prevents mucus from pooling in the eustachian tubes.
Feed infant in upright position.	Improves drainage and helps open nasal passages
Observe for irritability, shaking of head, or pulling at ears.	Early recognition of signs of otitis media promotes early diagnosis and treatment.

NURSING DIAGNOSIS

Anxiety by parents related to infant's illness

GOAL: *Family anxiety will be reduced*

OUTCOME CRITERIA

- The family caregivers demonstrate understanding of infant's condition and treatments.
- The family caregivers reflect confidence in the staff evidenced by cooperation and appropriate questions.

Nursing Interventions	Rationale
Actively listen to caregivers' concerns.	Family members gain confidence when they feel their concerns are being heard.
Provide reassurance and explain what you are doing and why you are doing it when working with infant.	Understanding the disease and treatment methods helps family to feel that infant's illness is under control.
Involve caregivers in caring for Chad. Teach them techniques of care that can be used at home.	Family caregivers feel valued and benefit from nursing care tips they can use at home.

are at risk for additional episodes and may be at risk for SIDS. Infants are usually kept on home apnea monitors until they are 1 year old. This is a stressful time for the family because someone who is trained in infant cardiopulmonary resuscitation must be with the infant at all times (Fig. 11-10).

EMOTIONAL SUPPORT FOR CAREGIVERS AND FAMILIES

The effects of SIDS on caregivers and families are devastating. Grief is coupled with guilt, even though SIDS cannot be predicted or prevented. Disbelief, hostility, and anger

are common reactions that families exhibit. An autopsy must be done and the results promptly made known to the family. Even though the family caregivers are told that they are not to blame for the infant's death, it is difficult for most caregivers not to keep searching for evidence of some possible neglect on their part. Prolonged depression usually follows the initial shock and anguish over the infant's death.

The immediate response of the emergency department staff should be to allow the family to express their grief, encouraging them to say goodbye to their baby and providing a quiet, private place for them to do so. Compassionate

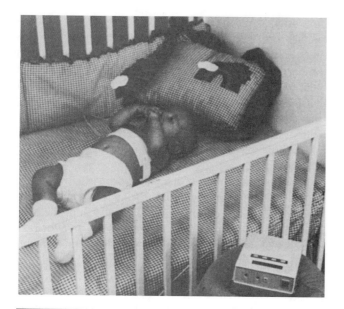

Figure 11-10
An apnea monitor for home monitoring.

care of the family caregivers includes helping to find someone to accompany them home or to meet them there. Referrals should be made to the local chapter of the National SIDS Foundation immediately. Sudden Infant Death Alliance is another resource for help. In some states, specially trained community health nurses who are knowledgeable about SIDS are available. These nurses are prepared to help families and can provide written materials as well as information, guidance, and support in the family's home. They maintain contact with the family as long as necessary and will provide support in a subsequent pregnancy.

One concern of the caregivers is how to tell other children in the family what has happened. "What Will I Tell the Children?" is a booklet written by Jacques Bell and Linda Esterling that provides sound advice with guidance at each age level.[3]

Caregivers are particularly concerned about subsequent infants. Data previously had suggested that these infants were at greater risk, but more recent studies have indicated that this risk is no greater than in the general population. However, many physicians continue to recommend monitoring these infants for the first few months of life to help reduce the family's stress. This is a decision that each physician and family must make together after looking at all the pros and cons. Monitoring is usually maintained until the new infant is past the age of the SIDS infant's death.

Grief waxes and wanes for months and years for these caregivers. Having another child by no means causes them to forget the one they lost. Mothers often relate that they think they are healing, only to have some small incident set them off again. Friends and acquaintances must be sensitive to their needs. Comments such as, "You are young; you can always have more children," "God must have

needed a little angel," and "Well, you have the other children" are inappropriate. The best way to interact with these caregivers is by actively listening and showing compassionate concern.

GENITOURINARY DISORDERS

A few conditions may affect the genitourinary system of the infant in the first year of life. Two structural defects, hydrocele (fluid in the saclike cavity around the testes) and cryptorchidism (undescended testes), occur in a few male infants. Urinary tract infections (UTIs) may occur when poor hygiene exists in infants wearing diapers. The most common type of renal cancer, Wilms' tumor (nephroblastoma), may first be seen in infancy. Each of these conditions is briefly discussed in this section.

Hydrocele

Hydrocele is a collection of peritoneal fluid that accumulates in the scrotum through a small passage called the processus vaginalis. This processus is a fingerlike projection in the inguinal canal through which the testes descend. Usually the processus closes soon after birth, but if it does not close, fluid from the peritoneal cavity passes through, causing hydrocele. This is the same passage through which intestines may slip, causing an inguinal hernia. If the hydrocele remains by the end of the first year, corrective surgery is performed.

Cryptorchidism

Shortly before or soon after birth, the male gonads (testes) descend from the abdominal cavity into their normal position in the scrotum. Occasionally, one or both of the testes do not descend, a condition called cryptorchidism. The testes are usually normal in size; the cause for failure to descend is not clearly understood.

In most infants with cryptorchidism, the testes descend by the time the infant is 1 year old. If one or both testes have not descended by this age, treatment is recommended. If both testes remain undescended, the male will be sterile.

A surgical procedure called **orchiopexy** is used to bring the testis down into the scrotum and anchor it there. Some physicians prefer to try medical treatment—injections of human chorionic gonadotropic hormone—before doing surgery. If this is unsuccessful in bringing the testis down, orchiopexy is performed. Surgery usually is performed when the child is 1 to 2 years of age. Prognosis for a normal functioning testicle is good when the surgery is performed at this young age and no degenerative action has taken place before treatment.

Urinary Tract Infections

Infections of the urinary tract are fairly common in the "diaper age," in infancy, and again between the ages of 2 and 6 years. The condition is more common in girls than in boys, except in the first 4 months of life, when it is more common in boys. Although many different bacteria may infect the urinary tract, intestinal bacteria, particularly *Escherichia coli*, account for about 80% of acute episodes. The female urethra is shorter and straighter than the male urethra; thus, it is more easily contaminated with feces. Inflammation may extend into the bladder, ureters, and kidney.

CLINICAL MANIFESTATIONS

In infants, the symptoms may be fever, nausea, vomiting, foul-smelling urine, weight loss, and increased urination. Occasionally, there is little or no fever. Vomiting is common, and diarrhea may occur. The infant is irritable. In acute pyelonephritis (inflammation of the kidney and renal pelvis), the onset is abrupt, with a high fever for 1 or 2 days. Convulsions may occur during the period of high fever. In preschool children, bedwetting may be a symptom.

DIAGNOSIS

Diagnosis is based on the finding of pus in the urine under microscopic examination. The urine specimen must be fresh and uncontaminated. A "clean catch" voided urine, properly performed, is essential for microscopic examination. If a culture is needed, the infant may be catheterized, but this is usually avoided if possible. A suprapubic aspiration also may be done to obtain a sterile specimen. In the cooperative, toilet-trained child, a clean midstream urine may be used successfully.

TREATMENT

Simple UTIs may be treated with antibiotics (usually sulfisoxazole or ampicillin) at home. The child with acute pyelonephritis is hospitalized. Fluids are given freely. The symptoms usually subside within a few days after antibiotic therapy has been initiated, but this is not an indication that the infection is completely cleared. Medication must be continued after symptoms disappear. An intravenous pyelogram or ultrasonographic study may be performed to assess the possibility of structural defects if the child has recurring infections.

🔎 ✒ *Nursing Process for the Child With* ✒ 🔎 *a Urinary Tract Infection*

ASSESSMENT

During the interview with the family caregiver, include basic information about the child, such as feeding and sleeping patterns and history of other illnesses. Gather information about the present illness: when the fever started and its course thus far, signs of pain or discomfort on voiding, recent change in feeding pattern, presence of vomiting or diarrhea, irritability, lethargy, abdominal pain, unusual odor to urine, chronic diaper rash, and signs of febrile convulsions. If the child is toilet-trained, ask the caregivers about toileting habits (how does the child wipe? does the child wash the hands when toileting?). Also ask about the use of bubble baths and the type of soap used, especially for girls.

Physical assessment of the child includes temperature; pulse (be alert for tachycardia) and respiration rates; weight and height; observation of a wet diaper or the urine in an older child; inspection of the perineal area for rash; presence of irritability and lethargy; and general skin condition, color, and turgor. A urine specimen is needed on admission. A midstream urine collection method is desirable, and catheterization is avoided if possible. Record and report any indications of urinary burning, frequency, urgency, or pain.

In the child who has repeated UTIs, observe the interaction between the child and the family caregivers to detect any indications that the infection may be caused by sexual abuse. Look for possible indications of sexual abuse, such as bruising, bleeding, and lacerations of the external genitalia in the child who is extremely shy and frightened.

NURSING DIAGNOSES

Nursing diagnoses vary with the age and condition of the child. Nursing diagnoses concerning development and safety are common to most nursing care plans for infants and children. Some specific nursing diagnoses that may be used are:

- Altered Urinary Elimination related to pain and burning on urination
- Health Seeking Behaviors by the parents related to the UTI

OUTCOME IDENTIFICATION AND PLANNING

Major goals for the infant with a UTI include reducing infection, encouraging normal elimination, and increasing fluid intake. An important goal for the family is improving knowledge about infection control to help prevent recurrent infections. Base the nursing plan of care on these goals, with adjustments appropriate for the child's age. To promote normal elimination, plan nursing care that helps relieve pain and fever. Be sure to include family teaching that focuses on infection prevention at home.

IMPLEMENTATION

MAINTAINING NORMAL ELIMINATION. Because of pain and burning on urination, the toilet-trained child may try to hold urine and not void. Encourage the child to void every 3 or 4 hours to prevent recurrent infection. Assess the child for burning, pain, and frequency. If possible, observe the voiding pattern to note trickling or other signs that the bladder is not being emptied completely. Carefully monitor and measure urine output. An infant's diaper can be weighed for accuracy. Accurate intake and output measurements are important.

Administer antibiotics as ordered and observe the child for signs of any reactions to the antibiotics. Prepare the family caregivers and the child for any other procedures that may be ordered, and give appropriate explanations.

Increasing the child's fluid intake is necessary to help dilute the urine and flush the bladder. An increase in fluid intake also helps decrease the pain experienced on urination. Frequent, small amounts of fluids, such as glucose water and liquid gelatin, for the infant are usually well accepted. However, it is often difficult to get the infant to accept fluids. It may be helpful to enlist the aid of the family caregivers, but if they are unsuccessful, the nurse must persevere. Most infants and children like apple juice, which helps acidify the urine. Cranberry juice is a good choice for the older child, if he or she tolerates it. Administer analgesics and antispasmodics as ordered.

PROVIDING FAMILY TEACHING. The family caregivers are the key people in helping prevent recurring infections. See Family Teaching Tips for Urinary Tract Infection.

EVALUATION: GOALS AND OUTCOME CRITERIA

- *Goal*: Normal elimination will be maintained.
  Criteria: The infant produces 2 to 3 mL/kg of urine per hour; the older child voids every 3 to 4 hours, emptying the bladder each time without apprehension.

Family Teaching
Tips for Urinary Tract Infection

1. Change infant's diaper when soiled, and clean baby with mild soap and water. Dry completely.
2. Teach girls to wipe from front to back.
3. Teach child to wash hands before and after going to the toilet.
4. Bubble baths create a climate that encourages bacteria to grow, especially in young girls.
5. Teach young girls to take showers. Avoid using water softeners in tub baths.
6. Encourage child to try to urinate every 3 or 4 hours and to empty the bladder.
7. Girls should wear cotton underpants to provide air circulation to perineal area.
8. Encourage child to drink fluids, especially cranberry juice.
9. Older girls should avoid whirlpools or hot tubs.

- *Goal*: Family caregivers will demonstrate an understanding of the genitourinary system and good hygiene habits.
  Criteria: Family caregivers verbalize signs and symptoms of a UTI, methods to prevent a recurrence, and when to contact a health practitioner.

Wilms' Tumor (Nephroblastoma)

Wilms' tumor, an adenosarcoma in the kidney region, is one of the most common abdominal neoplasms of early childhood. The tumor arises from bits of embryonic tissue that remain after birth. This tissue can spark rapid cancerous growth in the area of the kidney. The tumor is rarely discovered until it is large enough to be palpated through the abdominal wall. As the tumor grows, it invades the kidney or the renal vein and disseminates to other parts of the body. When the child is being evaluated and treated, a sign must be visibly posted stating that abdominal palpation should be avoided because cells may break loose and spread the tumor. Treatment consists of surgical removal as soon as possible after the growth is discovered, combined with radiation and chemotherapy.

Prognosis is best for the child younger than 2 years of age but has improved markedly for others with improved chemotherapy. Follow-up consists of regular evaluation for metastasis to the lungs or other sites. All long-term implications for chemotherapy apply to this child.

NERVOUS SYSTEM DISORDERS

Acute or Nonrecurrent Seizures

A seizure (convulsion) may be a symptom of a wide variety of disorders. In infants and children between the age of 6 months and 3 years, **febrile seizures** are the most common. Febrile seizures usually occur in the form of a generalized seizure early in the course of a fever. Although commonly associated with high fever (102°–106°F [38.9°–41.1°C]), some children appear to have a low seizure threshold and convulse when a fever of 100° to 102°F (37.8°–38.9°C) is present. These seizures are often one of the initial symptoms of an acute infection somewhere in the body.

Less common causes of convulsions are intracranial infections such as meningitis, toxic reactions to certain drugs or minerals such as lead, metabolic disorders, and various brain disorders.

CLINICAL MANIFESTATIONS

A seizure may occur suddenly, without warning; however, restlessness and irritability may precede an episode. The body stiffens and the infant loses consciousness. In a few seconds, clonic movements occur. These movements are quick, jerking movements of the arms, legs, and facial muscles. Breathing is irregular and the child cannot swallow saliva.

DIAGNOSIS

Immediate treatment is based on the presenting symptoms. Further evaluation is made after the urgency of the seizure has passed.

TREATMENT

Emergency care to protect the child during the seizure is the primary concern. Diazepam (Valium), the drug of choice, is usually administered IV if necessary. Acetaminophen is administered to reduce the temperature.

★ ↖ *Nursing Process for the Child at Risk* ↙ ↘ *for Seizures*

ASSESSMENT

During the family caregiver interview, ask about any history of seizure activity. Have the caregivers describe any previous episodes, including the infant's temperature, how the infant behaved immediately before the seizure, movements during the seizure, and any other information they believe to be relevant. Ask about the presence of any fever during the present illness and any indications of seizure activity before this admission. Promptly institute seizure precautions. An infant or child whose fever or other symptoms indicate that a seizure may be anticipated should be placed under constant observation.

During the physical assessment, carefully evaluate temperature and make a neurologic assessment and other assessments appropriate for the present illness.

NURSING DIAGNOSES

In addition to nursing diagnoses related to the presenting symptoms, those specific to anticipated seizure activity are suggested in this section. If the seizure is preceded by fever, nursing diagnoses and measures for fever reduction also are included. Some of the diagnoses specific to possible seizure activity are:

- Ineffective Airway Clearance during seizure related to loss of consciousness

- Risk for Injury related to uncontrolled muscular activity during seizure

- Ineffective Family Coping: Compromised related to the child's seizure activity

- Health Seeking Behaviors by the parents related to seizure prevention and precautions during seizures

OUTCOME IDENTIFICATION AND PLANNING

The immediate goals for the infant during a seizure are maintaining airway clearance and preventing injury. Goals for the family include relieving anxiety and increasing knowledge about seizures. With safety in mind, develop the nursing plan of care according to these goals.

IMPLEMENTATION

PREVENTING ASPIRATION.   When convulsions begin, position the infant to one side to prevent aspiration of saliva or vomitus. Do not put *anything* in the child's mouth. Remove blankets, pillows, or other items that may block the child's airway. Oxygen and suction equipment must be readily available for emergency use.

PROMOTING SAFETY PRACTICES.   Keep the child who has a history of seizures under close observation. Pad the crib sides, and keep sharp or hard items out of the crib. However, do not completely hide the view of the surroundings outside the crib, as this could make the child feel isolated. During the seizure, stay with the child to protect but not restrain him or her. Loosen any tight clothing. If the child is not in bed when the seizure starts, move him or her to a flat surface.

Document the seizure completely after the episode. Document the type of movements (rigidity, jerking, twitching), the parts of the body involved, the duration of the seizure, pulse and respirations, the child's color, and any deviant eye movements or other notable signs.

PROMOTING FAMILY COPING.   A convulsion or seizure is very frightening to family caregivers. With a calm, confident attitude, reassure caregivers that the child is in good hands. Explain that febrile seizures are not uncommon in small children. Reassure caregivers that the physician will evaluate the child to determine if the seizure has any cause other than nervous system irritation resulting from the high fever.

PROVIDING FAMILY TEACHING.   Teach family caregivers seizure precautions so that they can handle a seizure that occurs at home. Also instruct them on what observations to make during a seizure so that they can report these to the physician to help in evaluating the child. Explain methods to control fever, cautioning caregivers to avoid using aspirin for fever reduction. When teaching about tepid sponge baths, explain that when the child shivers, the body is working to conserve its temperature, and sponging should be stopped until shivering stops because this could increase temperature. See Family Teaching Tips on Ways to Reduce Fever.

EVALUATION: GOALS AND OUTCOME CRITERIA

- *Goal*: Airway will remain patent throughout the seizure. *Criteria*: The child's airway remains patent, with no aspiration of saliva or vomitus.

Family Teaching
Tips on Ways to Reduce Fever

If temperature is above 103°F (39.4°C) or child "acts sick," call the physician.
1. Use infant tub for baby or regular tub for child.
2. Use clean washcloths and towels.
3. Use about 2 inches of water, lukewarm to your wrist.
4. Place child in tub or on padded surface.
5. Sponge child's body with wet washcloths, using long, soothing strokes, rubbing lightly. Start with face, neck, arms, and chest. Get underarms as well.
6. Sponge abdomen, back, and legs. Include groin and diaper area.
7. Sponge 20 minutes; remove child and cover lightly.
8. Take temperature after 30 minutes. Repeat until temperature is below 101°F (38.3°C).

Note
If child shivers, stop sponging. When shivering stops, begin sponging again. Encourage child to drink as much water or juice as possible. Ice popsicles are good, too. Check with doctor about giving child acetaminophen (Tylenol). **Never give aspirin. Do not use alcohol or ice water to sponge child.**

■ *Goal*: The child will remain free from injury during the seizure.
Criteria: The child is free from bruises, abrasions, concussions, or fractures after the seizure.

■ *Goal*: Family caregiver anxiety will be reduced.
Criteria: The family caregivers verbalize their concerns and relate an understanding of febrile seizures.

■ *Goal*: The family caregivers will demonstrate an understanding of seizure precautions.
Criteria: Family caregivers verbalize methods to reduce fevers and handle seizures at home.

Haemophilus influenzae Meningitis

Purulent meningitis in infancy and childhood is caused by a variety of agents, including meningococci, the tubercle bacillus, and the *Haemophilus influenzae* type B bacillus. The most common form is *H influenzae* meningitis. Meningococcal meningitis is spread by means of droplet infection from an infected person; all other forms are contracted by invasion of the meninges via the bloodstream from an infection elsewhere.

Peak occurrence of *H influenzae* meningitis is between the ages of 6 and 12 months. It is rare during the first 2 months of life and is seldom seen after the fourth year. Purulent meningitis is an infectious disease. In addition to standard precautions, droplet transmission precautions should be observed for 24 hours after the start of effective antimicrobial therapy, or until pathogens can no longer be cultured from nasopharyngeal secretions. Current immunizations include the HbCV, which is given at 2 months and repeated at 4, 6, and 15 months (see Table 10-4 in Chap. 10).

CLINICAL MANIFESTATIONS

The onset may be either gradual or abrupt following an upper respiratory infection. Young infants with meningitis may have a characteristic high-pitched cry, fever, and irritability. Other symptoms include headache, **nuchal rigidity** (stiff neck) that may progress to **opisthotonos** (arching of the back), and delirium. Projectile vomiting may be present. Generalized convulsions are common in infants. Coma may occur early, particularly in the older child. Meningococcal meningitis, which tends to occur as epidemics in older children, produces a **purpuric rash** (caused by bleeding under the skin) in addition to the other symptoms.

DIAGNOSIS

Early diagnosis and treatment are essential for uncomplicated recovery. A spinal tap is performed promptly whenever symptoms raise a suspicion of meningitis. For accurate results, the spinal tap is done before antibiotics are administered. The nurse assists by holding the infant during the spinal tap (Fig. 11-11). The spinal fluid is under increased pressure, and laboratory examination of the fluid reveals increased protein and decreased glucose content. Early in the disease, the spinal fluid may be clear, but it rapidly becomes purulent. The causative organism usually can be determined from stained smears of the spinal fluid, enabling specific medication to be started early without waiting for growths of organisms on culture media.

TREATMENT

Treatment consists initially of IV administration of antibiotics in an effective dose. Third-generation cephalosporins, such as ceftazidime (Fortaz) or ceftriaxone (Rocephin), are commonly used. Later in the disease, medications may be given orally. Treatment depends on the progress of the condition and continues as long as there is fever or signs of subdural effusion or otitis media. The administration of IV steroids early in the course has decreased the incidence of deafness as a complication.

Subdural effusion may complicate the condition in infants during the course of the disease. Fluid accumulates in the subdural space between the dura and the brain. Needle aspiration through the infant's open suture lines or bur holes (in the skull of the older child) is used to remove the fluid. Repeated aspirations may be required.

Complications of *H influenzae* meningitis with long-term implications are hydrocephalus, nerve deafness, mental retardation, and paralysis. The risk of complications is lessened when appropriate medication is started early in the disease.

Figure 11-11

Two positions for a spinal tap. (A) Knee-chest position for young infant. The nurse can hold the infant securely. (B) Sitting position. Small infant is held in a sitting position, the knees flexed on the abdomen, and the nurse holds the elbow and knee in each hand, flexing the spine.

★⮢ Nursing Process for the Child
⮢⮞ With Meningitis

ASSESSMENT

The infant or child with meningitis is obviously extremely sick, and the anxiety level of the family caregivers is understandably high. Be patient and sensitive to their feelings when doing the assessment interview. Obtain a complete history, with particular emphasis on the present illness, including any recent upper respiratory infection or middle ear infection. Information on other children in the family and their ages is also important.

The physical assessment of the infant includes temperature, pulse, and respirations and a neurologic evaluation, which includes the level of consciousness (see the section on neurologic evaluation, Chp. 3). Examine the young infant for a bulging fontanelle, and measure the head circumference for a baseline. Perform this assessment after the spinal tap is completed and IV fluids and antibiotics are initiated, because these procedures take precedence over everything else.

NURSING DIAGNOSES

The following nursing diagnoses are some that may be used in planning the care of the child with meningitis:

- Risk for Injury related to presence of infection

- Risk for Fluid Volume Deficit related to vomiting, fever, and fluid restrictions

- Fluid Volume Excess related to syndrome of inappropriate antidiuretic hormone

- Risk for Ineffective Airway Clearance related to level of consciousness

- Risk for Infection related to airborne transmission exposure to others

- Ineffective Family Coping: Compromised related to the child's condition and prognosis

OUTCOME IDENTIFICATION AND PLANNING

The goals for the infant with meningitis include maintaining normal vital signs, normal neurologic status, fluid balance, and effective airway clearance. The goals for the family include preventing the transmission of infection and reducing anxiety. Plan the nursing care according to these goals. Include interventions such as eliminating the infection by administering antibiotics and observing for signs of increased intracranial pressure (increased head size, headache, bulging fontanelle, decreased pulse, seizures, high-pitched cry, increased blood pressure, change in level of consciousness, and irritability or other behavioral changes).

IMPLEMENTATION

MONITORING TO PREVENT COMPLICATIONS. The child may have signs of cerebral edema (see previous paragraph). Implement seizure precautions. Observe the child for seizure activity, vital signs, neurologic changes, and change in level of consciousness every 2 hours. An increase in blood pressure, decrease in pulse, change in neurologic signs, or signs of respiratory distress must be reported at once. Measure the infant's head circumference at least every 4 hours to detect complications of subdural effusion or obstructive hydrocephalus. The child's room should be quiet and darkened to decrease stimulation that may cause seizures. While in the room, speak softly, avoid sudden movements, move quietly, and raise and lower side rails carefully. The head of the bed can be elevated.

MAINTAINING FLUID INTAKE. Fluid balance is an important aspect of the care of this child. Strict intake and output measurements are critical. Methods of reducing fever may be used as needed. Administer IV fluids, while observing and monitoring the IV infusion site and following safety precautions to maintain the site.

MONITORING FLUID VOLUME. Secretion of the antidiuretic hormone that is produced by the posterior pituitary gland may be increased by the infectious process. As a result, the child may not excrete urine adequately, and a body fluid excess will occur. Strictly measure intake and output and monitor daily weight and electrolytes. Signs for concern that must be reported immediately are decreased urinary output, hyponatremia, increased weight, nausea, and irritability. Place the child on fluid restrictions if these signs occur.

PREVENTING ASPIRATION. Position the child in a side-lying position with the neck supported for comfort and the head elevated. Remove pillows, blankets, and soft toys that might obstruct the airway. Watch for and remove excessive mucus as much as possible. Use suction sparingly.

PREVENTING TRANSMISSION OF INFECTION. *H influenzae* is a highly contagious organism that may spread to other people by means of droplet transmission. Droplet transmission precautions must be maintained for the first 24 hours after the antibiotic is administered. Staff members and family caregivers must follow proper precautions. Other children in the family may need to be assessed to determine if they should receive prophylactic antibiotics.

PROMOTING FAMILY COPING. Teach the caregivers isolation and good handwashing technique and encourage them to stay with their child, if possible. Support family caregivers through every step of the process. Their anxiety about procedures, the child's seizures and condition, and the possible complications are all serious concerns. Family caregivers must be included and made to feel useful. If they are not too apprehensive, help them find small things they can do for their child. Keep them advised about the child's progress at all times.

EVALUATION: GOALS AND OUTCOME CRITERIA

- *Goal*: There will be no symptoms of cerebral edema, seizure activity, or respiratory distress.
  Criteria: The child's vital signs are within normal limits, neurologic status is stable, and there is no seizure activity. The infant's head circumference is not increased.

- *Goal*: Normal fluid balance will be maintained.
  Criteria: The child's fluid and electrolyte levels are within normal limits; hourly urine output is 2 to 3 mL/kg; temperature is 98.6° to 100°F (37°–37.8°C); there are no signs of dehydration.

- *Goal*: The child's airway will be kept clear.
  Criteria: The child does not aspirate.

- *Goal*: The *H influenzae* bacteria will not be transmitted to others.
  Criteria: Family members verbalize safety measures for preventing the spread of bacteria and relate the need for isolation of the ill child.

- *Goal*: The family caregivers' anxiety will decrease.
  Criteria: Family caregivers verbalize understanding of the disease process and relate the child's progress throughout the crisis.

SKIN AND MUCOUS MEMBRANE DISORDERS

Miliaria Rubra

Miliaria rubra, often called prickly heat, is common in infants who are exposed to summer heat or are overdressed. It also may appear in febrile illnesses and may be mistaken for the rash of one of the communicable diseases. The rash appears as pinhead-sized erythematous (reddened) papules. It is most noticeable in areas where sweat glands are concentrated, such as folds of the skin, the chest, and about the neck. It usually causes itching, making the infant uncomfortable and fretful.

Treatment primarily should be preventive. Family caregivers should be taught to avoid bundling their infants in layers of clothing in hot weather—a diaper may be all the child needs. Tepid baths without soap help control the itching. A thin sprinkling of cornstarch at diaper changes helps relieve the discomfort. The cornstarch should be carefully applied and brushed off so that it does not cake in the folds, but simply makes a smooth, soothing surface on the skin. Cornstarch is preferred over talc because talc may contain asbestos fibers that can cause aspiration pneumonia in the infant or young child if inhaled. Cornstarch has been associated with the promotion of growth of *Candida albicans*, but a 1984 study by Leyden found that neither talc nor cornstarch supported growth of *C albicans* under the conditions normally found in the diaper area.[4]

Diaper Rash

Diaper rash is common in infancy, causing the baby discomfort and fretfulness. Bacterial decomposition of urine produces ammonia, which is irritating to an infant's tender skin. Diarrheal stools also produce a burning erythematous area in the anal region. Some infants seem to be more susceptible than others, possibly due to inherited sensitive skin. Prolonged exposure to wet or soiled diapers, use of plastic or rubber pants, infrequently changed disposable diapers, inadequate cleansing of the diaper area (especially after bowel movements), sensitivity to some soaps or disposable diaper perfumes, and the use of strong laundry detergents without thorough rinsing are considered to be causes. Yeast infections, notably candidiasis, are also causative factors.

TREATMENT AND NURSING CARE

Caregivers should be taught that the primary treatment is prevention. Diapers must be changed frequently, without waiting for obvious leaking. Regular checking is necessary. Manufacturers of disposable diapers are constantly trying to improve the ability of disposable diapers to wick the wetness away from the infant's skin. Diapers washed at commercial laundries are sterilized, preventing the growth of ammonia-forming bacteria. However, caregivers may be unable to afford disposable diapers or a commercial diaper service. Diapers washed at home should be presoaked (good commercial products are available, such as Diaperene), washed in hot water with a mild soap, and rinsed thoroughly, with an antiseptic added to the final rinse. Drying diapers in the sun or in a dryer also helps destroy bacteria.

Exposing the diaper area to the air helps clear up the dermatitis. The use of baby powder when diapering is discouraged, as caked powder helps create an environment in which organisms love to grow. Cleaning the diaper area from front to back with warm water and drying thoroughly with each diaper change helps improve or prevent the condition. If soap is necessary when cleaning stool from the infant's buttocks and rectal area, be certain that the soap is completely rinsed before diapering. The use of commercial wet wipes may aggravate the condition. If the area becomes excoriated and sore, the health care provider may prescribe an ointment. See Family Teaching Tips for Diaper Rash.

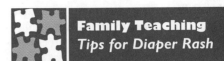

Family Teaching
Tips for Diaper Rash

1. Rinse all baby's clothes thoroughly to eliminate soap or detergent residue that may irritate baby's skin.
2. Rinse diapers two times in clear water. Do not use fabric softeners, because they can cause a skin reaction.
3. Use plastic or rubber diaper covers only when necessary. They hold moisture, which makes rash worse.
4. Change diapers as soon as wet or soiled. Disposable diapers hold moisture the same as plastic or rubber covers.
5. Avoid fastening diaper too tight, irritating baby's skin.
6. Expose baby's bottom to air without diapers as much as possible to help rash heal.
7. Do not overdress or overcover baby. Sweating makes rash worse.
8. Wash baby's bottom with lukewarm water only, using wet cotton balls or pouring over bath basin or sink. Pat dry with soft cloth. Do not use commercial baby wipes. Do not rub rash.
9. A cool, wet cloth placed over red diaper rash is very soothing. Try this for 5 minutes three or four times a day.
10. Use ointment only as recommended by health care provider. Apply very thin layer only. Wash off at each diaper change.
11. Dry diaper area thoroughly before rediapering. A hair dryer on low warm setting used after patting dry may help.

Candidiasis

C albicans is the causative agent for thrush and some cases of diaper rash. Newborns can be exposed to a candidiasis vaginal infection in the mother during delivery. Thrush appears in the infant's mouth as a white coating that looks like milk curds. Poor handwashing practices and inadequate washing of bottles and nipples are contributing factors. In addition, infants and toddlers may experience episodes of thrush or diaper rash after antibiotic therapy caused by the upset of the normal intestinal flora that allows an overgrowth of *Candida*.

Treatment for diaper rash caused by *Candida* is the application of nystatin ointment or cream to the affected area. Application of nystatin (Mycostatin, Nilstat) to the oral lesions every 6 hours is an effective treatment. A reliable—if unsightly—treatment for thrush is painting the infant's mouth with 1% gentian violet three times a day. Good hygiene practices should be reinforced.

Seborrheic Dermatitis

Seborrheic dermatitis (cradle cap) can usually be prevented by daily washing of the infant's hair and scalp. Characterized by yellowish, scaly, or crusted patches on the scalp, it occurs in newborns and in older infants possibly as a result

of excessive sebaceous gland activity. Family caregivers may be afraid to wash vigorously over the "soft spot." However, they need to understand that this is where cradle cap often begins and that careful but vigorous washing of the area with a washcloth can prevent this disorder. Using a fine-toothed baby comb after shampooing is also a helpful preventive measure. These principles are stressed during teaching about care of the newborn.

Once the condition exists, daily application of mineral oil helps loosen the crust. No attempt should be made to loosen it all at once, however, as the delicate skin on the scalp may break and bleed and can easily become infected.

Impetigo

Impetigo is a superficial bacterial skin infection (Fig. 11-12). In the newborn, the primary causative organism is *Staphylococcus aureus*. In the older child, the most common causative organism is group A beta-hemolytic streptococci. Impetigo in the newborn is usually bullous (blisterlike); in the older child, the lesions are nonbullous.

Impetigo in the newborn nursery is cause for immediate concern, as the condition is highly contagious and can spread through a nursery quickly. The nurse caring for an

Figure 11-12
Typical lesion of impetigo.

infant who has impetigo must follow contact (skin and wound) precautions, including wearing a cover gown and gloves. The infant should be segregated from other infants in the nursery to deter spread of the disease. Crusts can be soaked off with warm water followed by an application of topical antibiotics, such as bacitracin and neosporin. The infant's hands must be covered or elbow restraints applied to prevent scratching of lesions. Careful handwashing by nursing personnel and family members is essential.

The older child with impetigo is treated at home. The family caregivers must be taught hygiene practices to prevent the spread of impetigo to other children in the household or other contacts of the child in the day care center, nursery school, or elementary school. Lesions occur primarily on the face but may spread to any part of the body. The crusts and drainage are contagious. Because the lesions are pruritic (itchy), the child must learn to keep his or her fingers and hands away from the lesions. Nails should be trimmed to prevent scratching of lesions. Family members should be taught not to share towels and washcloths. Medical treatment includes oral penicillin or erythromycin for 10 days. Daily washing of the crusts helps speed the healing process. Mupirocin (Bactroban) ointment may be used.

Because this is commonly a streptococcal infection in the older child, rheumatic fever or acute glomerulonephritis may follow. Family caregivers should be alerted to this rare possibility.

Acute Infantile Eczema

Infantile eczema is an atopic dermatitis considered to be at least in part an allergic reaction to an irritant. It is fairly common during the first year of life after the age of 3 months. It is uncommon in breast-fed babies before they are given additional foods.

Infantile eczema is characterized by three factors:

- Hereditary predisposition
- Hypersensitivity of the deeper layers of the skin to protein or proteinlike allergens
- Allergens to which the child is sensitive that may be inhaled, ingested, or absorbed through direct contact, such as house dust, egg white, or wool.

Infants who have eczema tend to have hay fever or asthma later in life.

CLINICAL MANIFESTATIONS

Eczema usually starts on the cheeks and spreads to the extensor surfaces of the arms and legs. Eventually the entire trunk may become involved. The initial reddening of the skin is quickly followed by papule and vesicle formation. Itching is intense, and the infant's scratching makes the skin weep and crust. The areas easily become infected by hemolytic streptococci or by staphylococci.

DIAGNOSIS

The most common allergens involved in eczema are:

- Foods: egg white, cow's milk, wheat products, orange and tomato juice
- Inhalants: house dust, pollens, animal dander
- Materials: wool, nylon, plastic

However, diagnosis is not simple. Often, trial by elimination is as effective as any other diagnostic tool. Skin testing on a young infant generally is not considered valid, so it is discouraged as a means of diagnosis.

Diagnostic Diet   An elimination diet may be helpful in ruling out offending foods. A hypoallergenic diet consisting of a milk substitute such as soy formula, vitamin supplement, and other foods known to be hypoallergenic is given. If the skin condition shows improvement, other foods are added one at a time, at an interval of about 1 week, noting effects and eliminating any foods that cause a reaction. The protein of egg white is such a common offender that most pediatricians advise against feeding whole eggs to infants until late in the first year of life (see Table 11-1).

Great care must be taken to prevent the child from becoming undernourished. An elimination program must always be initiated under the supervision of a competent pediatric nurse practitioner, dietitian, or physician.

TREATMENT

Smallpox vaccination is *definitely contraindicated* for the child with eczema. In fact, such a child must be kept away from anyone who has recently been vaccinated. A serious condition called *eczema vaccinatum* results when an infant with eczema is vaccinated or is exposed to the vaccination of another person. The infant becomes seriously ill, and mortality rates have been high. Fortunately, because smallpox vaccination is no longer required, this is not a major concern, but it could occur if the child is exposed to someone preparing to go overseas.

Of greater current concern is protecting the child from anyone with a herpes simplex infection (cold sore). If the lesions become infected with herpes simplex, a generalized reaction may occur. In the child with severe eczema with many lesions, body fluid loss from oozing through the lesions can be serious. The infant may have severe pain and be gravely ill with this complication.

Oral antibiotics may be ordered for a coexistent infection such as staphylococci, streptococci, or viral infections. Oral antihistamines and sedatives may help relieve the itching and allow rest. If no infection exists, topical hydrocortisone ointments may be used to relieve inflammation. Wet soaks or colloidal baths also may be prescribed for their soothing effects. The water should be tepid for further soothing, and soap may not be used because of its drying effect. Some physicians recommend the use of a mild soap, such as Dove or Neutrogena, or a soap substitute. Lubrication is essential to retain moisture and prevent evaporation after the bath. Emollients containing lanolin or petrolatum, such as Eucerin, may be prescribed.

Inhalant and contact allergens should be avoided as far as possible. In the infant's bedroom, window drapes or curtains, dresser scarves, and rugs should be removed or made of washable fabric that can be frequently laundered. Furniture should be washed off frequently. The mattress of the crib should have a nonallergenic covering and be washed frequently, cleaning carefully along the binding. Feather pillows must be eliminated, and stuffed toys should be washable. It may be necessary to provide new homes for household pets. However, dander from the pets can remain in carpets, crevices, and overstuffed furniture for a long time. Carpets and area rugs may need to be removed. A home, especially an older one with a damp basement, may be harboring molds that shed allergenic spores. Bathrooms are also places for molds and mildews to hide, especially in warm, humid climates.

◤◥ Nursing Process for the Child With
◣◢ Infantile Eczema

ASSESSMENT

The family caregivers of the child with infantile eczema are often frustrated and exhausted. Although the caregiver can be assured that most cases of infant eczema clear up by the age of 2, this does little to relieve the present situation. Hospitalization is avoided whenever possible because these infants are highly susceptible to infections. Sometimes, however, admission seems to be the only answer to provide more intensive therapy or to relieve an exhausted caregiver.

During the interview with the family caregivers, cover the history of the condition, including treatments that have been tried already and foods that have been ruled out as allergens. Include a thorough review of the home environment. Evaluate the caregivers' knowledge of the condition.

The assessment of the infant includes vital signs, general nutritional state, and a complete examination of all body parts, with careful documentation of the eruptions and their location and size. Areas that are weeping and crusted should be indicated, as well as areas that are unaffected.

NURSING DIAGNOSES

Regardless of the severity of the eczema, the nursing diagnoses are much the same. In addition to Altered Growth and Development, nursing diagnoses that may be used are:

- Impaired Skin Integrity related to lesions and inflammatory process

- Sleep Pattern Disturbance related to itching and discomfort

- Risk for Altered Nutrition: Less than Body Requirements related to elimination diet

- Risk for Infection related to skin lesions

- Health Seeking Behaviors by the parents related to disease condition and treatment

OUTCOME IDENTIFICATION AND PLANNING

The major goals for the infant with eczema are maintaining comfort, preserving skin integrity, improving sleep patterns, maintaining good nutrition (within the constraints of allergens), and preventing infection of skin lesions. A family goal is increasing knowledge about the disease process. Base the nursing plan of care on these goals.

IMPLEMENTATION

MAINTAINING SKIN INTEGRITY. Cover the lesions with light clothing. Especially appropriate are the one-piece, loose-fitting terry pajamas or one-piece cotton underwear known as "onesies." This type of clothing helps keep the infant from scratching. In addition, the nails must be kept closely cut, and mittenlike hand coverings can be used. Use restraints only if necessary. Elbow restraints may sometimes be used. Remove restraints at least every 4 hours—more often, if feasible—but do not allow the child to rub or scratch while the restraints are off. If ointments or wet dressings must be kept in place on the infant's face, a mask may be made by cutting holes into a cotton stockinette-type material to correspond to eyes, nose, and mouth. Wet dressings on the rest of the body can be kept in place by wrapping the infant "mummy" fashion. Dressings may be left on for an extended period but should not be allowed to dry, because that can create open areas when they are removed.

PROVIDING COMFORT MEASURES. Plan soothing baths, such as a colloidal bath (Aveeno), just before naptime or bedtime. Time medications such as sedatives or antihistamines so that they will be effective immediately after the bath, when the infant is most relaxed.

MAINTAINING ADEQUATE NUTRITION. Weigh the child on admission and daily thereafter. This procedure gives some indication of weight gain. If an elimination diet is being used, the diet should be carefully balanced, within the framework of the foods permitted, and supplemented with vitamin and mineral preparations as needed. Fluids are encouraged to prevent dehydration.

PREVENTING INFECTION. As stated earlier, usually these children are kept out of the health care facility because of the concern about infection. However, they can also become infected at home. Whether in the health care facility or at home, the infant should be placed in a room alone, or in a room where there is no other child with any type of infection. Administer antibiotics as ordered. For open lesions, aseptic techniques are necessary to prevent infection.

PROVIDING FAMILY TEACHING. Help the family caregivers understand the condition and possible food, contact, or inhalant allergens. Teach them ways to soothe the infant. They should avoid overdressing and overheating the infant, since perspiration causes itching, and should use a mild detergent to launder the infant's clothing and bedding. Help them determine ways to encourage normal growth and development. Teach them to read labels of prepared foods, watching carefully for hidden allergens. Family caregivers may feel apprehensive or repulsed by this unsightly infant. Support them in expressing their feelings, and help them view this as a distressing but temporary skin condition.

Children with eczema are frequently active and "behaviorally itchy." Assist caregivers in handling challenging behavior. Help caregivers develop a strong self-image in the child to protect against strangers' openly negative reactions.

EVALUATION: GOALS AND OUTCOME CRITERIA

- *Goal*: The child's sleep pattern will not be disturbed.
  Criteria: The child sleeps an adequate amount for his or her age, after comfort measures are provided.

- *Goal*: The child's nutrition will meet the needs for growth and development.
  Criteria: The child has no weight loss and has weight gain appropriate for age.

- *Goal*: The child's skin lesions will not become infected.

Criteria: The infant does not scratch lesions; lesions do not become infected.

- *Goal*: Family caregivers will understand the disease and its treatment.
  Criteria: Caregivers demonstrate an acceptance of the infant and the condition by interacting in a positive fashion with the child.

■ KEY POINTS

- Small anatomic structures and immature systems contribute to the vulnerability of the infant in the first year of life.
- Infants need adequate nutrition for healthy development.
- Infants can quickly become seriously dehydrated from a bout of vomiting or diarrhea.
- Iron deficiency anemia occurs in infants who have an inadequate iron intake.
- Otitis media is a common complication of upper respiratory infections in infants.
- Immunizations can now eliminate the danger of *H influenzae*, a bacteria that can cause serious respiratory illnesses and complications in infants.
- Safety precautions must be included in any nursing care plan for infants.
- Sudden infant death syndrome, the leading cause of death in infants over 1 month of age, is devastating to the infant's family.
- Febrile seizures commonly occur in infants and children between 6 months and 3 years of age.
- Many infant skin conditions can be avoided with good preventive care.

? CRITICAL THINKING

1. You are caring for Jared, a 3-month-old infant with the diagnosis of NFTT. What observations will you make? What might you expect to find? Identify some nursing practices you can incorporate into your nursing care plan. Describe how you will work with his 16-year-old mother, Darcy, to help her set positive parenting behaviors.

2. Kayleen is your neighbor. Her 2-month-old infant, Jamal, has been very fretful and cries a lot. Jamal's health care provider has told Kayleen that Jamal has colic. Kayleen is overwhelmed and almost frantic. Discuss what you can say to her and suggestions you can make to help her cope.

3. Four-month-old Nicky is admitted with bronchiolitis, suspected to be caused by RSV. Describe the observations you will make during your assessment. He is placed in a mist tent. Discuss nursing care, including measures that may help ease his breathing.

4. Nine-month-old Tina has severe diarrhea. What symptoms and physical assessment characteristics would you look for in her? What documentation is especially important in her care?

5. James, a 6-month-old infant, has a fever of 102.8°F. While you are visiting him, he begins to have a seizure. Describe your actions and appropriate teaching for his caregivers.

6. Identify the relation between *Candida albicans* and some cases of diaper rash. Detail the teaching you would provide for a mother concerning diaper rash.

REFERENCES

1. Kline MK. Otitis media. In Oski FA, ed. Principles and practices of pediatrics. Philadelphia: JB Lippincott, 1994.

2. Carroll JL, Loughlin GM. Sudden unexplained death and apparent life-threatening events. In Oski FA, ed. Principles and practices of pediatrics. Philadelphia: JB Lippincott, 1994.

3. Bell J, Esterling LS. What will I tell the children? Omaha: University of Nebraska Medical Center Child Life Department and Meyer Children's Rehabilitation Institute, 1986.

4. Leyden JJ. Cornstarch, *Candida albicans*, and diaper rash. Pediatr Dermatol 1(4):322–325, 1984.

BIBLIOGRAPHY

Day S, Dancy R, Kelly K, Wang W. Iron overload in sickle cell disease? MCN 18(6):330–335, 1993.

Demmler GJ. Rotaviruses. In Oski FA, ed. Principles and practices of pediatrics. Philadelphia: JB Lippincott, 1994.

Engel NS. Phenobarbital for pediatric febrile seizures: Risk-benefit update. MCN 15(4):257, 1990.

Facione N. Otitis media: An overview of acute and chronic disease. Nurse Pract 15(10):11–20, 1990.

Janai H, Stutman HR, Marks MI. Invasive *Haemophilus influenzae* type B infections: A continuing challenge. Am J Infect Control 18(3):160–166, 1990.

Jury DL. More on RSV and ribavirin. Pediatr Nurs 19(1):89–91, 1993.

Klein MJA. The home health nurse clinician's role in the prevention of nonorganic failure to thrive. J Pediatr Nurs 5(2): 129–135, 1990.

Lerner H. Sleep position of infants: Applying research in practice. MCN 18(5):275–277, 1993.

Pillitteri A. Maternal and child health nursing, 2nd ed. Philadelphia: JB Lippincott, 1995.

Romeo SP. Atopic dermatitis: The itch that rashes. Pediatr Nurs 21(2):157–163, 1995.

Sharts-Hopko NC. The newest in vaccines. MCN 19(1):56, 1994.

Wong DL. Whaley and Wong's nursing care of infants and children, 5th ed. St. Louis: Mosby, 1995.

Chapter 12

Growth and Development of the Toddler: 1 to 3 Years

PHYSICAL DEVELOPMENT
PSYCHOSOCIAL DEVELOPMENT
    Play
    Discipline
    Sharing With a Sibling
NUTRITION

HEALTH PROMOTION AND MAINTENANCE
    Routine Checkups
    Family Teaching
    Accident Prevention
THE TODDLER IN THE HEALTH CARE FACILITY
    Special Considerations

STUDENT OBJECTIVES

On completion of this chapter, the student will be able to:

1. Identify the age group known as the toddler.
2. State why parenting a toddler is often frustrating.
3. Describe physical growth that occurs during toddlerhood.
4. Define the following terms as they relate to the psychosocial development of the toddler: a) negativism, b) ritualism, c) dawdling.
5. List three reasons why eating problems often appear in this age group.
6. Describe the progression of the toddler's self-feeding skills.
7. State the age at which a child should be taught toothbrushing, and explain why this is an appropriate age.
8. Describe the relation between sweet foods and plaque formation on the teeth.
9. Discuss the purpose of the toddler's first dental visit and the ideal age for it.
10. Describe the elements in timing of the beginning of toilet training.
11. Identify six suggestions to aid in bowel training.
12. State when complete bowel and bladder control might be achieved.
13. State why accident prevention is a primary concern when caring for a toddler.
14. State the four leading causes of accidental death of toddlers; list preventive measures for each.
15. List eight types of medications most commonly involved in childhood poisonings.
16. List desirable information to be gathered in a social assessment when a toddler is admitted to the hospital.

KEY TERMS

autonomy	parallel play
dawdling	punishment
discipline	ritualism
negativism	temper tantrum

Soon after a child's first birthday, important and sometimes dramatic changes take place. Physical growth slows considerably, mobility and communication skills improve rapidly, and a determined, often stubborn little person begins to create a new set of challenges for the caregivers. "No" and "want" are favorite words. Temper tantrums appear.

During this transition from infancy to early childhood, the child learns many new physical and social skills. With additional teeth and better motor skills, the toddler's self-feeding abilities improve and include the addition of a new assortment of foods. Left unsupervised, the toddler also may taste many nonfood items that may be harmful, even fatal.

This transition is a time of unpredictability: one moment, the toddler insists on "me do it"; the next moment, the child reverts to dependence on the mother or other caregiver. As the toddler seeks to assert independence and achieve autonomy, fear of separation develops. The toddler's curiosity about the world increases, as does his or her ability to explore. Family caregivers soon discover that this exploration can wreak havoc on orderly routine and a well-kept house and that the toddler requires close supervi-

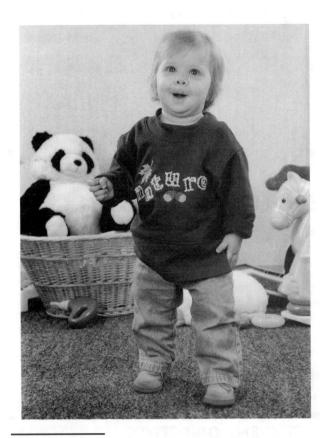

Figure 12-2
The toddler is proud of her ability to stand.

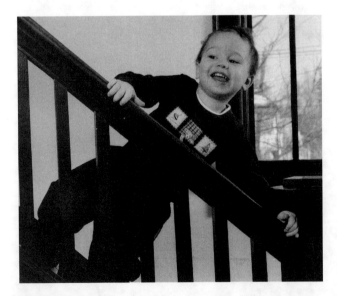

Figure 12-1
Playing on the stairs is a daring and fun activity for the toddler. It can also get him into big trouble.

sion to prevent injury to self or objects in the environment (Fig. 12-1). The toddler justly earns the title of "explorer."

Toddlerhood can be a difficult time for family caregivers. Just as they are beginning to feel confident in their ability to care for and understand their infant, the toddler changes into a walking, talking person whose attitudes and behaviors disrupt the entire family. Accident-proofing, safety measures, and firm but gentle discipline are primary tasks for caregivers of toddlers. Learning to discipline with patience and understanding is difficult but eventually rewarding. At the end of the toddlerhood stage, the child's behavior generally becomes more acceptable and predictable.

Erikson's psychosocial developmental task for this age group is **autonomy** (independence) while overcoming doubt and shame. As the infant's task was one of building trust, the toddler seeks independence, wavering between dependence and freedom, gaining self-awareness. This behavior is so common that the stage is commonly referred to as the "terrible twos," but it is just as often referred to as the "terrific twos" because of the toddler's exciting language development, the exuberance with which he or she greets the world, and a newfound sense of accomplishment. Both aspects of being 2 years old are essential to the child's development, and caregivers must learn how to manage the fast-paced switches between anxiety and enthusiasm.

PHYSICAL DEVELOPMENT

Toddlerhood is a time of slowed growth and rapid development. Each year the toddler gains 5 to 10 lb (2.26–4.53 kg) and about 3″ (7.62 cm). Continued eruption of teeth, particularly the molars, helps the toddler learn to chew food. The toddler learns to stand alone (Fig. 12-2) and to walk between the ages of 1 and 2 years. During this time, most children say their first words and continue to improve and refine their language skills. By the end of this period, the toddler may have learned partial or total toilet training.

The rate of development varies with each child, depending on the individual personality and the opportunities available to test, explore, and learn. Significant landmarks in growth and development of the toddler are summarized in Table 12-1.

TABLE 12-1. Growth and Development: The Toddler

Age (months)	Personal–Social	Fine Motor	Gross Motor	Language	Cognition
12–15	Begins Erikson's stage of "autonomy versus shame and doubt" Seeks novel ways to pursue new experiences Imitations of people are more advanced	Builds with blocks, finger paints Able to reach out with the hands and bring food to the mouth Holds a spoon Drinks from a cup	Movements become more voluntary Postural control improves; able to stand and may take few independent steps	First words are not generally classified as true language. They are generally associated with the concrete and are usually activity-oriented.	Begins to accomodate to the environment, and the adaptive process evolves
18	Extremely curious Becomes a communicative social being Parallel play Fleeting contacts with other children "Make-believe" play begins	Better control of spoon; good control when drinking from cup Turns page of a book Places objects in holes or slots	Walks alone; gait may still be a bit unsteady Begin to walk sideways and backward	Begins to use language in a symbolic form to represent images or ideas that reflect the thinking process Uses some meaningful words such as "hi," "bye-bye," and "all gone" Comprehension is significantly greater	Demonstrates foresight and can discover solutions to problems without excessive trial-and-error procedures Can imitate without the presence of a model (deferred imitation)
24	Language facilitates autonomy Sense of power from saying "no" and "mine" Increased independence from mother	Turns pages of a book singly Adept at building a tower of 6 or 7 cubes When drawing, attempts to enclose a space	Runs well with little falling Throws and kicks a ball Walks up and down stairs one step at a time	Begins to use words to explain past events or to discuss objects not observably present Rapidly expands vocabulary to about 300 words; uses plurals	Enters preconceptual phase of cognitive development State of continuous investigations Primary focus is egocentric
36	Basic concepts of sexuality are established Separates from mother more easily Attends to toilet needs	Copies a circle and a straight line Grasps spoon between thumb and index finger Holds cup by handle	Balances on one foot; jumps in place; pedals tricycle	Quest for information furthered by questions like "why," "when," "where," and "how" Has acquired the language that will be used in the course of simple conversation during the adult years	Preconceptual phase continues; can think of only one idea at a time; cannot think of all parts in terms of the whole

From Wieczorek RR, Natapoff JN. A conceptual approach to the nursing care of children: Health care from birth through adolescence. Philadelphia: JB Lippincott, 1981.

PSYCHOSOCIAL DEVELOPMENT

The toddler develops a growing awareness of self as a being, separate from other people or objects. Intoxicated with newly discovered powers and lacking experience, the child tends to test personal independence to the limit. This age has been called an age of **negativism**. Certainly, the toddler's response to nearly everything is a firm "no," but this is more an assertion of individuality than of an intention to disobey.

Ritualism, dawdling, and temper tantrums also characterize this age. **Ritualism** is a practice employed by the young child to help develop security. A certain routine must be followed, making rituals of simple tasks. At bedtime, all toys must be in accustomed places, and the caregiver must follow a habitual practice. This passion for a set routine is not found in every child to the same degree, but it does provide a comfortable base from which to step out into new and potentially dangerous paths. These practices often become more evident when a sitter is in the home, especially at bedtime. This gives the child some measure of security when the primary caregiver is absent.

Dawdling serves much the same purpose. The young child must decide between following the wishes and routines of the caregiver and asserting independence by following personal desires. Because he or she is incapable of making such a choice, the toddler compromises and tries both. If the matter is of any importance, the caregiver should help the child to follow along the way he or she should go, in a firm and friendly manner; otherwise, dawdling can be ignored, within reasonable limits.

Temper tantrums spring from frustration. The child's urge to be independent naturally results in many frustrations. Add to this the fact that the child is reluctant to leave the scene for necessary rest, and one can see that frequently the frustrations become too great. Even the best of caregivers may lose patience, showing a temporary lack of understanding. The child reacts with enthusiastic rebellion, but this, too, is a phase that must be lived through while the child works toward becoming a person.

Reasoning, scolding, or punishing during the tantrum is useless. A trusted person who remains calm and patient needs to be nearby until the child gains self-control. After the tantrum is over, help the child relax by diverting attention with a toy or some other interesting distraction. However, do not yield the point or give in to the child's whim. That would tell the child that to get whatever one wants, one need only throw oneself on the floor and scream. The child would have to learn, painfully, later in life that others cannot be controlled in this manner.

Admittedly, it is not easy to handle a small child who drops to the floor screaming and kicking in rage in the middle of the supermarket or the sidewalk, nor are comments from onlookers at all helpful. The best a caregiver can do is pick up the out-of-control child as calmly as possible and carry the child to a quiet, neutral place to regain self-control. These tantrums can be accompanied by head-banging and breath-holding. Breath-holding can be frightening to the caregiver, but the child will shortly lose consciousness and begin breathing. Head-banging can cause injury to the child, so the caregiver needs to provide protection.

The caregiver should try to be calm when dealing with a toddler having a tantrum. The child is out of control and needs help to regain control; the adult must maintain self-control to reassure the child and provide security.

Play

The play of the toddler moves from the solitary play of the infant to **parallel play,** in which the toddler plays alongside other children but not with them (Fig. 12-3). Much of the play time is filled with imitation of the people the child sees as role models: adults around him or her, siblings, and other children. Toys that involve the toddler's new gross motor skills, such as push-pull toys, rocking horses, large blocks, and balls, are popular. Fine motor skills are developed by use of thick crayons, Play-Dough, finger paints, wooden puzzles with large pieces, toys that fit pieces into shaped holes, and cloth books. Toddlers enjoy talking on a play telephone and like pots, pans, and toys such as brooms, dishes, and lawnmowers that help them imitate the adults in their environment, promoting socialization. The toddler cannot share toys until the later stage of toddlerhood, and adults should not make an issue of sharing at this early stage.

Toys should be carefully checked for loose pieces and

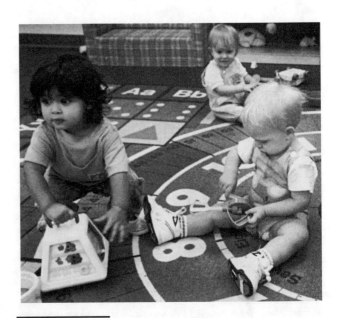

Figure 12-3
Toddlers engaged in parallel play.

sharp edges to ensure the toddler's safety. Toddlers still put a lot of things into their mouths; therefore, small pieces that may come loose, such as small beads and buttons, must be avoided.

For an adult, just staying quietly on the sidelines and observing the toddler play can be a fascinating revelation of what is going on in the child's world. However, the adult must intervene only if necessary to avoid injury.

Discipline

The word "discipline" has come to mean punishment to many people, but the concepts are not the same. To **discipline** means to train or instruct to produce a particular behavior pattern, especially moral or mental improvement, and self-control. **Punishment** means penalizing someone for wrongdoing. Although all small children need discipline, the need for punishment occurs much less frequently.

The toddler learns self-control gradually. The development from an egotistic being, whose world exists only to give self-satisfaction, into a person who understands and respects the rights of others is a long, involved process. The child cannot do this alone but must be taught.

Two-year-old children begin to show some signs of accepting responsibility for their own actions, but because of their egocentricity, they lack inner controls. The toddler still wants the forbidden thing but may repeat "no, no, mustn't" while reaching for a desired treasure, recognizing the act is not approved. Although the child understands the act is not approved, the desire is too strong to resist. Even at this age, children want and need limits. With no limits set, the child develops a feeling of insecurity and fear. With proper guidance, the child gradually absorbs the restraints and develops self-control or conscience.

Consistency and timing are important in the approach that the caregiver uses when disciplining the child. People caring for the child should agree on the methods of discipline and should be consistent. The adults should all operate by the same rules, so the child knows what is expected. This need for consistency can cause disagreement for family caregivers who have experienced different types of child-rearing themselves. The toddler needs a lot of help during this time. The caregivers may be confused by this child who had been a sweet, loving baby and has now turned into a belligerent little being who throws tantrums at will.

This period can be challenging to adults. The child needs to learn that the adults are in control and will help the child gain self-control while learning to be independent. When the toddler hits or bites another child, calmly remove the offender from the situation. Negative messages such as "You are a bad boy for hitting Jamal" or "Bad girl! You don't bite people" are not helpful. Instead, use messages that do not label the child as bad but label the act as unacceptable, such as "Biting hurts—be gentle."

Another method that can be used with a child who is not cooperating or who is out of control is to send the child to a "time out" chair. This should be a place where the child can be alone, but observed, without other distractions. The duration of the isolation should be limited—1 minute per year of age is usually adequate. Warn the child in advance of this possibility, but only one warning per event is necessary. Praise children for good behavior and, when possible, ignore the negative behavior.

"Extinction" is another technique of discipline that is effective with this age group. If the child has certain undesirable behaviors that occur frequently, ignore the behavior. Do not react to the child as long as the behavior is not harmful to the child or others. Be consistent, and never react in any way to that particular behavior. Act as though you do not hear the child. However, when the child responds acceptably in a situation in which the undesirable behavior was the usual response, be sure to compliment the child. For example, say that the child screams or makes a scene when you won't buy cookies in the grocery store. If at another time at the grocery store, after you have practiced extinction, the child talks in a normal voice, compliment the child's "grown-up" behavior.

Spanking or other physical punishment usually does not work well because the child is merely taught that hitting or other physical violence is acceptable, and the child who is spanked frequently becomes immune to it.

Sharing With a Sibling

The first child has the caregivers' undivided attention until a new baby arrives, often when the first child is a toddler. It is difficult to prepare a child just emerging from babyhood for this arrival. Although the toddler can feel the mother's abdomen and understand that this is where the new baby lives, it does not give adequate preparation for the baby's arrival. This real baby represents a rival for the mother's affection.

As in many stressful situations, the toddler frequently regresses to more infantile behavior. The toddler who no longer takes milk from a bottle may need or want a bottle when the new baby is being fed. Toilet training, which may have been moving along well, may regress, with the toddler having episodes of soiling and wetting.

The new infant creates considerable change in the home, whether he or she is the first child or the fifth. In homes in which the previous baby is being displaced by the newcomer, however, some special preparation is necessary. Moving the older child to a larger bed some time before the new baby appears lets the toddler take pride in being "grown up" now.

Preparation of the toddler for a new brother or sister is helpful but should not be intense until just before the expected birth. Many hospitals have sibling classes for new siblings-to-be, scheduled shortly before the anticipated delivery. These classes, geared to the young child, give the child some tasks to do for the new baby and discuss both

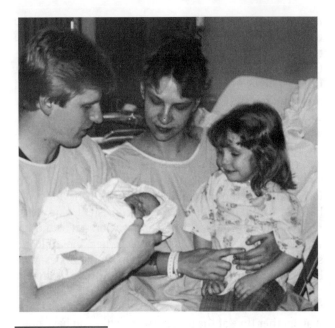

Figure 12-4
This toddler is meeting her new baby sister.

negative and positive aspects of having a new baby in the home. There are many books available that can help prepare the young child for birth and that also discuss sibling rivalry.

Probably the greatest help in preparing the child of any age to accept the new baby is to help the child feel that this is "our baby," not just "mommy's baby" (Fig. 12-4). Helping to care for the baby, according to the child's ability, contributes to a feeling of continuing importance and self-worth.

The displaced toddler almost certainly will feel some jealousy. With careful planning, however, the mother can reserve some time for cuddling and playing with the toddler just as before. Perhaps the toddler may profit from a little extra parental attention for a time. The toddler needs to feel that parental love is just as great as ever and that there is plenty of room in the parents' lives for both children.

The child should not be made to grow up too soon. The toddler should not be shamed or reproved for reverting to babyish behavior, but should receive understanding and a bit more love and attention. Perhaps the father or other family member can occasionally take over the care of the new baby while the mother devotes herself to the toddler. The mother also may plan special times with the toddler when the new infant is sleeping and she has no interruptions. This approach helps the toddler feel special.

NUTRITION

Between the ages of 1 and 3 years, eating problems commonly appear. These problems occur for a number of reasons, such as:

1. The child's growth rate has slowed; therefore, he or she may want and need less food than before. Family caregivers need to know that this is normal.
2. The child's strong drive for independence and autonomy compels an assertion of will to prove his or her individuality, both to self and others.
3. A child's appetite varies according to the kind of foods offered. "Food jags" are common, with a desire for only one kind of food for a while.

To minimize these eating problems and ensure that the child gets a balanced diet with all the proteins, carbohydrates, minerals, and vitamins essential for health and well-being, meals should be planned with an understanding of the toddler's developing feeding skills. Family Teaching

 Family Teaching
Tips for Feeding Toddlers

1. Serve small portions, and provide a second serving when the first has been eaten. 1 or 2 tbsp is an adequate serving for the toddler. Too much food on the dish may overwhelm the child.
2. There is no *one* food essential to health. Allow substitution for a disliked food. Food jags in which toddlers prefer one food for days on end are common and not harmful. If the child refuses a particular food, such as milk, use appropriate substitutes such as pudding, cheese, yogurt, and cottage cheese. Avoid a battle of wills at mealtime.
3. Toddlers like simply prepared foods, served warm or cool, *not* hot or cold.
4. Provide a social atmosphere at mealtimes; allow the toddler to eat with others in the family. Toddlers learn by imitating the acceptance or rejection of foods by other family members.
5. Toddlers prefer foods they can pick up with their fingers; however, they should be allowed to use a spoon or fork when they want to try.
6. Try to plan regular mealtimes with small nutritious snacks planned between meals. Do not attach too much importance to food by urging the child to choose what to eat.
7. Dawdling at mealtime is common with this age group and can be ignored unless it stretches on to unreasonable lengths or becomes a play for power. Mealtime for the toddler should not exceed 20 minutes. Calmly remove food without comment.
8. Do not make desserts a reward for good eating habits. It gives unfair value to the dessert and makes vegetables or other foods seem less desirable.
9. Offer regularly planned nutritious snacks, such as milk, crackers and peanut butter, cheese cubes, and pieces of fruit. Plan snacks midway between meals and at bedtime.
10. Remember that the total amount eaten each day is more important than the amount eaten at a specific meal.

Tips for Feeding Toddlers offers guidance for toddler mealtimes. Messiness is to be expected and prepared for when learning begins, but it gradually diminishes as the child gains skill in self-feeding. At 15 months, the toddler can sit through meals. The 15-month-old prefers finger feeding and wants to self-feed. He or she tries to use a spoon but has difficulty with scooping and spilling. The 15-month-old grasps the cup with the thumb and forefinger, but tilts the cup instead of the head. By 18 months, the toddler's appetite decreases. The 18-month-old has improved control of the spoon, puts spilled food back on the spoon, holds the cup with both hands, spills less often, and may throw

the cup when finished if no one is there to take it. At 24 months, the toddler's appetite is fair to moderate. The toddler at this age has clearly defined likes and dislikes and food jags. The 24-month-old grasps the spoon between the thumb and forefinger, can put food on the spoon with one hand, continues to spill, and accepts no help ("Me do!"). By 30 months, refusals and preferences are less evident. Some toddlers at this age hold the spoon like an adult, with the palm turned inward. The cup, too, may be handled in an adultlike manner. The 30-month-old tilts the head back to get the very last drop. A sample daily food plan is provided in Table 12-2.

TABLE 12-2. Suggested Daily Food Guidelines for the Toddler

Food Items	Daily Amounts*	Comments/Rationale
Cooked eggs†	3–5/wk	Good source of protein; moderate use is recommended because of high cholesterol content in egg yolk
Breads, grains, and cereals: whole-grain or enriched	4 or more servings (eg, ½ slice bread, ¼ cup cereal, 2 crackers, ¼ cup noodles)	Provides thiamine, niacin, and, if enriched, riboflavin and iron. Encourage the child to identify and appreciate a wide variety of foods
Fruit juices; fruit—canned or small pieces	3 or 4 child-sized servings (eg, ½ cup juice, ¼–½ cup fruit pieces)	Use those rich in vitamins A and C; also source of iron and calcium. Self-feeding enhances the child's sense of independence
Vegetables	1 or 2 child-sized servings (eg, ¼–⅓ cup)	Include at least 1 dark-green or yellow vegetable every other day for vitamin A
Meat, fish, chicken, casseroles, cottage cheese, peanut butter, dried peas and beans	2 child-sized servings (eg, 1 oz meat, 1 egg, ½ cup casserole, ¼ cup cottage cheese, 1–2 tbsp peanut butter)	Source of complete protein, iron, thiamine, riboflavin, niacin, and vitamin B₁₂. Nuts and seeds should not be offered until after age 3 when the risk of choking is minimal
Milk, yogurt, cheese	4–6 child-sized servings (eg, 4–6 oz milk, ½ cup yogurt, 1 oz cheese)	Cheese, cottage cheese, and yogurt are good calcium and riboflavin sources; also sources of calcium, phosphorus, complete protein, riboflavin, and niacin; also vitamin D if fortified milk used
Fats and sweets	In moderation	May interfere with consumption of nutrient-rich foods. Chocolate should be delayed until the child is 1 year old.
Salt and other seasonings	In moderation	Children's taste buds are more sensitive than those of adults. Salt is a learned taste, and high intakes are related to hypertension.

* Amounts are daily totals and goals to be achieved gradually.
† New food item for the age group.
Adapted from Eschleman MM. Introductory nutrition and diet therapy, 2d ed. Philadelphia: JB Lippincott, 1991, pp. 286–287.

HEALTH PROMOTION AND MAINTENANCE

Two important aspects of health promotion and maintenance for the toddler are routine checkups and accident prevention. Routine checkups help protect the toddler's health and ensure continuing growth and development. The nurse can encourage good health through family teaching, support of positive parenting behaviors, and reinforcement of the toddler's achievements. Toddlers need a stimulating environment and the opportunity to explore it. This environment, however, must be safe to help prevent accidents and infection. Give caregivers information regarding accident prevention and home safety.

Routine Checkups

In the second year of life, the child is seen at 15 and 18 months for immunization boosters and at least annually thereafter. Routine physical checkups include assessment of growth and development, oral hygiene, toilet training, daily health care, the caregiver–toddler relationship, and parenting skills. Interviews with caregivers, observations of the toddler, observations of the caregiver–toddler interaction, and communication with the toddler are all effective means to elicit this information. Remember that care-

TABLE 12-3. Guidelines for Health Promotion in the Toddler

Developmental Characteristics of Toddler (2–3 yr)	Possible Deviations from Health	Nursing Measures to Ensure Optimal Health Practices

Self-feeding (foods and objects more accessible for mouthing, handling, and eating)	Inadequate nutritional intake
	Accidental poisoning
	Gastrointestinal disturbances:
	  Instability of gastrointestinal tract
	  Infection from parasites (pinworm)
		Diet teaching
		Childproofing the home
		Careful handwashing (before meals, after toileting)
		  Avoidance of rich foods
		  Observe for perianal itching (Scotch tape test, administer anthelmintic)

Toilet training	Constipation (if training procedures are too rigid) Urinary tract infection (especially prevalent in girls due to anatomic structure and poor toilet habits)	Teaching regarding toileting procedures Urinalysis when indicated (eg, burning) Teaching hygiene (at the onset of training, instruct girls to wipe from front to back, and wash hands to prevent cross-infection)
Increased socialization	Increased prevalence of upper respiratory infections (immune levels still at immature levels)	Hygienic practices (eg, use of tissue or handkerchief, not drinking from same glass) Immunizations for passive immunity against communicable disease (MMR; boosters of HbCV, DPT, OPV)
Primary dentition	Caries with resultant infection or loss of primary as well as beginning permanent teeth	Oral hygiene, regular toothbrushing, dental exmination at 21½ months–3 years Proper nutrition to ensure dentition
Sleep disturbances	Lack of sleep may cause irritability, lethargy, decreased resistance to infection	Teaching regarding recommended amounts of sleep (12–14 h in first year, decreasing to 10–12 h by age 3); need for rituals to enhance the transition process to bedtime; possibility of need for nap; setting bedtime limits

MMR, meals, mumps, rubella; *HbCV*, hepatitis B conjugate vaccine; *DPT* diptheria, pertussis, tetanus; *OPV*, oral polio vaccine.
Adapted from Wieczorek RR, Natapoff JN. A conceptual approach to the nursing of children: Health care from birth through adolescence. Philadelphia: JB Lippincott, 1981.

giver interpretations may not be completely accurate. Communicate with the toddler on his or her level and offer only realistic options.

Current immunizations should be administered (see Table 10-4 in Chap. 10). Table 12-3 details nursing measure that may be implemented to ensure optimal health practices.

Family Teaching

The toddler is learning about the world in which she or he lives at a rapid pace. As part of that process, the toddler learns about everyday care needed for healthy growth and development. The toddler's urge for independence and the caregiver's response to that urge play an important part in everyday life with the toddler. Some of these activities are included in the following discussion.

BATHING

Toddlers generally love to take a tub bath. Setting a regular time each day for the bath helps give the toddler a sense of security about what to expect. Although the toddler can sit well in the tub, he or she should never be left alone. An adult must supervise the bath continuously to prevent an accident. The toddler enjoys having tub toys to play with. Avoid using bubble bath, especially for little girls, because it can create an environment that encourages the growth of organisms that cause bladder infections. A bath often is relaxing and may help the toddler quiet down before bedtime.

DRESSING

By their second birthday, toddlers take an active interest in helping to put their clothes on. They often begin around 18 months by removing their socks and shoes whenever they chose. This can be frustrating to the caregiver, but if it is accepted as another small step in development, the level of frustration may be lessened. Between the ages of 2 and 3 years, the toddler can begin by putting on underpants and shirts (Fig. 12-5). Often they end up backwards, but the important thing is that the toddler accomplished the task. Encourage the caregiver to take a relaxed attitude as the toddler learns to dress himself or herself. If clothes must be put on correctly, the caregiver should try to do it without criticizing the toddler's job. The caregiver should warmly acknowledge the toddler's accomplishment of putting on a piece of clothing that he or she may have struggled with for some time. Roomy clothing with easy buttons, large, smooth-running zippers, or Velcro is easier for the toddler to handle.

As in late infancy, shoes need to be worn, primarily to protect the toddler's feet from harsh surfaces. Sneakers are still a good choice. Avoid hard-soled shoes. High-topped shoes are unnecessary.

Figure 12-5
Getting dressed by himself is a fun morning activity for this 3-year-old.

DENTAL CARE

Dental caries (cavities) are a major health problem in children and young adults. Although sound teeth depend in part on sound nutrition, the process of dental caries is linked to the effect of diet on the oral environment.

Tooth decay is caused by bacteria that act in the presence of sugar and form a film, or dental plaque, on the teeth. People who eat sweet foods frequently accumulate plaque easily and are prone to dental caries. Sugars eaten at mealtime appear to be neutralized by the presence of other foods and therefore are not as damaging as between-meal sweets and bedtime bottles. Foods consisting of hard or sticky sugars, such as lollipops and caramels, that remain in the mouth for longer periods tend to cause more dental caries than those that are eaten quickly. Sugarless gum or candies are not as harmful.

When the child is about 2 years of age, he or she should be taught to brush the teeth or at least to rinse the mouth after each meal or snack. Because this is the period in which the toddler likes to imitate others, the child is best taught by example. Plain water should be used until the child has learned how to spit out toothpaste or tooth powder. An adult should also brush the toddler's teeth until the child becomes experienced. One good method is to stand behind the child in front of a mirror and brush the child's teeth. In addition to cleaning adequately, this also helps the child learn how it feels to have the teeth thoroughly brushed.

The use of a fluoride toothpaste strengthens tooth enamel and helps prevent tooth decay, particularly in communities where the water is not fluoridated. An adult should supervise the use of fluoride toothpaste; the child should use only a small pea-sized amount. Supplemental fluoride may be recommended by the physician, but those on limited incomes may find this difficult to afford. A fluoride supplement is a medication and should be treated and stored as such. Fluoride also can be applied during regular visits to the dentist, but the greatest benefit to the tooth enamel occurs before the eruption of the teeth.

The first visit to the dentist should occur at about 2 years of age, just to get acquainted with the dentist, staff, and office. A second visit might be a good time for a preliminary examination, and subsequent visits twice a year for checkups are recommended. If there are older siblings, the toddler can go along on a visit with them to help overcome the fears of a strange setting. Some clinics are recommending earlier visits to check the child and give dietary guidance. Children of low-income families often have poor dental hygiene and care, both because of the cost of care and parental lack of knowledge about proper care and nutrition. Some caregivers may believe it is unnecessary to take proper care of baby teeth because "they just fall out anyway." Nurses have a great responsibility to teach and guide these caregivers.

TOILET TRAINING

Learning control of the bowel and bladder is an important part of the socialization process. In Western culture, a great sense of shame and disgust has been associated with body waste products. To function successfully in this culture, one must learn to dispose of body waste products in a place considered proper by society.

The toddler has been operating on the pleasure principle, simply emptying the bowel and bladder when the urge is present without any thought of anything but personal comfort. During toilet training, the child, who is just learning about control of the personal environment, finds that some of that control must be given up to please those most important people, the caregivers. The toddler must now learn to conform not only to please those special loved ones but, to preserve self-integrity, must persuade himself or herself that this acceptance of the dictates of society is voluntary. These new routines make little sense to the child.

Timing   To be able to cooperate in toilet training, the child's sphincter muscles must have developed to the stage at which the child can control them. Control of the rectal sphincter develops first. The child also must be able to postpone the urge to defecate until reaching the toilet or potty and must be able to signal the need *before* the event. This level of maturation seldom takes place before the age of 18 to 24 months.

Bowel Training   At the start of training, the child has no understanding of the uses of the potty chair, but to please the caregiver the child will sit there for a short time.

Figure 12-6
Mom encourages her 18-month-old to use the potty.

If the child's bowel movements occur at about the same time every day, one day a bowel movement will occur while sitting on the potty. Although there is no sense of special achievement as yet, the child does like the praise and approval. Eventually, the child will connect this approval with the bowel movement in the potty, and the child will be happy that the caregiver is pleased (Fig. 12-6).

Suggestions for bowel training include:

1. A potty chair in which a child can comfortably sit with the feet on the floor is preferable. Most small children are afraid of a flush toilet.
2. The child should be left on the potty chair for only a short time. The caregiver should be readily available but should not hover anxiously over the child. If a bowel movement occurs, approval is in order; if not, no comment is necessary.
3. During the beginning stages of training, the child is likely to have a movement soon after leaving the potty. This is not willful defiance and need not be mentioned.
4. The potty should be emptied unobtrusively after the child has resumed playing. The child has cooperated and produced the product desired. If it is immediately thrown away, the child may be confused and not so eager to please the next time.
5. The ability to feel shame and self-doubt appears at this age. Therefore, the child should not be teased about reluctance or inability to conform. This teasing can shake the child's confidence and cause feelings of doubt in self-worth.
6. The caregiver should not expect perfection, even after control has been achieved. Lapses inevitably

COMMUNICATIONS BOX

Conversation about toilet training with Mike (father of 2-year-old Josh).

INEFFECTIVE COMMUNICATION

Mike: I don't get it. Josh doesn't let me know when he has to pee. He just goes off to a corner and wets himself.

Nurse: Why don't you just pick him up and run for the bathroom when he does that?

Mike: It's already too late. He's wet and I just get mad.

Nurse: Don't get mad at him. He's just a little guy. He's not doing it to be mean.

Mike: Well, it seems to me like he is. I know he knows better.

Nurse: Maybe he does, but he's not just doing it to be mean. Sooner or later he'll learn what he's supposed to do. You just have to be patient with him.

During this conversation, the nurse does not acknowledge Mike's feelings. Telling him not to get mad does not help him ventilate his own feelings. Telling him he must just be patient with Josh contributes to Mike's feelings of inadequacy.

EFFECTIVE COMMUNICATION

Mike: I don't get it. Josh doesn't let me know when he has to pee. He just goes off to a corner and wets himself.

Nurse: You get disgusted with Josh because he doesn't let you know when he has to urinate.

Mike: Well, yeah. I mean, if he knows enough to go off to the corner—why doesn't he just tell me?

Nurse: You are puzzled that he doesn't let you know ahead of time.

Mike: Yeah. I think he's just being stubborn.

Nurse: When Josh goes to the corner, he is indicating that he knows he is going to urinate. Perhaps you could quickly take him to his potty chair at that time, if you notice him.

Mike: Well, I suppose so. But how long is this going to go on?

Nurse: You feel like he will never learn. Toilet training can be a rather long and frustrating experience with some children. Josh needs continued positive support and praise when he "gets it right." Try to use a positive approach. Avoid punishing him for his mistakes. Eventually he will be successful and be very proud of himself.

Mike: Well, OK. I'll give that a try.

Nurse: Good. And if you continue to have problems, don't hesitate to seek guidance. Toddlers are challenging, but amazing when you think of all they accomplish in that period of their development.

By acknowledging to Mike that toilet training is one of the frustrating aspects of parenting a toddler, the nurse helps him understand that his feelings are not unusual and that Josh is behaving like a normal toddler. Offering him concrete ideas to help, and further support if needed, is a positive way to communicate.

occur, perhaps because the child is completely absorbed in play or because of a temporary episode of loose stools. Occasionally, a child feels aggression, frustration, or anger and may use this method to "get even." As long as the lapses are occasional, they should be ignored. If the lapses are frequent and persistent, however, the cause should be sought.

Bladder Training Generally, the first indication of readiness for bladder training is when the child makes a connection between the puddle on the floor and something he or she did. In the next stage, the child runs to the caregiver and indicates a need to urinate, but only after it has happened. There is not much benefit to be gained from a serious program of training until the child is sufficiently mature to control the bladder sphincter and reach the desired place. When the child stays dry for about 2 hours at a time during the day, sufficient maturity may be indicated.

Each child follows an individual pattern of development. No caregiver should feel embarrassed or ashamed because the child is still having accidents. No one should expect the child to accomplish self-training, and family caregivers should be alert to the signs of readiness. Patience and understanding by the caregivers are essential. Complete control, especially at night, may not be achieved until the fourth or fifth year of age. Each child should be taught a term or phrase to use for toileting that is recognizable to others, clearly understood, and socially acceptable. This is especially true for children who are cared for outside the home.

SLEEP

The toddler's sleep needs change gradually between the ages of 1 and 3 years. A total need for 12 to 14 hours of sleep is to be expected in the first year of toddlerhood, decreasing to 10 to 12 hours by 3 years. The toddler soon gives up a morning nap, but most continue to need an afternoon nap until sometime toward the third birthday.

Rituals are a common part of bedtime procedures. A bedtime ritual provides structure and a feeling of security because the toddler knows what to expect and what is expected of him or her. The separation anxiety that is common in the toddler may contribute to some of the toddler's reluctance to go to bed. Family caregivers must be careful that the toddler does not use this to manipulate them and delay bedtime. Gentle, firm consistency by caregivers is ultimately reassuring to the toddler. Regular schedules, with set bedtimes and a story time or quiet time beforehand, often help the toddler settle for the night. There are many wonderful stories to be read to the toddler that can provide a calming end to a busy day.

Accident Prevention

Toddlers are explorers who require constant supervision in a controlled environment to encourage autonomy and prevent injury. When supervision is inadequate or the envi-

A Personal Glimpse

One day I came home from work and my wife told me an amazing (and frightening) story about our 2-year-old son. I have a rifle cabinet in our living room. It is always locked, and only my wife and I know where the key is, or so we thought. My wife was at the sink doing dishes. While she was busy, Richie pulled a chair up to the wall and somehow reached up to the shelves where the keys were kept. By the time Becky noticed what he was up to, he was putting the key in the lock of the drawer where the pistols are kept. Of course, none of them are ever loaded, and the bullets are nowhere near where the weapons are kept. Anyway, she took the key from him and figured that was that. Well, he had other ideas! Somehow, without her knowing it, he had gotten two keys and gave her the wrong one on purpose (or maybe not, we'll never know). Luckily, his second attempt was also unsuccessful. We don't know how 2-year-olds think, but I wonder what comes after 2. I guess 3.

Max

ronment is unsafe, tragedy often results, making accidents the leading cause of death for children between the ages of 1 and 4 years. Accidents involving motor vehicles, drowning, burns, poisoning, and falls are the most common causes of death. The number of deaths caused by burns and drownings is similar, but motor vehicle deaths in this age group are more than three times greater than either of these causes. Family teaching can help minimize the risk for accident and injury.

MOTOR VEHICLE ACCIDENTS

Many childhood deaths or injuries resulting from motor vehicle accidents can be prevented by proper use of restraints. Federally approved child safety seats are designed to give the child maximum protection if used correctly. Children need to be taught that they must be securely fastened in the car seat before the car starts. Adults must be responsible for teaching the child that seat belts are required for safe car travel. Adults in the car with a child should set the example by also using seat belts. Many toddlers are killed or injured by moving vehicles while playing in their own driveway or garage. Caregivers need to be aware that these tragedies can occur and must take proper precautions at all times. See Family Teaching Tips to Prevent Motor Vehicle Accidents.

DROWNING

Although drowning of young children is often associated with bathtubs, the increased number of home swimming pools has added significantly to the number of accidental drownings. Often, these pools are fenced on three sides to keep out nonresidents but are bordered on one side by the family home, making the pool accessible to infants and toddlers. Even small plastic wading pools hold enough water to drown an unsupervised toddler. Any family living near a body of water, no matter how small, must not leave a mobile infant or toddler unattended, even for a moment. Even a small amount of water, such as that in a bucket, may be enough to drown a small child.

BURNS

Burn accidents occur most often as scalds from immersions and spills and from exposure to uninsulated electrical wires or live extension-cord plugs. Children also are burned while playing with matches or while left unattended in a home where a fire breaks out. Whether the fire results from a child's mischief, an adult's carelessness, or some

Family Teaching
Tips to Prevent Burns

1. Do not let electrical cords dangle over a counter or table. Repair cords if frayed. Newer small appliances have shorter cords to prevent dangling.
2. Cover electrical wall outlets with safety caps.
3. Turn handles of pans on the stove toward the back of the stove. If possible, place pans on back burners out of the toddler's reach.
4. Place cups of hot liquid out of reach. Do not use overhanging tablecloths that toddlers can pull.
5. Use caution when serving foods heated in the microwave—they can be hotter than apparent.
6. Supervise small children at all times while in the bathtub so they cannot turn on the hot water tap.
7. Turn thermostat on home water heater down so that the water temperature is no higher than 120°F.
8. Place matches in metal containers, out of reach of small children. Keep lighters out of reach of children.
9. Never leave small children unattended by an adult or responsible teenager.

unforeseeable event, the injuries, even if not fatal, can have long-term or permanent effects. Many burns can be prevented by following simple safety practices (see Family Teaching Tips to Prevent Burns).

INGESTION OF TOXIC SUBSTANCES

The curious toddler wants to touch and taste everything. Left unsupervised, the toddler may sample household cleaners, prescription or over-the-counter drugs, kerosene, gasoline, or peeling lead-based paint chips or dust particles. Poisoning is still the most common medical emergency in children, with the highest incidence between the ages of 1 and 4 years.

Caregivers need continual reminders about the possibility of childhood poisoning. Even with precautionary labeling and "child-resistant" packaging of medication and household cleaners, children display amazing ingenuity in opening bottles and packages that catch their curiosity. Mr. Yuk labels are available from the nearest poison control center. The child can be taught that products are harmful if they have the Mr. Yuk label on them. However, labeling is not sufficient: all items that are in any way toxic to the child must be placed under lock and key or totally out of the child's reach.

Preventive measures that should be observed by all caregivers of small children are listed in Family Teaching Tips for Prevention of Poisoning.

The following medications are most commonly involved in cases of childhood poisoning:

Acetaminophen
Salicylates (aspirin)

Family Teaching
Tips to Prevent Motor Vehicle Accidents

1. Never start the car until the child is securely in the car seat.
2. If the child manages to get out of the car seat or unfasten it, pull over to the curb or side of the road as soon as possible, turn off the car, and tell the child the car will not go until the child is safely in the seat. Children love to go in the car, and if they learn that they cannot go unless in the car seat, they will comply.
3. Never permit a child to stand in a car while it is in motion.
4. Teach the toddler to stop at a curb and wait for an adult escort to cross the street. An older child should be taught to look both ways for traffic. Start this as a game with toddlers, and continually reinforce it.
5. Teach the child to cross only at corners.
6. Begin in toddlerhood to teach awareness of traffic signals and their meaning. As soon as color recognition is achieved, the child can tell you when it is all right to cross.
7. Never let a child run into the street after a ball.
8. Teach a child never to walk between parked cars to cross.
9. As a driver, always be on the alert for children running into the street when in a residential area.

1. Keep medicines in their original containers in a locked cupboard. Do not rely on a high shelf being out of a child's reach.
2. Never refer to medicines as candy.
3. Discard unused medicines by a method that eliminates any possibility of access by children, other persons, or animals (eg, flush them down the toilet).
4. Replace safety caps properly, but do not depend on them to be childproof. Children can sometimes open them more easily than adults can.
5. Keep a bottle of syrup of ipecac in a locked cupboard to induce vomiting if needed.
6. Keep the telephone number of the nearest poison control center posted near the telephone.
7. Keep a chart with emergency treatment for poisoning in a handy permanent spot.
8. Store household cleaning and laundry products out of reach of children.
9. Never put kerosene or other household fluids in soda bottles or other drink containers.

Laxatives
Sedatives
Tranquilizers
Analgesics
Antihistamines
Cold medicines
Birth-control pills.

The importance of careful, continuous supervision of toddlers and other young children cannot be overemphasized.

THE TODDLER IN THE HEALTH CARE FACILITY

Although hospitalization is difficult and frightening for a child of any age, the developmental stage of the toddler intensifies these problems. When planning care, the nurse caring for the toddler must keep in mind the developmental tasks and needs of the toddler. The toddler, engaged in trying to establish self-control and autonomy, finds that strangers seem to have total power, eliminating any control on his or her part. Add these fears to the inability to communicate well, discomfort from pain, separation from family, the presence of unfamiliar people and surroundings, physical restraint, and uncomfortable or frightening procedures, and the toddler's reaction can be clearly understood.

As part of the admission procedure for the child, a social assessment survey should be completed by interviewing the family caregiver who has accompanied the child to the facility. Usually part of the standard pediatric nursing assessment form, the social assessment covers eating habits and food preferences, toileting habits and terms used for toileting, family members and the names the child calls them, the name the child is called by family members, pets and their names, favorite toys, sleeping or napping patterns and rituals, and other significant information that helps the staff better plan care for the toddler (see Fig. 4-4 in Chap. 4). This information should become an indispensable part of the nursing care plan. Using this information, the nurse should develop a nursing care plan that provides opportunities for independence for the toddler whenever possible.

Separation anxiety is high during the toddler age. As discussed in detail in Chapter 2, the stages of protest and despair are common. Acknowledge these stages and communicate to the child that it is acceptable to feel angry and anxious at being separated from the primary family caregiver, the person foremost in the child's life. *Never* interpret the toddler's angry protest as a personal attack. Many facilities encourage family involvement in the care of the child to minimize separation anxiety. The mother is often the family member who stays with the child, but in many families other members who are close to the child may take turns staying. Having a family caregiver with the toddler can be extremely helpful. However, do not neglect caring for the toddler who has a loved one present. In many families, it is impossible for the family caregiver to stay with the child, for any of a number of reasons. These children need extra attention and care. All children should be assigned a constant caregiver while in the facility, but this is especially important for the toddler who is alone.

The nurse assigned to the toddler will become a surrogate parent while caring for the child. Maintaining as much as possible the pattern, schedule, and rituals that the toddler is used to helps provide some measure of security to the child. This is a time when the toddler needs the security of a beloved thumb or other "lovey," a favorite stuffed animal or blanket. The nurse needs to recognize that the toddler uses this to provide self-comfort. The lovey may be well worn and dirty, but the toddler finds great reassurance in having it to snuggle or cuddle. Do not ridicule the child for its unkempt appearance, and make every effort to allow the toddler to have it whenever desired.

When the family caregiver must leave the toddler, it may be helpful for the adult to give the child some personal item to keep until the adult returns. The caregiver can tell the child he or she will return "when the cartoons come on TV" or "when your lunch comes." These are concrete times that the toddler will probably understand.

Special Considerations

The busy toddler just learning to use the toilet, self-feed, and be disciplined presents a unique challenge to the staff nurse. The nurse must maintain control on the pediatric unit, promote safety, and help establish the toddler's sense of security while allowing the toddler's development to continue.

The toddler learning sphincter control is still dependent on familiar surroundings and the family caregiver's support. For this reason, some pediatric personnel automatically put toddlers back in diapers when they are admitted. This practice should be discouraged. Under the right circumstances, and especially with the caregiver's help, many of these children can maintain control. They at least should be given a chance to try. Potty chairs can be provided for the child when appropriate. The nursing staff must know the method and times of accomplishing toilet training that were used at home and must try to comply with them as closely as possible in the hospital.

Some limits are needed for the toddler, but be careful when setting them. Toddlers, like children of any age, need to feel that someone is in control and need limits that are set with love and understanding. A child who has been overindulged for a long time may need firm, calm statements of limits, delivered in a no-nonsense but kind manner. Explaining what is going to be done, what is expected of the toddler, and what the toddler can expect from the nurse may be helpful. Sometimes the nurse may give some tactful guidance to the family caregiver to help set limits for the toddler. This is an area in which experience helps the nurse solve difficult problems. Discipline on the pediatric unit is discussed in Chapter 4.

A toddler's eating habit may loom large in the nurse's mind as a potential problem. In the hospital or clinic, as at home, food can assume an importance out of proportion to its value and create unnecessary problems. Some helpful hints to minimize potential problems are:

- Viewing mealtime as a social event
- Encouraging self-feeding
- Not pushing food
- Allowing others to eat with the child
- Offering familiar foods
- Providing fluids in small but frequent amounts.

Eating concerns for the pediatric patient are fully discussed in Chapter 4.

Safety is a concern with all hospitalized children, but safety promotion for a toddler may be particularly challenging. The curious toddler needs to be watched with extra care but should not be unnecessarily prohibited from exploring and moving about freely. Safety in the hospital setting is discussed in detail in Chapter 4.

■ KEY POINTS

- The toddler's physical growth slows while motor, social, and language development rapidly increases.

- Autonomy versus doubt and shame is the development task identified by Erikson for the toddler.

- During the toddler period, toilet training, ritualistic behavior, dawdling, negativism, temper tantrums, discipline, and separation anxiety are challenging issues. These issues are best met by caretakers who are understanding, patient, and consistent in their approach.

- As a result of the exploring nature of the toddler, safety concerns are extremely important. Caregivers must provide a safe environment, protecting the toddler from motor vehicle accidents, burns, and ingestion of poisonous substances.

- The toddler's language development proceeds from a few words to the ability to form short sentences by age 2. Verbal language increases rapidly between the toddler's second and third birthday.

- When caring for a toddler, the nurse provides for age-appropriate developmental tasks, encouraging autonomy while protecting the toddler from harm.

? CRITICAL THINKING

1. Jack is the father of 2 1/2-year-old Jimmy, who likes to go to his daddy's workshop with him. Construct a teaching plan to help Jack make this a safe experience for Jimmy.

2. Marti complains to you that 2-year-old Tasha is very difficult to put to bed at night. Marti often just gives up and lets Tasha fall asleep in front of the television. Create a parent teaching plan with suggestions to help Marti ease the bedtime scene.

3. You are in the supermarket with your 2-year-old niece, Lauren. She is having a loud, screaming temper tantrum because you won't buy some expensive cookies she wants. Based on your knowledge of toddlers and tantrums, describe how you will handle the situation.

4. You are caring for 18-month-old Reggie, who has a respiratory condition. Identify the social information you will gather from Reggie's caregiver. Describe how you will include this information in your plan of care for Reggie.

5. Jed is a 26-month-old whose family caregivers work outside the home. He goes to a day care center 3 days a week and is kept by his grandmother the other 2 days. Explain the guidance you would give his family caregiver to assist in toilet training in this situation.

6. Addie is the mother of 14-month-old Kaitlin. This is Addie's first child and she hovers over Kaitlin. She quickly jumps in and completes tasks for Kaitlin before Kaitlin has a chance to try to accomplish the task herself. Addie also frequently cries out, "Stop, Kaitlin, you're going to get hurt!", "Kaitlin, don't do that! You'll fall," and other warnings of this sort. Analyze this situa-

tion and describe what you think is happening. Identify the danger inherent in this situation.

BIBLIOGRAPHY

Brazelton TB. To listen to a child. New York: Addison-Wesley, 1984.

Brazelton TB. What every baby knows. New York: Ballantine Books, 1987.

Castiglia PT, Harbin RE. Child health care: Process and practice. Philadelphia: JB Lippincott, 1992.

Eschleman MM. Introductory nutrition and diet therapy, 2d ed. Philadelphia: JB Lippincott, 1991.

Greenspan SI. Development and behavior: The very young child. Pediatr Clin North Am 38(6):1370–1383, 1991.

Pillitteri A. Maternal and child health nursing, 2d ed. Philadelphia: JB Lippincott, 1995.

Schuster CS, Ashburn SS. The process of human development, 3d ed. Philadelphia: JB Lippincott, 1992.

Spock B, Rothenberg MB. Dr. Spock's baby and child care. New York: Pocket Books, 1992.

Wong DL. Whaley and Wong's nursing care of infants and children, 5th ed. St. Louis: Mosby, 1995.

Health Problems of the Toddler

STUDENT OBJECTIVES

On completion of this chapter, the student will be able to:

1. Describe four characteristics of infantile autism.
2. Identify four goals of treatment of infantile autism.
3. Describe treatment for bacterial conjunctivitis.
4. Describe the diagnosis of celiac disease.
5. Describe the usual treatment for spasmodic laryngitis.
6. Discuss acute laryngotracheobronchitis, including the symptoms and treatment.
7. Identify the basic defect in cystic fibrosis.
8. State the major organs affected by cystic fibrosis.
9. Name the most common type of complication in cystic fibrosis.
10. List the diagnostic procedures used to diagnose cystic fibrosis.
11. Describe the dietary and pulmonary treatment of cystic fibrosis.
12. State the most common cause of poisoning in toddlers.
13. List five common substances children ingest.
14. List seven sources of lead that may cause chronic lead poisoning.
15. Describe the symptoms, diagnosis, treatment, and prognosis of lead poisoning.
16. Discuss the incidence of burns in small children.
17. State the three major causes of burns in small children.
18. Differentiate between first-, second-, and third-degree burns.
19. Describe emergency treatment of a minor burn and of a moderate or severe burn.
20. State why hypovolemic shock occurs in the first 48 hours after a burn.
21. Describe the treatment of a child who has swallowed a foreign object.

KEY TERMS

achylia	eschar
allograft	esotropia
amblyopia	exotropia
autograft	external hordeolum
binocular vision	goniotomy
cataract	heterograft
celiac syndrome	homograft
chelating agent	hydrotherapy
conjunctivitis	hypervolemic
contractures	hypochylia
coryza	lacrimation
croup	orthoptics
débridement	photophobia
diplopia	pica
dysphagia	steatorrhea
echolalia	strabismus
emetic	stridor
encephalopathy	

Children from ages 1 to 3 years are likely to have a number of minor health problems, many of them caused by infection or environmental hazards. Most of these health problems can be managed at home after a visit to the pediatrician's office or clinic. Some of the problems, however, are serious enough to require hospitalization, thus separating the toddler from his or her family caregivers. This separation increases the seriousness of the health problem and the need for loving and understanding attention to the child's emotional needs as well as physical condition.

PSYCHOLOGICAL PROBLEMS

Autism

Although often called *infantile autism* because it is thought to be present from birth, autism usually is not conclusively diagnosed until after 12 months of age. The word *autism* comes from the Greek word *auto* meaning "self" and was first used by Dr. Leo Kanner in 1943 to describe a group of behavioral symptoms in children. The term *pervasive developmental disorder* was introduced in 1980 when the terminology was revised by the American Psychiatric Association. Disorders in this category are characterized by severe behavioral disturbance that affects the practical use of language as a means of communication, interpersonal interaction, attention, perception, and motor activity. Autistic children are totally self-centered and unable to relate to others, often exhibit bizarre behaviors, and often are destructive to themselves and others.

Autism occurs in about 4.5 in 10,000 births and four times as often in males as in females. Several theories exist about its cause as well as its treatment or management.

Originally thought to result from an unsatisfactory early mother–child relationship (emotionally cold, detached mothers, sometimes described as "refrigerator mothers"), autism now appears to have organic, and perhaps genetic, causes instead. Researchers suggest that autism may result from a disturbance in language comprehension, a biochemical problem involving neurotransmitters, or abnormalities in the central nervous system, probably brain metabolism. These children score poorly on intelligence tests but may have good memories and good intellectual potential.

Because the cause of autism is not understood, treatment attempts have met with limited success. These children experience the normal health problems of childhood in addition to those that result from their behaviors. Therefore, it is important that nurses understand this unexplained disorder and how it affects children and families.

CLINICAL MANIFESTATIONS

The characteristics of autism are divided into three categories: inability to relate to others, inability to communicate with others, and obviously limited activities and interests. Children with autism do not develop a smiling response to others or an interest in being touched or cuddled. In fact, they can react violently at attempts to hold them. Their blank expressions and lack of response to verbal stimulation can suggest deafness. They do not show the normal fear of separation from parents that most toddlers exhibit. Often they seem not to notice when family caregivers are present.

During their second year, autistic children become completely absorbed in strange repetitive behaviors, such as spinning an object, flipping an electrical switch on and off, or walking around the room feeling the walls. Their bodily movements are bizarre: rocking, twirling, flapping arms and hands, walking on tiptoe, twisting and turning fingers. If these movements are interrupted, or if objects in the environment are moved, a violent temper tantrum may result. These tantrums may include self-destructive acts such as hand biting and head banging. Although infants and toddlers normally are self-centered, ritualistic, and prone to displays of temper, autistic children show these characteristics to an extreme degree, coupled with an almost total lack of response to other people.

The autistic child is slow to develop speech, and any that does develop is primitive and ineffective in its ability to communicate. **Echolalia** ("parrot speech") is typical of autistic children; they echo words they have heard, such as a television commercial, but offer no indication that they understand the words. Although autistic children are self-centered, their speech indicates that they seem to have no sense of self because they never use the pronouns "I" or "me."

Standard intelligence tests that count on verbal ability usually indicate that these children are mentally deficient.

However, many of these children also demonstrate unusual memory and mathematic, artistic, and musical abilities.

DIAGNOSIS

To confirm a diagnosis of autism, at least eight of 16 identified characteristics must be present, and all three of the categories must be represented. The symptoms of autism can suggest other disorders such as lead poisoning, phenylketonuria, congenital rubella, and measles encephalitis. Therefore, a complete pediatric physical and neurologic examination is necessary, including vision and hearing testing, electroencephalography, radiographic studies of the skull, urine screening, and other laboratory studies. In addition, the nurse usually takes a complete prenatal, natal, and postnatal history, including development, nutrition, and family dynamics. Other members of the health team may be involved in the evaluation and treatment of the autistic child, including audiologists, psychiatrists, psychologists, special education teachers, speech and language therapists, and social workers.

TREATMENT

The treatment of an autistic child is extremely challenging. The child is mentally retarded but may demonstrate exceptional talent in areas such as factual memory and art or music. Four goals toward which treatment is geared are:

- Promotion of normal development
- Specific language development
- Social interaction
- Learning

The treatment must be individually planned and is highly structured. Behavioral modification, pharmacotherapeutics, and other techniques are used. Mixed results occur, and no one technique has met with resounding success. The family needs therapy to help relieve guilt and help them understand this puzzling child. The overall long-term prognosis for these children is not optimistic, but the earlier treatment is started, the better the long-term outlook is. Facilitated communication involves working with language development of autistic children by helping them express themselves in language through use of a computer keyboard. This method is viewed as controversial and unproved by the American Psychological Association.

NURSING CARE

Caring for the autistic child means recognizing that autism creates great stresses for the entire family. The problems that cause family caregivers to seek diagnosis are difficult to live with; diagnosis itself is usually a lengthy and expensive process, and the hope for successful treatment is slight. Most caregivers of autistic children feel guilty, despite the fact that current theories accept organic rather than psychological causes for this disorder. The possibility of genetic factors adds to this guilt. Often, there are other children in the family who are normal but who suffer from a lack of attention because the caregivers' energies are almost totally directed to solving the problems of the autistic youngster.

Nurses who care for these children should consider the family caregivers their most valuable source of information about the child's habits and communication skills. The nurse must learn what techniques have been used by the caregivers to communicate with the child and gain his or her cooperation. Establishing a relationship of trust between the child and the nurse is essential. This child should be cared for by a constant primary nurse to provide consistency.

In the hospital setting, a private or semiprivate room is generally preferred; visual and auditory stimulation should be minimized. Familiar toys or other valued objects from home reduce the child's anxiety about the strange environment.

SENSORY DISORDERS

As toddlers explore their environment, they use all their senses to gather information. As they grow, their senses become more fully developed. Vision screening is part of routine health maintenance; the following section discusses some eye conditions and injuries seen in toddlers.

Eye Conditions

Cataracts, congenital infantile glaucoma, and strabismus are disease conditions that may need to be dealt with during the toddler years. Eye injuries can occur in this exploring stage. In addition, eye infections may occur because exploring hands can easily carry infectious organisms to the eyes.

CATARACTS

A **cataract** is a development of opacity in the crystalline lens that prevents light rays from entering the eye. Congenital cataracts may be hereditary, or they may be complications of maternal rubella during the first trimester of pregnancy. Cataracts also may develop later in infancy or childhood from eye injury or from metabolic disturbances, such as galactosemia and diabetes.

Surgical extraction of the cataracts is performed at an early age. With early removal, the prognosis for good vision is improved. The infant or child is fitted with contact lens, and if only one eye is affected, the "good" eye is patched to prevent amblyopia (see discussion in the section on strabismus). Numerous lens changes are needed to change the strength as the child gets older.

GLAUCOMA

Glaucoma may be of the congenital infantile type, occurring in children younger than age 3 years; juvenile glaucoma, showing clinical manifestations after age 3; or secondary glaucoma, resulting from injury or disease. Increased intraocular pressure due to overproduction of aqueous fluid causes the eyeball to enlarge and the cornea to become large, thin, and sometimes cloudy. Untreated, the disease slowly progresses to blindness. Pain may be present. **Goniotomy** (surgical opening into Schlemm's canal), which provides drainage of the aqueous humor, is often effective in relieving intraocular pressure. Goniotomy may need to be performed multiple times to control intraocular pressure. Surgery is performed as early as possible to prevent permanent damage.

STRABISMUS

Strabismus is the failure of the two eyes to direct their gaze at the same object simultaneously, commonly called "squint" or "crossed eyes." **Binocular** (normal) **vision** is maintained through the muscular coordination of eye movements, so that a single vision results. In strabismus, the visual axes are not parallel, and **diplopia** (double vision) results. In an effort to avoid seeing two images, the child's central nervous system suppresses vision in the deviant eye, causing **amblyopia** (dimness of vision from disuse of the eye), sometimes called "lazy eye."

A wide variation in the manifestation of strabismus exists; there are lateral, vertical, and mixed lateral and vertical types. There may be monocular strabismus, in which one eye deviates while the other eye is used, or alternating strabismus, in which deviation alternates from one eye to the other. The term **esotropia** is used when the eye deviates toward the other eye; **exotropia** denotes a turning away from the other eye (Fig. 13-1).

Treatment depends on the type of strabismus present. In monocular strabismus, occlusion of the better eye by patching to force the use of the deviating eye should be initiated at an early age. Patching is continued for weeks or months. The younger the child, the more rapid the improvement. The patching may be for set periods or continuous, depending on the child's age. The older child needs continuous periods of patching, whereas the younger one may respond quickly to short periods of patching. The child should be stimulated to use the unpatched eye by occupa-

tions such as puzzles, drawing, sewing, and similar activities.

Glasses can correct a refractive error if amblyopia is not present. **Orthoptics** (therapeutic ocular muscle exercises) to improve the quality of vision may be prescribed to supplement the use of glasses or surgery.

Surgery on the eye muscle to correct the defect is necessary for children who do not respond to glasses and exercises. Many children need surgery after amblyopia has been corrected. Early detection and treatment of strabismus is essential for a successful outcome. The correction is believed to be necessary before the child reaches age 6 years, or the visual damage may be permanent; however, some authorities believe that correction can be successful even up to age 10 years.

EYE INJURY AND FOREIGN OBJECTS IN THE EYE

Eye injuries are fairly common, particularly in older children. Ecchymosis of the eye (black eye) is of no great importance unless the eyeball is involved. A penetrating wound of the eyeball is potentially serious—BB shots in particular are dangerous—and requires the attention of an ophthalmologist. With any history of an injury, a thorough examination of the entire eye is necessary.

Sympathetic ophthalmia may follow perforation wounds of the globe, even if the perforations are small. Sympathetic ophthalmia, an inflammatory reaction of the uninjured eye, often includes **photophobia** (intolerance to light), **lacrimation** (secretion of tears), pain, and some dimness of vision. The retina may finally become detached, and atrophy of the eyeball may occur. Prompt and skillful treatment at the time of the injury is essential to avoid involvement of the other eye.

Small foreign objects, such as specks of dust, that have lodged inside the eyelid may be removed by rolling the lid back and exposing the object. Cotton-tipped applicators should not be used for this purpose because of the danger of sudden movement and of possible perforation of the eye. If the object cannot be easily removed with a small piece of moistened cotton or soft clean cloth, or flushed out with saline solution, the child should be taken to the physician.

EYE INFECTIONS

External hordeolum, known commonly as a stye, is a purulent infection of the follicle of an eyelash, generally caused by *Staphylococcus aureus*. Localized swelling, tenderness,

A   B

Figure 13-1
Strabismus. (A) Esotropia. (B) Exotropia.

and pain are present, with a reddened lid edge. The maximal tenderness is over the infected site. The lesion progresses to suppuration, with eventual discharge of the purulent material. Warm saline compresses applied for about 15 minutes three or four times daily give some relief and hasten resolution, but recurrence is common. The stye should never be squeezed. Antibiotic ointment may help prevent accompanying conjunctivitis and recurrence.

Conjunctivitis is an acute inflammation of the conjunctiva. In children, conjunctivitis may be caused by a virus, bacteria, allergy, or foreign body. Conjunctivitis caused by bacteria is the most common type. The purulent drainage, a common characteristic, can be cultured to determine the causative organism. Bacterial conjunctivitis is treated with ophthalmic antibacterial agents such as erythromycin, bacitracin, sulfacetamide, and polymyxin due to the danger of spreading infection. Because ointments blur vision, eye drops are used during the day and ointments at night. Before applying medication, warm moist compresses can be used to remove the crusts that form on the eyes. The child who has bacterial conjunctivitis should be kept separate from other young children until the condition has been treated. The use of separate washcloths and towels and disposable tissues is important to prevent spread of infection among family members.

Nursing Care for the Child Undergoing Eye Surgery

Anyone experiencing sensory deprivation finds it difficult to stay in touch with reality, and a child whose eyes are covered is particularly vulnerable. The implications of not being able to see are not always appreciated by nurses who have not themselves experienced this. A young child who wakens from surgery to total darkness may well go into a state of panic. Observation of the child returning from surgery may reveal the panic and anxiety as evidenced by trembling and nervousness. The child needs a family caregiver or loved one to stay during the time when vision is restricted.

Of course, the child should be as well prepared for the event as possible, but the small child has no experience to help in understanding what actually is going to happen. The darkness, pain, and total strangeness of the situation can be overwhelming. One preoperative preparation might be to play a game with a blindfold to help the child become used to having his or her eyes covered (Fig. 13-2).

Restraints should not be used indiscriminately, but most small children need some reminder to keep their hands away from the sore eye, unless someone is beside them to prevent them from rubbing or from removing eye dressings. Elbow restraints are useful, although they do not prevent rubbing the eye with the arm. Flannel strips applied to the wrists in clove-hitch fashion can be tied to the crib sides in such a manner as to allow freedom of arm

Figure 13-2
Pretending to be a pirate enables this toddler to find enjoyment in wearing an eye patch.

movement but to prevent the child from causing damage to the operative site.

To alert the child, the nurse should speak when approaching. The child needs tactile stimulation; therefore, after speaking, the nurse would do well to stroke or pat the child. If permitted, the nurse may hold the child for additional reassurance.

GASTROINTESTINAL SYSTEM DISORDERS

Celiac Syndrome

Intestinal malabsorption with **steatorrhea** (fatty stools) is a condition brought about by various causes, the most common being cystic fibrosis and gluten-induced enteropathy, the so-called idiopathic celiac disease. The term **celiac syndrome** is used to designate the complex of malabsorptive disorders.

GLUTEN-INDUCED ENTEROPATHY

Idiopathic celiac disease is a basic defect of metabolism precipitated by the ingestion of wheat gluten or rye gluten, leading to impaired fat absorption. The exact cause is not known; the most acceptable theory is that of an inborn error of metabolism with an allergic reaction to the gliadin fraction of gluten (a protein factor in wheat) as a contributing or, possibly, the sole factor.

Severe manifestations of the disorder have become rare in the United States and in western Europe, but mild disturbances in intestinal absorption of rye, wheat, and sometimes oat gluten are common, occurring in about 1 in 2,000 children.

Clinical Manifestations   Signs generally do not appear before age 6 months and may be delayed until age 1 year or later. Manifestations include chronic diarrhea with foul, bulky, greasy stools and progressive malnutrition. Anorexia and a fretful, unhappy disposition are typical. The onset is generally insidious, with failure to thrive, bouts of diarrhea, and frequent respiratory infections. If the condition becomes severe, the effects of malnutrition are prominent. Retarded growth and development, a distended abdomen, and thin, wasted buttocks and legs are characteristic signs (Fig. 13-3).

Figure 13-3
A child with celiac disease. Notice the protruding abdomen.

The chronic course of this disease may be interrupted by a celiac crisis, an emergency situation. Frequently, this is triggered by an upper respiratory infection. The child vomits copiously, has large, watery stools, and becomes severely dehydrated. As the child becomes drowsy and prostrate, an acute medical emergency develops. Parenteral fluid therapy is essential to combat acidosis and to achieve normal fluid balance.

Diagnosis and Treatment   One way to determine if a small child's failure to thrive is caused by celiac disease is to initiate a trial gluten-free diet and to evaluate the results. Improvement in the nature of the stools and general well-being with a gain in weight should follow, although several weeks may elapse before clear-cut manifestations can be confirmed. Conclusive diagnosis can be made by a biopsy of the jejunum through endoscopy that shows changes in the villi. Serum screening of IgG and IgA antigliaden antibodies shows the presence of the condition and also aids in monitoring the progress of therapy.

Response to a diet from which rye, wheat, and oats are excluded is generally good, although probably no cure can be expected, and dietary indiscretions or respiratory infections may bring relapses. The omission of wheat products, in particular, should continue through adolescence because the ingestion of wheat appears to inhibit growth in sensitive people.

Dietary Program   The young child is usually started on a starch-free, low-fat diet. If the condition is severe, this consists of skim milk, glucose, and banana flakes. Bananas contain invert sugar and are usually well tolerated. Lean meats, puréed vegetables, and fruits are gradually added to the diet. Eventually, fats may be added, and the child can be maintained on a regular diet with the exception of all wheat, rye, and oat products.

Commercially canned creamed soups, cold cuts, frankfurters, and pudding mixes generally contain wheat products. The forbidden list also includes malted milk drinks, some candies, many baby foods, and breads, cakes, pastries, and biscuits, unless they are made from corn flour or cornmeal. Vitamins A and D in water-miscible (able to be mixed with water) solutions are needed in double amounts to supplement the deficient diet.

Nursing Care   The primary focus of nursing care is to help caregivers maintain a restrictive diet for the child. Family teaching should include information regarding the disease and the need for long-term management, as well as guidelines for a gluten-free diet. Caregivers must learn to read the list of ingredients on packaged foods carefully before purchasing anything. The diet of the young child may be monitored fairly easily, but when the child goes to school, monitoring the diet becomes a much greater challenge. As the child grows, caregivers and children might need additional nursing support to help them make dietary modifications.

RESPIRATORY SYSTEM DISORDERS

Croup

Croup is not a disease but a group of disorders typically involving a barking cough, hoarseness, and inspiratory **stridor** (shrill, harsh respiratory sound). The disorders are named for the respiratory structures involved. For instance, acute laryngotracheobronchitis affects the larynx, trachea, and major bronchi.

SPASMODIC LARYNGITIS

Spasmodic laryngitis occurs in children between ages 1 and 3 years. The cause is undetermined; it may be of infectious or allergic origin, but certain children seem to develop severe laryngospasm with little, if any, apparent cause. The attack may be preceded by **coryza** (runny nose) and hoarseness or by no apparent signs of respiratory irregularity during the evening. The child awakens after a few hours of sleep with a barklike cough, increasing respiratory difficulty, and stridor. The child becomes anxious and restless, and there is marked hoarseness. There may be a low-grade fever and mild upper respiratory infection.

This condition is not serious but is frightening, both to the child and the family. The episode subsides after a few hours; little evidence remains the next day when an anxious caregiver takes the child to the physician. Attacks frequently occur two or three nights in succession.

Treatment Humidified air is helpful in reducing laryngospasm. Taking the child into the bathroom and opening the hot water taps, with the door closed, is a quick method for providing moist air, if the water runs hot enough. The physician may prescribe an **emetic** (an agent that causes vomiting), such as syrup of ipecac, in a dosage less than that needed to produce vomiting; this usually gives relief by helping to reduce spasms of the larynx. Humidifiers may be used in the child's bedroom to provide high humidity. Cool humidifiers are recommended, but vaporizers may be used. If a vaporizer is used, caution must be taken to place it out of the child's reach to protect the child from being burned. Cool-mist humidifiers provide safe humidity. Humidifiers and vaporizers must be cleaned regularly to prevent the growth of undesirable organisms. Sometimes the spasm is relieved by exposure to cold air—for instance, when the child is taken out into the night to go to the emergency department or to see the physician.

ACUTE LARYNGOTRACHEOBRONCHITIS

Laryngeal infections are common in small children, and they often involve tracheobronchial areas as well. Acute laryngotracheobronchitis (bacterial tracheitis or laryngotracheobronchitis) may progress rapidly and become a serious problem within a matter of hours. The toddler is the most frequently affected member of the 1- to 4-year age group. This condition is usually of viral origin, but bacterial invasion, usually staphylococcal, follows the original infection. It generally occurs after an upper respiratory infection with fairly mild rhinitis and pharyngitis.

The child develops hoarseness and a barking cough, with a fever that may reach 104° to 105°F (40°–40.6°C). As the disease progresses, marked laryngeal edema occurs and the child's breathing becomes difficult; the pulse is rapid, and cyanosis may appear. Congestive heart failure and acute respiratory embarrassment can result.

Treatment The major goal of treatment for acute laryngotracheobronchitis is to maintain an airway and adequate air exchange, followed by antimicrobial therapy. The child is placed in a supersaturated atmosphere such as a croupette or some other kind of mist tent that also can include the administration of oxygen. To effect bronchodilation, racemic epinephrine (Vaponefrin) may be administered by means of a nebulizer, usually by a respiratory therapist. Rapid improvement may be seen because of vasoconstriction, but the child must be carefully watched for reappearance of symptoms. Nebulization is usually administered every 3 or 4 hours. Nebulization often produces relief, but if necessary intubation with a nasotracheal tube may be performed for a child with severe distress unrelieved by other measures. Tracheostomies, once performed frequently, are rarely performed today; intubation is preferred. Antibiotics are administered parenterally initially and continued after the temperature has normalized.

Close and careful observation of the child is important. Observation includes checking the pulse, respirations, and color, listening for hoarseness and stridor, and noting any restlessness that may indicate an impending respiratory crisis. Pulse oximetry is used to determine the degree of hypoxia.

EPIGLOTTITIS

Epiglottitis is acute inflammation of the epiglottis (the cartilaginous flap that protects the opening of the larynx). Commonly caused by *Haemophilus influenzae* type B, it most often affects children ages 2 to 7 years. The epiglottis becomes inflamed and swollen with edema. The edema decreases the ability of the epiglottis to move freely, which results in blockage of the airway, creating an emergency.

The child may have been well or may have had a mild upper respiratory infection before the development of a sore throat, **dysphagia** (difficulty swallowing), and a high fever of 102.2° to 104°F (39°–40°C). The dysphagia may cause drooling. A tongue blade should *never* be used to initiate a gag reflex because complete obstruction may occur. The child is very anxious, preferring to sit up and leaning forward to breathe. Immediate emergency attention is necessary.

The child may need endotracheal intubation or a tracheostomy if the epiglottis is so swollen that intubation cannot be performed. Moist air is necessary to help reduce the inflammation of the epiglottis. Pulse oximetry is required to evaluate oxygen requirements. Antibiotics are administered intravenously (IV). After 24 to 48 hours of antibiotic therapy, the child may be extubated. Antibiotics are usually continued for 10 days. Although this condition is not common, it is extremely frightening for the child and the family.

Nursing Process for the Toddler With an Upper Respiratory Disorder

ASSESSMENT

Conduct a thorough interview with the caregiver. In addition to standard information, include specific data such as when the symptoms were first noticed, if the child has had a fever, a description of respiratory difficulties, signs of hoarseness, the character of any cough, and any other information that can be determined about the condition.

Conduct a physical assessment, including vital signs. Carefully assess the child's respiratory effort. Inspect the accessory muscles; assess lung sounds and signs of impending respiratory obstruction; observe for circumoral pallor, cyanotic nail beds, irritability, or mental confusion. If the child is old enough to communicate verbally, ask questions to determine how the child feels.

NURSING DIAGNOSES

The nursing diagnoses depend on the assessment of the child and the severity of the respiratory distress. The following nursing diagnoses may be appropriate:

- Ineffective Airway Clearance, related to obstruction associated with edema and mucous secretions of the upper airway

- Risk for Fluid Volume Deficit, related to respiratory fluid loss, fever, and difficulty swallowing

- Anxiety, related to dyspnea, invasive procedures, and separation from caregiver

- Family Coping, Ineffective: Compromised, related to child's respiratory symptoms

- Health Seeking Behaviors, related to child's condition and home care

OUTCOME IDENTIFICATION AND PLANNING

The major goals for the young child with an upper respiratory disorder are maintaining respiratory or cardiac status, preventing fluid deficit, and relieving anxiety. Goals for the family include relieving anxiety and improving caregiver knowledge. The need for immediate intubation is always a possibility; thus, vigilance is essential. The child's energy must be conserved to reduce oxygen requirements.

IMPLEMENTATION

MONITORING RESPIRATORY FUNCTION.   Be continuously alert for warning signs of airway obstruction. Monitor the child at least every hour; uncover the child's chest and observe the child's breathing efforts, noting the amount of chest movement, shallow breathing, and retractions. Listen with a stethoscope for breath sounds, particularly noting the amount of stridor, which indicates difficult breathing. Increasing hoarseness should be reported. In addition, observe for pallor, listlessness, circumoral cyanosis, cyanotic nail beds, and restlessness; these are indications of impaired oxygenation and should be reported at once. Evaluate the heart beat for rate, strength, and regularity. A rapid, weak pulse may indicate impending cardiac problems. Cool, high humidity provides relief. Oxygen may be administered. Pulse oximetry may be used to evaluate oxygen requirements.

MONITORING ADEQUATE FLUID INTAKE.   Adequate hydration helps reduce thick mucus. Maintaining adequate fluid intake may be a problem, as the child may be too ill to want to eat. Offer warm, clear fluids to encourage oral intake. Observe carefully for aspiration, especially in severe respiratory distress. The child may need to be kept NPO to prevent this threat. Parenteral fluids may be administered to replace those lost through respiratory loss, fever, and anorexia. Follow all safety measures for administration of parenteral fluids. Fluid needs are determined by the amount needed to maintain body weight with sufficient amounts added to replace the additional losses. Monitor daily weights and accurately record intake and output. Monitor serum electrolyte levels to ensure they are within normal limits. Observe and record skin turgor and the condition of mucous membranes at least once per shift.

REDUCING THE CHILD'S ANXIETY.   When frightened or upset and crying, the child with croup or a related upper respiratory condition may hyperventilate, causing additional respiratory distress. For this reason, maintain a calm, soothing manner while caring for the child. When possible, the child should be cared for by a constant caregiver with whom a trusting relationship has been achieved. Avoid any nonessential invasive procedures to help decrease the child's anxiety. The family can provide the child with a favorite blanket or toy. The family caregiver is encouraged to stay with the child if possible to provide reassurance and avoid separation anxiety in the child. Plan care so as to minimize interrupting the child's much-needed rest. Give the child age-appropriate explanations of treatment and procedures. As the child improves, provide age-appropriate diversional activities to help relieve anxiety and boredom. Make extra efforts to relieve the child's feelings of loneliness while in respiratory isolation.

PROMOTING FAMILY COPING. For the parent or family caregiver, watching a child with severe respiratory symptoms is frightening. The parent or caregiver may feel helpless, and these feelings of anxiety and helplessness may be exhibited in a variety of ways. To alleviate these feelings, encourage the caregiver to discuss these feelings. Explain procedures, treatments, the illness, and the prognosis to the caregiver, using easily understood terminology. Include the caregiver in the care of the child as much as possible, and encourage him or her to soothe and comfort the child.

PROVIDING FAMILY TEACHING. Provide the caregiver with thorough explanations of the signs and symptoms of the condition. Explain the symptoms that can be handled at home (hoarseness, croupy cough, and inspiratory stridor when disturbed) and those that indicate the child needs to be seen by the physician (continuous stridor, use of accessory muscles, labored breathing, lower rib retractions, restlessness, pallor, and rapid respirations). The family must be aware that recurrence of these conditions is common. Teach the use of cool humidifiers or vaporizers, including cleaning methods and safety measures to avoid burns when using a steam vaporizer. Explain the effects, administration, dosage, and side effects of medications. To be certain the information was understood, have the parent relate back specific facts. Write the information down in a simple way so that it can be clearly understood; determine that the parent can actually read and understand the written material. When appropriate, observe the caregiver demonstrate care of equipment and any treatments to be done at home.

EVALUATION: GOALS AND OUTCOME CRITERIA

- *Goal*: The child's airway will remain clear.
  Criteria: The child's airway is clear, with no evidence of retractions, stridor, hoarseness, or cyanosis.

- *Goal*: The child's fluid intake will be adequate for age and weight.
  Criteria: The child exhibits good skin turgor and moist, pink mucous membranes. Urine output is 1 mL/kg/hr.

- *Goal*: The child will experience a reduction in anxiety.
  Criteria: The child rests quietly, with no evidence of hyperventilation; cooperates with care; cuddles a favorite toy for reassurance; smiles; and plays contentedly.

- *Goal*: The family caregiver will demonstrate coping mechanisms.

Criteria: The caregiver cooperates with and participates in the child's care, appears more relaxed, verbalizes his or her feelings, and soothes the child.

- *Goal*: The family caregiver will demonstrate understanding of the child's home care.
  Criteria: The family caregiver accurately describes facts about the child's condition, asks appropriate questions, relates signs and symptoms to observe in the child, and names the effects, side effects, dosage, and administration of medications.

Cystic Fibrosis

When first described, cystic fibrosis (CF) was called "fibrocystic disease of the pancreas." Further research has revealed that this disorder represents a major dysfunction of all exocrine glands. The major organs affected are the lungs, pancreas, and liver. Because about half of all children with CF have pulmonary complications, this disorder is discussed here with other respiratory conditions.

Cystic fibrosis is hereditary and transmitted as an autosomal recessive trait. Both parents must be carriers of the gene for CF to appear. With each pregnancy, the chance is one in four that the child will have the disease. The incidence is about 1 in 2,000 in white children in the United States; the incidence in black children is 1 in 17,000.

Recent studies have determined that the gene involved in CF normally produces a protein, cystic fibrosis transmembrane conductance regulator, that serves as a channel through which chloride enters and leaves cells. When mutated, the gene blocks chloride movement, bringing on the apparent signs of CF. The blocking of chloride transport results in a change in sodium transport; this in turn results in abnormal secretions of the exocrine (mucus-producing) glands, which produce thick, tenacious mucus rather than the thin, free-flowing secretion normally produced. This abnormal mucus leads to obstruction of the secretory ducts of the pancreas, liver, and reproductive organs. Thick mucus obstructs the respiratory passages, causing air trapping and overinflation of the lungs. In addition, the sweat and salivary glands excrete excessive electrolytes, specifically sodium and chloride.

CLINICAL MANIFESTATIONS

Meconium ileus is the presenting symptom of CF in 5% to 10% of the newborns who later develop additional manifestations. Depletion or absence of pancreatic enzymes before birth results in impaired digestive activity, and the meconium becomes viscid (thick) and mucilaginous (sticky). The inspissated (thickened) meconium fills the small intestine, causing complete obstruction. Clinical manifestations are bile-stained emesis, a distended abdomen, and an absence of stool. Intestinal perforation with symptoms of shock may occur. These newborns taste salty when kissed because of the high sodium chloride concentration in their sweat.

Initial symptoms of CF may occur at varying ages during infancy, childhood, or adolescence. A hard, nonproductive chronic cough may be the first sign. Later, frequent bronchial infections occur. Development of a barrel chest and clubbing of fingers indicate chronic lack of oxygen. Despite an excellent appetite, malnutrition is apparent and becomes increasingly severe. The abdomen becomes distended, and body muscles become flabby.

Pancreatic Involvement Thick, tenacious mucus obstructs the pancreatic ducts, causing **hypochylia** (diminished flow of pancreatic enzymes) or **achylia** (absence of pancreatic enzymes). This achylia or hypochylia leads to intestinal malabsorption and severe malnutrition. The pancreatic enzymes that are deficient are lipase, trypsin, and amylase. Malabsorption of fats causes frequent steatorrhea. Anemia or rectal prolapse is common if the pancreatic condition remains untreated. The incidence of diabetes is greater in these children than in the general population, possibly due to changes in the pancreas. The incidence of diabetes in patients with CF is expected to increase because of their increasing life expectancy.

Pulmonary Involvement The degree of lung involvement determines the prognosis for survival. The severity of pulmonary involvement differs in individual children, a few showing only minor involvement. More than half of children with CF are now expected to live beyond age 18, with increasing numbers living into their late 20s and even 30s.

Respiratory complications pose the greatest threat to children with CF. Abnormal amounts of thick, viscid mucus clog the bronchioles and provide an ideal medium for bacterial growth. *S aureus* coagulase can be cultured from the nasopharynx and sputum of most patients. *Pseudomonas aeruginosa* and *H influenzae* also are found frequently. The basic infection, however, appears most often to be caused by *S aureus*.

Numerous complications arise from severe respiratory infections. Atelectasis and small lung abscesses are common early complications. Bronchiectasis and emphysema may develop, with pulmonary fibrosis and pneumonitis, eventually leading to severe ventilatory insufficiency. These children often have barrel chests and clubbing of the fingers. In advanced disease, pneumothorax, right ventricular hypertrophy, and cor pulmonale are common complications. Cor pulmonale is a common cause of death.

Other Affected Organs The tears, saliva, and sweat of children with CF contain abnormally high concentrations of electrolytes, and the submaxillary salivary glands are enlarged in most of these children. In hot weather, the loss of sodium chloride and fluid through sweating produces frequent heat prostration. Additional fluid and

salt should be given in the diet as a preventive measure. In addition, males with CF who reach adulthood will most likely be sterile because of the blockage or absence of the vas deferens or other ducts. Females often have thick cervical secretions that prohibit the passage of sperm.

DIAGNOSIS

Diagnosis is based on family history, elevated sodium chloride levels in the sweat, analysis of duodenal secretions (via a nasogastric [NG] tube) for trypsin content, a history of failure to thrive, chronic or recurrent respiratory infections, and radiologic findings of hyperinflation and bronchial wall thickening. In the event of a positive sodium chloride sweat test, at least one other criterion must be met to make a conclusive diagnosis.

The principal diagnostic test to confirm CF is a sweat chloride test using the pilocarpine iontophoresis method. This method induces sweating by using a small electric current that carries topically applied pilocarpine into a localized area of the skin. Elevations of 60 mEq/L or more are diagnostic, with values of 50 to 60 mEq/L highly suspect. Although the test itself is fairly simple, false-positive results do occur, and conducting the test on an infant is difficult.

TREATMENT

In the newborn, meconium ileus is treated nonoperatively with hyperosmolar enemas administered gently. If this does not resolve the blockage of thick, gummy meconium, surgery is necessary. During surgery, a mucolytic such as Mucomyst may be used to liquefy the meconium. If this procedure is successful, resection may not be necessary. Most of these infants develop CF of varying degrees of severity.

In the older child, treatment is aimed at correcting pancreatic deficiency, improving pulmonary function, and preventing respiratory infections. If bowel obstruction does occur (meconium ileus equivalent), the preferred management includes hyperosmolar enemas and an increase in fluids and dietary fiber, oral mucolytics, lactulose, and mineral oil.

The overall treatment goals are to improve the child's quality of life and to provide for long-term survival. A health care team is needed, including a physician, a nurse, a respiratory therapist, a dietitian, and a social worker, to work together with the child and family. Treatment centers with a staff of specialists are becoming more common, particularly in larger medical centers. With improved treatment, it is not unusual for a child with CF to grow into adulthood and reach age 30.

Dietary Treatment Commercially prepared pancreatic enzymes given during meals or snacks aid digestion and absorption of fat and protein. Because pancreatic enzymes are inactivated in the acidic environment of the stomach, microencapsulated capsules that deliver the enzymes to the duodenum, where they are needed, are preferred. These enzymes come in capsules that can be swallowed or opened and sprinkled on the child's food. A powdered preparation is used for infants.

The child's diet should be high in carbohydrates and protein, with no restriction of fats. The child may need 1.5 to 2 times the normal caloric intake to promote growth. Unless acutely ill, these children have large appetites, but they can receive little nourishment without a pancreatic supplement. With proper diet and enzyme supplements, these children show evidence of improved nutrition and their stools become relatively normal. Enteric-coated pancreatic enzymes essentially eliminate the need for dietary restriction of fat.

Because of the increased loss of sodium chloride, these children are allowed to use as much salt as they wish, even though onlookers may think it is too much. During hot weather, additional salt may be provided with pretzels, salted bread sticks, and saltine crackers.

Supplements of fat-soluble vitamins A, D, and E are necessary because of the poor digestion of fats. Vitamin K may be supplemented if the child has coagulation problems or is scheduled for surgery. Water-miscible preparations can be given to provided the needed supplement.

Pulmonary Treatment   The goal of treatment is to prevent and treat respiratory infections. Respiratory drainage is provided by thinning the secretions and by mechanical means, such as postural drainage and clapping, to loosen and drain the secretions from the lungs. Antibacterial drugs for the treatment of infection are necessary as indicated. Some physicians prescribe a prophylactic antibiotic regimen when the child is diagnosed. Antibiotics may be administered orally or parenterally, even in the home. With home parenteral administration of antibiotic therapy, a central venous access device is used. Immunization against childhood communicable diseases is extremely important for these chronically ill children. All immunization measures may be used and should be maintained at appropriate intervals. Physical activity is essential because it improves mucous secretion and helps the child feel good. The child can be encouraged to participate in any aerobic activity he or she enjoys. Activity, along with physical therapy, should be limited only by the child's endurance.

Inhalation therapy can be preventive or therapeutic. Hand-held nebulizers are easy to use and convenient for the ambulatory child. A bronchodilator drug such as theophylline or a beta-adrenergic agonist (metaproterenol, terbutaline, or albuterol) may be administered either orally or through nebulization. Recombinant human DNA (DNase, Pulmozyme) breaks down DNA molecules in sputum, breaking up the thick mucus in the airways. A mucolytic such as Mucomyst may be prescribed during acute infection.

A humidified atmosphere can be provided with humidifiers. In summer, a room air conditioner can help provide comfort and controlled humidity.

Chest physical therapy, a combination of postural drainage and chest percussion, is performed routinely at least every morning and evening, even if little drainage is apparent (Fig. 13-4). Chest percussion (clapping and vibrating of the affected areas) if performed correctly helps loosen and move the secretions out of the lungs. The physical therapist usually performs this procedure in the hospital and teaches it to the family because it is an essential part of home care. Chest physical therapy, although time-consuming, should be carried out long term.

HOME CARE

The home care for a child with CF places a tremendous burden on the family. This is not a one-time hospital treatment, nor is there a prospect of cure to brighten the horizon. Each day, much time is spent performing treatments. Family caregivers must learn to perform chest physical therapy and how to operate respiratory equipment and administer IV antibiotics when necessary. The child's diet must be planned, with additional enzymes regulated according to need. Great care is needed to prevent exposure to infections.

Family caregivers must guard against overprotection and against undue limitation of their child's physical activity. Somehow, a good family relationship must be preserved, with time and attention given to other members of the family.

Physical activity is an important adjunct to the child's well-being and is necessary in getting rid of secretions. Capacity for exercise is soon learned, and the child can be trusted to become self-limiting as necessary, especially if given an opportunity to learn the nature of the disease. The child may find postural drainage fun when a caregiver raises the child's feet in the air and walks the child around "wheelbarrow" fashion, or the older child can learn to hang from a monkey bar by the knees. Providing as much normalcy as possible is always desirable. Hot-weather activity should be watched a little more closely, with additional attention to increased salt and fluid intake during exercise.

Caring for a child with CF places great stress on a family's financial resources. The expense of daily medications, frequent clinic or office visits, and sometimes lengthy hospitalizations can be devastating to an ordinary family budget, even with medical insurance coverage. The Cystic Fibrosis Foundation, with chapters throughout the United States, is helpful in providing education and services. Some assistance may be available through local agencies or community groups.

◤ ◥ *Nursing Process for the Child With*
◣ ◢ *Cystic Fibrosis*

ASSESSMENT

The assessment of the child with CF varies with the child's age and the circumstances of the admission. Conduct a complete parent interview that includes the standard infor-

Figure 13-4
Bronchial drainage positions for the main segments of all lobes of children. **(A)** Apical segment of right upper lobe and apical subsegment of apical-posterior segment of left upper lobe. **(B)** Posterior segment of right upper lobe and posterior subsegment of apical-posterior segment of left upper lobe. **(C)** Anterior segments of both upper lobes. **(D)** Superior segments of both lower lobes. **(E)** Posterior basal segments of both lower lobes. **(F)** Lateral basal segment of right lower lobe. **(G)** Anterior basal segment of left lower lobe. **(H)** Right middle lobe. **(I)** Lingual segments of left upper lobe.

mation as well as data concerning respiratory infections, the child's appetite and eating habits, stools, noticeable salty perspiration, history of bowel obstruction as an infant, and family history for CF, if known. Also assess the caregiver's knowledge of the condition.

Include in the assessment routine vital signs; observation of respirations, including cough, breath sounds, and barrel chest; respiratory effort, such as retractions and nasal flaring; clubbing of the fingers; and signs of pancreatic involvement, such as failure to thrive and steatorrhea. Examine the skin around the rectum for irritation and breakdown from frequent foul stools. Ask the child age-appropriate questions, involve the child in the assessment, and determine the child's perception of the disease and this current illness.

NURSING DIAGNOSES

The nursing diagnoses for CF may be many and varied. The reason for the present admission, the child's age, the progression of the condition, the level of understanding that the child and the caregiver have about the condition, and the current illness all merge to determine the pertinent nursing diagnoses for this admission. For the child who has just been diagnosed, the nursing diagnoses may be much more complex than for the child who has complications of a longstanding condition. The family caregiver and the child, as suitable for age, should be included in the determination of current nursing diagnoses. Some of the diagnoses that may be appropriate include:

- Ineffective Airway Clearance, related to thick, tenacious mucous production
- Ineffective Breathing Pattern, related to tracheobronchial obstruction
- Risk for Infection, related to bacterial growth medium provided by pulmonary mucus and impaired body defenses
- Risk for Altered Nutrition: Less Than Body Requirements, related to impaired absorption of nutrients
- Anxiety, related to hospitalization
- Altered Family Processes, related to child's chronic illness and its demands on caregivers

OUTCOME IDENTIFICATION AND PLANNING

As stated before much depends on the reason for the specific admission and other factors discussed under the nursing diagnosis. The child's age and ability for self-expression affect any goal-setting the child can do. The major goals for the child are relieving immediate respiratory distress, remaining free from infection, improving nutritional status, and relieving anxiety. The caregivers' primary goal may include relieving problems related to this admission. Other goals, however, may include concerns about stress on the family related to the illness, as well as a need for additional information about the disease.

IMPLEMENTATION

IMPROVING AIRWAY CLEARANCE. The mucus causes obstruction of the airways and diminishes gas exchange. Assess the child for signs of respiratory distress, monitoring dyspnea, tachypnea, labored respirations with or without activity, retractions, nasal flaring, and color of nail beds. Perform aerosol treatments. Perform chest physical therapy every 2 to 4 hours as ordered. If these treatments are done by respiratory therapy technicians or physical therapists, observe the child after the treatment to assess effectiveness and determine if more frequent treatments may be needed. Supervise the child who can self-administer nebulizer treatments to ensure correct use. Teach the child to cough effectively. Examine and document the mucus produced, noting the color, consistency, and odor. Send cultures to the laboratory as appropriate. Increase fluid intake to help thin mucous secretions. Encourage the child to drink extra fluids and ask the child (or the caregiver if the child is too young) what favorite drinks might be appealing. Intravenous fluids may be necessary. Provide humidified air, either in the form of a cool mist humidifier or mist tent as prescribed.

IMPROVING BREATHING. Maintain the child in a semi-Fowler's or high Fowler's position to promote maximal lung expansion. Pulse oximetry may be used. Maintain oxygen saturation higher than 90%. Administer oxygen if the oxygen saturation falls below this level for an extended period. Administer mouth care every 2 to 4 hours, especially when oxygen is administered. Conserve the child's energy. Plan nursing and therapeutic activities so that maximal rest time is provided for the child. Note dyspnea and respiratory distress in relation to any activities. Plan quiet diversional activities as the child's physical condition warrants. Help the child and family understand that activity is excellent for the child when not in an acute situation. Teach them that exercise helps loosen the thick mucus and also improves the child's self-image.

PREVENTING INFECTION. The child with CF has low resistance, especially to respiratory infections. For this reason, take care to protect the child from any exposure to infectious organisms. Good handwashing techniques should be practiced by all; teach the child and family the importance of this first line of defense. Practice and teach other good hygiene habits. Carefully follow medical asepsis when caring for the child and the equipment. Monitor vital signs every 4 hours for any indication of an infectious process. Restrict people with an infection, including staff, family members, other patients, and visitors, from contact with the child. Advise the family to keep the child's immunizations up to date. Administer antibiotics as prescribed, and teach the child or caregiver home administration as needed. Also teach the family the signs and symptoms of an impending infection so they can begin prophylactic measures at once.

MAINTAINING ADEQUATE NUTRITION. Adequate nutrition helps the child resist infections. Greatly increase the child's caloric intake to compensate for impaired absorption of nutrients and to provide adequate growth and development. In addition to increased caloric intake at meals, provide the child with high-calorie, high-protein snacks, such as peanut butter and cheese. Newer low-fat products can be selected, if desired. Administer pancreatic enzymes with all meals and snacks. In addition, multiple vitamins and iron may be prescribed. Reinforce the need for these supplements to both the child and the family. The child also may require additional salt in the diet. Encourage the child to eat salty snacks. If the child has bouts of diarrhea or constipation, the dosage of enzymes may need to be adjusted. Report any change in bowel movements. Weigh and measure the child. Plot growth on a chart so that progress can easily be visualized.

REDUCING THE CHILD'S ANXIETY. Provide age-appropriate activities to help alleviate anxiety and the boredom that can result from enforced hospitalization. Choose activities such as reading or arts and crafts according to age. Schoolwork may help ease some anxiety. Some older children may enjoy a video game, if available, but watch the child for overexcitement. Encourage the family caregiver to stay with the child to help diminish some of the child's anxiety. Allow the child to have familiar toys or mementos from home. Stay with the child during acute episodes of coughing and dyspnea to reduce anxiety. Give the child age-appropriate information about CF. Quiz the child in a relaxed, friendly manner to help determine what the child knows and what teaching may be needed. Learning about CF can be turned into a game for some children, making it much more enjoyable.

PROVIDING TEACHING AND FAMILY SUPPORT. The family is faced with a long-term illness and may have already seen a deterioration in the child's health. Evaluate the family's knowledge about CF to determine their teaching needs. The family may need to have all the information repeated, or they may have just a few areas of need. Demonstrate an interest and willingness to talk to the family; do not make them feel as though they are intruding on time needed to do other things. Provide information for resources, such as the Cystic Fibrosis Foundation, the American Lung Association, and other local organizations. Give the family and the child opportunities to voice fears and anxieties. Respond with active-listening techniques to help authenticate their feelings. The family may have questions about genetic counseling and may need referrals for counseling. Provide emotional support throughout the entire hospital stay. The nurse is the person who can best provide overall support.

EVALUATION: GOALS AND OUTCOME CRITERIA

- *Goal*: The child's airway will be clear.
  Criteria: The child cooperates with chest physical therapy; the child effectively clears mucus from the airway.

- *Goal*: The child will exhibit normal respiratory function. *Criteria*: The child rests quietly with no dyspnea; the respiratory rate is even and appropriate for age.

- *Goal*: The child will exhibit no signs of infection. *Criteria*: The child's vital signs are within normal limits for age. The child and family follow infection-control practices.

- *Goal*: The child will have an adequate intake. *Criteria*: The child's growth chart shows normal growth.

- *Goal*: The child's anxiety will subside. *Criteria*: The child engages in age-appropriate activities and appears relaxed with no signs of distress.

- *Goal*: The family will demonstrate ability to cope. *Criteria*: The family demonstrates an understanding of the child's illness and therapy and becomes involved in available support groups.

ACCIDENTS

Toddlers are natural explorers, examining their environment to learn all they can about it. As a result of their lack of experience and judgment, however, toddlers are prone to accidents. Accidents are the leading cause of death in children over age 1 year. Nurses can contribute to safety education by providing information to families of young children pertaining to accident prevention and appropriate emergency responses.

Ingestion of Toxic Substances

One of the ways in which toddlers find out about their environment is to taste the world around them. Toddlers and preschoolers are developing autonomy and initiative, which add to their tendency to examine their environment on their own. Substances that would repel an adult because of taste or smell are ingested by young children because their senses of taste and smell are not yet refined. This makes these age groups prime targets for ingestion of poisonous substances. The ordinary household has an abundance of poisonous substances in almost every room. The kitchen, bathroom, bedroom, and garage are the most common sites harboring substances that are poisonous when ingested. Although most poisonings occur in the child's home, grandparents' homes offer many temptations to the young child as well. Grandparents tend to be less concerned about placing dangerous substances out of children's reach simply because the children are not part of the household, or the grandparents may place supplies where they are convenient, never giving the young grandchild's developmental stage and exploratory nature a thought.

A Personal Glimpse

While peeling apples, I stopped to get the ringing phone. My 3-year-old, Kasey, thought this was the perfect time to be a mother's helper. She managed to get on top of the table and tried to peel an apple herself.

I had to take her to the emergency room for a badly cut finger. The doctor on staff was not personable with children or with their parents! After going through a barrage of questions on why I would GIVE a child a knife to play with, things got worse. He did not want me in the room with her, which caused Kasey to become hysterical. He had to put her in a restraint. I had to assure her I was not leaving.

The doctor grabbed Kasey's hand and a small scissors. She was screaming that he was going to cut her fingers off. Of course I was questioned again. The doctor asked me if I often trimmed Kasey's fingers. I had to explain that she didn't even like to have her fingernails clipped and that he was what was making her more scared. I guess he was unaware that not all accidents are child abuse.

This entire experience made me angry and my daughter frightened.

Daria

When a child is found with a container whose contents he or she has obviously sampled, action can be taken immediately. When a child manifests symptoms that are difficult to assess or that do not appear to relate specifically to any known cause, the possibility of poisoning should be suspected. Ingestion of a poisonous substance can produce symptoms that simulate an attack of an acute disease—vomiting, abdominal pain, diarrhea, shock, cyanosis, coma, and convulsions. If evidence of such a disease is lacking, acute poisoning should be suspected.

In instances of apparent poisoning, the family caregivers are asked to consider all medications in their home, if the substance is unknown. Is it possible that any medication could have been available to the child, or did an older child or other person possibly give the child the container to play with? Is it possible that a parent inadvertently gave a wrong dose or wrong medication to a child? All such

possibilities need to be considered. In the meantime, the most important priority is treatment for the child who shows symptoms of poisoning.

EMERGENCY TREATMENT

The first step the caregiver should take when poison ingestion is suspected is to call the local poison control center. Most localities have a toll-free number available to those in remote areas. This number can be found in the local telephone directory, and all homes with young children should have this number posted by every telephone for quick reference. Any obvious poison should be removed from the child's mouth before calling. The poison control center evaluates the situation and tells the caller whether the child can be treated at home or if the child needs to be transported to a hospital or treatment center.

Except when corrosive or highly irritant poisons have been swallowed, the first measure is to induce vomiting. If the child is convulsing or unconscious, however, vomiting should not be induced because of the danger of aspiration.

The approved method for producing vomiting is to have the child swallow 15 mL of syrup of ipecac. A second 15-mL dose can be given if vomiting does not occur within 15 to 30 minutes. Vomiting also may be induced by stimulating the child's posterior pharynx with the adult's finger. The child's head should be allowed to droop forward or should be turned to the side to avoid aspiration of the vomitus.

If the substance is unknown, all material vomited at home or on the way to the hospital or treatment center should be saved for analysis. If the substance that the child swallowed is known, the container should be taken along. If the container is left behind in the panic and confusion, someone will need to go to the home and retrieve it.

If the substance the child has swallowed is known, the ingredients can be found on the label. The poison control center can suggest an antidote if the name of the drug or other substance is known. If the substance is a prescription drug, the pharmacist who filled the prescription or who is familiar with the drug also can be contacted for information. In some instances, it is necessary to analyze the residual stomach contents.

There are specific antidotes for certain poisons, but not for all. Some antidotes react chemically with the poison to render it harmless; others prevent absorption of the poison. Activated charcoal given after vomiting absorbs many poisons. It is given in 6 to 8 ounces of water in a dose of 5 to 10 g per gram of ingested poison. This may be given through an NG tube, if necessary.

Treatment Steps in Order of Importance The treatment steps in order of importance are:

1. Remove the obvious remnants of the poison.
2. Call the poison control center.

3. Prevent further absorption.
4. Administer appropriate antidote if known.
5. Administer general supportive and symptomatic care.

Further specific treatment is given according to the kind and amount of the toxic substance ingested. Common types of poisoning and general treatment are described in Table 13-1. Complete listings of poisonous substances with the specific treatment for each are available from poison control centers, clinics, and pharmacies.

LEAD POISONING (PLUMBISM)

Chronic lead poisoning has been a serious problem among children for many years. It is responsible for neurologic handicaps, including mental retardation, because of its effect on the central nervous system. Infants and toddlers are potential victims because of their tendency to put in their mouths any object within their reach. In some children, this habit leads to **pica** (the ingestion of nonfood substances such as laundry starch, clay, paper, and paint). The unborn fetus of a pregnant mother who is exposed to lead (such as lead dust from renovation of an older home) also can be affected by lead contamination. Screening for lead poisoning is part of a complete well-baby checkup between ages 6 months and 6 years.

Causes of Chronic Lead Poisoning The most common causes of lead poisoning are:

- Lead-containing paint used on the outside or the inside of older houses
- Furniture and toys painted with lead-containing paint, including inexpensive mini-blinds
- Drinking water contaminated by lead pipes or copper pipes with lead-soldered joints
- Dust containing lead salts from automotive exhaust, lead paint, or emission from lead smelters
- Storage of fruit juices or other food in improperly glazed earthenware
- Inhalation of motor fumes containing lead or burning of storage batteries
- Exposure to industrial areas with smelteries or chemical plants
- Exposure to hobbyists using lead, such as in stained glass

There are other causes, but the most common cause has been the lead in paint. Children tend to nibble on fallen plaster, painted wooden furniture (including cribs), or painted toys because they have a sweet taste. Fine dust that results from removing lead paint in remodeling also can cause harm to the young children in the household without parents becoming aware of it. When the danger of lead poisoning became apparent, attempts were made to control the sale of lead-based paint. In 1973, federal regulations banned the sale of paint containing more than 0.5% lead

for interior residential use or use on toys. This has not eliminated the problem, however, because many homes built before the 1960s were painted with lead-based paint, and they still exist, not only in inner-city areas but also in small towns and suburbs. Older mansions in which upper-income families may live also may have lead paint because of their age. Only contractors experienced in lead-based paint removal should do renovation.

Clinical Manifestations The onset of chronic lead poisoning is insidious. Some early indications may be irritability, hyperactivity, aggression, impulsiveness, or disinterest in play. Short attention span, lethargy, learning difficulties, and distractibility also are signs of poisoning.

The condition may progress to **encephalopathy** (degenerative disease of the brain) because of intracranial pressure. Acute manifestations include convulsions, mental retardation, blindness, paralysis, coma, and death. Acute episodes sometimes develop sporadically and early in the condition.

Diagnosis The nonspecific nature of the presenting symptoms makes examination of the environmental history of the child important. Testing of erythrocyte protoporphyrin levels has been used as a screening method, but it is not accurate in identifying children with blood levels lower than 25 μg/dL; therefore, it is no longer an adequate method of screening. Finger sticks, or heel sticks for infants, can be used to collect a sample for lead level screening. In 1991, the Centers for Disease Control in Atlanta revised the blood lead level criteria to repeat testing on all children with blood levels greater than 10 μg/dL, with emphasis on primary prevention to reflect new information regarding safe levels.

Treatment The most important aspect of treatment of a child with lead poisoning is to remove the lead from the child's system and environment. The use of a **chelating agent** (an agent that binds with metal) increases the urinary excretion of lead. Several chelating agents are available; individual circumstances and the physician's choice determine the particular drug used. Edetate disodium, known as EDTA, is usually given IV; intramuscular administration is painful. Renal failure can occur with inappropriate dosage. Dimercaptopropanol (dimercaprol), also known as BAL, causes excretion of lead through bile and urine; it may be administered intramuscularly. Because of its peanut oil base, BAL should not be used in children allergic to peanuts. These two drugs may be used together in children with extremely high levels of lead.

The oral drug D-penicillamine can be used to treat children with blood lead levels lower than 45 μg/dL. The capsules can be opened and sprinkled on food or mixed in liquid for administration. This drug should not be administered to children allergic to penicillin. In 1991, the Food and Drug Administration approved succimer (Chemet), a

TABLE 13-1. Commonly Ingested Toxic Substances

Agent	Symptoms	Treatment
acetaminophen	Under 6 y—vomiting is the earliest sign Adolescents—vomiting, diaphoresis, general malaise. Liver damage can result in 48–96 hr if not treated	Induce vomiting with syrup of ipecac. Gastric lavage may be necessary. Administer acetylcysteine (Mucomyst) diluted with cola, fruit juice, or water if plasma level elevated. Mucomyst may be administered by gavage, especially because its odor of rotten eggs makes it objectionable.
acetylsalicyclic acid (aspirin)	Hyperpnea (abnormal increase in depth and rate of breathing), metabolic acidosis, hyperventilation, tinnitus, vertigo are initial symptoms. Dehydration, coma, convulsions, and death follow untreated heavy dosage.	Induce vomiting with syrup of ipecac. Gastric lavage may be necessary. Activated charcoal may be administered. IV fluids, sodium bicarbonate to combat acidosis, and dialysis for renal failure may be necessary when large amounts are ingested.
ibuprofen (Motrin, Advil)	Similar to aspirin; metabolic acidosis, GI bleeding, renal damage	Induce vomiting. Activated charcoal is administered in emergency department. Observe for and treat GI bleeding. Electrolyte determination is done to detect acidosis. IV fluids are given.
ferrous sulfate (iron)	Vomiting, lethargy, diarrhea, weak rapid pulse, hypotension are common symptoms. Massive dose may produce shock, erosion of small intestine, black, tarry stools, bronchial pneumonia.	Induce vomiting with syrup of ipecac. Deferoxamine, a chelating agent that combines with iron, may be used when child has ingested a toxic dose.
barbiturates	Respiratory, circulatory, and renal depression may occur. Child may become comatose.	Establish airway; administer oxygen if needed; perform gastric lavage. Close observation of level of consciousness is needed.

corrosives
  alkali: lye, bleaches
  acid: drain cleaners, toilet bowl cleaners, iodine, silver nitrate
	Intense burning and pain with first mouthful; severe burns of mouth and esophageal tract; shock, possible death	*Never have child vomit.*
		  Alkali corrosives are treated initially with quantities of water, diluted acid fruit juices, or diluted vinegar.
		  Acid corrosives are treated with alkaline drinks such as milk, olive oil, mineral oil, or egg white.
		Lavage or emetics are never used.
		  Continuing treatment includes antidotes, gastrostomy or IV feedings, and specialized care. A tracheostomy may be needed.

hydrocarbons kerosene, gasoline, furniture polish, lighter fluid, turpentine	Damage to the respiratory system is the primary concern. Vomiting often occurs spontaneously, possibly causing additional damage to the respiratory system. Pneumonia, bronchopneumonia, or lipoid pneumonia may occur.	Emergency treatment and assessment are necessary. Vital signs are monitored; oxygen is administered as needed. Gastric lavage is performed only if the ingested substance contains other toxic chemicals that may threaten other body systems, such as the liver, kidneys, or cardiovascular system.

1. If you live in an older home, make sure your child does not get any chips of paint or chew any surface painted with lead-based paint. Look for paint dust on window sills, and clean with a high-phosphate sodium cleaner like Spic 'n Span.
2. Wet-mop hard-surfaced floors and woodwork with the cleaner at least once a week. Vacuuming hard surfaces scatters dust.
3. Wash child's hands and face before eating.
4. Wash toys and pacifiers frequently.
5. Prevent child from playing in dust near an old lead-painted house.
6. Prevent child from playing in dust near a busy highway. Lead from gasoline fumes will remain near an old lead-painted house.
7. If your water supply has a high lead content, fully flush faucets before using for cooking, drinking, or making formula.
8. Avoid contamination from hobbies or work.
9. Make sure your child eats regular meals. Food slows absorption of lead.
10. Encourage your child to eat foods high in iron and calcium.

From Centers for Disease Control and Prevention: Preventing lead poisoning in young children: a statement by The Centers for Disease Control. Atlanta, 1991.

new oral drug for treating children with blood lead levels higher than 45 μg/dL. Succimer comes in capsules that can be opened and mixed with applesauce or other soft foods.

All the chelating drugs may have toxic side effects, and children being treated must be carefully monitored with frequent urinalysis, blood cell counts, and renal function tests. Any child receiving chelation therapy should be under the care of an experienced health care team.

Outcome   The prognosis after lead poisoning is uncertain. Early detection of the condition and removal of the child from the lead-containing surroundings offer the best hope. Follow-up should include routine examinations to prevent recurrence and to assess any residual brain damage not immediately apparent.

Although the incidence of lead poisoning has decreased, it is still prevalent. Measures to educate the public on the importance of preventing this disorder are essential if the problem is to be eliminated. Education of the family caregivers is an essential aspect of the treatment (see Family Teaching: Tips to Prevent Lead Poisoning).

Ingestion of Foreign Objects

Young children are apt to put any small objects into their mouths, and these objects are too often swallowed. Normally, many of these objects pass smoothly through the digestive tract and are expelled in the feces. Occasionally, however, something such as an open safety pin, a coin, a button, or a marble may lodge in the esophagus and need to be extracted. Foods such as hot dogs, peanuts, carrots, popcorn kernels, apple pieces, and round candy are frequent offenders.

Unless symptoms of choking, gagging, or pain are present, it is usually safe to wait and watch the feces carefully for 3 or 4 days. Any object, however, may pass safely through the esophagus and stomach only to become fixed in one of the curves of the intestine, causing an obstruction or fever due to infection. Also, sharp objects present the danger of perforation somewhere in the digestive tract.

Diagnosis of a swallowed solid object is often, but not always, made from the history. If a foreign object in the digestive tract is suspected, fluoroscopic and radiographic studies may be required.

TREATMENT

If a caregiver has seen an infant swallow an object and begin choking, the infant should be held along the rescuer's forearm with the head lower than the chest and given several back blows. After the back blows are delivered, the infant's back and head should be supported and the infant should be turned over onto the opposite thigh. Up to five quick downward chest thrusts should be delivered. The foreign body should be removed if it is visualized. A child older than age 1 year can be encouraged to continue to cough as long as the cough remains forceful. If the cough becomes ineffective (no sound with cough) or respirations become more difficult and stridor is present, the Heimlich maneuver can be attempted (Fig. 13-5).

If the child is not having respiratory problems and coughing has not resulted in removal of the object, the child needs to be transported to an emergency department to be assessed by a physician. Objects in the esophagus are removed by direct vision through an esophagoscope. Attempts to push the object down into the stomach or to extract it blindly can be dangerous. Some objects may need to be removed surgically. If the object is small and the physician believes that there is little danger to the gastrointestinal tract, the caregiver may be advised to take the child home and watch the child's bowel movements over the next several days to confirm that the object has passed through the system.

Increasing respiratory difficulties indicate that the object has been aspirated rather than swallowed. Foreign objects aspirated into the larynx or bronchial tree may become lodged in the trachea or larynx. Back blows and chest thrusts or the Heimlich maneuver should be delivered as described. The child's airway should be opened and rescue breathing attempted. If the child's chest does not rise, the child should be repositioned and rescue breathing tried again. If the airway is still obstructed, these steps should be repeated until the object is removed and respirations

Figure 13-5

(A) Back blows (top) and chest thrusts (bottom) to relieve foreign-body airway obstruction in infant. Hold infant over arm as illustrated, supporting head by firmly holding jaw. Deliver up to 5 back blows. Turn infant over while supporting head, neck, jaw, and chest with one hand and back with other hand. Keep head lower than trunk. Give 5 quick chest thrusts with one finger below intermammary line. If foreign body not removed and airway remains obstructed, attempt rescue breathing. Repeat these 2 steps until successful. **(B)** Abdominal thrusts with child standing or sitting can be performed when child is conscious. Standing behind child, place thumb side of one fist against child's abdomen in midline slightly above navel and well below xiphoid process. Grab fist with other hand and deliver 5 quick upward thrusts. Continue until successful or child loses consciousness. **(C)** Abdominal thrusts with child lying can be performed on a conscious or unconscious child. Place heel of hand on child's abdomen slightly above the navel and below the xiphoid process and rib cage. Place other hand on top of first hand. Deliver 5 separate, distinct thrusts. Open airway and attempt rescue breathing if object not removed. Repeat until successful. **(D)** Combined jaw thrust-spine stabilization maneuver for a child trauma victim with possible head or neck injury. To protect from damage to cervical spine the neck is maintained in a neutral position and traction on or movement of neck is avoided.

are established. The child should be transported to the emergency department as quickly as possible. The caregiver should get emergency assistance while continuing to try to remove the offending object.

Adults must be aware of the power of example. A child who sees an adult hold pins or nails in his or her mouth may well follow this example, with disastrous and often fatal results.

Insertion of Foreign Bodies Into the Ear or Nose

Children may insert small objects, such as peas or beans, crumpled paper, beads, and small toys, into their ears or noses. Irrigation of the ear may remove small objects, except paper, which becomes impacted as it absorbs moisture. The physician generally uses small forceps to remove objects not dislodged by irrigation.

A foreign body in the nose may have been placed just inside the nares by the child, but manipulation may push it in further. If the object remains in the nose for any length of time, infection may occur. Inspection with a speculum and removal of the object by a physician should be done promptly when discovered.

Drownings

Drowning is the second leading cause of accidental death in children. Toddlers and older adolescents have the highest actual rate of death from drowning. Drownings in young children occur when the child has been left unattended in a body of water. Infants more commonly drown in a bathtub; toddlers and preschoolers drown in pools or small bodies of water. A pail of water that becomes something for the toddler to investigate can lead to accidental death. Many deaths in this age group occur in home pools, including spas, hot tubs, and whirlpools.

All infants and young children must be continuously

TABLE 13-2.   Summary of Basic Life Support Maneuvers in Infants and Children

Maneuver	Infant (<1 y)	Child (1 to 8 y)
Airway	Head tilt–chin lift (unless trauma present)	Head tilt–chin lift (unless trauma present)
	Jaw thrust	Jaw thrust
Breathing	2 breaths at 1 to 1½ s/breath	2 breaths at 1 to 1½ s/breath
Initial	20 breaths/min	20 breaths/min
Subsequent		
Circulation	Brachial/femoral	Carotid
Pulse check	Lower third of sternum	Lower third of sternum
Compression area	2 or 3 fingers	Heel of 1 hand
Compression width	About ½" to 1"	About 1" to 1½"
Depth		
Rate	At least 100/min	100/min
Compression–ventilation ratio	5:1 (pause for ventilation)	5:1 (pause for ventilation)
Foreign body airway obstruction	Back blows/chest thrusts	Heimlich maneuver

From Pediatric basic life support. JAMA 268(16):2257, 1992.

supervised by a responsible adult when near any source of water. Older children and adolescents should not play alone around any body of water. Swimming in undesignated swimming areas such as creeks, quarries, and rivers is hazardous for older children and adolescents.

When a drowning victim of any age is discovered, cardiopulmonary resuscitation (CPR) should be started immediately and continued until the victim can be transported to a medical facility for further care. Intensive care is carried out according to the patient's needs. All adults who care for children in any capacity must learn CPR and be ready to perform it immediately (Table 13-2, Fig. 13-6).

Burns

Among the many accidents that occur in the lives of children, burns are the most frightening. More than 70% of burn accidents happen to children younger than age 5 years. Nearly all childhood burns are preventable, which causes considerable guilt for families and the child. Adult carelessness, the child's exploring and curious nature, and failure to supervise the child adequately all contribute to the high incidence of burns in children. In addition, burns are a common form of child abuse.

CAUSES

Scalds from Hot Liquids   This type of burn, common in small children, results from a dangling electric coffee-maker cord, pans of hot liquid on the stove with handles turned out, cups of hot tea or coffee, bowls of soup or other hot liquids, or small children left alone in bathtubs. Dangerous, sometimes fatal, burns can occur from these conditions.

Burns from Fire   The second most common kind of burn results from children playing with matches or being left alone in buildings that catch fire. Careless use of smoking materials is a common cause of house fires. Children are fascinated by fires and must be carefully supervised around fireplaces, campfires, room heaters, and outside barbecues. Cigarette lighters are currently being produced with a "child-safe" lighting mechanism, but they should still be kept away from children.

Electricity   Although uncommon in children, infants and toddlers can suffer severe facial or mouth burns requiring extensive plastic surgery from biting on electrical cords plugged into a socket. These burns may be more serious than they first appear because of the damage to underlying tissues.

TYPES OF BURNS

Burns are divided into types according to the depth of tissue involvement: superficial, partial thickness, or total thickness (Table 13-3, Fig. 13-7).

Superficial or First-Degree Burns   The epidermis is injured, but there is no destruction of tissue or nerve endings. Thus, there is erythema, edema, and pain but prompt regeneration.

Partial-Thickness or Second-Degree Burns   The epidermis and underlying dermis are both injured and devitalized or destroyed. There is generally blistering, with an escape of body plasma, but regeneration of the skin occurs from the remaining viable epithelial cells in the dermis.

A. Opening the airway with the head tilt-chin lift maneuver. One hand is used to tilt the head, extending the neck. The index finger of the rescuer's other hand lifts the mandible outward by lifting on the chin. Head tilt should not be performed if cervical spine injury is suspected.

B. Opening the airway with the jaw-thrust maneuver. The airway is opened by lifting the angle of the mandible. The rescuer uses two or three fingers of each hand to lift the jaw while other fingers guide the jaw upward and outward.

C. Rescue breathing in an infant. The rescuer's mouth covers the infant's nose and mouth, creating a seal. One hand performs head tilt while the other hand lifts the infant's jaw. Avoid head tilt if the infant has sustained head or neck trauma.

D. Rescue breathing in a child. The rescuer's mouth covers the mouth of the child, creating a mouth-to-mouth seal. One hand maintains the head tilt; the thumb and forefinger of the same hand are used to pinch the child's nose.

E. Locating and palpating the carotid artery pulse in the child.

F. Palpating the brachial artery pulse.

G. Cardiac compressions. Top: Infant supine on palm of the rescuer's hand. Bottom: Performing CPR while carrying the infant or small child. Note that the head is kept level with the torso. (Compare with **H**).

H. Locating proper finger position for chest compression in infant. Note that the rescuer's other hand is used to maintain head position to facilitate ventilation.

I. Locating hand position for chest compression in child. Note that the rescuer's other hand is used to maintain head position to facilitate ventilation.

Figure 13-6
Cardiopulmonary resuscitation.

Degree	Cause	Surface Appearance	Color	Pain Level	Histologic Depth	Healing Time
First (superficial) All are considered minor unless under 18 mo, over 65 y, or with severe loss of fluids	Flash, flame, ultraviolet (sunburn)	Dry, no blisters, edema	Erythematous	Painful	Epidermal layers only	2 to 5 days with peeling, no scarring, may have discoloration
Second (partial thickness) Minor—less than 15% in adults, less than 10% in children; Moderate—15% to 30% in adults, or less than 15% with involvement of face, hands, feet, or perineum; minor chemical or electrical; in children, 10% to 30%; Severe—more than 30%	Contact with hot liquids or solids, flash flame to clothing, direct flame, chemical	Moist blebs, blisters	Mottled white to pink, cherry red	Very painful	Epidermis, papillary, and reticular layers of dermis; may include fat domes of subcutaneous layer	Superficial—5 to 21 days with no grafting Deep with no infection—21 to 35 days If infected, convert to full thickness
Third (full thickness) Minor—less than 2%; Moderate—2% to 10%, any involvement of face, hands, feet, or perineum; Severe—more than 10% and major chemical or electrical	Contact with hot liquids or solids, flame, chemical, electricity	Dry with leathery eschar until débridement; charred blood vessels visible under eschar	Mixed white (waxy or pearly), dark (khaki or mahogany), charred	Little or no pain; hair pulls out easily	Down to and including subcutaneous tissue; may include fascia, muscle, and bone	Large areas require grafting that may take many months. Small areas may heal from the edges after weeks.

Adapted from Wagner MM. Emergency care of the burned patient. Am J Nurs 77:1788–1791, 1977.

Figure 13-7
Cross section of the skin showing the relative depths of the types of burn injury.

Total-Thickness or Third-Degree Burns   The epidermis, dermis, and nerve endings are all destroyed. Pain is minimal, and there is no longer any barrier to infection or any remaining viable epithelial cells. Fourth-, fifth-, and sixth-degree burns have been described that are extensions of full-thickness burns with involvement of fat, muscle, and bone, respectively.

EMERGENCY TREATMENT

Cool water is an excellent emergency treatment for burns involving small areas. The immediate application of cool compresses or cool water to burn areas appears to inhibit capillary permeability and thus suppress edema, blister formation, and tissue destruction. Ice water or ice packs must not be used because of the danger of increased tissue damage. Immersing a burned extremity in cool water alleviates pain and may prevent further thermal injury. This can be done after the airway, breathing, and circulation have been assessed but should not be done when large areas are involved because of the danger of hypothermia.

In the case of a fire victim, special attention should be given to the airway to assess for smoke inhalation and respiratory passage burns. Clothing should be removed to inspect the whole body for burned areas; also, clothing may retain heat, causing further tissue damage. The child should be transported to a medical facility for assessment. If transported to a special burn unit, the child may be wrapped in a sterile sheet and the burn treated on arrival.

Superficial Burns   Superficial burns can usually be treated on an outpatient basis because they heal readily unless infected. The area is cleaned, an anesthetic ointment is applied, and the burn is covered with a sterile gauze bandage or dressing. An analgesic may be needed to relieve pain. Blisters should not be intentionally broken because of the risk of infection, but blisters that are already broken may be débrided (cut away). The child is seen again in 2 days to inspect for infection. The caregiver is instructed to keep the area clean and dry (no bathing the area) until the burn is healed, usually about a week to 10 days.

Partial- and Full-Thickness Burns   It is not always possible to distinguish between partial- and full-thickness burns. In the presence of infection, a partial-thickness burn may be converted into full thickness; also, with extensive burns, there is often a greater amount of full-thickness burn than had been estimated.

Full-thickness burns require the attention, skill, and conscientious care of a team of specialists. Children with mixed second- and third-degree burns, or with third-degree burns involving 15% or more of the body surface, require hospitalization. Burns are classified according to criteria of the American Burn Association (Table 13-4).

TREATMENT OF MODERATE TO SEVERE BURNS: FIRST PHASE—48 TO 72 HOURS

Hypovolemic shock is the major manifestation in the first 48 hours in massive burns. As extracellular fluid pours into the burned area, it collects in enormous quantities, dehydrating the body. Edema becomes noticeable, and symptoms of severe shock appear. Intense pain seldom is a major factor. Symptoms of shock are low blood pressure, rapid pulse, pallor, and often considerable apprehension.

Intravenous Fluids   The primary concern is to replace body fluids that have been lost or immobilized at the

TABLE 13-4. Classification of Burns

Classification	Description
Minor	First-degree burn or second degree <10% of body surface or third degree <2% of body surface; no area of the face, feet, hand, or genitalia is burned
Moderate	Second-degree burn 10% to 20% body surface or on the face, hands, feet, or genitalia, or third-degree burn <10% body surface or if smoke inhalation has occurred
Severe	Second-degree burn >20% body surface or third-degree burn >10% body surface

Oral Fluids   The administration of oral fluids should be omitted or minimized for 1 or 2 days. Delayed gastric emptying, causing acute gastric dilatation, is a common complication of burns and can become a serious problem, resulting in vomiting and anorexia. An NG tube on low suction prevents vomiting. The child's thirst, which is usually severe, should be relieved by IV fluids, and sips of water may be allowed. Oral feedings can be started when bowel sounds are heard. Nasogastric feedings may be needed to supplement intake. The child's caloric and nutritional requirements are two or three times those needed for normal growth; thus, nutritional supplements will most likely be needed.

Diuresis   Urinary output must be monitored closely. The output may be decreased by the decrease in blood volume. Renal shutdown may be a threat. An output of 1 to 2 mL/kg/hr for children weighing 30 kg (66 lb) or less or 30 to 50 mL/hr for those over 30 kg is desirable. An indwelling catheter facilitates the accurate measurement of urine and

burn areas. Because there is a distinct relation between the extent of the surface area burned and the amount of fluid lost, the percentage of the skin area affected as well as the classification of the burns must be estimated to determine the medical treatment (Fig. 13-8). The extent and depth of the burn and the expertise available within the hospital determine whether the child is treated at the general hospital or immediately transported to a burn unit.

An IV infusion site must be selected and fluids started, most often lactated Ringer's solution, isotonic saline, or plasma, using a large-bore catheter to administer replacement fluids and maintain total parenteral nutrition (TPN). Intravenous fluids for maintenance and replacement of lost body fluids are estimated for the first 24 hours, with half of this calculated requirement given during the first 8 hours. The patient's needs may change rapidly, however, necessitating a change in the rate of flow or the amount or type of fluid. The patient's urinary output, vital signs, and general appearance are all part of the information that the physician needs to determine the fluid requirements. With TPN, fluids can be administered to provide needed amino acids, glucose, fats, vitamins, and minerals so that large amounts of food do not need to be consumed orally. This nutrition is essential for tissue repair and healing.

Airway   The adequacy of the airway must be assessed in case an endotracheal tube needs to be inserted or (rarely) a tracheostomy performed. Inhalation injury is a leading cause of complications in burns. If there are burns around the face and neck, or if the burns occurred in a small enclosed space, inhalation injury should be suspected. In fires, toxic substances and the heat produced can cause damage to the respiratory tract. All these possibilities must be assessed.

Relative Percentages of Areas Affected by Growth			
Area	Age 0	1	5
A = $\frac{1}{2}$ of head	$9\frac{1}{2}$	$8\frac{1}{2}$	$6\frac{1}{2}$
B = $\frac{1}{2}$ of one thigh	$2\frac{3}{4}$	$3\frac{1}{4}$	4
C = $\frac{1}{2}$ of one leg	$2\frac{1}{2}$	$2\frac{1}{2}$	$2\frac{3}{4}$

Figure 13-8

Determination of extent of burns in children.

specific gravity. After the first hour, the volume of urine should be relatively constant. Any change in volume or specific gravity should be reported.

After the initial fluid therapy has brought the burn shock under control, and after the extracellular fluid deficit has been made up, the patient faces another hazard with the onset of the diuretic phase. This occurs within 24 to 96 hours after the accident. The plasmalike fluid is picked up and reabsorbed from the third space in the burn areas, and the patient may rapidly become **hypervolemic** (exhibit an abnormal increase in the blood volume in the circulatory system), even to the point of pulmonary edema. This is the principal reason for the extremely close check on all vital signs and for the close monitoring of IV fluids, which must now be slowed or stopped entirely.

The nurse must notify the physician at once if any of the following signs of the onset of this phase occur:

- Rapid rise in urinary output; may increase to 250 mL/hr or higher
- Tachypnea, followed by dyspnea
- Increase in pulse pressure; mean blood pressure also may increase. Central venous pressure, if measured, is elevated.

Infection Control   The child has lost a portion of the integumentary system, which is a primary defense against infection. For this reason, measures must be taken to protect the child from infection. Antibiotics are not considered very effective in controlling infection of this type, most likely because the injured capillaries cannot carry the antibiotic to the site. If used, antibiotics are usually added to the IV fluids. Tetanus antitoxin or toxoid should be ordered according to the status of the child's previous immunization. If inoculations are up to date, a booster dose of tetanus toxoid is all that is required.

To protect the child from infection introduced into the burn, sterile equipment must be used in the child's care. People caring for the child must wear a gown, a mask, and a head cover. Visitors are required to scrub, gown, and mask as well. Burn units are designed to be self-contained, with treatment and operating areas, hydrotherapy units, and patient care areas. In hospitals where there is no specific burn unit, a private room with a door that can be closed should be set up as a burn unit. The strictest aseptic technique must be observed.

Wound Care   Two types of burn care are generally used: the open method and the closed method. The open method of burn care is most often used for superficial burns, burns of the face, and burns of the perineum. In open burn care, the wound is not covered, but antimicrobial ointment is applied topically. This type of care requires strict aseptic precautions. In the closed burn method of burn care, nonadherent gauze is used to cover the burn. The child can be moved more easily, and there is less dan-

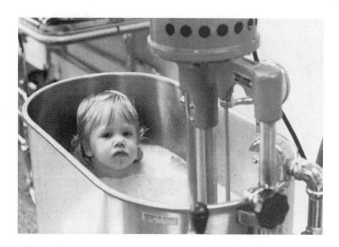

Figure 13-9
Child receiving hydrotherapy.

ger of added injury or pain. In the closed method, dressing changes are very painful, and infection may occur under the dressings. Occlusive dressings help minimize pain because of the reduced exposure to air.

In both methods, daily **débridement** (removal of necrotic tissue), usually preceded by **hydrotherapy** (use of water in treatment) is performed. Débridement is extremely painful, and the child must have an analgesic administered before the therapy. The child is placed in the tub of water to soak the dressings, which helps remove any sloughing tissue, **eschar** (hard crust or scab), exudate, and old medication (Fig. 13-9). Often, the tissue is trapped in the mesh gauze of the dressing, easing its removal. Loose tissue is trimmed before the burn is redressed. Hosing instead of tub soaking is being used in some centers to reduce the risk of infection. Débridement is difficult emotionally for the child and the nurse. Diversionary activities may be used to help distract the child. Researchers also have found that children who are encouraged to participate actively in their burn care, even to help change dressings, experience healthy control over their situation and often suffer less anxiety than those who are completely dependent on the nurse. The child should never be scolded or reprimanded for uncooperative behavior. Praise for cooperation should be used generously.

Topical medications that may be used to reduce invading organisms are silver nitrate, mafenide acetate (Sulfamylon), silver sulfadiazine (Silvadene), gentamicin sulfate (Garamycin), and povidone-iodine (Betadine). Each of these agents has advantages and disadvantages. The choice of agent is made by the physician and is determined, at least partially, by the organisms found in cultures of the burn area.

Grafting   Grafts may be **homografts, heterografts** (xenografts), or **autografts.** Homografts and heterografts are temporary grafts. A homograft consists of skin taken from another person and is eventually rejected by the recipient tissue, sloughing off after 3 to 6 weeks. Skin from cadavers is often used, a procedure called an **allograft**; this skin can be stored and used up to several weeks, and permission for this use is seldom refused.

A heterograft is skin obtained from animals, usually pigs (porcine). Both homografts and heterografts provide a temporary dressing after débridement and have proved to be lifesaving measures for children with extensive burns.

An autograft, consisting of skin taken from the child's own body, is the only kind of skin accepted permanently by recipient tissues, except for the skin from an identical twin. It is usually impossible to obtain enough healthy skin to cover a large area; therefore, homografts are of great value for immediate covering. If the donor site is kept free from infection and grafts of sufficient thinness are taken, the site should be ready for use again in 10 to 12 days.

After grafting, the donor and the graft sites are kept covered with sterile dressings.

COMPLICATIONS

Curling's ulcer (also called a stress ulcer) is a gastric or duodenal ulcer that often occurs after serious skin burns. It can easily be overlooked when the attention of nurses and physicians is directed toward the treatment of the burn area and the prevention of infection. Symptoms are those of any gastric ulcer but usually are vague, concerned with abdominal discomfort, with or without localization, or related to eating. Ulcers appear during the first 6 weeks. Blood in the stools, combined with abdominal discomfort, may be the basis for diagnosis. If desired, roentgenograms can confirm the diagnosis. Treatment consists of a bland diet and the use of antacids and antispasmodics.

The health care team must guard carefully against the complication of **contractures**. If the burn extends over a movable body part, fibrous scarring that forms in the healing process can cause serious deformities and limit movement. Joints must be positioned, possibly in overextension, so that maximal flexibility is maintained. Splinting, exercise, and pressure also are used to prevent contractures. In severe burns, pressure garments, which help decrease hypertrophy of scar tissue, may need to be worn for 12 to 18 months (Fig. 13-10). The child must wear these garments continuously, except when bathing.

LONG-TERM CARE

The rehabilitative phase of care for the child is often long and difficult. Even after discharge from the health care facility, the child needs to return for further treatment or plastic surgery to release the contractures and revise the scar tissue. The emotional scars of the family and the child must be evaluated, and therapy must be initiated or continued. The impact of scarring and disfigurement may need to be resolved by both the child and members of the family. If the child is of school age, school work and social interaction must be considered.

Nursing Process for the Child With a Burn

ASSESSMENT

Assessment of the child with a burn is complex and varies with the extent and depth of the burn, the stage of healing, and the age and general condition of the child. Initially, the primary concerns are the cardiac and respiratory state, the assessment of shock, and an evaluation of the burns.

(text continues on page 288)

Figure 13-10
Child continues to wear pressure garment for one year after burns occurred to avoid the contractures and scar formation. New suit required as child grows. (A) Front view; (B) side view; (C) back view.

Nursing Care Plan
for the Toddler with a Burn

Two-year-old Jed was watching his mother fix dinner. She turned away from the stove where she had vegetables cooking. Jed climbed on his chair and grabbed the handle of the pan. Before his mother could react, the boiling liquid from the vegetables poured down over his right arm, the right side of his torso, and his right groin and leg. He is now in the pediatric unit for care of second- and third-degree burns of his right arm, right torso and groin, and right leg.

NURSING DIAGNOSIS

Risk for Infection related to the loss of a protective layer secondary to burn injury

GOAL: *Jed's burns will show no signs of infection*

OUTCOME CRITERIA

- Jed's burns show no signs of foul smelling drainage
- Jed's vital signs remain within normal limits: pulse ranging between 80–110, respirations 20–30, and temperature ranging between 98.6°–101°F (37°–38.4°C)

Nursing Interventions	Rationale
Carry out conscientious handwashing and follow other infection control precautions, including the use of sterile equipment and supplies. Wear sterile gown, mask and cap and use sterile gloves when giving direct care to the burned area.	Sterile technique decreases the introduction of microorganisms. Handwashing is the foundation of good medical asepsis. These procedures reduce the risk of infection.
Teach family and visitors sterile techniques, especially handwashing.	Infection control procedures must include all who enters the child's room in order to be effective.
Screen visitors for signs of upper respiratory or skin infections.	The child with severe burns may be easily susceptible to upper respiratory and skin infections.
Note and document all drainage and any unusual odor; take regular cultures.	Early detection and prompt treatment of infection is essential as severe infection places an additional burden on the child's already stressed system.

NURSING DIAGNOSIS

Altered Nutrition: Less than Body Requirements related to increased caloric needs secondary to burns and anorexia

GOAL:

Jed's nutrition will meet his needs for tissue repair and growth

OUTCOME CRITERIA:

- Jed consumes at least 80% of diet high in calories and protein
- Jed's output is 1–2 mL/kg/h
- Jed maintains his preburn weight

(continued)

Nursing Care Plan (Continued)
for the Toddler with a Burn

Nursing Interventions	Rationale
Offer Jed a high-calorie, high-protein, bland diet.	Plan appealing meals offered in small servings catering to Jed's food likes and dislikes. Give Jed choices.
Weigh Jed daily in the morning with only underpanties on.	Increased calories and high-protein are required to promote wound healing.
Small servings are more appealing to a child. Allowing Jed to make choices gives him some feeling of control and encourages his cooperation.	Daily or weekly weights provides information to determine nutritional needs.

NURSING DIAGNOSIS

Pain related to tissue destruction and painful procedures

GOAL: *Jed will experience reduction of pain to an acceptable level*

OUTCOME CRITERIA

- Jed rests quietly, pupils not dilated, pulse between 80-110 bpm and respirations 20-30 and regular
- Jed uses the faces pain rating scale to indicate his pain level (Chapter 4)
- Analgesics are administered before dressing changes and débridement procedures

Nursing Interventions	Rationale
Monitor Jed every two to four hours to assess his comfort level, vital signs and to determine whether he is restless.	Each individual reacts differently to pain and analgesics. Learning Jed's responses helps to effectively plan to reduce his pain.
Administer analgesics 20 to 30 minutes before dressing changes and débridement.	This gives the analgesics time to reach optimum effectiveness for pain relief during procedures.
Support and comfort Jed during procedures. Plan a favorite activity after procedures to give Jed something pleasant to anticipate.	Acknowledging that the procedures are painful and his cooperation deserves a reward may help the child accept the inevitable.
Give Jed opportunities to exercise some control when possible over timing, what gets done first or other details.	A feeling of control over some aspects of his care and situation helps offset feelings of powerlessness.

NURSING DIAGNOSIS

Risk for Impaired Physical Mobility related to pain and scarring

GOAL: *Contractures will be minimal; mobility will be maintained*

OUTCOME CRITERIA

- Jed participates in range-of-motion activities; uses both arms and legs
- Splints, pressure suit, and positions are maintained
- Contractures are not evidenced
- Jed participates in ambulatory activities

(continued)

Nursing Care Plan (Continued)
for the Toddler with a Burn

Nursing Interventions	Rationale
Position Jed so that no two skin surfaces touch; give special attention to right armpit, right elbow, wrist and hand, right groin and right knee.	When any two skin surfaces touch scarring will occur, resulting in contractures and limited movement.
Maintain splints and pressure dressings to hyperextend joints.	Hyperextension and limits the formation of contractures.
Plan self-care activities which give Jed some control and also will encourage movement of the affected joints.	Encouraging Jed to do small activities to help himself promotes movement and decreases contractures.
Encourage active play and ambulation.	A child is more likely to cooperate in exercise and movement which is fun.

NURSING DIAGNOSIS

Parental Health Seeking Behaviors regarding the long-term care required by the child

GOAL: *Jed's mother and other family caregivers will demonstrate understanding of long-term home care*

OUTCOME CRITERIA

- Family caregivers demonstrate knowledge of the care needed to treat Jed's burns
- Family caregivers verbalize an understanding of the long-term management of Jed's care
- Jed's family secures the home care equipment needed for his care
- Jed's family plans for follow-up care and utilizes social service assistance

Nursing Interventions	Rationale
Explain to Jed's mother and other family caregivers what you are doing and why as you give care and perform procedures for Jed.	Having a child with a burn is an overwhelming experience. Providing explanations as you give care helps the family to begin to grasp the care process.
Provide information to Jed's mother and other family caregivers in small amounts, repeating information from one time to another. Allow for ample opportunity for questions.	Family caregivers can absorb only so much information at a time. Repetition and patient, careful answering of questions help the family understand the long-term view.
Teach Jed's family the importance of diet, infection control, exercise, rest, activity, pressure suit, and all aspects of Jed's care.	Jed's family needs to understand all aspects of care, including how the pressure suit is worn, the care of the suit, and the need to change the suit as Jed grows.
Teach signs and symptoms that are important to note and what may need to be reported promptly.	Learning what to observe for and which signs or symptoms need to be reported promptly give the family caregivers confidence in their ability and improve the level of home care that they give.
Provide Jed's mother with information and contacts for social services which will help her care for Jed.	Long-term care is improved and aided by contact and interaction with appropriate social services.

After the first phase (the first 24 to 48 hours), the healing of the child's burns must be evaluated and the child's nutrition, signs of infection, and pain must be assessed. The emotional condition of the child and the family also must be evaluated.

NURSING DIAGNOSES

Many nursing diagnoses may be identified over the extended hospitalization of the child. The following are a few that may be appropriate:

- Risk for Infection, related to the loss of a protective layer secondary to burn injury

- Altered Nutrition: Less Than Body Requirements, related to increased caloric needs secondary to burns and anorexia

- Pain, related to tissue destruction and painful procedures

- Risk for Impaired Physical Mobility, related to pain and scarring

- Anxiety, related to body image disturbance secondary to thermal injury

- Ineffective Family Coping: Compromised, related to the impact of the injury on the child's life

- Health Seeking Behaviors, regarding the long-term care required by the child

OUTCOME IDENTIFICATION AND PLANNING

During the first phase of care, the major goals relate to cardiopulmonary stabilization, fluid and electrolyte balance, and infection control. After the first 72 hours, in the phase sometimes called the management or subacute phase, more long-term goals are developed. The child's goals are limited by his or her age and ability to communicate. Goals related to the child include preventing infection, maintaining adequate nutrition, relieving fear and anxiety, reducing pain, and increasing mobility. The family goals include optimizing healing, decreasing complications with minimal permanent disability, and gaining an understanding of the long-term implications of care.

IMPLEMENTATION

PREVENTING INFECTION. The immaturity of the child's immune system, the destruction of the skin layer, and the presence of necrotic tissue (an ideal medium for bacterial growth) contribute to the significant danger of infection. Conscientious handwashing is necessary by anyone who has contact with the child. Observe rigid infection control precautions and use only sterile equipment and supplies. Monitor vital signs, including temperature, on a 1-, 2-, or 4-hour schedule. Screen all people who have any contact with the child, including visitors, family, or staff

caretakers, for any signs of upper respiratory or skin infection.

When caring for the burn, wear a sterile gown, mask, and cap. Wear sterile gloves or use a sterile tongue blade to apply ointment to the burn. Maintain the room temperature at around 80°F because water evaporates quickly through the denuded areas, and even through the leathery burn eschar, with thermal loss resulting. Note and document all drainage. Report immediately and document any unusual odor. Cultures are done regularly, usually several times a week. Avoid injury to the eschar and the donor site. Hair on the tissue adjacent to the burn area should be shaved.

ENSURING ADEQUATE NUTRITION. The child who has received extensive burns requires special attention regarding nutritional needs. The nutritional problem is much more complex than simply getting a seriously ill child to eat. The child is in negative caloric balance from a number of causes, including:

- Poor intake due to anorexia, ileus, Curling's ulcer, or diarrhea

- External loss due to exudative losses of protein through the burn wound

- Thermal losses due to the burn itself; heat loss from the radiation of heat and water loss, responsible for large caloric losses

- Hypermetabolism due to fever, infection, and the state of toxicity

A bland diet high in protein (for healing and replacement) and calories is an essential component of therapy. Use every effort possible to interest the child in foods essential for tissue building and repair. Do not serve large servings because of anorexia as well as the child's physical condition. Foods are of no value if the child refuses to eat them. Try using colorful trays, foods with eye appeal, and any special touches to spur a child's appetite. Allow the child to have some control to encourage cooperation. Foods that may appeal are flavored milk shakes, ice cream shakes, high-protein drinks containing eggs and extra dried protein milk, ice cream, milk and egg desserts, and puréed meats and vegetables.

Even with the best efforts of nurses, dietitians, and the child, the burn patient seldom can eat enough food to meet the increased needs. Hyperalimentation or tube feedings are often necessary as supplements to the oral intake. Commercial high-calorie formulas are available for tube feedings that meet the child's needs. Avoid using hyperalimentation or tube feedings as a threat to the child. Explain carefully to the child what is to be done and why, and make sure the child understands. Try demonstrating the tube feeding process with a doll to help the child grasp the idea.

Weigh the child daily at the same time and with the same coverings. Carefully monitor intake and output.

RELIEVING PAIN AND PROVIDING COMFORT MEASURES. The pain of a thermal injury can be severe. As a result of the pain, or the fear and anxiety that pain causes, the child may not sleep well, may suffer anorexia, and may be apprehensive and uncooperative during treatments and care. Analgesics must be administered to provide the most relief possible. Administer analgesics at least 20 to 30 minutes before dressing changes and débridement. Monitor the child's physiologic response to the pain and analgesics. Document the child's pupil reaction, heart and respiratory rates, and behavior in response to pain and analgesics. Schedule administration of pain medications so that the child is not too sedated at mealtimes.

Provide support and comfort during painful procedures. Use diversionary activities to help the child focus on something other than the pain. It is acceptable to promise a favorite activity after the dreaded procedure. Television may be helpful, but be cautious not to overuse it. The younger child may enjoy learning new songs, playing age-appropriate games, or listening to someone reading stories. The older child may enjoy video or computer games, tape recordings, books, and board or card games. The child should never be admonished for crying or behaving "like a baby." Acknowledge the child's pain, give the child as much control as possible, and work with the child and the family to minimize the pain and to bring about the greatest rewards for all involved.

PREVENTING CONTRACTURES. Care must be taken to avoid contractures and scarring that limit movement. Never permit two burned body surfaces, such as fingers, to touch. If the neck is involved, the child may have to be kept with the neck hyperextended; the arms may need to be placed in a brace to prevent underarm contractures; joints of the knee or elbow must be extended to prevent scar formation from causing contractures that limit movement. Pressure dressings and pressure suits may be used for this purpose and may need to be worn for more than a year. Physical therapy may be needed, and splints may be used to position the body part to prevent contractures. All these measures can add to the child's discomfort.

Encourage range of motion, early ambulation, and self-help activities as additional means of preventing contractures. Use creativity to devise ways to involve the child in enjoyable activities that encourage movement of the affected part.

REDUCING ANXIETY ABOUT CHANGED BODY IMAGE. The child's age and level of understanding influence the amount of anxiety that he or she has about scarring and disability related to the burn. If the child is in a burn unit with other children, seeing others may cause unrealistic fears. Encourage the child to explore his or her feelings about changes in body image. Use therapeutic play with puppets or dolls, if possible. Encourage both the family and the nursing staff to provide the child with continuous support.

PROMOTING FAMILY COPING. The family may feel guilty about the injury; one member may feel especially responsible. These feelings affect the family's coping abilities. Give both the family and the child opportunities to discuss and express their feelings. Suggest counseling if necessary to help family members handle their feelings. Put the family in touch with support groups if available to help the family work through problems. Explain the child's care to family members and involve them in the care when possible. Avoid saying anything that might add to the guilt or anxiety that the family members are feeling.

PROVIDING FAMILY TEACHING. Provide the family with explanations about the whole process of burns, the care, the healing process, and the long-term implications. Give information to the family as they are ready for it. Do not thrust it on them all at once. To prepare for home care, teach the family about wound care, dressing changes, signs and symptoms to observe and report, and the importance of diet, rest, and activity. Help the family find resources for any necessary supplies and equipment. Make a referral to social services to assist them in home care planning.

EVALUATION: GOALS AND OUTCOME CRITERIA

- *Goal*: The child will have no signs or symptoms of infection.
  Criteria: The child's pulse and respirations are within normal limits for age; temperature is 98.6° to 101°F (37° to 38.4°C); there is no malodorous drainage.

- *Goal*: The child's nutrition will meet tissue repair and growth needs.
  Criteria: The child consumes at least 80% of diet high in calories and protein; output is 1 to 2 mL/kg/hr if the child is 66 lb (30 kg) or less, or 30 to 50 mL/hr if heavier.

- *Goal*: Pain will be relieved promptly.
  Criteria: The child rests quietly, the pupils are not dilated, and the pulse and respiratory rate are regular and normal for age.

- *Goal*: Contractures will be minimal.
  Criteria: The child participates in range-of-motion activities; splints, pressure dressings and suits, and positions are maintained; there is no evidence of contractures.

- *Goal*: Child will accept body image changes.
  Criteria: The child expresses any fears about body image and demonstrates a positive attitude of acceptance.

- *Goal*: Caregivers will evidence healthy coping.
  Criteria: Family members express any guilt and anxieties, participate in the child's care, cooperate with counseling, and become involved in support groups when available.

- *Goal*: Family caregivers will demonstrate understanding of home care.

Criteria: Family members demonstrate knowledge of how to care for the child, verbalize an understanding of the long-term management of the child's care, secure needed home care equipment, and use social service assistance if appropriate.

Head Injuries

Head injuries are a significant cause of serious injury or death in children of all ages. The primary cause of a head injury varies with the child's age. Toddlers and young children may receive a head injury from a fall or child abuse; schoolchildren and adolescents usually experience such an injury as a result of a bicycling, in-line skating, or motor vehicle accident.

Toddlers seem to receive a lot of head injuries. Fortunately, most of them are not serious, but they are often frightening to the caregiver. If a scalp laceration is involved, the caregiver can be quite alarmed by the amount of bleeding that occurs due to the large blood supply to the head and scalp. The caregiver can apply an ice pack and pressure until the bleeding is controlled. Applying ice cubes in a zip-closure sandwich bag wrapped in a washcloth works well at home. An open wound should be cleaned with soap and water and a sterile dressing applied. For an injury without a break in the skin, the caregiver can apply ice for an hour or so to decrease the amount of swelling.

The caregiver should observe the child for at least 6 hours for vomiting or a change in the child's level of consciousness. If sleeping, the child is awakened to determine that the level of consciousness has not changed. No analgesics or sedatives should be administered during this period of observation. The child's pupils are checked for reaction to light every 4 hours for 48 hours. The caregiver should notify the health care provider immediately if the child vomits more than three times, has pupillary changes, has double or blurred vision, has a change in level of consciousness, acts strange or confused, has trouble walking, or has a headache that becomes more severe or wakes him or her from sleep; these instructions should be provided in written form to the caregiver.

Family caregivers are wise to take the child to a health care facility to have the injury evaluated if they have any doubt about its seriousness. Complications of head injuries, with or without skull fractures, can include cerebral hemorrhage, cerebral edema, and increased intracranial pressure. These conditions require highly skilled intensive care, and victims are usually cared for in a pediatric neurologic or intensive care unit.

■ KEY POINTS

- Toddlerhood is a time of exploring and learning, when mobility and communication influence what happens to the child.

- Autism may become evident if the child does not form relationships with parents and family.

- Respiratory infections may occur frequently in the toddler, causing anxiety for caregivers and possibly leading to respiratory emergencies.

- Hereditary diseases that affect nutrition include celiac syndrome and cystic fibrosis.

- Cystic fibrosis often causes respiratory involvement, contributing to the severity of the disease.

- Toddlers need constant supervision because their inquiring mind has not developed judgment about those things that are safe and those that are not. This trait sometimes results in accidents, which can be life-threatening or cause permanent damage.

- Toddlers like to experience many things by tasting them. Thus, toddlers may swallow poisons or objects that can cause serious systemic damage.

- Burns can cause lifelong damage.

? CRITICAL THINKING

1. Melanie, a toddler with two young siblings, has infectious conjunctivitis. Develop a teaching plan for infection control that you can use with her caregiver.
2. Carmella has idiopathic celiac disease. From the following list, select the foods that she may have in her meal plan. With the help of a nutrition text or by reading labels, identify the foods you will not recommend, and state why each of those foods is inappropriate:
   ice cream
   corn flakes
   grits
   rice pudding
   whole-wheat bread
   baked beans
   hamburger
   hot dog
   french fries
   fresh vegetables
   yogurt
   oatmeal
   Rice Krispies
   orange juice
   graham crackers
   corn chips
   peanut butter
   baked potato
   tuna salad
   pizza
3. Draw a diagram to explain the heredity pattern of cystic fibrosis.
4. You discover your 18-month-old child with an empty bottle of children's acetaminophen. Describe the actions

you should take. Using a drug reference, identify the specific antidote used in acetaminophen overdose.

5. Survey your house (or a house you select) and list the hazards for ingestion of poisonous substances, drowning, and burns. Include all types of burns. After the hazards are identified, formulate a plan to correct or lessen the hazards.

6. Two-year-old Omar has partial- and total-thickness burns from a wood stove accident. Develop a teaching plan covering the importance of infection control for Omar during his convalescence.

BIBLIOGRAPHY

Adler R. Burns are different: The child psychiatrist on the pediatric burns ward. J Burn Care Rehabil 13(1):28–32, 1992.

Anson A, Weizman Z, Zeevi N. Celiac disease: Parental knowledge and attitudes of dietary compliance. Pediatrics 85(1):98–103, 1990.

Attas AB, Orenstein SR, Orenstein DM. Pancreatitis in young children with cystic fibrosis. J Pediatr 120:756–759, 1992.

Campbell LS, Thomas DO. Pediatric trauma: When kids get hurt. RN 54(9):32–38, 1991.

DeRienzo-DeVivio S. Childhood lead poisoning: Shifting to primary prevention. Pediatr Nurs 18(6):565–567, 1992.

Gutteridge C, Kuhn RJ. Pulmozyme—dornase alfa. Pediatr Nurs 20(3):278, 1994.

Jones NE. Childhood residential injuries. MCN 18(3):168–172, 1993.

Kachoyeanos MK, Friedhoff M. Cognitive and behavior strategies to reduce children's pain. MCN 18(1):14–19, 1993.

Mitchell A, Steffenson N, Hogan H, Coleman R. Acute organophosphate pesticide poisoning in children. MCN 20(5):261–268, 1995.

Pillitteri A. Maternal and child health nursing, 2d ed. Philadelphia: JB Lippincott, 1995.

Spock B, Rothenberg MB. Dr. Spock's baby and child care. New York: Pocket Books, 1992.

Walsh EA, Ioli JG. Childhood near-drowning: Nursing care and primary prevention. Pediatr Nurs 20(3):265–269, 1994.

White KR, Munro CL, Pickler RH. Therapeutic implications of recent advances in cystic fibrosis. MCN 20(6):304–308, 1995.

Williams JK. Genetics and cystic fibrosis: A focus on carrier testing. Pediatr Nurs 21(5):444–448, 1995.

Wong DL. Whaley and Wong's nursing care of infants and children, 5th ed. St. Louis: Mosby, 1995.

Chapter 14

Growth and Development of the Preschool Child: 3 to 6 Years

PHYSICAL DEVELOPMENT
  Growth Rate
  Dentition
  Visual Development
  Skeletal Growth
PSYCHOSOCIAL DEVELOPMENT
  Language Development
  Development of Imagination
  Sexual Development
  Social Development

NUTRITION
HEALTH PROMOTION AND MAINTENANCE
  Routine Checkups
  Family Teaching
  Accident Prevention
  Infection Prevention
THE HOSPITALIZED PRESCHOOLER

STUDENT OBJECTIVES

On completion of this chapter, the student will be able to:

1. Briefly describe several social characteristics of the preschooler, and state the age group this includes.
2. Describe the growth rate of the preschooler.
3. State the age at which 20/20 vision usually is attained.
4. List four factors that may delay language development.
5. Discuss the role of magical thinking and imagination in the preschooler.
6. Describe the characteristics of dreams, nightmares, and imaginary playmates.
7. Discuss the nurse's role in helping parents understand their preschooler's sexual curiosity.
8. Discuss masturbation in the preschool age.
9. List six types of play in which preschoolers engage, and define each.
10. Discuss aggression in the preschooler: a) verbal aggression, b) physical aggression, c) parents' tasks, d) parents' example.
11. State the role of discipline for the preschooler: a) caregiver behavior, b) effect on child, c) effect on caregiver.
12. Discuss the special needs of the disadvantaged preschooler.
13. Discuss the value of Head Start programs.
14. State preschool nutritional needs, including a) daily minimum needs, b) appetite variations, c) suggested snacks, d) television commercials and other influences.
15. State the recommended health maintenance schedule for the preschooler.
16. List guidelines for accident prevention in the preschool-age population.
17. List nine health teachings for the preschooler concerning prevention of infection.
18. Identify the preschool social characteristic that increases the risk of infection.

KEY TERMS

associative play	onlooker play
cooperative play	parallel play
magical thinking	solitary independent play
noncommunicative	unoccupied behavior
language	

Preschoolers are fascinating creatures. As their social circles enlarge to include peers and adults outside the family, their language, play patterns, and appearance change markedly. Their curiosity about the world around them grows, as does their ability to explore the world in greater detail and see new meanings in what they find (Fig. 14-1). Preschoolers can be said to soak up information "like a sponge." "Why?" and "how?" are favorite words. This curiosity also means that accidents are still a serious concern.

At 3 years of age, the child still has the chubby, baby-faced look of a toddler, but by age 5, a leaner, taller, better coordinated social being has emerged. The child works and plays tirelessly, "making things" and telling everyone about it. Although the child has some problem separating fantasy from reality, exploring and learning go on continuously. According to Erikson, the developmental task of the preschool age is initiative versus guilt. Preschoolers often try to find ways to do things to help, but if they fail because of inexperience or lack of skill and get scolded, they may feel guilty.

PHYSICAL DEVELOPMENT

Growth Rate

The preschool period is one of slow growth. The child gains about 3 to 5 lb each year (1.4–2.3 kg) and grows about 2.5″ (6.3 cm). Because the increase in height is proportionately greater than the increase in weight, the 5-year-old child appears much thinner and less babyish than the 3-year-old does. Boys tend to be leaner than girls during this time. Gross and fine motor skills continue to develop rapidly. Balance improves, and with that improvement the confidence to try new activities emerges. By age 5 the child generally can throw and catch a ball well, climb effectively, and ride a bicycle. Important milestones for growth and development are summarized in Table 14-1.

Dentition

By 6 years of age, the child's skull is 90% of its adult size. The deciduous teeth have completely emerged by the beginning of the preschool period. Toward the end of the preschool stage, these teeth begin to be replaced by permanent teeth. This is an event that most children anticipate as an indication that they are "growing up." Pictures of smiling 5- and 6-year-olds typically show missing front teeth (Fig. 14-2).

The age at which teeth erupt varies with individual children and with various ethnic and economic groups. Perma-

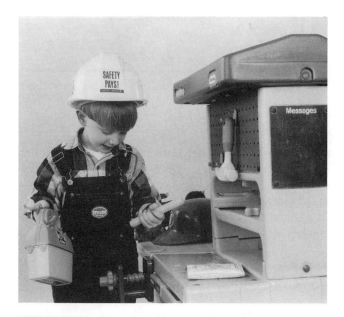

Figure 14-1
Preschoolers engage in meaningful play and are fascinated by what they find. They enjoy dressing up like the people they are playing.

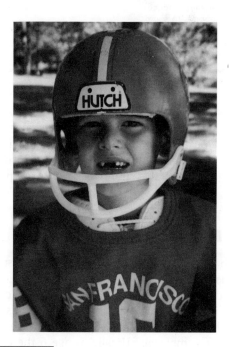

Figure 14-2
The smiling 6-year-old is often seen without his front teeth.

TABLE 14-1. Growth and Development: The Preschooler

Age (yr)	Personal–Social	Fine Motor	Gross Motor	Language	Cognition
3	Begins Erikson's stage of "initiative vs. guilt." Conscience develops. Shy with strangers and inept with peers. Sufficiently independent to be interested in group experiences with age mates (eg, nursery school)	Able to button clothes Copies ○ and + Uses pencils, crayons, paints Shows preference for right or left hand	Tends to watch motor activities before attempting them Can jump several feet Uses hands in broad movements Rides tricycle Negotiates stairs well	Vocabulary up to 1,000 words Articulates vowels accurately Talks a lot Sings and recites Asks many questions	Continues in preoperational stage (2–7 years) characterized by: 1. Centration, or the inability to attend to more than one aspect of a situation 2. Egocentricity, or the inability to consider the perception of others 3. The static and irreversible quality of thought that makes the child unable to perceive the processes of change
4	Boisterous and inflammatory Aggressive physically and verbally but developing behaviors to become socially acceptable Becomes socially acceptable Accepts punishment for wrongdoing because it relieves guilt	Can use scissors; copies a square Adds three parts to stick figures	Has some hesitation but tends to try feats beyond ability Greater powers of balance and accuracy Hops on one foot; can control movements of hands	Vocabulary of about 1,500 words Constant questions Sentences of 4 or 5 words Uses profanity Reports fantasies as truth	Reality and fantasy are not always clear to the preschooler Believes that words make things real—"magical thinking"
5	Initiates contacts with strangers and relates interesting little tales Interested in telling and comparing stories about self Peer relations are important ("best friends" abound) Responds to social values by assuming sex roles with rigidity	Ties shoelaces Copies a diamond and a triangle Prints a few letters or numbers May print first name Cuts food	Will not attempt feats beyond ability Throws and catches ball well Jumps rope Walks backward with heel to toe Skips and hops Adept on bicycle and climbing equipment	Vocabulary of 3,000 words Speech is intelligible Asks meanings of words Enjoys telling stories	Thinks feelings and thoughts can happen Intrusions into the body cause fear and anxiety (fear of mutilation and castration)

nent teeth of African-American children erupt at least 6 months earlier than those of American children of European ancestry. The central incisors are usually the first to go, just as they were the first to erupt in infancy.

Visual Development

Although the preschooler's senses of taste and smell are acute, visual development is still immature at age 3. Eye–hand coordination is good, but judgment of distances generally is faulty, leading to many bumps and falls. During the preschool years, the child's vision should be checked to screen for amblyopia. Usually by age 6 the child has achieved 20/20 vision, but mature depth perception may not occur in some children until 8 to 10 years of age.

Skeletal Growth

Between the third and sixth birthdays, the greatest amount of skeletal growth occurs in the feet and legs. This contributes to the change from the wide-gaited, pot-bellied look of the toddler into the slim, taller figure of the 6-year-old. In addition, the carpals and tarsals mature in the hands and feet, contributing to better hand and foot control.

PSYCHOSOCIAL DEVELOPMENT

Language Development

Between the ages of 3 and 5 years, language development is generally rapid. Most 3-year-olds can construct simple sentences, but they have many hesitations and repetitions as they search for the right word or try to make the right sound. Stuttering can develop during this period but usually disappears within 3 to 6 months. By the end of the fifth year, preschoolers use long, rather complex sentences; their vocabulary will have increased by more than 1,500 words since age 2.

Preschoolers' use of language changes during this period. Three-year-olds often talk to themselves or to their toys or pets without any apparent purpose other than the pleasure of using words. Piaget called this egocentric or **noncommunicative language**. By 4 years of age, children increase their use of communicative language, using words to transmit information other than their own needs and feelings.

Four- and 5-year-olds delight in using "naughty" words or swearing. Bathroom words become favorites, and taunts such as, "you're a big doo-doo" bring heady excitement to them. Caregivers may become concerned by this turn of events, but the child simply may be trying words out to test their impact. A calm, matter-of-fact response that lets the child know that this is not language to use in the company of others may help defuse some of its power. Development of preschoolers' verbal abilities is summarized in Table 14-2.

Delays or other difficulties in language development may be caused by one or more of the following:

- Hearing impairment or other physical problem
- Lack of stimulation
- Overprotection
- Lack of parental interest, or rejection by parents.

Good language skills are developed as the child is engaged regularly in conversation with caregivers and others. The conversation should be on a level that the child can understand. Reading to the child is an excellent method of contributing to language development. This can be enhanced by talking with the child about the pictures in the story books. Praise, approval, and encouragement are all part of supporting attempts at communication.

Family and cultural patterns also influence language development. Some children come from bilingual families and are trying to learn the rules of both languages. Others may come from geographic or social communities that have dialects different from the general population.

Development of Imagination

Preschoolers have learned to think about something without actually seeing it—to visualize or imagine. This normal development, sometimes called **magical thinking**, makes it difficult for them to separate fantasy from reality. Preschoolers believe that words or thoughts can make things real, and this belief can have either positive or negative results. For example, in a moment of anger, a child wishes that a parent or a sibling would die; if that person later is hurt, the child feels responsible and suffers guilt. The child needs reassurance that this is not so.

Imagination makes preschoolers good audiences for storytelling, simple plays, and television, as long as the characters and events are not too frightening or sad. When preschoolers see a television character die, they believe it is real and often cry. The child's television viewing should be supervised to avoid programs with negative impact or overstimulation.

During this stage, children often have imaginary playmates who are very real to them. This occurs particularly with only children, filling times of loneliness. The imaginary friend often has the characteristics that the child might wish for. Sometimes the child blames the imaginary friend for breaking a toy or engaging in another act the

TABLE 14-2. Verbal Mastery by Preschoolers

Age (yr)	Characteristics of Language Usage	Vocabulary Size, Pattern, Comprehension, Rhythm
3–4	Loves to talk; talks a lot; makes up words; sings or recites own version of song; likes new words; asks many questions and wants answers. Not always logical in sentences and concepts. Uses 4- or 5-word phrases. Aggressive with words rather than actions.	Vocabulary of 900–1500 words; at 3 understands up to 3,600 words, up to 5,600 words by 4. By 4 years, speech understandable, even with mispronunciations. May have hesitations, repetitions, and revisions while trying to imitate adult speech. Stuttering may occur, but disappears with 3–6 months; may continue up to 2 years without being permanent.
4–5	Understands out-of-context words. Speech highly emotional. Difficulty finding right word; tells function rather than name of item. Changes subject rapidly. Boasts, brags, quarrels; loves "naughty" words. Relates fanciful tales.	Vocabulary of 3,000 words; understands up to 9,600 words by 5 years. Speech completely understandable.

A Personal Glimpse

It was a beautiful day and the kids were in the sandbox, but Christine (5 years old) came in downstairs while I was vacuuming upstairs. I finished and lay down on my bed for a minute. Suddenly I heard a smashing noise. I said, "What was that?" "Nothing, Mom." I said again, "What WAS that?" Christine came running upstairs and went into her room. I went over to her room and the door was locked. I went downstairs and didn't see anything wrong in the kitchen. The noise sounded like the kid's big bin of Duplo blocks. I went into the family room and at first didn't see anything, and then I screamed. The TV was face down on the floor and the stand was knocked over too. It was still playing, or at least noise was coming out of it. Christine came down, and I said, "Christine, what happened?" She told me she was on the couch and the TV "just fell over." I sent her to her room until she could tell the truth. I unplugged the TV and got it upright, and got the stand up, but it was heavy. I was finally able to get it back on the stand and hooked up, but it didn't work. It is only by the grace of God that it didn't land on her or shatter into a million pieces or blow up. Christine finally told us she was lying on the floor with her feet on the stand pushing it when it fell over.

Dana

child does not want to take credit for. Caregivers need assurance that this is normal behavior.

The preschooler's active imagination often leads to a fear of the dark or nightmares. Consequently, problems with sleep are common (see the discussion on sleep needs later in this chapter).

Sexual Development

The preschool period is the stage that Freud termed the *oedipal* or *phallic* (genital) *period*. During these years, children become acutely aware of their sexuality, including sexual roles and organs. They generally develop a strong emotional attachment to the parent of the opposite sex. Curiosity about their own genitalia and those of peers and adults may make parents uncomfortable and evoke responses that indicate to the child that sex is dirty and something to be ashamed and guilty about.

Despite today's abundance of sexually oriented literature, many families find it difficult to deal with the questions and actions of the young child. Nurses can help caregivers understand that the child's sexual curiosity is a normal, natural part of total curiosity about oneself and the surrounding world. The informed, understanding parent can help children develop positive attitudes toward sexuality and toward themselves as sexual human beings.

In addition to responsible teaching of sexual information, the caregiver also should teach the child about "good touch" and "bad touch." The child needs to understand that no one should touch the child's body in a way that is unpleasant.

MASTURBATION

Exploration of the genitalia is just as natural for the preschooler as thumbsucking is for the infant. This is one way the child learns to perceive the body as a possible source of pleasure and is the beginning of acceptance of sex as natural and pleasurable.

Caregivers can be reassured that this is not uncommon behavior, and a calm, matter-of-fact response to the child is the most effective approach. The child should be helped to understand that masturbation is not an activity that is appropriate in public. If the child seems to be masturbating excessively, counseling may be needed, especially if the child's life has been unsettled in other aspects.

Social Development

Preschoolers are outgoing, imaginative, social beings. They play vigorously and, in the process, learn about the world in which they live. Preschoolers have been characterized as "sponges," soaking up all that goes on about them (whether positive or negative). As they gain control over their environment, preschoolers try to manipulate it, which may lead to conflict with caregivers. Preschool children are delightful to watch as they go about the business of growing and learning.

PLAY

Play activities are one way that children learn. Normally, by 3 years of age, children begin imitative play, pretending to be the mommy, the daddy, a policeman, a cowboy, an astronaut, or some well-known person or television character (Fig. 14-3). Caregivers can gain good insight into the way their child interprets family behavior by watching the child play. Listening to a preschooler scold a doll or stuffed animal for "bothering me while I'm busy talking on the phone" lets the adults hear how they sound to the child.

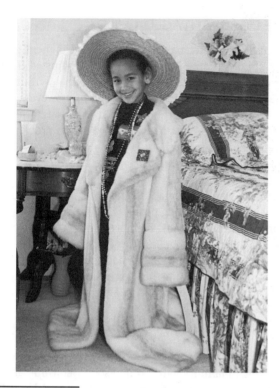

Figure 14-3
Preschoolers identify with adults. Dressing up like mommy is a favorite play activity.

Dramatic play allows a child to act out troubling situations and to control the solution to the problem. This is important to remember when teaching children who are going to be hospitalized. Using dolls and puppets to explain procedures makes the experience less threatening.

Drawing is another form of play through which children learn to express themselves. During the preschool years, as fine motor skills improve, children's drawings become much more complex and controlled and can be revealing about the child's self-concept and perception of the environment.

Preschoolers engage in various types of play: cooperative, associative, parallel, solitary independent, onlooker, and unoccupied behavior. In **cooperative play**, children play with each other, as in team sports. **Associative play** means being engaged in a common activity but without any sense of belonging. In **parallel play**, children play alongside each other, but independently. Although common among toddlers, parallel play exists in all age groups—for example, in a Scout troop where each member is working on an individual project or craft. **Solitary independent play** means playing apart from others without making an effort to be part of the group or their activity. Watching television is one form of **onlooker play**, in which there is observation without participation. In **unoccupied behavior**, the child may be daydreaming or fingering clothing or a toy without apparent purpose.

Children need all types of play to aid in their total devel-

opment. Too much of one kind may signal a problem; for example, a youngster who spends most of the time unoccupied may be troubled, depressed, or unstimulated. Cooperative play helps develop social interaction skills and often physical health as well.

Too much onlooker play, particularly television viewing, means that children are missing the benefits of other kinds of play and may be forming strong, highly inaccurate impressions of people and their behaviors. The amount of time that preschoolers spend watching television should be limited, and interactive play should be encouraged.

AGGRESSION

Temper tantrums are an early form of aggression. The preschooler with newly developed language skills uses words aggressively in name-calling and threats. Four-year-olds use physical aggression as well, pushing, hitting, and kicking in an effort to manipulate the environment. The family caregivers' task during these years is to help the child understand that the anger and frustration that result in aggressive behavior are normal but need to be handled differently because aggressive behavior is not socially acceptable.

Children who come from unhappy home situations are likely to be more aggressive than children from a comfortable family situation. Their caregivers have served as role models, and their aggressive behavior toward each other has said to the child, "this is acceptable."

DISCIPLINE

It is important for family caregivers to remember that preschoolers are developing initiative and a sense of guilt. They want to be good and follow instructions, and they feel bad when they do not, even though they are not physically punished. Discipline during this time should strive to teach the child a sense of responsibility and inner control. All the child's caregivers must understand and agree to the limits and discipline measures for the child. If one caregiver says "no" and another one says "yes," the child soon learns to play one against the other, leading to confusion about limits. Spanking and other forms of physical punishment remove the responsibility from the child. Taking away a privilege from a child who has misbehaved until he or she can demonstrate that there has been an improvement in behavior is much more effective. Because the child's concept of time is not clear, the period should be comparatively brief (Fig. 14-4). Table 14-3 presents some examples of the effects of positive and negative responses by caregivers.

NURSERY SCHOOL OR DAY CARE EXPERIENCE

Group experiences with peers and adults outside the immediate family are important to a child's development. However, the transition to new experiences, new people, and

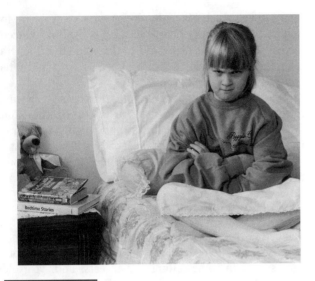

Figure 14-4
Although she may not like it, quiet solitude helps the preschooler develop inner control.

new surroundings can be threatening to some preschoolers. Children vary in their willingness or ability to handle new situations, but being introduced gradually, according to individual readiness, produces the most satisfactory adjustment. Some children spend only a few hours each week in a nursery school or other day care program; others, because the adult family members work outside the home, must spend a great deal more time away from home and family. The family should understand that this probably means the child will demand more of their attention during the hours when they are together. As the child grows older and the attachment to peers becomes stronger, family caregivers sense a decrease in the need for adult attention and a greater sense of independence in the child.

THE DISADVANTAGED CHILD

Discussions of normal growth and development assume that children come from a secure, well-adjusted home in which there is ample opportunity for social, cultural, and intellectual enrichment. Many children, however, are deprived of such a background, for many reasons. This population is the one most likely to have health problems and to need health services.

Children who have not been able to achieve a sense of security and trust, for whatever reason, need special understanding, warm acceptance, and intelligent guidance to grow into self-accepting people. Society is gradually awakening to the needs of these children and is trying to provide enriched nursery school and kindergarten experiences for those whose home life cannot do this for them, but much remains to be done. Further discussion of the problems of these children can be found in Unit IV: A Child in Crisis.

HEAD START PROGRAMS

Recognition that environmental enrichment is often unavailable in families with limited social, cultural, and economic resources led to the establishment of Head Start programs. Head Start programs are funded by federal and local money and are free to the children enrolled. Children in such programs have an opportunity to broaden their horizons through varied experiences, and their understanding of the world in which they live is increased. Family caregiver participation is a central component of the Head Start concept. Also, involvement of family caregivers often has a positive effect on other children in the household. In some programs, teachers go into the home to help the caregiver teach the young child motor, cognitive, self-help, and language skills. Counseling and referral services are also provided through Head Start programs. Children who have had a background of Head Start enrichment are better

TABLE 14-3. Effects of Positive and Negative Caregiver Behavior

Behavior	Effect on Child	Effect on Adult
Attending only to desired behaviors Calm reasoning with expression of dislike of behavior Physical restraint with adult present Isolation of child for a period of time equal to 1 min per year of age Withholding of desired treats, outings, presents	Development of inner control	Feelings of adequacy as a parent
Yelling, screaming, and implying guilt and punishment Telling child he or she is bad Physical punishment	Development of fears and compulsive behaviors	Feelings of guilt and inadequacy
Giving treats, presents, or food for lack of undesired behavior Physical punishment Threatening punishment from God or other authority figure	Development of control based on external forces	Feelings of being manipulated by child

prepared to enter kindergarten or first grade and compete successfully with their peers.

NUTRITION

The preschool period is not a time of rapid growth; therefore, children do not need large quantities of food. Nevertheless, protein needs continue to remain high to provide for muscle growth. The preschooler's appetite is erratic, however; at one sitting the preschooler may devour everything on the plate and at the next he or she may be satisfied with just a few bites. Portions are smaller than adult-sized portions. The child may need to have meals supplemented with nutritious snacks (Box 14-1). Note that certain snacks are recommended only for the older child to avoid any danger of choking. Frequent, small meals with snacks in between generally are best accepted by the preschooler.

Among the preschooler's favorites are soft foods, grain and dairy products, raw vegetables, and sweets. Television commercials for sugar-coated cereals, snacks, and fast foods of questionable nutritional value exert a powerful influence on the preschooler and can make supermarket shopping an emotional struggle between the caregiver and child. Caregivers should read labels carefully before making a purchase.

Preschoolers need guidance in choosing foods and are strongly influenced by the example of family members and peers. Food should never be used as a reward or bribe; otherwise, the child will continue to use food as a means to manipulate the environment and the behavior of others.

To meet the minimum daily requirements, the preschooler should have two or three glasses of milk each day and several small portions from each food group. Preschoolers have definite food preferences. They generally do not like highly spiced foods, often will eat raw vegetables but not cooked ones, and prefer plain foods rather than casseroles. New foods may be accepted but should be introduced one at a time to avoid overwhelming the child.

The preschooler shows growing independence and skill in eating. The 3-year-old tries to mimic adult behavior at the table but often reverts to eating with the fingers, spilling liquids, and squirming. The 4-year-old is more skilled with the use of utensils, but an occasional misjudgment of abilities results in a mess. The 5-year-old uses utensils well, even cutting his or her own food, and can be taught to practice sophisticated table manners. Rituals such as using the same plate, cereal bowl, cup, or placemat may become important to the child's mealtime happiness.

HEALTH PROMOTION AND MAINTENANCE

Routine Checkups

Preschoolers with up-to-date immunizations need boosters of diphtheria-tetanus-pertussis, oral polio vaccine, and measles-mumps-rubella (MMR) vaccine between 4 and 6 years of age. These are required as preschool boosters for entrance into kindergarten. The MMR booster, however, can be administered at age 10 to 12 instead, if desired.

An annual health examination is recommended to monitor the child's growth and development and to screen for potential health problems. Recommended screening procedures include urinalysis, hematocrit, lead level, tuberculin skin testing, and Denver Developmental Screening Test. The preschool child needs to be told in advance about the upcoming examination, with simple explanations and an opportunity to ask questions and voice anxieties. There are a number of books available through the public library that are excellent for this purpose. Children who attend nursery school or a day care program are required to have an annual examination, but children who stay at home may not have this advantage. Particular attention should be paid to the child's vision and hearing so that any problems can be treated before he or she enters school at age 6. A semiannual dental examination is also recommended.

Family Teaching

The nurse can use routine checkups and any other opportunities to teach the caregivers about common aspects of everyday life with a preschooler. Preschoolers are busy learning and showing initiative as they are involved in their day-to-day life. Preschoolers are usually a pleasure to be

Box 14-1. Suggested Snacks for the Preschooler

Raw vegetables: carrots,* cucumbers, celery,* green beans, green pepper, mushrooms, turnips, broccoli, cauliflower, tomatoes
Fresh fruits: apples, oranges, pears, peaches, grapes,* cherries,* melons
Unsalted whole-grain crackers
Whole-grain bread: cut to finger-sized sticks; plain, toasted, or with peanut butter
Small sandwiches: cut into quarters
Natural cheese: cut into cubes
Cooked meat: cut in small chunks or sliced thinly
*Nuts**
*Sunflower seeds**
Cookies: made with lightly sweetened whole grains
*Plain popcorn**
Yogurt: plain or with fresh fruit added

* Children younger than 2 years of age may choke on nuts, seeds, popcorn, celery strings, or carrot sticks. Avoid these until pre-school years.

around since they are so eager to learn anything new and are full of questions.

BATHING

Although preschoolers view themselves as "grown-up," they still need continual supervision while bathing. The caregiver should run the bath water. The hot water heater should be turned down to 120°F (49°C) to avoid the danger of burns. Children should be taught to leave the faucets alone. Preschoolers can generally wash themselves with supervision. Ears, necks, and faces are spots that often need extra attention. Hands and fingernails often get soaked clean in the tub, but fingernails do need to be checked by the caregiver.

Preschoolers cannot wash their own hair, and this can be a time of tension between the child and caregiver. Shampooing in the tub with a children's nonirritating shampoo may work out best. The child can lean the head back, looking at the ceiling and holding a washcloth on the forehead to keep water and soap from getting into the eyes. Shampoo protectors (a clear plastic brim with no crown) can be purchased if desired.

Bath time can be rather lengthy if the preschooler gets involved in playing with bath toys. This is something the caregiver can negotiate if limits need to be set. Some children this age are interested in taking a shower and may do so with adult supervision.

When washing their hands before meals or before or after going to the bathroom, preschoolers often wash only the fronts, totally ignoring the backs. If not supervised, the child may use only cold water and no soap. Again, the caregiver should turn the water on to a warm temperature to avoid burns.

DENTAL CARE

The preschool child needs to be supervised in toothbrushing. Although the preschooler can brush well, the caregiver should check the cleanliness of the child's teeth. The caregiver should be responsible for flossing because the preschooler does not have the necessary motor skills. To help prevent tooth decay, the preschooler should be encouraged to eat healthy snacks such as fruits, raw vegetables, and natural cheeses rather than candy, cakes, or sugar-filled gum. Fluoridated water or fluoride supplements should be continued.

DRESSING

The preschooler may have definite ideas about what he or she wants to wear. Giving the child the opportunity to choose what to wear each day is an excellent way to begin fostering a sense of control and to help the child learn to make decisions. Preschoolers do not have very good taste in what goes with what, so some interesting outfits may result! Nevertheless, the child should be permitted to make

these choices, and the caregivers (as well as older siblings and other adults) should accept the choices without negative comments. When it does matter—for the adults—how the child is dressed, the best plan is to give the child limited choices that will suit the occasion.

TOILETING

By the preschool years, almost all children have succeeded in toilet training, although an occasional accident may occur. When the child does have an accident, it is best to treat it in a matter-of-fact way and provide the child with clean, dry clothing. The preschooler needs continual reminders to wash the hands before and after toileting. Little girls should be taught to wipe from front to back. Preschoolers may still need to be checked for careful wiping, especially after a bowel movement.

It is not uncommon for young preschoolers to experience bedwetting. Bedwetting is not a concern until it goes past the age of 5 to 7 (see Chap. 17 for further discussion).

SLEEP NEEDS

Preschoolers are often ready to give up their nap. This may depend partially on whether they go to a preschool program that has a rest time. Often preschoolers will just curl up and fall asleep, on a chair, a couch, or the floor. Bedtime can still be a challenge, but leading up to it with a period of quiet activities or stories encourages the child to wind down for the day.

Dreams and nightmares are common during the preschool period. Caregivers need to explain that "it was only a dream" and offer love and understanding until the fear has subsided. Fear of the dark is another common problem during these years. Children may be afraid to go to sleep in a dark bedroom. These are very real fears to the child. A small nightlight may be reassuring to the child. One mother solved this problem in an interesting fashion. The child was afraid of a monster in the closet or under the bed. The mother acknowledged the child's fears and purchased a spray can of room air freshener. At bedtime she ceremoniously sprayed around the room, in the closet, and under the bed. She assured the child that it was a special spray to kill monsters, just like bug spray kills bugs. The child was reassured and slept without fear.

Accident Prevention

Adults caring for preschoolers need to be just as attentive as with toddlers because a child's curiosity at this stage still exceeds his or her judgment. Burns, poisoning, and falls are common accidents. Preschoolers are often victims of motor vehicle accidents, either because they dart into the street or driveway or fail to wear proper restraints. All states have laws that define safety seat and restraint requirements for children. Adults must teach and reinforce these rules. One primary responsibility of adults is always to wear seat belts themselves and to make certain that the child always is in a safety seat or has a seat belt on. A child can be calmly taught that the vehicle "won't go" unless the child is properly restrained.

By the age of 5 years, many preschoolers move from riding a tricycle to riding a bicycle. If the preschooler is not already wearing a bicycle helmet, it is important to educate caregivers that safety helmets are a necessary safety precaution. Lightweight, child-sized safety helmets that fit properly can be purchased, and the child should be taught that the helmet must be worn when riding a bike. Adults who wear helmets provide the best incentive to children. Safety rules for bicycle riding should be reinforced. The preschool child should be limited to protected areas for riding and should have adult supervision.

The preschool age is an excellent time to begin teaching safety rules. The rules for crossing the street and playing in an area near traffic are of vital importance. Adults who care for preschool children should be careful to serve as a good role model. These safety rules should extend into all aspects of the child's life. See Family Teaching: Preschooler Safety Teaching.

Infection Prevention

Preschoolers who enjoy sound nutrition and adequate rest, exercise, and shelter usually are not seriously affected by simple childhood infections. Children who live in less than adequate economic circumstances, however, can be severely threatened by even a simple illness, such as diarrhea or chickenpox. Immunizations are available for many childhood communicable diseases, but some caregivers do not have their children immunized until it is required for entrance to school. As a result, some children suffer unnecessary illnesses.

Family Teaching
Preschooler Safety Teaching

1. Look both ways before crossing the street.
2. Cross the street only with an adult.
3. Watch for cars coming out of driveways.
4. Never play behind a car or truck.
5. Watch for cars or trucks backing up.
6. Wear a safety helmet when bike riding.
7. Learn your name, address, and phone number.
8. Stay away from strange dogs.
9. Stay away from any dog while it's eating.
10. Take only medicine your caregiver gives you.
11. Don't play with matches or lighters.
12. Stay away from fires.
13. Don't run near a swimming pool.
14. Only swin when with an adult.
15. Don't go anywhere with someone you don't know.
16. Don't let anyone touch you in a way you don't like.

Family Teaching
Teaching to Prevent Infections

1. Cover your mouth when coughing or sneezing.
2. Throw away tissues used for nose blowing.
3. Wipe carefully after bowel movements (girls wipe front to back).
4. Wash hands after going to bathroom or blowing your nose.
5. Wash hands before eating.
6. Do not share food you've partly eaten.
7. If food or eating utensil falls on the floor, wash it right away.
8. Do not drink from another person's cup.
9. Do not share a toothbrush with someone else.

Preschoolers are just learning to share, and that can mean sharing infections with the entire family—and playmates as well. Teaching them basic precautions can help prevent the spread of infections. See Family Teaching: Teaching to Prevent Infections.

THE HOSPITALIZED PRESCHOOLER

The preschooler may view hospitalization as an exciting new adventure or a frightening, dangerous experience, depending on the preparation by caregivers and health professionals. As mentioned earlier, play is an effective way to let children act out their anxiety and to learn what to expect from the hospital situation. Preschoolers are frightened about intrusive procedures; therefore, it is usually preferable to take the temperature with an oral or tympanic thermometer, if available, rather than a rectal one. Children are less anxious about procedures if they are allowed to handle equipment beforehand and perhaps "use" it on a doll or another toy.

The hospitalized preschooler may revert to bedwetting but should not be scolded for it. The nurse should assure the family that this is normal. Explanations of where the bathrooms are and how to use the call light or bell to get help can help avoid problems with bedwetting. If a child is afraid of the dark, a nightlight can be provided.

Hospital routines should follow home routines as closely as possible. The child should be allowed to participate in the care, even though this may take longer. All procedures should be carefully explained to the child in words that are at an appropriate level for the child's age, repeating the information as necessary.

If the child is ambulatory and not on infection control precautions, the playroom can offer diversionary activities.

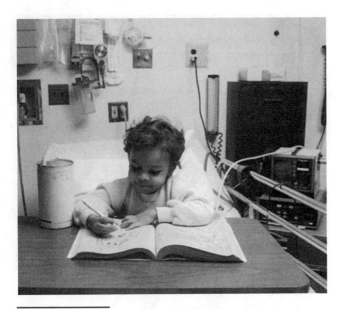

Figure 14-5
The preschooler's love for creating things makes coloring a
great diversional activity during hemodialysis.

If not, play materials can be provided for use in bed (Fig.
14-5).

KEY POINTS

- During the preschool years, psychosocial growth is sub-
stantial but physical growth slows.

- Endless questions, boundless energy, and an ongoing
struggle to separate fantasy from reality are characteristics of the preschooler.

- According to Erikson, the psychosocial developmental
task for the preschool-age group is initiative versus
guilt.

- Language develops rapidly during the preschool period,
progressing from the ability to use simple sentences at
age 3 to telling sometimes long and involved tales by
age 5.

- Magical thinking and imagination contribute to fears
and anxieties of the preschool child. These concerns
must be acknowledged by the caregiver. Patient explanations and reassurance by the caregiver are important.

- The child needs to have limits set by caregivers, within
which he or she can be free to explore and learn and to
assert autonomy and initiative.

- Caregivers must serve as models of the kind of person
they want the child to become, helping the child build
confidence and self-esteem.

- Permitting preschoolers to decide what clothes to wear
is a good way to begin helping them learn to make decisions.

- Safety promotion continues to be an important aspect
of the care of the preschool child, because the child's
curiosity still exceeds his or her judgment.

? CRITICAL THINKING

1. Four-year-olds are sometimes characterized as "the
frustrating fours." After reviewing the preschool growth
and development chart, identify the reasons you believe
this may occur.
2. The parent of $3\frac{1}{2}$-year-old Mario is worried that Mario
is stuttering. With your knowledge of language development, what should you say to the parent?
3. Rita must place her 3-year-old in a day care facility while
she works. Using your knowledge of preschool growth
and development, specify the guidance you can give her.
4. Jackson reports that his 4-year-old son, Chad, wakes up
screaming in the middle of the night. This is causing
the family to lose sleep. Develop a plan of action for
Jackson to use to ease the problem.
5. Clara has noticed her 4-year-old son Theo masturbating.
She is upset and comes to you for help. Detail what you
will tell her.
6. Describe the guidelines you would give a family to help
children develop good eating habits and encourage
trying new foods.

BIBLIOGRAPHY

Castiglia PT, Harbin RE. Child health care: Process and practice.
    Philadelphia: JB Lippincott, 1992.
Christopherson ER. Discipline. Pediatr Clin North Am 39(3):
    395–411, 1992.
Eschleman MM. Introductory nutrition and diet therapy, 3d ed.
    Philadelphia: Lippincott-Raven, 1996.
Howard BJ. Discipline in early childhood. Pediatr Clin North Am
    38(6):1351–1369, 1991.
Pillitteri A. Maternal and child health nursing, 2d ed. Philadel-
    phia: JB Lippincott, 1995.
Schmitt BD. Does your child have a stuttering problem? Contemp
    Pediatr 8(3):83–84, 1991.
Spock B, Rothenberg MB. Dr. Spock's baby and child care. New
    York: Pocket Books, 1992.
Wong DL. Whaley and Wong's nursing care of infants and chil-
    dren, 5th ed. St. Louis: Mosby, 1995.

Health Problems of the Preschool Child

COMMUNICABLE DISEASES
　Prevention
SENSORY DISORDERS
　Hearing Impairment
　Vision Impairment
CENTRAL NERVOUS SYSTEM DISORDERS
　Reye Syndrome
　Cerebral Palsy
　Mental Retardation
　Nursing Process for the Child with Cognitive Impairment
　Down Syndrome

RESPIRATORY SYSTEM DISORDERS
　Tonsillitis
　Nursing Process for the Child having a Tonsillectomy
BLOOD DISORDERS
　Acute Leukemia
　Nursing Process for the Child with Leukemia
　Idiopathic Thrombocytopenia Purpura
　Hemophilia
　Nursing Process for the Child with Hemophilia
GENITOURINARY SYSTEM DISORDERS
　Nephrotic Syndrome
　Nursing Process for the Child with Nephrotic Syndrome
　Acute Glomerulonephritis

STUDENT OBJECTIVES

On completion of this chapter, the student will be able to:

1. Differentiate between the child who is hard of hearing and one who is deaf.
2. Differentiate between rubella and rubeola: a) length of illness, b) signs and symptoms, c) complications.
3. State the contagious period for chickenpox.
4. List two nursing measures to increase comfort and decrease scarring in chickenpox.
5. Describe cerebral palsy.
6. Discuss the causes of cerebral palsy: a) prenatal, b) perinatal, c) postnatal.
7. Differentiate between spastic and athetoid cerebral palsy.
8. Identify the health care professionals involved in the care of the child with cerebral palsy.
9. List the causes of mental retardation: a) prenatal, b) perinatal, c) postnatal.
10. Explain why Down syndrome is also called trisomy 21.
11. List 10 signs and symptoms of Down syndrome.
12. Name the most common complication of a tonsillectomy, and list the signs to observe for.
13. List four drugs commonly used in the treatment of acute lymphatic leukemia.
14. Name the most common type of hemophilia, and state how it is inherited.
15. Describe the symptoms of nephrotic syndrome.
16. Identify the cause of acute glomerulonephritis.
17. Name the most common presenting symptom of acute glomerulonephritis.
18. Compare nephrotic syndrome with acute glomerulonephritis.

KEY TERMS

abdominal paracentesis	intercurrent infections
adenoids	intrathecal administration
adenopathy	leukemia
alopecia	leukopenia
ascites	lymphoblast
astigmatism	lymphocytes
ataxia	monocytes
brachycephaly	myopia
clonus	oliguria
dysarthria	petechiae
granulocytes	purpura
hemarthrosis	refraction
hyperlipidemia	striae
hyperopia	tonsils

Box 15-1. *Common Terms in Communicable Disease Nursing*

Antibody: a protective substance in the body produced in response to the introduction of an antigen

Antigen: a foreign protein that stimulates the formation of antibodies

Antitoxin: an antibody that unites with and neutralizes a specific toxin

Carrier: a person in apparently good health whose body harbors the specific organisms of a disease

Enanthem: an eruption on a mucous surface

Endemic: habitual presence of a disease within a given area

Epidemic: an outbreak in a community of a group of illnesses of similar nature in excess of the normal expectancy

Erythema: redness of the skin produced by congestion of the capillaries

Exanthem: an eruption appearing on the skin during an eruptive disease

Host: a human, animal, or plant that harbors or nourishes another organism

Immunity: passive—immunity acquired by administration of an antibody. Active—immunity acquired by an individual as the result of his or her own reactions to pathogens. Natural—resistance of the normal animal to infection.

Incubation period: the time interval between the infection and the appearance of the first symptoms of the disease

Macule: a discolored skin spot not elevated above the surface

Pandemic: a worldwide epidemic

Papule: a small, circumscribed, solid elevation of the skin

Pustule: a small elevation of epidermis filled with pus

Toxin: a poisonous substance produced by certain organisms, such as bacteria

Toxoid: a toxin that has been treated to destroy its toxicity but that retains its antigenic properties

Vaccine: a suspension of attenuated or killed microorganisms administered for the prevention of a specific infection

---

Today's preschoolers have a better opportunity for good health than ever before. Immunizations have dramatically reduced the threat of communicable childhood diseases. Antibiotics can minimize the dangers of infection. Early detection and proper nutrition can prevent certain kinds of mental retardation. Simpler, more effective screening techniques help identify vision and hearing problems that need early treatment. Surgical advances have made possible the early repair of life-threatening heart problems. However, serious health problems do occur during the preschool period. These problems must be recognized and treated as soon as possible so that the child can be in optimum physical and emotional health when it is time to enter school, a landmark in the child's total development.

COMMUNICABLE DISEASES

Half a century ago, growing up meant being able to survive measles, mumps, whooping cough, diphtheria, and often poliomyelitis. These diseases were expected almost as routinely as the loss of the deciduous teeth. Immunization has changed that outcome so drastically that some caregivers have become less conscientious about having their children immunized until the immunization is required for entrance to school. Nevertheless, the incidence of childhood diseases has decreased, with only an occasional outbreak in certain communities where many children are not immunized. One example of this is the measles epidemic among Amish children in the late 1980s.

Understanding the various communicable diseases and their prevention, symptoms, and treatment (Table 15-1, p. 306) requires knowledge of the terms in Box 15-1. Some communicable diseases require specific precautions to prevent spreading of the infection. Specific transmission precaution procedures can be found in the procedure manuals of individual institutions.

The nurse should explain to the child and the caregivers the reason for the transmission precautions, whether to protect the child from the threat of infection or to protect others from the infection the child has. Otherwise, the child may feel that the precautions are a form of punishment. Families are more likely to follow the correct procedures if they understand the need for them. Transmission precautions may intensify the normal loneliness of being ill, so the child needs extra attention and stimulation during this time.

Prevention

The recommended schedule of infant immunization is found in Chapter 10. Caregivers of children whose immunizations are incomplete must be urged to have the immunizations brought up to date. For families of limited means, free immunizations are available at clinics.

SENSORY DISORDERS

Hearing Impairment

Hearing loss is one of the most common disabilities in the United States, affecting an estimated 1 million children. Depending on the degree of hearing loss and the age at which it is detected, a child's development can be moderately to severely impaired. Development of speech, human relationships, and understanding of the environment all depend on the ability to hear. Infants at high risk for hearing loss should be screened when they are between 3 and 6 months of age.

Hearing loss ranges from mild (hard of hearing) to profound (deaf) (Table 15-2). A child who is hard of hearing has a loss of hearing acuity but can learn speech and language by imitating sounds. A deaf child has no hearing ability.

TYPES OF HEARING IMPAIRMENT

There are four types of hearing loss: conductive, sensorineural, mixed, and central.

Conductive Hearing Loss In this type of impairment, middle ear structures fail to carry sound waves to the inner ear. Most often, conductive hearing loss is the result of chronic serous otitis media or other infection, and it can make hearing levels fluctuate. Chronic middle ear infection can destroy part of the eardrum or the ossicles, leading to conductive deafness. This type of deafness is seldom complete and responds well to treatment.

Sensorineural (Perceptive) Hearing Loss This type of hearing loss may be caused by damage to the nerve endings in the cochlea or to the nerve pathways leading to the brain. It is generally severe and unresponsive to medical treatment. Diseases such as meningitis and encephalitis, hereditary or congenital factors, and toxic reactions to certain drugs (such as streptomycin) may cause sensorineural hearing loss. Maternal rubella is believed to be the most common cause of sensorineural deafness in children.

Mixed Hearing Loss Some children have both conductive and sensorineural hearing impairment. In these instances, the conduction level determines how well the child can hear.

Central Auditory Dysfunction Although this child may have normal hearing, damage to or faulty development of the proper brain centers makes the child unable to use the auditory information received.

CLINICAL MANIFESTATIONS

Mild to moderate hearing loss often remains undetected until the child moves outside the family circle into nursery school or kindergarten. The hearing loss may have been gradual, and the child may have become such a skilled lip reader that neither the child nor the family is aware of the partial deafness. Caregivers and teachers should be aware of the possibility of hearing loss in children who appear to be inattentive and noisy and who create disturbances in the classroom.

Certain reactions and mannerisms characterize a child with hearing loss. The child should be observed for an apparent inability to locate a sound and turning of the head to one side when listening. The child who fails to comprehend when spoken to, who gives inappropriate answers to questions, who consistently turns up the volume on the television or radio, or who cannot whisper or talk softly may have hearing loss.

DIAGNOSIS

Children who are profoundly deaf are more likely to be diagnosed before 1 year of age than are children with mild to moderate hearing losses. The child who is suspected of having a hearing loss should be referred for a complete audiologic assessment, including pure-tone audiometric, speech reception, and speech discrimination tests. Children with sensorineural impairment generally have a greater loss of hearing acuity in the high-pitched tones. The loss may vary from slight to complete. Children with a conductive loss are more likely to have equal losses over a wide range of frequencies.

A child's hearing should be tested at all frequencies by a pure-tone audiometer in a soundproof room. Speech reception and speech discrimination tests measure the amount of hearing impairment for both speech and communication. Accurate measurements usually can be made in children as young as 3 years of age if the test is introduced as a game (Fig. 15-1).

Infants and very young children must be tested in a different way. An infant with normal hearing should be able to locate a sound at 28 weeks, imitate sounds at 36 weeks, and associate sounds with people or objects at 1 year of age. A commonly used screening test for very young children uses noisemakers of varying intensity and pitch. The examiner stands beside or behind the child, who has been given a toy. As the examiner produces sounds with a rattle, buzzer, bell, or other noisemaker, a hearing child is distracted and turns to the source of the new sound, whereas a deaf child does not react in a particular way.

Deafness, mental retardation, and autism are sometimes incorrectly diagnosed because the symptoms can be similar. Deaf children may fail to respond to sound or fail to

(text continues on page 308)

TABLE 15-1. Infectious Diseases of Childhood

Disease/ Causative Organism	Incubation	Communicable Period; When/ How	Immunization/ Immunity	Symptoms	Treatment/Nursing Implications	Type of Precautions	Complications
Rubeola (measles) Measles virus	10–21 days	Fifth incubation day until after first few days after rash erupts Direct or indirect contact with droplets	Attenuated live vaccine (part of MMR vaccine); disease gives natural immunity	Occurs in winter or spring; high fever; coryza (runny nose); cough; enlarged lymph nodes (head and neck); Koplik spots (small red spots with blue-white centers on oral mucosa, specific to rubeola); conjunctivitis; photophobia; maculopapular rash starts at hairline and spreads to entire body	Soothing measures for rash include tepid baths, soothing lotion, maintaining dry skin; dimly lighted room for comfort; encouraging fluids	Airborne	Otitis media, pneumonia, encephalitis, airway obstruction
Rubella (German measles) Rubella virus	14–21 days	5–7 days before until about 5 days after rash appears Direct or indirect contact with droplets	Attenuated live vaccine (part of MMR vaccine); disease gives lasting natural immunity	Low-grade fever; malaise; lymph glands of neck and head enlarged; pale small rash, disappears in 3 days	Symptomatic relief	Droplet	Avoid contact with pregnant women; unborn fetus can suffer severe birth deformities if nonimmunized mother is exposed, especially in first trimester.
Parotitis (mumps) Paramyxovirus	14–21 days	Shortly before swelling appears until after it disappears Direct contact, droplet; indirect from contaminated articles	Attenuated live mumps vaccine (part of MMR vaccine); disease gives natural immunity Passive: mumps immune globulin	Parotid glands swollen, unilaterally or bilaterally; may have fever, headache, malaise, and complain of earache before swelling appears; angle of jaw obliterated on affected side	Chewing is painful, so liquids and soft foods are given; sour foods cause discomfort; analgesics for pain; antipyretics for fever; local compresses of heat or cold may be soothing	Droplet	In males past puberty, orchitis (inflammation of the testes); meningoencephalitis; may rarely cause severe hearing impairment

Disease/Organism	Incubation	Period of Communicability/Transmission	Immunity	Signs and Symptoms	Nursing Care/Treatment	Precautions	Complications
Varicella (chickenpox) Varicella zoster virus	10–21 days	1 day before rash appears for about 6 days (until all vesicles crusted over) Direct or indirect contact with saliva or uncrusted vesicles	Lasting natural immunity; may reactivate in adult as herpes zoster; active artificial immunity available	Low-grade fever; malaise; successive crops of macules, papules, vesicles, and crusts, all present at the same time; itching is intense; scarring may occur when scabs are picked off before ready to fall off	Antihistamines to reduce itching; soothing baths and lotions may help; prevent scratching with short fingernails, mittens; acyclovir has been given to shorten the course of the disease. **Aspirin must not be given.**	Airborne, contact	Reye syndrome can occur if child has had aspirin during illness; superinfection of lesions if scratched; encephalitis
Pertussis (whooping cough) Bordetella pertussis	5–21 days	About 4–6 weeks Direct contact, droplet; indirect from contaminated articles	Pertussis vaccine is part of the DPT vaccine; disease gives natural immunity	Begins with mild upper respiratory symptoms; in second week progresses to severe paroxysmal cough with inspiratory whoop, sometimes followed by vomiting; especially dangerous for young infants; may last 4–6 weeks	Bed rest; infants hospitalized; may need oxygen; observe for airway obstruction; provide high humidity; protect from secondary infections; encourage fluid intake; refeed child if vomiting occurs	Droplet	Pneumonia (can cause death of infant); otitis media; hemorrhage; convulsions
Diphtheria Corynebacterium diphtheriae	2–5 days	As long as bacilli are present—2–4 weeks or less with antibiotic therapy Direct contact with infected person, carrier, or contaminated article	Active immunity from diphtheria toxin in DPT vaccine; passive immunity with diphtheria antitoxin	Mucous membranes of nose and throat covered by gray membrane; purulent nasal discharge; brassy cough; toxin from organism passes through blood stream to heart and nervous system	Strict precautions maintained; intravenous antitoxin and antibiotics administered; bed rest; liquid to soft diet; analgesics for throat pain; nonimmunized contacts should be immunized	Contact, droplet	Neuritis; carditis; congestive heart failure; respiratory failure
Poliomyelitis (infantile paralysis) Poliovirus types 1, 2, 3	5–14 days	Variable; 1 week after symptoms for respiratory contact, up to 6 weeks for feces	Trivalent live oral polio vaccine; disease causes active immunity against specific strain	Fever, headache, nausea, vomiting, abdominal pain; stiff neck, pain and tenderness in lower extremities that proceeds to paralysis	Bed rest; moist hot packs to extremities; range-of-motion exercises; supportive care; long-term ventilation if respiratory muscles involved	Standard	Permanent paralysis; respiratory arrest

TABLE 15-2. Levels of Hearing Impairment

Decible Level	Hearing Level Present
Slight (<30 dB)	Unable to hear whispered word or faint speech No speech impairment present May not be aware of hearing difficulty Achieves well in school and home by compensating by leaning forward, speaking loudly
Mild (30–50 dB)	Beginning speech impairment may be present Difficulty hearing if not facing speaker; some difficulty with normal conversation
Moderate (55–75 dB)	Speech impairment present; may require speech therapy Difficulty with normal conversation
Severe (70–90 dB)	Difficulty with any but nearby loud voice Hears vowels easier than consonants Require speech therapy for clear speech May still hear loud sounds such as jets or whistles of a train
Profound (>90 dB)	Hears almost no sound

From Pillitteri A. Maternal and child health nursing. Philadelphia: JB Lippincott. 1995.

Figure 15-1
Hearing testing. Using a game-like model, the child is taught to respond to hearing a sound by taking a toy from the test assistant.

guage, and oral speech (Fig. 15-2). The family members are the child's first teachers, and they must be aware of all phases of development—physical, emotional, social, intellectual, and language—and then seek to aid this development.

A deaf child depends on sight to interpret the environment and to communicate. Thus, it is important to be sure

Figure 15-2
A young deaf boy (wearing hearing aids and an FM amplifier to increase the loudness of his teacher's voice) makes speech sounds into the microphone. As he changes the volume or pitch of the sound, the images on the Speech Viewer screen change. This gives him immediate feedback about his own voice and is very useful in speech development.

develop speech because they cannot hear. Mentally retarded or autistic children may show the same lack of response and development even though they do not have a hearing loss.

TREATMENT AND EDUCATION

When the type and degree of hearing loss have been established, the child, even an infant, may be fitted with a hearing aid. Hearing aids are helpful only in conductive deafness, not in sensorineural or central auditory dysfunction. These devices only amplify sound; they do not localize or clarify it. Many models are available, including those in the ear, behind the ear, incorporated in glasses, or on the body with a wire connection to the ear. FM receiver units are also available that can broadcast the speaker's voice from a greater distance, cutting out the background noise. When the FM transmitter is turned off, this type of unit functions as an ordinary hearing aid.

It is believed that deaf children can best be taught to communicate by a combination of lip reading, sign lanthat the child's vision is normal, and if not, to correct that problem. The probability is twice as great that the child with a hearing loss also will have some vision impairment. Training in the use of all the other senses—sight, smell, taste, and touch—makes the deaf child better able to use any available hearing. It is believed that most deaf children do have some hearing ability.

Preschool classes for deaf children exist in many large communities. These attempt to create an environment in which a deaf child can have the same experiences and activities that normal preschoolers have. Children are generally enrolled at age 2.5 years.

The John Tracy Clinic in Los Angeles, founded in 1943, is dedicated to young children (birth through age 5) born with a severe hearing loss or those who have lost hearing through illness before acquiring speech and language. The Clinic's purpose is "to find, encourage, guide, and train the parents of deaf and hard-of-hearing children, first in order to reach and help the children, and second to help the parents themselves." With early diagnosis and intervention, hearing-impaired children can develop language and communication skills in the critical preschool period that enable many of them to speech-read and to speak. All services to parents and children are free. Full audiologic testing, parent–infant education, demonstration nursery school, parent education classes, and parent groups are offered. Many medical residents, nurses, and allied health care professionals come to observe the model programs at the Clinic to see for themselves the benefits of early diagnosis.

The Clinic also provides a correspondence course for parents. There are three courses available in both English and Spanish: deaf infants, deaf preschoolers, and deaf–blind children. These courses, which include materials and videotapes, guide parents in encouraging their child to develop auditory awareness, speech-reading skills, and expressive language. Information about the Clinic can be obtained by calling toll-free (800) 522-4582.

Free and appropriate education for all disabled children is required by federal law. Children with a hearing loss who cannot successfully function in regular classrooms are provided with supplementary services (speech therapy, speech interpreter, signer) in special classrooms or in a residential school.

NURSING CARE FOR THE DEAF CHILD

When the deaf child is in a health care facility, the child's primary caregiver should be present during the stay, not as a convenience to the nursing staff but to help the child communicate needs and feelings.

The deaf child's anxiety about unfamiliar situations and procedures can be greater than that of the child with normal hearing. When speaking to the deaf child, stand or sit face to face on the child's level. Be certain that a deaf child can see you before you touch him or her. Demonstrate

each procedure before it is performed, showing the child the equipment or pictures of the equipment to be used. Follow demonstrations with explanations to be sure the child understands. Keep a nightlight in the child's room, because sight is a critical sense to the deaf child. To understand the helpless feeling of the child, imagine being in a dark room with no sound.

Hearing aids are expensive, so it is wise to learn how to take care of and maintain them. Put the aid in a safe place when the child is not wearing it. Check linens before putting them into the laundry so as not to discard a hearing aid along with the dirty linens.

Use family members as important resources to learn about the child's habits and communication patterns. Signing classes are available in many communities for those working with hearing-impaired children and adults.

Vision Impairment

Like hearing, good vision is essential to a child's normal development. How well a child sees affects his or her learning process, social development, coordination, and safety. One in 1,000 children of school age has a serious vision impairment. The sooner these impairments are corrected, the better a child's chances for normal or near-normal development.

Children with vision impairments are classified as sighted with eye problems, partially sighted, and legally blind.

TYPES OF VISION IMPAIRMENT

Eye Problems in Sighted Children Among sighted children with eye problems, errors of **refraction** (the way light rays bend as they pass through the lens to the retina) are the most common. About 10% of school-age children have **myopia** (nearsightedness), which means that the child can see objects clearly at close range but not at a distance. When proper lenses are fitted, vision is corrected to normal. If uncorrected, this defect may cause a child to be labeled inattentive or retarded. Myopia tends to be familial and often progresses into adolescence and then levels off.

Hyperopia (farsightedness) is a refractive condition in which the person can see objects better at a distance than close up. It is common in young children and often persists into the first grade or even later. Whether corrective lenses are needed must be decided on an individual basis by the ocular specialist examining the child. Usually, correction is not needed in a preschooler. Teachers and parents should be aware of the considerable eye fatigue that may result from efforts at accommodation for close work.

Astigmatism may occur with or without myopia or hyperopia and is caused by unequal curvatures in the cornea that bend the light rays in different directions, producing a blurred image. Slight astigmatism often does not require

Lighthouse flash-card vision test. This test may be obtained from the New York Association for the Blind, 111 East 59th Street, New York, New York 10022.

Figure 15-3
Home testing kit. This allows the very young preschooler to take the test in more familiar surroundings. The test may be obtained from the National Society to Prevent Blindness, 79 Madison Avenue, New York, NY 10016.

correction; moderate degrees usually require glasses for reading and watching television and movies; severe astigmatism requires glasses at all times.

Partial Sight   Children with partial sight have a visual acuity between 20/20 and 20/200 in the better eye after all necessary medical or surgical correction. These children also have a high incidence of refractive errors, particularly myopia. Eye injuries also cause loss of vision, as do conditions such as cataracts that can be improved by treatment but result in diminished sight.

Blindness   Blindness is legally defined as a corrected vision of 20/200 or less or peripheral vision of less than 20° in the better eye. Many of the causes of blindness have been reduced or eliminated, such as retrolental fibroplasia (due to excessive oxygen concentrations in newborns) and trachoma, a viral infection. Maternal infections are still a common cause of blindness, although the incidence of maternal rubella has decreased because of immunization.

Between the ages of 5 and 7 years, children begin to form and retain visual images; they have memory with pictures. Children who become blind before 5 years of age are missing this crucial element in their development. Blindness can seriously hamper the child's ability to form human attachments, learn coordination, balance, and locomotion, distinguish fantasy from reality, and interpret the surrounding world. How well the blind child learns to cope depends on the family's ability to communicate, teach, and foster a sense of independence in the child.

CLINICAL MANIFESTATIONS AND DIAGNOSIS

Squinting and frowning while trying to read a blackboard or other material at a distance, tearing, red-rimmed eyes, holding work too close to the eyes while reading or writing, and rubbing the eyes are all signs of possible vision impairment. Although blindness is likely to be detected in early infancy, partial sightedness or correctable vision problems may go unrecognized until a child enters school unless vision screening is part of routine health maintenance.

A simple test kit for preschoolers is available for home use by family caregivers or visiting nurses (Fig. 15-3). This kit is an adaptation of the Snellen E chart used for testing children who have not learned to read. The child covers one eye and then points the fingers in the same direction as the "fingers" on each E, beginning with the largest. Some examiners refer to these as "legs on a table."

The Snellen Chart   This is the familiar test in which the letters on each line are smaller than those on the line above. If the child can read the 20-ft line standing 20 ft away from the chart, visual acuity is stated as 20/20. If the child can read only the line marked 100, acuity is stated as 20/100. The chart should be placed at eye level with

good lighting and in a room free from distractions. One eye is tested at a time with the other eye covered. Normal preschool acuity is 20/30.

Picture charts for identification also are used but are not considered as accurate. An intelligent child can memorize the pictures and guess from the general shape without seeing distinctly.

TREATMENT AND EDUCATION

Significant medical and surgical advances have occurred in the treatment of cataracts, strabismus, and amblyopia. The earlier the treatment, the better the child's chances of adequate vision for normal development and function. Errors of refraction are usually correctable. Corrective lenses for minor vision impairments should be prescribed early and checked regularly to be sure they still provide adequate correction.

Children who are partially sighted or totally blind benefit from association with normally sighted children. In most communities, education for these special children is provided within the regular school or in special classes that offer the child more specialized equipment and instruction (Fig. 15-4).

Special equipment includes printed material with large

Figure 15-4
A trip to a farm provides this visually impaired child a chance to experience it—through touch, sound, and smell.

Figure 15-5
Interaction with a stimulating environment is necessary for every child's development. For visually impaired, developmentally delayed, or multi-impaired children, it is often necessary to create special environments to meet unique learning needs. Through the use of a realistic skills table, with a mailbox, door handle with lock and key, and rewired telephone, and various nooks and crannies filled with cherished objects, this child is developing the concept of spatial organization and receiving positive reinforcement about her ability to have an impact on what happens around her.

print, pencils with large leads for darker lines, tape recordings, magnifying glasses, and typewriters. For children with a serious impairment whose participation in regular activities is sharply curtailed, talking books, raised maps, and Braille equipment are needed as well (Fig. 15-5). These devices prevent isolation of the visually impaired child and minimize any differences from the other children.

NURSING CARE FOR THE VISUALLY IMPAIRED CHILD

Children with a visual impairment have the same needs as other children, and these should not be overlooked. The child who is blind needs emotional comfort and sensory stimulation, much of which must be communicated by touch, sound, and smell. It is important for the nurse to explain sounds and other sensations that are new to the child and to let him or her touch the equipment that will be used in procedures. A tactile tour of the room helps orient the child to the location of furniture and other facili-

ties. Awareness of safety hazards is particularly important when caring for the blind or partially sighted child.

Nurses and other personnel must identify themselves when they enter the room and must tell the child when they leave. Explanations of what is going to happen reduce the child's fear and anxiety and the possibility of being startled by an unexpected touch.

The child with a visual impairment should be involved with as many peers and their activities as possible. The child also should be encouraged to be as independent as possible. One step is to provide the child with finger foods and encourage self-feeding after orienting the child to the plate. A small bowl, instead of a plate, is useful so that food can be scooped against the side to get it on the spoon. Eating is a time-consuming and messy affair, but it is essential to the growth of independence in all children.

CENTRAL NERVOUS SYSTEM DISORDERS

Reye Syndrome

Reye syndrome (rhymes with "eye") is characterized by acute encephalopathy and fatty degeneration of the liver and other abdominal organs. It occurs in children of all ages but is seen more in young school-age children than in any other age group. Reye syndrome usually occurs after a viral illness, particularly after varicella (chickenpox) or an upper respiratory infection. Administration of aspirin during the viral illness has been implicated as a contributing factor. As a result, the American Academy of Pediatrics recommends that aspirin or aspirin compounds not be given to children with viral infections.

CLINICAL MANIFESTATIONS

The symptoms appear 1 to 3 weeks after the initial illness. The child is recuperating unremarkably when symptoms of severe vomiting, irritability, lethargy, and confusion occur. Immediate intervention is needed to prevent serious insult to the brain, including respiratory arrest (Table 15-3).

DIAGNOSIS

The history of a viral illness is an immediate clue. Liver function tests, including serum glutamic oxaloacetic transaminase, serum glutamic pyruvic transaminase, lactic dehydrogenase, and serum ammonia levels, are elevated because of poor liver function. The child is hypoglycemic.

TREATMENT AND NURSING CARE

The child with Reye syndrome is often cared for in the intensive care unit because the disease may rapidly progress. Medical management focuses on supportive mea-

TABLE 15-3. Staging of Reye Syndrome

Clinical Grade		Symptoms
I	Mild–moderate	Usually quiet or mild lethargy
II		Deep lethargy, confusion; possibly brief unconsciousness
III		Extreme lethargy or light coma lasting <2 hours; possibly seizures or agitation
IV	Severe	Seizures; possibly agitation and combativeness; usually protracted deep coma lasting >3 hours; intermittent decerebrate posturing
V		Seizures; deep coma; decerebrate posturing; fixed pupils

Adapted from Novak DA, Suchy FJ, Baliteri WF. Reye's syndrome. In Oski FA, DeAngelis CD, Feigin RD, McMillan JA, Warshaw JB, eds. Principles and practice of pediatrics, 2d ed. Philadelphia: JB Lippincott, 1994.

sures—improving respiratory function, reducing cerebral edema, and controlling hypoglycemia. The specific treatment is determined by the staging of the symptoms. The nurse carefully observes the child for overall physical status and any change in neurologic status. This is essential in evaluating the progression of the illness. Accurate intake and output determinations are necessary to determine when fluids need to be adjusted to control cerebral edema and prevent dehydration. Osmotic diuretics (eg, mannitol) may be administered to reduce cerebral edema. The nurse monitors the blood glucose level and bleeding time. Low blood glucose levels can lead to seizures quickly in young children, and a prolonged bleeding time can indicate coagulation problems as a result of liver dysfunction.

This hospitalization period is a traumatic time for the family. The nurse must give the family opportunities to deal with their feelings. In addition, the family must be kept well informed about the child's care. Having a child in intensive care is a frightening experience, and every effort must be made to reassure the family with sincerity and honesty.

Since the American Academy of Pediatrics made its recommendation to avoid giving aspirin to children, especially during viral illnesses, there has been a steady decrease in the number of cases of Reye syndrome. The prognosis of children with Reye syndrome is greatly improved with early diagnosis and vigorous treatment. The nurse is responsible for teaching families with young children to avoid the use of aspirin.

Cerebral Palsy

Cerebral palsy (CP) is a group of disorders arising from a malfunction of motor centers and neural pathways in the brain. It is one of the most complex of the common permanent disabling conditions and often can be accompanied by seizures, mental retardation, sensory defects, and behavior disorders. Research in this area is directed at adapting biomedical technology to help people with cerebral palsy cope with the activities of daily living and achieve maximum function and independence.

CAUSES

Although the cause of CP cannot be identified in many cases, there are several possible causes. It may be caused by damage to the parts of the brain that control movement; this damage generally occurs during the fetal or perinatal period, particularly in premature infants.

Common *prenatal* causes are:

- Any process that interferes with the oxygen supply to the brain, such as separation of the placenta, compression of the cord, or bleeding
- Maternal infection (eg, cytomegalovirus, toxoplasmosis, rubella)
- Nutritional deficiencies that may affect brain growth
- Kernicterus (brain damage caused by jaundice) resulting from Rh incompatibility
- Teratogenic factors such as drugs and radiation.

Common *perinatal* causes are:

- Anoxia immediately before, during, and after birth
- Intracranial bleeding
- Asphyxia or interference with respiratory function
- Maternal analgesia (eg, morphine) that depresses the sensitive neonate's respiratory center
- Birth trauma
- Prematurity, because immature blood vessels predispose the neonate to cerebral hemorrhage.

About 10% to 20% occur after birth. Common *postnatal* causes (responsible for 10%–20% of cases) are:

- Head trauma (eg, due to a fall, motor vehicle accident)
- Infection (eg, encephalitis, meningitis)
- Neoplasms
- Cerebrovascular accident.

PREVENTION

Because brain damage in CP is irreversible, prevention is the most important aspect of care. Prevention of CP focuses on:

- Prenatal care to improve nutrition, prevent infection, and decrease the incidence of prematurity
- Perinatal monitoring with appropriate interventions to decrease birth trauma

- Postnatal prevention of infection through breast-feeding, improved nutrition, and immunizations
- Protection from trauma of motor vehicle accidents, child abuse, and other childhood accidents.

CLINICAL MANIFESTATIONS AND TYPES

Difficulty in controlling voluntary muscle movements is one manifestation of the central nervous system damage. Seizures, mental retardation, hearing and vision impairments, and behavior disorders often accompany the major problem. Delayed gross motor development, abnormal motor performance (eg, poor sucking and feeding behaviors), abnormal postures, and persistence of primitive reflexes are other signs of CP. Diagnosis of CP seldom occurs before 2 months of age and may be delayed until the second or third year, until walking is attempted and an obvious lag in motor development is evident. Diagnosis is based on observations of delayed growth and development through a process that rules out other diagnoses.

There are several major types of CP, each with distinctive clinical manifestations.

Spastic Type   This is the most common type and is characterized by:

- A hyperactive stretch reflex in associated muscle groups
- Increased activity of the deep tendon reflexes
- Clonus (rapid involuntary muscle contraction and relaxation)
- Contractures affecting the extensor muscles, especially the heel cord
- Scissoring caused by severe hip adduction. When scissoring is present, the child's legs are crossed and the toes are pointed down, so the child is standing on the toes. It is difficult for this child to walk on the heels or run.

Athetoid Type   Athetoid CP is marked by involuntary, incoordinate motion with varying degrees of muscle tension. Children with this disorder are constantly in motion, and the whole body is in a state of slow, writhing muscle contractions whenever voluntary movement is attempted. Facial grimacing, poor swallowing, and tongue movements causing drooling and dysarthria (poor speech articulation) are also present. These children are likely to have average or above-average intelligence, despite their abnormal appearance. Hearing loss is most common in this group.

Ataxia Type   Ataxia is essentially a lack of coordination caused by disturbances in the kinesthetic and balance senses. The least common type of CP, ataxia may not be diagnosed until the child starts to walk: the gait is awkward and wide-based.

Rigidity Type   This type is uncommon and is characterized by rigid postures and lack of active movement.

Mixed Type   Children with signs of more than one type of CP are usually severely disabled. The disorder may have been caused by postnatal injury.

DIAGNOSIS

Children with CP may not be diagnosed with certainty until they have difficulties when attempting to walk. They may show signs of mental retardation, attention deficit disorder, or recurrent convulsions. Computed tomography, magnetic resonance imaging, and, in infants, before closure of skull sutures, ultrasonography may be used to help determine the cause of CP.

TREATMENT AND SPECIAL AIDS

Treatment of CP focuses on helping the child make the best use of residual abilities and achieve maximum satisfaction and enrichment in life. A team of health care professionals—physician, surgeon, physical therapist, occupational therapist, speech therapist, and perhaps a social worker—works with the family to set realistic goals. Dental care is important because enamel hypoplasia is common, and children whose seizure disorders are controlled with phenytoin (Dilantin) are likely to develop gingival hypertrophy. Medications such as baclofen, diazepam, and dantrolene may be used to help decrease spasticity.

Physical Therapy   Control of the body needed for purposeful physical activity is learned automatically by a normal child but must be consciously learned by a child who has problems with physical mobility (Fig. 15-6). Physical therapists attempt to teach the child activities of daily living that the child has been unable to accomplish. Methods must be suited to the needs of each child as well as to the general needs arising from the condition. These methods are based on principles of conditioning, relaxation, use of residual patterns, stimulation of contraction and relaxation of antagonistic muscles, and others. Various techniques are used. Because there are many variations in the disabilities caused by CP, each child must be evaluated individually and treated appropriately.

Orthopedic Management   Braces are used as supportive and control measures to facilitate muscle training, to reinforce weak or paralyzed muscles, or to counteract the pull of antagonistic muscles. Various types are available, each designed for a specific purpose. Orthopedic surgery sometimes is used to improve function and correct deformities, such as the release of contractures and the lengthening of tight heel cords.

Technologic Aids for Daily Living   Biomedical engineering, particularly in the field of electronics, has per-

Figure 15-6
During a physical therapy session, this boy with CP works hard to take a step forward. His mom stays by his side to encourage him.

fected a number of devices to help make the disabled person more functional and less dependent on others. The devices range from simple items, such as wheelchairs and specially constructed toilet seats, to completely electronic cottages furnished with a computer (even including a voice synthesizer), a tape recorder, a calculator, and other equipment that facilitates independence and useful study or work. Many of these devices can be controlled by a mouth stick, an extremely useful feature for people with poor hand coordination.

A child who has difficulty maintaining balance while sitting may need a high-backed chair with side pieces and a foot platform. Feeding may be a challenge. Feeding aids include spoons with enlarged handles for easy grasping or with bent handles that allow the spoon to be brought easily to the mouth (Fig. 15-7). Plates with high rims and suction devices to prevent slipping enable a child to eat with little assistance. Covered cups set in holders, with a hole in the lid to admit a straw, help a child who does not have hand control. A nasogastric or gastrostomy tube may be necessary for the severely disabled child.

Manual skill can be aided by games, such as pegboards and cards, that must be manipulated. Keyboarding is an ego-boosting alternative for a child whose disability is too severe to permit legible writing. Computer programs have been designed to enable these children to communicate and improve their learning skills. Special keyboards, joysticks, and electronic devices help the child have fun and gain a sense of achievement while learning. Computers also

Figure 15-7
Feeding techniques to promote jaw control.

have expanded the opportunities for future employment for these children.

NURSING CARE

The child with CP may be seen in the health care setting at any age level. Assess the child and the family to determine the child's needs, the level of development, and the stage of family acceptance and to set realistic long-range goals. The newly diagnosed child and family may have more potential nursing diagnoses than the child and family who have been successfully dealing with CP for a long time.

To ease the change of environment, the nurse needs to assess the family to learn as much as possible about the child's activities at home. The child should be encouraged to maintain current self-care activities and set goals for attaining new ones. Positioning to prevent contractures, providing modified feeding utensils, and suggesting appropriate educational play activities are all important aspects of the child's care. If the child has been admitted for surgery, the child and family need appropriate preoperative and postoperative teaching, emotional support, and assistance in setting realistic expectations. The family may need help in exploring educational opportunities for the child.

Like any chronic condition, CP can become a devastating drain on the family's emotional and financial resources. The child's future depends on many variables: family attitudes, economic and therapeutic resources, the child's intelligence, and the availability of competent, understanding health care professionals. Some children, given the emotional and physical support they need, can achieve a satisfactory degree of independence. Some have been able to attend college and find fulfilling work. Vocational training is also available to an increasing number of these young people. Some people with CP will always need a significant amount of nursing care, with the possibility of institutionalized care when their family can no longer care for them.

The outlook for these children and their families is improving, but a great deal of work must be done. Working as a community member, the health care professional can play a vital role in promoting educational opportunities, rehabilitation, and acceptance for disabled children.

Mental Retardation

Mental retardation is defined in the American Psychiatric Association's *Diagnostic and Statistical Manual, Fourth Edition, Revised* using two criteria: significantly subaverage general intellectual functioning—an intelligence quotient (IQ) of 70 or lower—and concurrent deficits in adaptive functioning. *Adaptive functioning* refers to how well people can meet the standards of independence (activities of daily living) and social responsibility expected of them for their age and the cultural group to which they belong. Mental retardation often occurs in combination with other physical disorders.

A Personal Glimpse

The mother of a developmentally delayed child knows her child has a problem before any doctor notices. Visually my son looked perfect. There were no outward signs of retardation. He was a beautiful baby but he was often ill—severe croup, pneumonia, bronchitis, grand mal seizures due to fever, hospital stays, EEGs, spinal taps, tests and more tests—but he always bounced back, much better than his parents recovered.

Slowly I started to notice that he was not the same as other kids his age. His vocabulary was Mom and DaDa where other 3-year-olds were starting to put words together into little sentences. Everyone said he didn't talk because I spoiled him and got him everything he needed before he asked for it. I would try to believe people, including doctors, who would say, "Don't worry; you are just being an overprotective mother. Your son will be fine." You try to hide from the truth but slowly you realize you have to get others to see what you see. You have to get help for your child—someone has to listen to you.

Finally I forced my pediatrician to try some physical dexterity tests. My son failed these tests. I heard the doctor say the words that broke my heart: "I am sorry. I thought you were just another hysterical mother—but there is something wrong with your child. We must schedule him for more testing." Then I cried.

Patricia

CAUSES

Many factors can cause mental retardation. *Prenatal* causes include:

- Inborn errors of metabolism, such as phenylketonuria, galactosemia, or congenital hypothyroidism. Damage often can be prevented by early detection and treatment.
- Prenatal infection, such as toxoplasmosis or cytomegalovirus. Microcephaly, hydrocephalus, cerebral palsy, and other brain damage can result from intrauterine infections.

- Teratogenic agents, such as drugs, radiation, and alcohol, can have devastating effects on the central nervous system of a developing fetus.
- Genetic factors—inborn variations of chromosomal patterns—result in a variety of deviations, the most common of which is Down syndrome.

Perinatal causes of mental retardation include birth trauma, anoxia from various causes, prematurity, and difficult birth. In some instances, prenatal factors may have influenced the perinatal complications.

Postnatal causes include:

- Poisoning, such as lead poisoning. Children who develop encephalopathy from chronic lead poisoning usually have significant brain damage.
- Infections and trauma, such as meningitis, convulsive disorders, and hydrocephalus
- Impoverished early environment, such as inadequate nutrition and a lack of sensory stimulation. Emotional rejection in early life may do irreparable damage to a child's ability to respond to the environment.

THE MENTALLY RETARDED CHILD

About 3% of all children born in the United States have some level of cognitive impairment. About 20% of these are so severely retarded that diagnosis is made at birth or during the first year. Most of the other children are diagnosed as retarded when they begin school.

The most common classification of mental retardation is based on IQ. Although controversy exists about the validity of tests that measure intelligence, this system is still the most useful for grouping these children.

The child with an IQ of 70 to 50 is considered mildly mentally retarded. This child is a slow learner but can acquire basic skills. The child can learn to read, write, and do arithmetic to a fourth- or fifth-grade level but is slower than average in learning to walk, talk, and feed himself or herself. Retardation may not be obvious to casual acquaintances. With support and guidance, this child usually can develop social and vocational skills that are adequate for self-maintenance. About 80% of retarded children are classified in this category.

The moderately retarded child, with an IQ of 55 to 35, has little, if any, ability to attain independence and academic skills and is referred to as *trainable*. Motor development and speech are noticeably delayed, but training in self-help activities is possible. This child may be able to learn repetitive skills in sheltered workshops. Some children may learn to travel alone, but few become capable of assuming complete self-maintenance. This category accounts for about 10% of retarded children.

The child considered severely retarded tests in the IQ range of 40 to 20. This child's development is markedly delayed during the first year of life. The child cannot learn academic skills but may be able to learn some self-care activities if sensorimotor stimulation is begun early. Eventually, this child will probably learn to walk and develop some speech; however, a sheltered environment and careful supervision always will be required.

The profoundly retarded child has an IQ lower than 20. This child has minimal capacity for functioning and needs continuing care. Eventually, the child may learn to walk and develop a primitive speech but will never be able to perform self-care activities. Only about 1% of retarded children are in this category.

TEACHING AND EDUCATION

Knowledge about teaching children with cognitive impairment has increased dramatically, and new teaching methods have been yielding encouraging results. Mildly and moderately retarded people are taught to perform tasks that enable them to achieve some degree of independence and usefulness. More and better services are being provided for all cognitively impaired children and adults.

The child with cognitive impairment may not be identified until well into the preschool stage. Slow development often can be excused in one way or another. The family may be the best judge of the child's development, and health care personnel must listen carefully to any concerns or questions they express.

When family members are faced with the fact that their child is retarded, they need to go through a grieving process, as do family members of any other child with a serious disorder. They need to mourn the loss of the normal child that was expected and resolve to give this child the best opportunities to develop his or her potential.

Early diagnosis and intervention are important tools to use in the care of the cognitively impaired child. Early infant tests are difficult to administer, and the results are inaccurate, but they may provide the family with some idea about the possible potential of the child. The family must be aware that these are only predictions based on unreliable test data.

The child is usually kept at home in the family environment. The current philosophy of care for such a child is to approach teaching in an aggressive manner, encouraging learning in a supportive home environment where the child can relate closely to a few people whose role is to stimulate and encourage maximum development. The individual attention, security, and sense of belonging to a family are important factors in every child's growth and development.

◥ ◤ *Nursing Process for the Child With* ◣ ◢ *Cognitive Impairment*

ASSESSMENT

The child who has a cognitive impairment is seen in the health care setting for diagnosis, treatment, and follow-up, as well as for the usual health maintenance visits that any child has. During these visits, health care personnel may be challenged to communicate with the child. A thorough assessment accomplished through an interview with the child's caregiver can be helpful. Listen carefully to the caregiver, paying particular attention to any comments or concerns he or she has.

The assessment may be lengthy and detailed, depending partially on the circumstances of the child's primary need for health care. Aside from the assessment dictated by the current health care needs, the nurse also needs information about the child's habits, routines, and personal terminology (such as nicknames and toileting terms). Be careful to communicate at the child's level of understanding, and do not talk down to the child during the assessment interview. Treat the child with respect. This approach helps gain cooperation from both the family and the child. Arrange the assessment interview so that it can be conducted in an unhurried atmosphere to avoid placing undue stress on the child or the family.

NURSING DIAGNOSES

The appropriate nursing diagnoses vary with the primary health care needs of the child. Often, the child with mental retardation also has physical disabilities that must be considered when a plan of care is being developed. Work with the child's caregiver to set goals that are realistic for the child. Some nursing diagnoses that are useful for the child with cognitive impairment are:

- Self Care Deficit in Bathing/Hygiene, Dressing/Grooming, Feeding, and Toileting related to cognitive or neuromuscular impairment (or both)
- Impaired Verbal Communication related to impaired receptive or expressive skills
- Altered Growth and Development related to physical and mental disability
- Risk for Injury related to physical or neurologic impairment (or both)
- Ineffective Family Coping: Compromised related to emotional stress or grief
- Risk for Social Isolation (family or child) related to fear of and embarrassment about the child's behavior or appearance

OUTCOME IDENTIFICATION AND PLANNING

The major goals for the cognitively impaired child depend entirely on the child's abilities, as assessed during the assessment interview. Common goals include learning self-care (within the child's ability), communicating with caregivers and nurses, and remaining free from injury. The goals for the family include learning new methods of working with the child, finding support and guidance, and learning about available resources.

IMPLEMENTATION

PROMOTING SELF-CARE. Teaching the mentally retarded child can be time-consuming, frustrating, challenging, and rewarding. When the child is admitted, design a teaching program that reflects his or her developmental level. Be certain that all personnel who care for the child and any involved family members are aware of the program. Break each element of care to be taught into small segments, and repeat them over and over. Patience is one of the most important aspects of teaching a mentally retarded child. Use praise generously, and give small material rewards as useful tools to aid in teaching. Challenge the child, but make the immediate small goals realistic and attainable. Brushing teeth, brushing or combing the hair, bathing, washing the hands and face, feeding oneself, dressing independently, and basic safety are all self-care areas in which the child needs instruction and positive reinforcement.

Teaching the cognitively impaired child requires the same principles used in teaching any child: work at a level appropriate to the stage of the child's maturation, not the chronologic age. If the child has physical disabilities in addition to retardation, the rate of physical development is also affected. One factor that makes the child with cognitive impairment different from the average child is the lack of ability to reason abstractly. This prevents transfer of learning or application of abstract principles to varied situations. Learning takes place by habit formation, emphasizing the "three R's": routine, repetition, and relaxation. Most cognitively impaired children increase in mental age, although slowly and to a limited level. Therefore, each child needs to be watched for evidence of readiness for a new skill.

Environmental stimulation is essential for development in all children, but the cognitively impaired child needs much more environmental enrichment than the average child. Suggested activities for providing this enrichment are summarized in Table 15-4.

Whether at home or in a health care facility, the child with cognitive impairment needs to know which behaviors are acceptable and which are unacceptable. Discipline is as important to this child as to any other. The limited ability of these children to adapt to varying circumstances makes it essential that discipline be consistent, with instructions given in simple, direct, concise language. Using a positive approach, with many examples and demonstrations, achieves better results than a constant stream of "don't touch" or "stop that."

Obedience is an important part of discipline, especially for the child with faulty reasoning ability, but the objectives of discipline should be much broader. The child needs to know what to expect and finds security and support in routines and consistency. Use kindness, love, understanding, and physical comforting as a major part of discipline.

If discipline is needed, be certain it follows the misdeed immediately so that the cause-and-effect relation is made

TABLE 15-4. Examples of Developmental Stimulation and Sensorimotor Teaching for Retarded Infants and Young Children

Developmental Sequence	Possible Activities to Encourage Development
Sitting	
1. Sit with support in caretaker's lap	Hold child in sitting position on lap, supporting under armpits. Do several times a day, gradually lessening the support.
2. Sit independently when propped	Place child in sitting position against firm surface with pillow behind the back and on either side. Leave the child alone several times a day.
3. Sit with increasingly less support	Allow child to sit on equipment that provides increasingly less support, such as baby swing, feeder, walker, high chair.
4. Sit in chair without assistance	Place child in a chair with arms. Provide balance support at first, then gradually withdraw. Leave for 10 minutes at a time.
5. Sit without support	Place child on floor. Gradually withdraw assistance.
Self-Feeding	
1. Sucking	Encourage child to suck by putting food on pacifier, putting a drop on tongue, and so forth.
2. Drink from a cup	Put small amount of fluid in a baby cup. Raise cup to mouth by placing hands under child.
3. Grasp piece of food and place in mouth	Place bit of favorite food in child's hand. Guide hand and food to mouth. Gradually reduce support.
4. Transfer food from spoon to mouth	Move spoon to child's mouth with hand supporting baby's. Gradually withdraw support.
5. Scoop up food and transfer to mouth	Have child hold spoon by handle, scoop up food, and transfer to mouth. Do not allow child to use fingers. Progress from bowl to flat plate.
Stimulation of Touch	
1. Body sensation	Hold, cuddle, rock child.
2. Explore environment through touch	Brush skin with objects of various textures (feathers, silk, sandpaper). Place objects of different textures near child. Move hand to object.
3. Explore environment through mouth	Give child objects that can be chewed. Guide hand to mouth at first.
4. Explore tactile sensations	Expose child to hard, soft, warm, and cold objects.
5. Explore with water	Place hands or feet in water.

Adapted from Johnson V, Werner R. A step-by-step learning guide for retarded infants and children. Syracuse: Syracuse University Press, 1975; and Eddington C, Lee T. Sensory-motor stimulation for slow to develop children. Am J Nurs 75(1):59–62, 1975.

clear. Taking the child away from the group for a short time may help restore self-control. Retaliation can confuse and anger the child. If the child is using misbehavior to get attention, praise and approval for good behavior may eliminate the need for wrongdoing.

FOSTERING COMMUNICATION SKILLS. The child with cognitive impairment often has major problems with language skills. The child may have problems forming various speech sounds because of an enlarged tongue or other physical deviations, including hearing impairment. These problems can frustrate attempts at communication. In addition, the child may not be able to process the words that have been spoken, which compounds communication problems. A speech therapist can evaluate the child and develop a program to help caregivers work with the child to improve both the child's understanding of what is said and the child's ability to use language.

PROMOTING GROWTH AND DEVELOPMENT. The child with cognitive impairment often has physical disabilities that affect growth and development. All but the most profoundly impaired children go through the sequence of normal development, with delays at each stage and leveling off of ability as they reach the limits of their capabilities. A cognitively impaired child proceeds according to mental age rather than chronologic age. Thus, an impaired 6-year-old may be functioning on a mental level of 2 years, and the expected behavior must be essentially that of a 2-year-old. Teach the family caregivers about the important landmarks of normal growth and development to help them understand the progressive nature of maturation and to improve planning for the child.

PREVENTING INJURY. The child with cognitive impairment has faulty reasoning ability and a short attention span. As a result, the caregivers must be responsible for protecting the child. The health care facility as well as the home must be made safe. Teach elementary safety rules and reinforce them continuously.

PROMOTING FAMILY COPING. Before effective treatment can begin, the family must accept the reality of the child's problem and must want to cope with the difficult task of helping the child develop his or her full potential. Diagnosis made at birth or during the first year affords the greatest hope of early acceptance and beginning education and training.

The family's first reaction to learning that the child may have cognitive impairment is grief—this is not the perfect child of their dreams. A parent may feel shame, assuming that he or she cannot produce a perfect child. Some rejection of the child is almost inevitable, at least in the initial stages, but this must be worked through for the family to cope. Some parents compensate for their early hostile feelings by overprotection or overconcern, making the child unnecessarily helpless and perhaps taking out their anger and frustration on the normal siblings. Only when the family accepts the child as another member of the family, to be helped, loved, and disciplined as the others, can they begin to function effectively.

PREVENTING SOCIAL ISOLATION. The family needs to know that their feelings are normal. Talking with other families of impaired children can offer some of the best support and guidance as they seek information to help them deal with the problem. One group that includes both families and health care professionals is the National Association of Retarded Citizens, a volunteer organization with chapters in many communities. The National Down Syndrome Society is an excellent resource for the family of a child with Down syndrome. Participating in the Special Olympics is a good way for children to begin to gain self-confidence.

EVALUATION: GOALS AND OUTCOME CRITERIA

- *Goal*: The child will practice basic hygiene habits.
  Criteria: The child practices basic hygiene habits within his or her abilities with support and supervision.

- *Goal*: The child's communication will improve.
  Criteria: The child can communicate basic needs to staff and family.

- *Goal*: Family caregivers will demonstrate knowledge of normal growth and development.
  Criteria: Family caregivers identify the child's developmental level and set realistic goals.

- *Goal*: The child will be protected from injury by caregivers and will learn basic safety rules.

Criteria: The child remains free from injury and cooperates with basic safety rules within his or her abilities.

- *Goal*: The family will effectively cope with the child's diagnosis.
  Criteria: The family verbalizes feelings to the nurse, mourns the loss of the "perfect child," and provides appropriate care to help the child reach optimum functioning.

- *Goal*: The family will interact with social groups and support networks.
  Criteria: The family freely voices feelings and concerns about the child to the staff, makes contact with support systems, and establishes relationships with families of other cognitively impaired children.

Down Syndrome

Down syndrome is the most common chromosomal anomaly, occurring in about one in 700 to 1,000 births. The condition was first described by Langdon Down in 1866, but its cause was a mystery for many years. In 1932, it was suggested that a chromosomal anomaly might be the cause, but the anomaly was not demonstrated until 1959.

Down syndrome has been observed in nearly all countries and races. The old term "mongolism" is inappropriate and no longer used. Most people with Down syndrome have trisomy 21 (see Fig. 6-6 in Chap. 6); a few have partial dislocation of chromosomes 15 and 21. Women older than 35 years of age are at a greater risk of bearing a child with Down syndrome, but children with Down syndrome are born to women of all ages. Older women are more likely to choose to have an amniocentesis to determine if they are carrying a child with Down syndrome and may decide to have an abortion. The growing trend toward routine screening of all pregnant women for an elevated maternal serum alpha-fetoprotein level may reduce the number of children with Down syndrome who are born because the parents have the option to abort the pregnancy.

CLINICAL MANIFESTATIONS

All forms of the condition show a variety of abnormal characteristics. Mental status is usually within the moderate to severe range of retardation, with most children being moderately retarded. The most common anomalies include:

- **Brachycephaly** (shortness of head)
- Retarded body growth
- Upward and outward slanted eyes (almond-shaped) with an epicanthic fold at the inner angle
- Short, flattened bridge of the nose
- Thick, fissured tongue
- Dry, cracked, fissured skin that may be mottled
- Hair may be dry and coarse

- Hands are short, with an incurved fifth finger
- A single palmar crease
- Wide space between the first and second toes
- Lax muscle tone (often referred to as "double jointed" by others)
- Heart and eye anomalies
- Susceptibility to leukemia greater than in the general population.

Not all of these physical signs are present in all people with Down syndrome. Some may have only one or two characteristics; others may show nearly all of them (Fig. 15-8).

TREATMENT AND CARE

The physical characteristics of the child with Down syndrome determine the medical and nursing management. Lax muscles, congenital heart defects, and dry skin contribute to a large variety of problems. The child's relaxed muscle tone may contribute to respiratory complications as a result of decreased respiratory expansion. The relaxed skeletal muscles contribute to late motor development. Gastric motility is also decreased, leading to problems with constipation. Congenital heart defects and vision or hearing problems add to the complexities of the child's care.

In infancy, the child's large tongue and poor muscle tone may contribute to difficulty breast-feeding or ingesting formula and can cause great problems when the time comes to introduce solid foods. The family caregivers need support during these trying times. As the child gets older, concerns about excessive weight gain become a primary consideration.

Figure 15-8
Typical facial features of a child with Down syndrome.

The family caregivers of the Down syndrome child and other children who are cognitively impaired need strong support and guidance from the time the child is born. Early intervention programs have yielded some encouraging results, but the family must decide whether they can manage the child at home. A cognitively impaired child who is undisciplined or improperly supervised may threaten the safety of others in the home and the neighborhood. Caring for the child may demand so much sacrifice from other family members that the family eventually disintegrates.

RESPIRATORY SYSTEM DISORDERS

Tonsillitis

Tonsillitis is a common illness in childhood, resulting from pharyngitis. A brief description of the location and functions of the tonsils and adenoids serves as an introduction to the discussion of their infection and medical and surgical treatment.

A ring of lymphoid tissue encircles the pharynx, forming a protective barrier against upper respiratory infection. This ring consists of groups of lymphoid tonsils.

The faucial tonsils, the commonly known **tonsils**, are two oval masses attached to the side walls of the back of the mouth between the anterior and posterior pillars. The pharyngeal tonsils, known as the **adenoids**, are masses of lymphoid tissue in the nasal pharynx, extending from the roof of the nasal pharynx to the free edge of the soft palate. The lingual tonsils are two masses of lymphoid tissue at the base of the tongue.

There is a normal progression of enlargement of lymphoid tissue in childhood between the ages of 2 and 10 years and reduction during preadolescence. If the tissue itself becomes a site of acute or chronic infection, it may become hypertrophied and can interfere with breathing, may cause partial deafness, or may become a source of infection in itself.

CLINICAL MANIFESTATIONS AND DIAGNOSIS

The child with tonsillitis may have a fever of 101°F (38.4°C) or more, a sore throat, often with dysphagia (difficulty swallowing), hypertrophied tonsils, and erythema of the soft palate. There may be exudate visible on the tonsils. The symptoms vary somewhat with the causative organism. Throat cultures are performed to diagnose tonsillitis and the causative organism. Frequently, the cause of tonsillitis is viral, although β-hemolytic streptococcal infection also may be the cause.

TREATMENT

Medical treatment of tonsillitis consists of analgesics for pain, antipyretics for fever, and, in the case of streptococcal infection, an antibiotic. A standard 10-day course of antibiotics is recommended. Stress the importance of completing the full prescription of antibiotic to ensure that the streptococcal infection is eliminated. A soft or liquid diet is easier to swallow, and the child should be encouraged to maintain good fluid intake. A cool-mist vaporizer may be used to ease respirations.

Tonsillectomies and adenoidectomies are controversial. One can be performed independent of the other, but they are often done together. No conclusive evidence has been found that a tonsillectomy, in itself, improves a child's health by reducing the number of respiratory infections, increasing the appetite, or improving general well-being. Currently, tonsillectomies generally are not performed unless other measures are ineffective or the tonsils are so hypertrophied that breathing and eating are difficult. Tonsillectomies are not performed while the tonsils are infected.

The adenoids are more susceptible to chronic infection. An indication for adenoidectomy is hypertrophy of the tissue to the extent of impairing hearing or interfering with breathing. An increasingly common practice is to perform only an adenoidectomy if the tonsil tissue appears to be healthy.

Tonsillectomy is postponed until after the age of 4 or 5 years, except in the rare instance when it appears urgently needed. Often, when a child has reached the acceptable age, the apparent need for the tonsillectomy has disappeared.

⬥⬥ Nursing Process for the Child Having a Tonsillectomy

ASSESSMENT

Much of the presurgical preparation, including complete blood count, bleeding and clotting time, and urinalysis, is often done on a preadmission outpatient basis. In many facilities, the child is admitted on the day of surgery. Psychological preparation is often accomplished through preadmission orientation. Acting out the forthcoming experience, particularly in a group, with the use of puppets, dolls, and play-doctor or play-nurse material helps the child develop security. The amount and the timing of preparation before admission depend on the child's age. The child may become frightened about losing a body part. Telling the child that the troublesome tonsils are going to be "fixed" is a much better choice than saying that they are going to be "taken out."

Include the child and the caregiver in the admission assessment. Ask about any bleeding tendencies, since postoperative bleeding is a concern. Carefully explain all procedures to the child, and be sensitive to the child's apprehension. Take and record vital signs to establish a baseline for postoperative monitoring. The temperature is an important part of the assessment to determine that the child has no upper respiratory infection. Assess the child for loose teeth that could cause a problem during administration of anesthesia.

NURSING DIAGNOSES

Use the information gathered in the assessment to determine appropriate nursing diagnoses. Preoperative nursing diagnoses are generally those for any child undergoing a surgical procedure. Postoperative nursing diagnoses may include:

- Risk for Aspiration postoperatively related to unswallowed saliva and bleeding at the operative site
- Risk for Fluid Volume Deficit related to inadequate oral intake secondary to painful swallowing
- Pain related to surgical procedure
- Risk for Altered Health Maintenance related to caregivers' knowledge deficit about postdischarge care

OUTCOME IDENTIFICATION AND PLANNING

The major postoperative goals for the child include preventing aspiration, improving fluid intake, and relieving pain, especially while swallowing. The major goal for the family is to increase knowledge and understanding of postdischarge care. Design the plan of care with these goals in mind.

IMPLEMENTATION

PREVENTING ASPIRATION POSTOPERATIVELY.
Immediately after a tonsillectomy, place the child in a partially prone position, head turned to one side, until the child is completely awake. This position can be accomplished by turning the child partially over and by flexing the knee on which the child is not resting to help maintain the position. Avoid placing pillows under the chest and abdomen, as this may hamper respiration. Encourage the child to expectorate all secretions, and provide an ample supply of tissues and a waste container close by. Discourage the child from coughing. Check vital signs every 10 to 15 minutes until the child is fully awake, then every 30 minutes or 1 hour. Note the child's preoperative baseline vital signs to interpret the vital signs correctly.

Hemorrhage is the most common complication of tonsillectomy. Observe, document, and report any unusual restlessness or anxiety, frequent swallowing, or rapid pulse, which may indicate bleeding. Vomiting of dark, old blood may be expected, but bright, red-flecked emesis or oozing indicates fresh bleeding. Observe the pharynx with a flashlight each time vital signs are checked.

ENCOURAGING FLUID INTAKE. When the child is fully awake from surgery, give small amounts of clear fluids or ice chips. Synthetic juices, carbonated beverages that are "flat," and juice popsicles are good choices. Avoid red liquids to eliminate confusion with bloody discharge. Also avoid irritating liquids such as orange juice and lemonade. Milk and ice cream products tend to cling to the surgical site and make swallowing more difficult; thus, they are poor choices, despite the old tradition of offering ice cream after a tonsillectomy. Continue administration of intravenous fluid and record intake and output until adequate oral intake is established.

PROVIDING COMFORT AND RELIEVING PAIN. Apply an ice collar postoperatively; however, if the child is uncomfortable with it, remove the collar. Administer pain medication as ordered. Liquid acetaminophen with codeine is often prescribed. Rectal or intravenous analgesics may be used. Encourage the caregiver to remain at the bedside to provide soothing reassurance. Crying irritates the raw throat and increases the child's discomfort; thus, it should be avoided, if possible. Tell the caregiver what may be expected in drainage and signs that should be reported immediately to the nursing staff.

PROVIDING FAMILY TEACHING. The child is typically discharged on the day after surgery if no complications are present. Instruct the caregiver to keep the child relatively quiet for a few days after discharge. Recommend giving soft foods and nonirritating liquids for the first few days. Advise the caregivers that a transient earache may be expected about the third day. See Nursing Care Plan for the Child Having a Tonsillectomy.

EVALUATION: GOALS AND OUTCOME CRITERIA

- *Goal*: The child will not aspirate postoperatively.
  Criteria: The child expectorates saliva and drainage with no breathing difficulties. No evidence of bleeding is noted.

- *Goal*: The child will have an adequate fluid intake.
  Criteria: The child's skin turgor is good, mucous membranes are moist, and hourly urinary output is at least 50 mL. Parenteral fluids are maintained until the child's oral fluid intake is adequate.

- *Goal*: The child's pain will be reduced to a level acceptable to the child.
  Goal: The child rests with minimal discomfort and states that pain is lessened.

- *Goal*: Caregivers will demonstrate an understanding of postdischarge care.
  Criteria: Family caregivers give appropriate responses when questioned about care at home and ask appropriate questions for clarification.

BLOOD DISORDERS

Several blood dyscrasias, or abnormalities of the blood, may manifest themselves in the preschooler. Although leukemia, purpura, and hemophilia may be diagnosed at either an earlier or a later age, they are commonly associated with the preschool years. Children with these disorders are often chronically ill and require long-term care.

Acute Leukemia

Leukemia is the most common type of cancer in children, accounting for about 30% of all childhood cancers. *Acute lymphatic leukemia* (ALL) is responsible for about 70% to 75% of the childhood leukemias, *acute myeloid leukemia* (AML) for almost all the rest. Fortunately, ALL is also the most curable of all the major forms of leukemia. The cure rate for AML is about 40%. The incidence of ALL is greatest between the ages of 3 and 5 years and is higher in boys; ALL is more common in white children than in African-American children. This discussion focuses on ALL.

PATHOPHYSIOLOGY

Leukemia is the uncontrolled reproduction of deformed white blood cells. Despite intensive research, its cause is unknown. Mature leukocytes (white blood cells) are made up of three types of cells:

- **Monocytes** (5%–10% of white blood cells) defend the body against infection.
- **Granulocytes** are divided into eosinophils, basophils, and neutrophils. Neutrophils (60% of the white blood cells) can pass through capillary walls to surround and destroy bacteria.
- **Lymphocytes** (30% of white blood cells) are divided into T cells, which attack and destroy virus-infected cells, foreign tissue, and cancer cells, and B cells, which produce antibodies (proteins that help destroy foreign matter).

An immature lymphocyte is called a **lymphoblast.** Leukemia occurs when lymphocytes reproduce so quickly that they are mostly in the blast, or immature, stage. This rapid increase in lymphocytes causes crowding, which in turn decreases the production of red blood cells and platelets. The decrease in red blood cells, platelets, and normal white blood cells causes the child to become easily fatigued and susceptible to infection and increased bleeding.

CLINICAL MANIFESTATIONS

Clinical manifestations of leukemia appear with surprising abruptness in many affected children, with few, if any, warning signs. The symptoms result from the proliferation of lymphoblasts. Presenting manifestations are often lassitude, pallor, and low-grade fever caused by anemia. Other early or presenting symptoms are bone and joint pain caused by invasion of the periosteum by lymphocytes, widespread **petechiae** (pinpoint hemorrhages beneath the skin), and **purpura** (hemorrhages into the skin or mucous membranes) as a result of a low thrombocyte count.

Anorexia, nausea and vomiting, headache, diarrhea, and abdominal pain, although seldom presenting signs, often occur during the course of the disease as a result of enlargement of the liver and spleen. Easy bruising is a constant problem. Ulceration of the gums and throat develops as a result of bacterial invasion and contributes to anorexia. Intracranial hemorrhages are not uncommon. Anemia becomes increasingly severe.

DIAGNOSIS

In addition to the history, symptoms, and laboratory blood studies, a bone marrow aspiration must be done to confirm the diagnosis of leukemia. The preferred site for bone marrow aspiration in children is the iliac crest. Radiographs of the long bones demonstrate changes caused by the invasion of the lymphoblasts.

TREATMENT

The advances in the treatment of ALL have dramatically improved long-term survival. In children whose initial prognosis is good, about 90% have long-term survival. For children who have a relapse, survival rates are greatly reduced. Each succeeding relapse reduces the probability of survival.

Intensive chemotherapy is initially divided into three phases:

- *Induction*—geared to achieving a complete remission with no leukemia cells
- *Sanctuary*—preventing invasion of the central nervous system by leukemia cells (no sanctuary is given to the leukemia cells)
- *Maintenance*—maintaining the remission.

A combination of drugs is used during the induction phase to bring about remission; among the drugs used are vincristine, prednisone, and asparaginase. During the sanctuary phase, **intrathecal administration** (drugs injected into the cerebrospinal fluid by lumbar puncture) of methotrexate is used to eradicate leukemia cells in the central nervous system. The maintenance phase may last 2 or 3 years and includes treatment with methotrexate, vincristine, prednisone, and 6-mercaptopurine. The drugs are often administered through a double-lumen catheter (Broviac) placed in the subclavian vein.

Two additional phases are instituted for children who suffer a relapse:

- *Reinduction*—the drugs previously used, plus additional drugs, are administered

- *Bone marrow transplant*—usually recommended after the second remission in children with ALL.

▶❚ *Nursing Process for the Child* ◀❚ *With Leukemia*

ASSESSMENT

The nursing assessment of the child with leukemia varies according to the stage of the illness. Conduct the assessment interview with both the family caregiver and the child. Do not allow the caregiver to monopolize the interview; give the child an opportunity to express feelings and fears and answer the questions.

The physical assessment should include examination for **adenopathy** (enlarged lymph glands), vital signs (especially a low-grade fever), signs of bruising, petechiae, bleeding from or ulcerations of mucous membranes, abdominal pain or tenderness, and bone or joint pain. Observe the child for lethargic behavior, and question the caregiver about this. Note signs of local infection, including edema, redness, and swelling, or any indication of systemic infection.

Assess the emotional state of the child and the family. The diagnosis of leukemia is devastating. Evaluate the child's and family's emotional states so that the nursing care plan can include helping them discuss and resolve their feelings and fears.

NURSING DIAGNOSES

Develop nursing diagnoses as a result of the nursing assessment and the interview with both the child and the caregiver. Some appropriate diagnoses may be:

- Risk for Infection related to increased susceptibility secondary to leukemic process and side effects of chemotherapy
- Risk for Injury related to bleeding tendencies
- Pain related to the effects of chemotherapy and the disease process
- Activity Intolerance related to fatigue
- Risk for Altered Growth and Development related to impaired ability to achieve developmental tasks secondary to limitations of disease and treatment
- Body Image Disturbance related to alopecia and weight loss
- Anticipatory Grieving by the family related to the prognosis

OUTCOME IDENTIFICATION AND PLANNING

Goals for the child with leukemia vary depending on individual circumstances. Preventing infection, relieving fatigue, preventing injury, and relieving pain are major goals. Another important goal for the child may be improving body image. The goal for the family may be relieving anxiety and increasing coping abilities.

IMPLEMENTATION

PREVENTING INFECTION. The immune system is weakened by the uncontrolled growth of lymphoblasts that overpower the normal production of granulocytes (particularly neutrophils) and monocytes. In addition, the chemotherapy that is necessary to inhibit this proliferation of lymphoblasts causes immunosuppression. Thus, these children are susceptible to infection, especially during chemotherapy. Infections such as meningitis, septicemia, and pneumonia are the most common causes of death. The organism most often responsible is *Pseudomonas*. Other organisms that can be dangerous for the child are *Escherichia coli, Staphylococcus aureus, Klebsiella, Pneumocystis carinii, Candida albicans*, and *Histoplasmosis*. These infectious organisms can threaten the child's life.

To protect the child from infectious organisms, follow standard guidelines for protective isolation. Carefully screen staff, family, and visitors to eliminate any known infection. Enforce handwashing, gowning, and masking. The social isolation that this imposes on the child can be difficult for the child to understand and tolerate, so spend time with the child in addition to the time that is necessary for direct care. Playing games, coloring, reading stories, and doing puzzles are all good activities that the child will enjoy. This also provides the caregiver, who may be staying with the child, a much-needed break.

PREVENTING BLEEDING. The mucous membranes bleed easily, so be gentle when doing oral hygiene. Use a soft, sponge-type brush or gauze strips wrapped around your finger. Mouthwash composed of one part hydrogen peroxide to four parts saline solution or normal saline solution may be used. Epistaxis (nosebleed) is a common problem that can usually be handled by applying external pressure to the nose. Apply pressure to sites of injections or venipunctures to prevent excessive bleeding. At least every 4 hours, assess the child for other signs of bleeding, such as petechiae, ecchymosis, hematemesis (bloody emesis), tarry stools, and swelling and tenderness of the joints. Protect the child from injury by external forces to prevent the possibility of hemorrhage from the injury. Take extra caution when the child's platelet count is especially low.

REDUCING PAIN. Pain from the invasion of lymphoblasts into the periosteum and bleeding into the joints can be excruciating. Use gentle handling, sheepskin pads under bony prominences, and positioning to help relieve discomfort and skin breakdown. Painful procedures are also a concern. Explain to the child that these procedures are necessary to help and are not in any way a form of punishment. Provide a pain scale to help the child rate the pain and communicate its intensity. The Oucher Scale[1] and the Faces Scale[2] are useful with children 3 years of age and older (see Fig. 4-5 in Chap. 4). Administer analgesics as ordered to achieve maximum comfort.

PROMOTING ENERGY CONSERVATION AND RELIEVING ANXIETY. As a result of anemia, the child is fatigued. Pace procedures so that the child has as much uninterrupted rest as possible. Stress adds to the child's feelings of exhaustion; therefore, help the child deal with the stress caused by the illness and treatments to decrease fatigue. Encourage the child to talk about feelings, and acknowledge the child's feelings as valid to help relieve anxiety.

PROMOTING NORMAL GROWTH AND DEVELOPMENT. During treatment, the child may be prevented from participating in normal activity much of the time. The social isolation that accompanies reverse isolation often interferes with normal development. Physical activities often are limited simply because of the child's lack of energy. Knowledge of normal growth and development expectations is important to consider when planning developmental activities. Stimulate growth and development, within the child's physical capabilities. Stress positive developmental tasks—for example, practicing or improving reading skills and learning or increasing computer skills. Encourage the family to help the child return to normal activities as much as possible during the maintenance phase of the treatment when the child has been discharged from the hospital.

PROMOTING A POSITIVE BODY IMAGE. The drugs administered in chemotherapy cause **alopecia** (loss of hair). Prepare the child and the family psychologically for this change in appearance. The child may want to wear a wig, especially when returning to school. Encourage the family to chose the wig before chemotherapy is started so that it matches the child's hair and the child has time to get used to it. A cap or scarf often is appealing to a child, particularly if it carries a special meaning for him or her. Reassure the child and family that the hair will grow back in about 3 to 6 months. Wash the scalp regularly to avoid cradle cap.

Prednisone therapy may cause the child to have a moon-faced appearance, which may be upsetting to either the child or the family. Reassure them that this is temporary and will disappear when the drug is no longer needed.

The child may be hesitant for peers to see these changes. Encourage visits from peers before discharge, if possible, so the child can be prepared to handle their reactions and questions. A schoolteacher can be invaluable in preparing classmates to welcome the child back with minimal reaction to the child's physical changes. Encourage the family to enlist the assistance of the child's teacher, school nurse, and pediatrician to ease the transition. Meeting other children who are undergoing chemotherapy and are in various stages of recovery is often helpful to the child and helps relieve the feeling that no one else has ever looked like this. Provide the child and the family opportunities to express their feelings and apprehensions.

PROMOTING FAMILY COPING. Family members often are devastated when they first learn that their child has leukemia. Provide support from the moment of the first diagnosis, through the hospitalization, and continuing through the maintenance phase. Families live one day at a time, hoping that the remission will not end and that their child will be one who does not have a relapse and is finally considered cured. Provide opportunities for the family to freely express their feelings about the illness and treatment. The family will find comfort in having one nurse caring for the child consistently. This consistency helps give them a feeling of stability.

Involve the caregivers in the care of the child during hospitalization, and give them complete information about what to expect when caring for the child at home during the maintenance phase. Identify a contact person for the family to call to answer questions during this phase. Help the family work through feelings of overprotectiveness toward the child so that the child can lead as normal a life as possible.

Encourage the family to consider how siblings can fit into the child's return home. Siblings may have many questions about the seriousness of the illness and about the possible death of their brother or sister. Provide support for families to deal with these concerns. Most hospitals that provide care for pediatric oncology patients have caregiver support groups that meet regularly. Candlelighters is a national organization for parents of young cancer patients.

EVALUATION: GOALS AND OUTCOME CRITERIA

- *Goal*: The child will remain free of superimposed infection.
  Criteria: The child's temperature will not exceed 100°F (37.8°C), with no inflammation, discharge, or other signs of infection.
- *Goal*: The child will remain free from injury related to bleeding.
  Criteria: The child will have no signs of petechiae, ecchymosis, hematemesis, tarry stools, and swelling and tenderness of the joints.
- *Goal*: The child will not experience pain.
  Criteria: The child rests quietly and indicates, through use of a pain scale, that the pain is tolerable.
- *Goal*: The child will have adequate rest.
  Criteria: Activities and procedures are paced so that the child has adequate rest. The child can express anxieties.
- *Goal*: The child will accomplish growth and development milestones, within the limits of the condition.
  Criteria: The child is involved in age-appropriate activities provided by staff and family.
- *Goal*: The child will accept changes in physical appearance.

Criteria: The child will evidence acceptance of physical appearance by demonstrating pride and adjustments in grooming.
- *Goal*: The family will develop coping mechanisms.
  Criteria: The family expresses feelings and fears about the child's prognosis and accepts counseling and support as needed.

Idiopathic Thrombocytopenic Purpura

Purpura is a blood disorder associated with a deficit of platelets in the circulatory system. The most common type of purpura is idiopathic thrombocytopenic purpura (ITP). Purpura is preceded by a viral infection in about half the diagnosed cases.

CLINICAL MANIFESTATIONS AND DIAGNOSIS

The onset of ITP is often acute. Bruising and a generalized rash occur. In severe cases, hemorrhage may occur in the mucous membranes; hematuria or difficult-to-control epistaxis may be present. Rarely, the serious complication of intracranial hemorrhage occurs. In most cases, symptoms disappear in a few weeks without serious hemorrhage. A few cases may continue in a chronic form of the disease.

In ITP, the platelet count may be 20,000/mm³ (normal 150,000–300,000/mm³) or lower. The bleeding time is prolonged, and the clot retraction time is abnormal. The white blood cell count remains normal, and anemia is not present unless excessive bleeding has occurred.

TREATMENT AND NURSING CARE

Corticosteroids are useful in reducing the severity and shortening the duration of the disease in some, but not all, cases of ITP. Intravenous gamma globulin has been used to increase the production of platelets until recovery occurs spontaneously. If the platelet count is higher than 20,000/mm³, treatment may be delayed to see if a spontaneous remission will occur.

Nursing care consists of protecting the child from falls and trauma, observing for signs of external or internal bleeding, and providing a regular diet and general supportive care.

Hemophilia

Hemophilia is one of the oldest known hereditary diseases. Recent research has demonstrated that hemophilia is a syndrome of several distinct inborn errors of metabolism, all resulting in the delayed coagulation of blood. Defects in the synthesis of protein lead to deficiencies in any of the factors in the blood plasma needed for thromboplastic activity. The principal factors involved are factors VIII, IX, and XI.

MECHANISM OF CLOT FORMATION

The mechanism of clot formation is complex. In a simplified form, it can best be described as occurring in three stages:

1. Prothrombin is formed through plasma–platelet interaction.
2. Prothrombin is converted to thrombin.
3. Fibrinogen is converted into fibrin by thrombin.

Fibrin forms a mesh that traps red and white blood cells and platelets into a clot, closing the defect in the injured vessel. A deficiency in one of the thromboplastin precursors may lead to hemophilia. This progression of events is shown in Figure 15-9. Refer to a specialized text on the circulatory system for a detailed discussion of the clot-forming mechanism.

CLINICAL MANIFESTATIONS

Hemophilia is characterized by prolonged bleeding, with frequent hemorrhages externally and into the skin, the joint spaces, and the intramuscular tissues. Bleeding from tooth extractions, brain hemorrhages, and crippling disabilities are serious complications. Death during infancy or early childhood is not unusual in severe hemophilia and results from a great loss of blood, intracranial bleeding, or respiratory obstruction caused by bleeding into the neck tissues.

An infant with hemophilia who is beginning to creep or walk bruises easily, and serious hemorrhages may result from minor lacerations. Bleeding often occurs from lip biting or from sharp objects put in the mouth. Tooth eruption seldom causes bleeding, but extractions require specialized handling and should be avoided by preventive care, if possi-

ble. Family caregivers must avoid overprotecting the child, however. The preschooler is active and plays hard, and injuries are practically unavoidable.

Clinical manifestations in any type of hemophilia are similar and are treated by administration of the deficient factor and by measures to prevent or treat complications. In severe bleeding, the quantities of fresh blood or frozen plasma needed may easily overload the circulatory system. Administration of factor VIII concentrate eliminates this problem.

DIAGNOSIS

A careful examination of the family history and the type of bleeding present is conducted. Abnormal bleeding beginning in infancy, in combination with a positive family history, suggests hemophilia. A markedly prolonged clotting time is characteristic of severe factor VIII or IX deficiency, but mild conditions may have only a slightly prolonged clotting time. The partial prothrombin time is the test that most clearly demonstrates that factor VIII is low.

COMMON TYPES OF HEMOPHILIA

The two most common types of hemophilia are factor VIII deficiency and factor IX deficiency. These two types are briefly presented here.

Factor VIII Deficiency (Hemophilia A; Antihemophilic Globulin Deficiency; Classic Hemophilia)

Classic hemophilia is inherited as a sex-linked recessive mendelian trait with transmission to affected males by carrier females. Hemophilia A (classic hemophilia) is the most common type, occurring in about one in 10,000 people, and is also the most severe. It is caused by a deficiency of antihemophilic globulin—the factor VIII necessary for blood clotting.

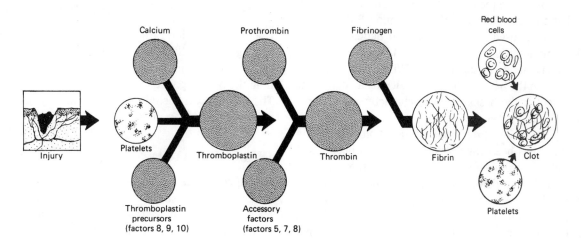

Figure 15-9

The mechanism of the formation of a blood clot is complex.

Factor IX Deficiency (Hemophilia B; Plasma Thromboplastin Component Deficiency; Christmas Disease) Christmas disease was named after a 5-year-old boy who was one of the first patients diagnosed as having a deficiency of factor IX. This deficiency constitutes about 15% of the hemophilias. It is a sex-linked recessive trait appearing in male offspring of carrier females and is caused by a deficiency of one of the necessary thromboplastin precursors, factor IX, the plasma thromboplastin component. Hemophilia B is indistinguishable from classic hemophilia in its clinical manifestations, particularly in its severe form. It also may exist in a mild form, probably more commonly than in hemophilia A.

In either hemophilia A or B, 25% or more of the affected people can trace no family history of the disease; it is assumed that spontaneous mutations have occurred in some of these cases.

TREATMENT

For many years, the only treatment for bleeding in hemophilia was the use of fresh blood or plasma. When fresh-frozen plasma came into use, it became the mainstay in hemophilia management. It has been particularly helpful in emergencies. Frozen plasma does, however, have several shortcomings. One major problem has been the large volumes needed to control bleeding. Another is the danger that injections of large amounts of plasma may lead to congestive heart failure. In addition, plasma must be given within 30 minutes because factor VIII loses its potency at room temperature.

Commercial preparations are now available that supply higher-potency factor VIII than previous preparations. These concentrates are supplied in dried form together with diluent for reconstitution. Directions for mixing and administration are included with the package. The preparations can be stored for a long time but have the disadvantage of exposing the recipient to a large number of donors. A synthetic preparation, DDAVP (1-deamino-8-D-arginine vasopressin), is used in mild factor VIII deficiencies and von Willebrand disease. Von Willebrand Disease (Vascular Hemophilia; Pseudohemophilia) von Willebrand disease is classified with the hemophilias. It is a Mendelian dominant trait present in both sexes and is characterized by prolonged bleeding times.

One of the serious problems with using blood products of any kind has been the risk of exposure to hepatitis B and human immunodeficiency virus (HIV), the causative organism of acquired immunodeficiency syndrome (AIDS). Currently, blood is screened thoroughly for viral contamination, greatly diminishing the danger of transmission of HIV. However, large numbers of hemophiliacs treated before the late 1980s were exposed to HIV and now test positive for HIV antibodies. Researchers continue to explore new ways to replace the missing factor while protecting the recipient from the threat of contracting an unknown illness.

Nursing Process for the Child With Hemophilia

ASSESSMENT

Begin the nursing assessment by reviewing the child's history with the caregiver. Include previous episodes of bleeding, the usual treatment, medications the child takes, and the current episode of bleeding. Include the child in the interview if he or she is old enough to answer questions. Carefully observe the child for any signs of bleeding. Inspect the mucous membranes, examine the joints for tenderness and swelling, and check the skin for evidence of bruising. Question the child or caregiver about hematuria, hematemesis, headache, or black tarry stools.

NURSING DIAGNOSES

After conducting a careful nursing assessment, select appropriate nursing diagnoses, such as:

- Pain related to joint swelling and limitations secondary to hemarthrosis
- Impaired Physical Mobility related to pain and tenderness of joints
- Risk for Injury related to hemorrhage secondary to trauma
- Risk for Altered Health Maintenance related to insufficient knowledge of condition, treatments, and hazards
- Risk for Ineffective Family Coping: Compromised related to treatment and care of the child

OUTCOME IDENTIFICATION AND PLANNING

Use the information gathered from the nursing assessment to set goals with the cooperation and input of the caregiver and the child. The major goals for the child include stopping the bleeding, decreasing pain, and preventing injury. The family goals include increasing knowledge about the child's condition and care.

IMPLEMENTATION

RELIEVING PAIN. Bleeding into the joint cavities often occurs after some slight injury and seems nearly unavoidable if the child is allowed to lead a normal life. Pain, caused by the pressure of the confined fluid in the narrow joint spaces, is extreme, requiring the use of sedatives or narcotics. Promptly immobilize the involved extremity to prevent contractures of soft tissues and the destruction of the bone

Figure 15-10
The hemophiliac can suffer from bleeding into the joints and painful swollen knees.

and joint tissues (Fig. 15-10). Immobilization helps relieve pain and decrease bleeding. A bivalve plaster cast may be applied in the hospital to immobilize the affected part. Do not administer aspirin (or drugs containing aspirin) or other nonsteroidal antiinflammatory drugs (NSAIDs), such as phenylbutazone and indomethacin, because of the danger of prolonging bleeding. Conversely, ibuprofen, also an NSAID, has been proven safe for these children. Use of cold packs to stop bleeding is acceptable. The affected limb may be elevated above the level of the heart to slow blood flow. Use age-appropriate diversionary activities to help the child deal with the pain. Handle the affected joints carefully to prevent additional pain.

PREVENTING JOINT CONTRACTURES. Passive range-of-motion exercises help prevent the development of joint contractures. Do not use them, however, after an acute episode, because stretching of the joint capsule may cause bleeding. Encourage the child to do active range-of-motion exercises, as he or she can recognize his or her own pain tolerance. Many patients who have had repeated episodes of **hemarthrosis** (bleeding into the joints) develop functional impairment of the joints despite careful treatment. Use splints and devices to position the limb in a functional position. Physical therapy is helpful after the bleeding episode is under control. Joint contractures are a serious risk, so make every effort to avoid them.

PREVENTING INJURY. The child with hemophilia is continuously at risk for additional injury. Protect the child from trauma caused by necessary procedures. Limit invasive procedures as much as possible; if possible, collect blood samples by a finger stick. Avoid intramuscular injections. When an invasive procedure must be done, compress the site for 5 minutes or longer after the procedure, and apply cold compresses.

Remove any sharp objects from the child's environment.

If the child is young, pad the crib sides to prevent bumping and bruising. Examine toys for sharp edges and hard surfaces. Soft toys are best for the young child. For mouth care, use a soft toothbrush or sponge-type brush to decrease the danger of bleeding gums. During daily hygiene, trim the nails to prevent scratching, and give adequate skin care to prevent irritation.

PROVIDING FAMILY TEACHING. Provide the family with a thorough explanation of hemophilia or reinforce information they have already received. Review the family's knowledge about the disease and give additional information when needed. A child with hemophilia is healthy between bleeding episodes, but the fact that bleeding may occur as the result of slight trauma, or often without any known injury, causes considerable anxiety. For an unknown reason, bleeding episodes are more common in the spring and fall. There is some evidence that emotional stress can initiate bleeding episodes.

Topical fluoride applications to the teeth are particularly important in these children. Pay particular attention to proper oral hygiene, a well-balanced diet, and proper dental treatment, and teach the family about these considerations. Advise the family to select a dentist who understands the problems presented and who will set up an appropriate program of preventive dentistry.

Discuss safety measures for the home and the child's lifestyle. A young child may need a protective helmet and elbow and knee pads for everyday wear, especially when first becoming mobile. Installing carpeting in the home, when possible, helps soften the falls of a toddler just learning to walk. An older child may need to wear the protective devices when playing outdoors. Playground areas can be treacherous for these children, but, within reason, normalcy should be maintained.

Instruct the family about medications, range-of-motion exercises, emergency measures to stop or limit bleeding, and all aspects of the child's care. Emergency splints should be kept in the home of every person with hemophilia. Ice packs also should be available for instant use. If possible, the bleeding area can be raised above the level of the heart. Before leaving for the health care facility, the caregiver should apply a splint and cold packs and give factor replacement, according to the protocol established with the child's physician.

The family experiences continuous anxiety over how much activity to allow their child, how to keep from overprotecting him or her, and how to help the child achieve a healthy mental attitude, all the while preventing mishaps that may cause serious bleeding episodes. They must help the child toward autonomy and independence within the framework of necessary limitations. At times, the emotional effect of social deprivation and restrained activity must be weighed against possible physical harm.

The financial strain on the family is considerable, as it is with most families with a child who has a chronic condition. Children who have had several episodes of hemarthrosis may be disabled to the extent of needing crutches and braces or wheelchairs. Measures toward rehabilitation require hospitalization, with possible surgery, casts, and other orthopedic appliances.

A hemophiliac child usually loses much school time. Any child who must frequently interrupt schooling, for whatever reason, experiences a considerable setback. Each child should be considered individually and provided with as normal an environment as possible.

PROMOTING FAMILY COPING. Both the child and family must accept the limitations and yet realize the importance of normal social experiences. School, health, and community agencies can offer the family counseling and encouragement and can help them raise the affected child in a healthy manner, both emotionally and physically. The National Hemophilia Foundation is a resource for services and publications. Give the family information about other support systems that may be available.

Review all these concerns with the family, and through discussion, questions, and demonstrations, confirm that the family understands the information provided. Counseling may be required for the family to learn to cope with the child's needs. Encourage the family to express their feelings about the impact the disease has on their lifestyle. The family may fear that the child will die from hemorrhaging. Guilt may play an important part in the family's reactions to the child. Recognizing and validating these feelings are important aspects of active listening. During hospitalization, involve the family in the care of the child so they can learn how to help the child without causing additional pain.

EVALUATION: GOALS AND OUTCOME CRITERIA

- *Goal*: The child will experience diminished pain.
  Criteria: The child rests quietly with minimal pain, as evidenced by the child's reporting of pain using a pain scale.
- *Goal*: The child will move freely with minimal pain.
  Criteria: There is no evidence of new joint contractures. The child can maintain range of motion.
- *Goal*: The child will not experience any new injuries.
  Criteria: No injuries or bleeding episodes occur as a result of procedures or treatments.
- *Goal*: The family will gain knowledge of the disease.
  Criteria: The family demonstrates knowledge of the disease and discusses the child's home care, asking and answering appropriate questions.
- *Goal*: The family will learn coping mechanisms.
  Criteria: Family members express their feelings and demonstrate good coping mechanisms by seeking help from appropriate support systems.

GENITOURINARY SYSTEM DISORDERS

Nephrotic Syndrome

Several different types of nephrosis have been identified in the nephrotic syndrome. The most common type in children is called *lipoid nephrosis, idiopathic nephrotic syndrome*, or *minimal change nephrotic syndrome* (MCNS). All forms of nephrosis have early characteristics of edema and proteinuria; therefore, definite clinical differentiation cannot be made early in the disease.

Nephrotic syndrome has a course of remissions and exacerbations, usually lasting for months. The recovery rate is generally good with the use of intensive steroid therapy and protection against infection.

The cause of MCNS is unknown. In rare cases, it is associated with other specific diseases. The nephrotic syndrome is present in as many as seven children per 100,000 population younger than 9 years of age. The average age of onset is 2.5 years, with most cases occurring between the ages of 2 and 6 years.

CLINICAL MANIFESTATIONS

Edema is usually the presenting symptom, appearing first around the eyes and ankles. As the swelling advances, the edema becomes generalized, with a pendulous abdomen full of fluid (Fig. 15-11). Respiratory embarrassment may be severe, and edema of the scrotum on the male is characteristic. The edema shifts when the child changes position when lying quietly or walking about. Anorexia, irritability, and loss of appetite develop. Malnutrition may become severe. However, the generalized edema masks the loss of body tissue, causing the child to present a chubby appearance and to double his or her weight. After diuresis, the malnutrition becomes quite apparent. These children are usually susceptible to infection, and repeated acute respiratory conditions are the usual pattern. This is intensified by the immunosuppression caused by the administration of prednisone.

DIAGNOSIS

Laboratory findings include marked proteinuria, especially albumin, with large numbers of hyaline and granular casts in the urine. Hematuria is not usually present, although a few red blood cells may appear in the urine. The blood serum protein level is reduced, and there is an increase in the level of cholesterol in the blood (**hyperlipidemia**).

TREATMENT

The management of nephrotic syndrome is a long process, with remissions and recurrence of symptoms. The use of corticosteroids has induced remissions in most cases and

Figure 15-11
A child with nephrotic syndrome. Notice the distended abdomen caused by ascites and the edematous labia.

has reduced recurrences. Corticosteroid therapy usually produces diuresis in about 7 to 14 days, but the drug is continued until a remission occurs. Prednisone is the drug most commonly used. After the diuresis occurs, intermittent therapy is continued every other day, or for 3 days a week. Daily urine testing for protein is continued whether the child is at home or in the hospital.

Diuretics may not be necessary when diuresis can be induced with steroids. Diuretics have not been effective in reducing the edema of nephrotic syndrome, although a loop diuretic (furosemide) may be administered if the edema causes respiratory embarrassment.

Immunosuppressant therapy may be used to reduce symptoms and prevent further relapses in children who do not respond adequately to corticosteroids. Cyclophosphamide (Cytoxan) is the drug most commonly used. Because cyclophosphamide has serious side effects, the family caregivers must be fully informed before therapy is started. **Leukopenia** (leukocyte count less than $5,000/mm^3$) can be expected, as well as the other common side effects of immunosuppressant therapy, such as gastrointestinal symptoms, hematuria, and alopecia. The length of therapy is usually a brief period of 2 or 3 months.

A general diet is recommended, appealing to the child's poor appetite with frequent, small feedings if necessary. The addition of salt is discouraged. Family caregivers need encouragement and support for the long months ahead. Relapses usually become less frequent as the child gets older.

Nursing Process for the Child With Nephrotic Syndrome

ASSESSMENT

Evaluate for edema when performing the nursing assessment of the child with nephrotic syndrome. Weigh the child and record the abdominal measurements to serve as a baseline. Assess vital signs, including blood pressure. Note any swelling about the eyes or the ankles and other dependent parts, and record the degree of pitting. Inspect the skin for pallor, irritation, or breakdown. Examine the scrotal area of the young boy for swelling, redness, and irritation. Question the caregiver about the onset of symptoms, the child's appetite, urine output, and signs of fatigue or irritability.

NURSING DIAGNOSES

The nursing diagnoses vary with the outcome of the nursing assessment. Consult the caregiver and child when determining suitable diagnoses so that their needs are met. Among the nursing diagnoses that may be included are:

- Fluid Volume Excess related to fluid accumulation in tissues and third spaces
- Risk for Altered Nutrition: Less than Body Requirements related to anorexia
- Risk for Impaired Skin Integrity related to edema
- Activity Intolerance related to fatigue
- Risk for Infection related to immunosuppression
- Altered Family Processes related to care of a child with chronic illness

OUTCOME IDENTIFICATION AND PLANNING

The major goals for the child with nephrotic syndrome are relieving edema, balancing fluid intake, maintaining skin integrity, conserving energy, and preventing infection. The family goal may be learning to cope with the long-term care of the child. Design the nursing care plan to include all these goals.

MONITORING FLUID INTAKE AND OUTPUT. Accurately assess and document intake and output. Weigh the child at the same time every day, on the same scale, wearing the same clothing. Measure the child's abdomen daily at the level of the umbilicus, and make certain that all staff personnel are measuring at the same level. Note the desired location for measuring on the nursing care plan so that everyone follows the same practice. Test the urine regularly for albumin and specific gravity. Albumin can be tested with reagent strips that are dipped into the urine and read by comparison with a color chart on the container.

The abdomen may be greatly enlarged with **ascites** (edema in the peritoneal cavity). The abdomen can even become marked with **striae** (stretch marks). Before the use of corticosteroids became common, an **abdominal paracentesis** (surgical puncture into the abdomen to drain fluid) was frequently necessary to drain the fluid. This was traumatic for the child and is rarely needed with current therapy.

IMPROVING NUTRITIONAL INTAKE.   Although the child may look plump, underneath the edema is a thin, possibly malnourished child. The child's appetite is poor for several reasons:

- The ascites diminishes the appetite because of the full feeling in the abdomen.
- The child may be lethargic and apathetic and simply not interested in eating.
- A no-added-salt diet may be unappealing to the child.
- Corticosteroid therapy may decrease the appetite.

Offer a visually appealing and nutritious diet. Consult the child and the family to learn which foods are appealing to the child. Cater to the child's wishes as much as possible to perk up a lagging appetite. A dietitian can help plan appealing meals for the child. Serving six small meals may help increase the child's total intake better than the customary three meals a day.

PROMOTING SKIN INTEGRITY.   The child's skin is stretched with edema and becomes thin and fragile. Inspect all skin surfaces regularly for breakdown. Turn and position the child every 2 hours, because the child is lethargic. Protect skin surfaces from pressure by means of pillows and padding. Protect overlapping skin surfaces from rubbing by careful placement of cotton gauze. Bathe the child regularly. Wash thoroughly the skin surfaces that touch each other with soap and water and dry them completely. A sheer dusting of cornstarch may be soothing. If the scrotum is edematous, use a soft cotton support to provide comfort.

PROMOTING ENERGY CONSERVATION AND SENSORY STIMULATION.   Bed rest is common during the edema stage of the condition. The child rarely protests because of his or her fatigue. The sheer bulk of the edema makes movement difficult. When diuresis occurs, several days after beginning prednisone, the child may be allowed more activity, but balance the activity with rest periods and encourage the child to rest when fatigued. Plan quiet, age-appropriate activities that interest the child. Most children love having someone read to them. Coloring books, dominoes, puzzles, and some kinds of computer and board games are quiet activities that many children enjoy. Involve the family in providing some of these activities. Avoid using television excessively as a diversion.

PREVENTING INFECTION.   The child with nephrotic syndrome is especially at risk for respiratory infections because the edema and the corticosteroid therapy lower the body's defenses. Protect the child from anyone with an infection—staff, family, visitors, and other children. Handwashing and strict medical asepsis are essential. Monitor vital signs every 4 hours and evaluate for any early signs of infection.

PROVIDING FAMILY SUPPORT AND TEACHING.
Children with nephrotic syndrome are usually hospitalized for diagnosis, thorough evaluation of their general health and specific condition, and institution of therapy. If the child has an infection, a course of antibiotic therapy may be given, and unless unforeseen complications develop, the child is discharged with complete instructions for management. Provide a written plan to help family caregivers follow the program successfully. They must keep a careful record of home treatment for the health care provider to review at regular intervals.

Teach the family caregivers reactions that may occur with the use of steroids and the adverse effects of abrupt discontinuance of these drugs. If the family understands these aspects well, the incidence of forgetting to give the medication or of neglecting to refill the prescription may be reduced or eliminated. Encourage the family caregivers to report promptly any symptoms that they consider caused by the medication.

Teach the family that special care necessary to keep the child in optimum health is important, and that **intercurrent infections** (those occurring during the course of an already existing disease) must be reported promptly. Also, teach them that exacerbations are common, and they need to understand that these will probably occur. Stress the information that they should report, including rapidly increasing weight, increased proteinuria, or signs of infections. Any of these may be a reason for altering the therapeutic regimen or changing the specific antibiotic agents used.

Provide the family caring for the child at home with the home care information appropriate for any chronically ill child. Bed rest is not indicated, except during an intercurrent illness. Activity is restricted only by edema, which may slow the child down considerably, but otherwise normal activity is beneficial. Sufficient food intake may be a problem, as in other types of chronic illness. Fortunately, there are usually no food restrictions, and the appetite can be tempted by attractive, appealing foods.

As the name implies, MCNS causes few changes in the kidneys, and these children have a good prognosis. Complications from kidney damage alter the course of treatment. Failure to achieve satisfactory diuresis, or the need to discontinue steroids because of adverse reactions, requires a reevaluation of treatment. The presence of gross hematuria suggests renal damage. In a few children, the persistence of abnormal urinary findings after diuresis presents a less hopeful outlook. A child who has frequent relapses lasting into adolescence or adulthood may develop renal failure and eventually be a candidate for a kidney transplant.

EVALUATION: GOALS AND OUTCOME CRITERIA

■ *Goal*: The child's edema will be decreased.
Criteria: Edema is decreased, as evidenced by weight loss and decreased abdominal girth.

■ *Goal*: The child's nutritional needs will be met.
Criteria: The child eats 80% or more of his or her meals.

■ *Goal*: The child's skin integrity will be maintained.
Criteria: The child's skin remains free of breakdown, as evidenced by absence of redness and irritation.

■ *Goal*: The child will conserve energy.
Criteria: The child rests as needed and engages in quiet diversional activities.

■ *Goal*: The child will not experience any infection.
Criteria: The child has no signs or symptoms of infection, as evidenced by normal vital signs, no respiratory symptoms, and no gastrointestinal symptoms.

■ *Goal*: The family will receive adequate support and teaching.
Criteria: The family demonstrates an understanding of the disease and home care, asking and answering appropriate questions.

Acute Glomerulonephritis

Acute glomerulonephritis is a condition that appears to be an allergic reaction to a specific infection, most often group A β-hemolytic streptococcal infection, as in rheumatic fever. The antigen–antibody reaction causes a response that blocks the glomeruli, permitting red blood cells and protein to escape into the urine. Acute glomerulonephritis has a peak incidence in children 6 and 7 years of age and occurs twice as often in boys. The disease is discussed in this chapter so it can be compared with nephrotic syndrome (Table 15-5). The prognosis is usually excellent, but a few children develop chronic nephritis.

CLINICAL MANIFESTATIONS

Presenting symptoms appear 1 to 3 weeks after the onset of a streptococcal infection, such as strep throat, otitis media, tonsillitis, or impetigo. Usually, the presenting symptom is grossly bloody urine. The caregiver may describe the urine as smoky or bloody. Periorbital edema may accompany or precede hematuria. Fever may be 103° to 104°F (39.4°–40°C) at the onset but decreases in a few days to about 100°F (37.8°C). Slight headache and malaise are usual, and there may be vomiting. Hypertension appears in 60% to 70% of patients during the first 4 or 5 days. Both hematuria and hypertension disappear within 3 weeks.

Oliguria (production of a subnormal volume of urine) is usually present, and the urine has a high specific gravity and contains albumin, red and white blood cells, and casts. The blood urea nitrogen and serum creatinine levels and sedimentation rates are elevated.

TABLE 15-5. Comparison of Features of Acute Glomerulonephritis and Nephrotic Syndrome

Assessment Factor	Acute Glomerulonephritis	Nephrotic Syndrome
Cause	Immune reaction to group A β-hemolytic streptococcal infection	Idiopathic; possibly a hypersensitivity reaction
Onset	Abrupt	Insidious
Hematuria	Grossly bloody	Rare
Proteinuria	3+ or 4+, but not massive	Massive
Edema	Mild	Extreme
Hypertension	Marked	Mild
Hyperlipidemia	Rare or mild	Marked
Peak age frequency	5–10 y	2–3 y
Interventions	Limited activity; antihypertensives as needed; symptomatic therapy if congestive heart failure occurs	Bed rest during edema stage; Corticosteroid administration; Possible cyclophosphamide administration
Diet	Normal for age; no added salt if child is hypertensive	Nutritious for age; no added salt; small, frequent meals may be desirable
Prevention	Prevention through treatment of group A β-hemolytic streptococcal infections	None known
Course	Acute—up to 2–3 weeks	Chronic—may have relapses

Adapted from Pillitteri A. Maternal and child health nursing, 2nd ed. Philadelphia: JB Lippincott, 1994.

Cerebral symptoms, consisting mainly of headache, drowsiness, convulsions, and vomiting, occur in connection with hypertension in a few cases. When the blood pressure is reduced, these symptoms disappear. Cardiovascular disturbance may be revealed in electrocardiogram tracings, but few children have clinical signs. In most children, this condition is short term, but in some it progresses to congestive heart failure.

TREATMENT

Although the child usually feels well in a few days, activities should be limited until the clinical manifestations subside, generally 2 to 4 weeks after the onset. Penicillin may be given during the acute stage to eradicate any existing infection; however, it does not affect the recovery from the disease because the condition is an immunologic response. The diet is generally not restricted, but additional salt may be limited if edema is excessive. Treatment of complications is symptomatic.

NURSING CARE

Bed rest should be maintained until acute symptoms and gross hematuria have disappeared. The child must be protected from chilling and contact with people with infections. When the child is allowed out of bed, he or she must not become fatigued.

Urinary output should be checked and recorded every 8 hours. The child must be weighed daily at the same time, on the same scale, wearing the same clothes. The amount of fluid the child is allowed may be based on output as well as on evidence of continued hypertension and oliguria. Fluid intake should be carefully recorded; special attention is needed to keep the intake within prescribed limits.

Blood pressure should be monitored regularly using the same arm and a properly fitting cuff. If hypertension develops, a diuretic may help reduce the blood pressure to normal levels. An antihypertensive drug may be added if the diastolic pressure is 90 mmHg or higher. The urine must be tested regularly for protein and hematuria using dipstick tests.

Traces of protein in the urine may persist for months after the acute symptoms disappear, and an elevated Addis count, indicating red blood cells in the urine, persists as well. Family caregivers must learn to test for urinary protein routinely. If the urinary signs persist for more than 1 year, the disease has probably assumed a chronic form.

■ KEY POINTS

■ The preschooler may view any illness as punishment for wrongdoing and must be reassured that this is not so.

■ The preschooler can begin to understand simple explanations.

■ Fear of bodily harm is common, so the child needs to be reassured about necessary procedures. Allowing the child to handle the equipment and act out procedures with dolls when possible can be helpful. Nurses must choose their words carefully so that the child does not misunderstand the explanation and perceive it as threatening.

■ Magical thinking can cause anxieties and fears that are real to the child. Nurses must be alert for these perceptions so they can help the child acknowledge and deal with them.

■ During hospitalization, the child may regress to bedwetting, thumb sucking, and fussiness.

■ Encouraging and involving the child in bathing, dressing, feeding, and other activities of daily living can help preserve his or her developing independence.

■ Many children are affected by hearing disabilities. The disability can range from mild to severe and can affect the child's speech development, social development, and learning.

■ When working with a mentally retarded child, the nurse must be aware of the child's cognitive level and adjust the care plan accordingly.

■ Illnesses that require isolation procedures, either to protect the child (as in leukemia and nephrotic syndrome) or to prevent infection of other children (as in infectious diseases), cause feelings of rejection and separation. Thoughtful nursing care can decrease the trauma that children suffer when they are isolated for any reason.

❓ CRITICAL THINKING

1. You are caring for 3½-year-old Missy, who has a mild hearing impairment. Describe how you will adapt your nursing care to improve your communication with her.
2. Four-year-old Todd is blind. You are helping with his care. Explain how you will orient him to the unit and prepare him for his hospital stay.
3. Your friend asks you if cerebral palsy is inherited. Give a complete answer about the causes of cerebral palsy.
4. Jerome, a 6-year-old with Down syndrome, has the mental age of a 3-year-old. Develop a plan to prepare him for a tonsillectomy.
5. The family of Sean, a 3-year-old with hemophilia, is concerned that Sean might get AIDS from his treatments. Give them an explanation that will reassure them.
6. Make a list of safety measures to protect Sean from injury in the hospital and at home.

REFERENCES

1. Beyer JE. The Oucher: A user's manual and technical report. Denver: University of Colorado, 1988.
2. Wong D, Baker C. Pain in children: Comparison of assessment scales. Pediatr Nurs 14(1):9–17, 1988.

BIBLIOGRAPHY

Bossert E, Martinson IM. Kinetic drawings—revised: A method of determining the impact of cancer on the family as perceived by the child with cancer. J Pediatr Nurs 5(3):204–213, 1990.

Garvin JM. Reye's syndrome. Emerg Med Serv 19(3):33, 1990.

Hockenberry MJ, Coody DK, Bennett BS. Childhood cancers: Incidence, diagnosis, and treatment. Pediatr Nurs 16(3):234–246, 256–257, 1990.

Munet Vilaro F, Vessey JA. Children's explanation of leukemia: A Hispanic perspective. J Pediatr Nurs 5(4):274–282, 1990.

Norinkavich KM, Howie G, Cariofiles P. Quality improvement study of day surgery for tonsillectomy and adenoidectomy patients. Pediatr Nurs 21(4):341–344, 1995.

Pillitteri A. Maternal and child health nursing, 2d ed. Philadelphia: JB Lippincott, 1995.

Ragab A. Growth factors in leukemia: How it all begins. J Pediatr Oncol Nurs 7(2):56, 1990.

Suderman JR. Pain relief during routine procedures for children with leukemia. MCN 15(3):163–166, 1990.

Weinstein BD, De Neffe LS. Hemophilia, AIDS, and occupational therapy. Am J Occup Ther 44(3):228–232, 1990.

Wong DL. Whaley and Wong's nursing care of infants and children, 5th ed. St. Louis: Mosby–Year Book, 1995.

Yasukasa A. Upper extremity casting: Adjunct treatment for a child with cerebral palsy. Am J Occup Ther 44(9):480–486, 1990.

Chapter 16

Growth and Development of the School-Age Child: 6 to 10 Years

PHYSICAL DEVELOPMENT
  Growth
  Dentition
  Skeletal Growth

PSYCHOSOCIAL DEVELOPMENT
  The Child From Ages 6 to 7 Years
  The Child From Ages 7 to 10 Years

NUTRITION

HEALTH PROMOTION AND MAINTENANCE
  Routine Checkups
  Family Teaching
  Health Education
  Accident Prevention

THE SCHOOL-AGE CHILD IN THE HEALTH CARE FACILITY

STUDENT OBJECTIVES

On completion of this chapter, the student will be able to:

1. State the major developmental task of the school-age group according to Erikson.
2. Discuss the physical growth patterns during the school-age years for a) girls and b) boys.
3. Describe dentition in this age group.
4. State factors that may deter successful completion of the developmental task of industry versus inferiority.
5. Describe the psychosocial characteristics of the 6- to 7-year-old child.
6. Discuss the importance of "gangs" in the 7- to 8-year-old child.
7. Briefly describe the progression in the 6- to 10-year-old child's concept of biology: a) birth, b) death, c) human body, d) health, e) illness.
8. Identify nutritional influences on the school-age child, including a) family attitudes, b) mealtime atmosphere, c) snacks, d) school's role.
9. List three factors that contribute to obesity in the school-age child.
10. State two appropriate ways to help an obese child control weight.
11. State the usual amount of sleep the school-age child needs.
12. Describe practices that contribute to good dental hygiene for this age group.
13. Discuss the need for sex education in the school-age group: a) family's role, b) school's role, c) others.
14. Identify common inhalant products that children may use as deliriants.
15. Discuss principles that a family caregiver can use to teach children about substance abuse.
16. Describe safety education appropriate for the school-age group.
17. State several factors that may influence the school-age child's hospital experience.

KEY TERMS

classification
conservation
decentration
deliriants
epiphyses

hierarchical arrangement
inhalants
reversibility
scoliosis

The first day of school marks a major milestone in a child's development, opening a new world of learning and growth. Between the ages of 6 and 10 years, dramatic changes occur in the child's thinking process, social skills, activities, attitudes, and use of language. The squirmy, boisterous 6-year-old child with a limited attention span bears little resemblance to the more reserved 10-year-old child who can become absorbed in a solitary craft activity for several hours.

Moving from the small circle of family into school and community, children begin to see differences in their own lives and the lives of others. They constantly compare their families with other children's families and observe the way other children are disciplined, the foods they eat, the way they dress, and the houses they live in. Every aspect of lifestyle is subject to comparison with that of other children.

Most children reach school age with the necessary skills, abilities, and independence to function successfully in this new environment. They can feed and dress themselves, use the primary language of their culture to communicate their needs and feelings, and separate from their caregivers for extended periods. They show increasing interest in group activities and in making things. Children of this age work at many activities, involving motor, cognitive, and social skills. Success in these activities provides the child with self-confidence and a feeling of competence. Children who are unsuccessful during this stage, whether from physical, social, or cognitive disadvantages, develop a feeling of inferiority.

The health of the school-age child is no longer the exclusive concern of the family but of the community. Before entrance, most schools require that children have a physical examination and that immunizations meet state requirements. Generally, this is a healthy period in the child's life, although minor respiratory disorders and other communicable diseases can spread quickly within a classroom. Few major diseases have their onset during this period. Accidents still pose a serious hazard; therefore, safety measures are an important part of learning.

PHYSICAL DEVELOPMENT

Growth

Between the ages of 6 and 10 years, growth is slow and steady. Average annual weight gain is about 7 lb (3 kg). By age 7, the child weighs about seven times as much as at birth. Annual height increase is about 2.5″ (6 cm). This period ends in the preadolescent growth spurt in girls at about age 10 and in boys at about age 12.

Dentition

At about age 6, the child starts to lose the deciduous ("baby") teeth, usually beginning with the lower incisors. At about the same time, the first permanent teeth, the 6-year molars, appear directly behind the deciduous molars (Fig. 16-1). These 6-year molars are of the utmost importance: they are the key or pivot teeth that help to shape the jaw and affect the alignment of the permanent teeth. If they are allowed to decay so severely that they must be removed, the child will have dental problems later. (More information on care of the teeth is given later in this chapter.)

Skeletal Growth

The 6-year-old's silhouette is characterized by a protruding abdomen and lordosis ("swayback"). By the time the child has reached the age of 10 years, the spine is straighter, the

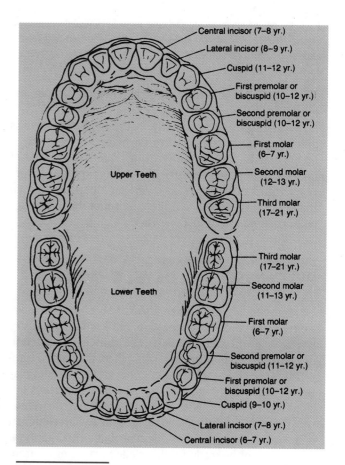

Figure 16-1
Chart showing the sequence of eruption of permanent teeth.

Figure 16-2
Left, Profile of a 6-year-old showing protuberant abdomen.
Right, Profile of a 10-year-old showing flat abdomen and four curves of adultlike spine.

abdomen flatter, and the body generally more slender and long-legged (Fig. 16-2).

Bone growth occurs mostly in the long bones and is gradual during the school years. Cartilage is being replaced by bone at the **epiphyses** (growth centers at the end of long bones and at the wrists). Skeletal maturation is more rapid in girls than in boys and in African-American children than in whites. Growth and development of the school-age child is summarized in Table 16-1.

PSYCHOSOCIAL DEVELOPMENT

The sense of duty and accomplishment occupies the years from 6 to 12 years. This is the period Erikson calls *industry versus inferiority,* during which the child is interested in engaging in real projects and seeing them through to completion. The child applies the energies earlier put into play toward accomplishing tasks, often spending numerous sessions on one project. With these attempts come the refinement of motor, cognitive, and social skills and development of a positive sense of self. Some school-age children, however, may not be ready for this stage because of environmental deprivation, a dysfunctional family, insecure attachment to parents, immaturity, or other reasons.

Entering school at a disadvantage, these children may not be ready to be productive. Excessive or unrealistic goals set by a teacher or caregiver who is insensitive to the child's needs will defeat such a child, possibly leading to a feeling of inferiority rather than self-confidence.

Several personality development tasks should be completed during these years, providing that environmental support is adequate. These tasks include developing coping mechanisms, a sense of right and wrong, a feeling of self-esteem, and an ability to care for oneself.

During the school-age years, the child's cognitive skills develop, and at about the age of 7 years, the child enters the concrete operational stage identified by Piaget. Significant in this stage are the skills of **conservation** (the ability to recognize that a change in shape does not necessarily mean a change in amount or mass). This begins with the conservation of numbers, when the child understands that the number of cookies does not change, even though they may be rearranged, to the conservation of mass, when the child can see that an amount of cookie dough is the same whether it is in a ball or flattened out for baking. This is followed by conservation of weight, in which the child recognizes that a pound is a pound, regardless of whether plastic or bricks are being weighed. Conservation of volume (for instance, a half-cup of water is the same amount regardless of the shape of the container) does not come until late in the concrete operational stage, at about 11 or 12 years of age.

Each child is a product of personal heredity, environment, cognitive ability, and physical health. Every child needs love and acceptance, with understanding, support, and concern when mistakes are made. Children thrive on praise and will work to earn more praise and recognition (see Family Teaching: Guiding Your School-Age Child).

The Child From Ages 6 to 7 Years

Children in the age group of 6 to 7 years are still characterized by magical thinking—the tooth fairy, Santa Claus, the Easter bunny, and others. Keen imaginations contribute to fears, especially at night, about remote, fanciful, or imaginary events. Trouble distinguishing fantasy from reality can contribute to lying to escape punishment or boost self-confidence.

Children who have attended a day care center, preschool, kindergarten, or a Head Start program usually make the transition into first grade with pleasure, excitement, and little anxiety. Those who have not may find it helpful to visit the school, to experience separation from home and caregivers, and to try getting along with other children on a trial basis. Most 6-year-old children can sit still for short periods and understand about taking turns. Those who have not matured sufficiently for this experience will find school unpleasant and may not do well.

Group activities are important to most 6-year-old children, even if the groups include only two or three children. They delight in learning and show an intense interest in

TABLE 16-1.   Developmental Milestones for the School-Age Child

Age (yr)	Physical	Motor	Social	Language	Perceptual	Cognitive
6	Average height 45" (116 cm) Average weight 46 lb (21 kg) Loses first tooth (upper incisors) Six-year molars erupt Food "jags" Appetite increased	Ties shoes Can use scissors Runs, jumps, climbs, skips Can ride bicycle Can't sit for long periods Cuts, pastes, prints, draws with some detail	Increased need to socialize with same sex Egocentric— believes everyone thinks as they do Still in preoperational stage until age 7	Uses every form of sentence structure Vocabulary of 2,500 words Sentence length about 5 words	Knows right from left May reverse letters Can discriminate vertical, horizontal, and oblique Perceives pictures in parts or in whole but not in both	Recognizes simple words Conservation of number Defines objects by use Can group according to an attribute to form subclasses
7	Weight is seven times birth weight Gains 4.4–6.6 lb/yr (2–3 kg) Grows 2"–2.5"/yr (5–6 cm)	More cautious Swims Printing smaller than 6-year-old's Activity level lower than 6-year-old's	More cooperative Same-sex play group and friends Less egocentric	Can name day, month, season Produces all language sounds	b, p, d, q confusion resolved Can copy a diamond	Begins to use simple logic Can group in ascending order Grasps basic idea of addition and subtraction Conservation of substance Can tell time
8	Average height 49.5" (127 cm) Averge weight 55 lb (25 kg)	Movements more graceful Writes in cursive Can throw and hit a baseball Has symmetric balance and can hop	Adheres to simple rules Hero worship begins Same-sex peer group	Gives precise definitions Articulation near adult level	Can catch a ball Visual acuity 20/20 Perceives pictures in parts and whole	Increasing memory span Interest in causal relation Conservation of length Seriation
9–10	Average height 51.5"–53.5" (132–137 cm) Average weight 59.5–77 lb (27–35 kg)	Good coordination Can achieve the strength and speed needed for most sports	Enjoys team competition Moves from group to best friend Hero worship intensifies	Can use language to convey thoughts and look at other's point of view	Eye–hand coordination almost perfect	Classifies objects Understands explanations Conservation of area and weight Describes characteristics of objects Can group in descending order

Adapted from Castiglia PT, Harbin RE. Child health care: Practice and process. Philadelphia: JB Lippincott, 1992, p. 321.

every experience. Judgment about acceptable and unacceptable behavior is not well developed, possibly resulting in name calling and the use of vulgar words.

Between the ages of 6 and 8 years, children begin to enjoy participating in real-life activities, helping with gardening, housework, and other chores (Fig. 16-3). They love making things, such as drawings, paintings, and craft projects.

The Child From Ages 7 to 10 Years

Between the seventh and eighth birthdays, children begin to shake off their acceptance of parental standards as the ultimate authority and become more impressed by the behavior of their peers. Interest in group play increases, and acceptance by the group or gang is tremendously important. These groups quickly become all-boy or all-girl

Family Teaching
Guiding Your School-Age Child

- Give your child consistent love and attention. Try to see the situation through your child's eyes. Do your best to avoid a hostile or angry reaction toward your child.
- Know where your child is at all times and who his or her friends are. Never leave your child home alone.
- Encourage your child to become involved in school and community activities. Become involved with your child's activities whenever possible. Encourage fair play and good sportsmanship.
- Set good examples for your children by your behavior toward others.
- Never hit your children. Physical punishment shows them that it's alright to hit others and that they can solve problems in that way.
- Use positive nonphysical methods of discipline, such as:
  —"Time out"—1 minute per year is an appropriate amount of time.
  —"Grounding"—don't permit them to play with friends or take part in a special activity.
  —Take away a special privilege.
  Set these limits for brief periods only. Consistency is extremely important in setting these restrictions.
- Be consistent. Make a reasonable rule, let your child know the rule, and then stick with it. You can involve your child in helping to set rules.
- Treat your child with love and respect. Always try to find the "positives" and praise the child for those behaviors. Don't treat your child in a manner that you would not use with an adult friend.
- Let the child know what you expect of him or her. Children who have responsibilities (age-appropriate) learn self-discipline and self-control.
- When you have a problem with your child, try to sit down and solve it together. Help him or her figure out ways to solve problems nonviolently.

Figure 16-4
These 8-year-olds gain a sense of belonging by huddling as a team.

groups and are often project-oriented, such as Scout troops and athletic teams. Private clubs with homemade clubhouses, secret codes, and languages are popular. Individual friendships also are formed, and "best friends" are intensely loyal, if only for short periods. Table games, arts and crafts requiring skill and dexterity, computer games, school science projects, and science fairs are popular, as are more active pursuits. This period includes the beginning of many neighborhood team sports, including Little League, softball, football, and soccer. Both boys and girls are actively involved in many of these sports (Fig. 16-4).

Even though parents are no longer considered the ultimate authority, their standards have become part of the child's personality and conscience. Although the child may cheat, lie, or steal on occasion, he or she suffers considerable guilt if he or she learns that these are unacceptable behaviors.

Important changes occur in a child's thinking processes at about age 7 years, when there is movement from pre-operational, egocentric thinking to concrete, operational, decentered thought. For the first time, children can see the world from someone else's point of view. **Decentration** means being able to see several aspects of a problem at the same time and to understand the relation of various parts to the whole situation. Cause-and-effect relations become clear; consequently, magical thinking begins to disappear.

During the seventh or eighth year, children have an increased understanding of the conservation of continuous quantity. Understanding conservation depends on **reversibility**, the ability to think in either direction. Seven-year-olds can add and subtract, count forward and backward, and see how it is possible to put something back the way it was. A 7- or 8-year-old can understand that illness is probably only temporary, whereas a 6-year-old may think it is permanent.

Another important change in thinking during this period is **classification**, the ability to group objects into a

Figure 16-3
A 7-year-old helps his grandfather sift compost.

hierarchical arrangement (grouping by some common system). Children in this age group love to collect sports cards, pogs, insects, rocks, stamps, coins, or anything else that strikes their fancy. These collections may be only a short-term interest, but some can develop into lifetime hobbies.

NUTRITION

As coordination improves, the child becomes increasingly active and requires more food to supply the necessary energy. Increased appetite and a tendency to go on food "jags" are typical of the 6-year-old child. This stage soon passes and is unimportant if the child generally gets the necessary nutrients. Allowing the child to express food dislikes and permitting refusal of the disliked food item are usually the best ways to handle this phase. As the child's tastes develop, once-disliked foods may become favorites unless earlier battles have been waged over the food. Children are more likely to learn to eat most foods if everyone else accepts them in a matter-of-fact way.

Children learn by the examples caregivers and others set for them. They will accept more readily the importance of manners, calm voices, appropriate table conversation, and courtesy if they see them carried out consistently at home. Mealtime should never be used for nagging, finding fault, correcting manners, or discussing a poor report card. Hygiene should be taught in a cheerful but firm manner, even if the child must leave the table more than once to wash his or her hands adequately.

Most children prefer simple, plain foods and are good judges of their own needs if they are not coaxed, nagged, bribed, rewarded, or influenced by television commercials. Disease or strong emotions may cause loss of appetite, but force helps little and can have harmful effects.

Caregivers must carefully supervise children's snacking habits to be sure that snacks are nutritious and not too frequent. Children should avoid junk food and continual nibbling that can cause lack of interest at mealtime. Children should be encouraged to eat a good breakfast to provide the energy and nutrients needed to perform well in school. Children need a clearly planned schedule that allows time for a good breakfast and toothbrushing before leaving for school.

Obesity can be a concern during this age. Some children may have a genetic tendency to obesity; environment and a sedentary lifestyle also play a part. In many families, children are urged to "clean your plate" or are encouraged to belong to the "clean plate club." In addition, many families now eat fast foods several times a week, which reinforces the problem because fast foods tend to have high fat and calorie content, contributing to obesity. Other children, especially in the later elementary grades, can be unkind to overweight children, teasing them, not choosing them in games, or avoiding them as friends. The child who becomes

sensitive to being overweight is often miserable. Encouraging physical activity and limiting dietary fat intake to 35% of total calories will help control the child's weight. Popular fad diets must be avoided because they do not supply adequate nutrients for the growing child. Caregivers must avoid nagging and creating feelings of inferiority or guilt, because the child may simply rebel. The child who is pressured too much to lose weight may become a food sneak, setting up patterns that will be harmful later in life. In addition, anorexia nervosa (see Chap. 19) has become a problem for some girls in the older school-age group.

Health teaching at school should reinforce the importance of a proper diet (Table 16-2). Family and cultural food

TABLE 16-2. Foods to Meet the Nutritional Needs of the 6- to 10-Year-Old

Food	Serving Size
Milk, vitamin D-fortified	2–3 cups
Eggs	3 or 4 per wk
Meat, poultry, fish	2–3 oz (small serving)
Dried beans, peas, or peanut butter	2 servings each week. If used as an alternative for meat, allow ½ cup cooked beans or peas or 2 tbsp peanut butter for 1 oz meat.
Potatoes, white or sweet (occasionally spaghetti, macaroni, rice, noodles, etc.)	1 small or ⅓ cup
Other cooked vegetables (green leafy or deep yellow 3 or 4 times per wk)	¼ cup
Raw vegetables (salad greens, cabbage, celery, carrots, etc.)	¼ cup
Vitamin C food (citrus fruit, tomato, cantaloupe, etc.)	1 medium orange or equivalent
Other fruits	1 portion or more as: 1 apple, 1 banana, 1 peach, 1 pear, ½ cup cooked fruit
Bread, enriched or whole-grain	3 slices or more
Cereal, enriched or whole-grain	½ cup
Additional foods	Butter or margarine, desserts, etc., to satisfy energy needs

Adapted from Robinson CH, Lawler MR, Chenoweth WL, et al. Normal and therapeutic nutrition, 17th ed. New York: Macmillan, 1986.

patterns are strong, however, and tend to persist despite nutrition education. Some families are making a positive effort to reduce fat and cholesterol when preparing meals. Most schools have subsidized lunch programs for eligible children, and some have breakfast programs. These provide well-balanced meals, but often children eat only part of what they are offered. Some families post the school lunch menu on the refrigerator or kitchen bulletin board so that children can decide whether to eat the school's lunch or pack their own on any particular day. This way the child can avoid lunches he or she dislikes or simply refuses to eat. School-age children are old enough to be at least partially responsible for preparing their own lunch.

HEALTH PROMOTION AND MAINTENANCE

The school years are generally healthy years for most children. However, routine health care and health education, including health habits, safety, sex education, and substance abuse, are very important aspects of well-planned health promotion and maintenance programs for school-age children.

Routine Checkups

The school-age child should have a physical examination by a physician or other health care provider every year. Additional visits are commonly made throughout the year for minor illness. The school-age child should visit the dentist at least twice a year for a cleaning and application of fluoride.

Most states have immunization requirements that must be met when the child enters school. A booster of tetanus–diphtheria vaccine is recommended every 10 years lifelong. In addition, physical and dental examinations may be required at specific intervals during the elementary school years. During a physical examination at about the age of 10 to 11 years, the child is examined for signs of **scoliosis** (lateral curvature of the spine) (Fig. 16-5). Vision and hearing screening should be performed before entrance to school and on a periodic basis (annual or biannual) thereafter. These examinations often are conducted by the school nurse.

Elementary school children generally are healthy, with

A   B

Figure 16-5
Scoliosis checkup. (A) Viewing from the back, the examiner checks the symmetry of the girl's shoulders. She will also look for a prominent shoulder blade, an unequal distance between the girl's arms and waist; a higher or more prominent hip; and curvature of the spinal column. (B) With the child bending over and touching her toes, the examiner checks for a curvature of the spinal column. She will also look for a rib hump.

only minor illnesses, usually respiratory or gastrointestinal in nature. The leading cause of death in this age group continues to be accidents.

Family Teaching

The school-age child generally incorporates healthy habits into his or her daily routine, but reinforcement by caregivers is still needed. Education for the care of the teeth, with particular attention to the 6-year molars, is important. Proper dental hygiene includes a routine inspection and conscientious brushing after meals. A well-balanced diet with plenty of calcium and phosphorus and minimal sugar is important to healthy teeth. Foods containing sugar should be eaten only at mealtimes and should be followed immediately by proper brushing (Fig. 16-6).

Exercise and sufficient rest are also important during this period. Caregivers need to help school-age children to balance their rest needs and their extracurricular activities. Extracurricular activities help the child remain fit, bond with peers, and establish positive, lifelong attitudes toward exercise. The school-age child needs 10 to 12 hours of sleep per night. The 6-year-old needs 12 hours of sleep and should be provided with a quiet time after school to recharge after a busy day in the classroom. The nurse should take an opportunity to highlight these important aspects of daily health care to both the caregivers and child.

Health Education

Health teaching, both in the home and at school, is essential. Caregivers have a responsibility to teach the child about basic hygiene, sexual functioning, substance abuse,

Figure 16-6
The school-age child needs encouragement to brush after meals and at bedtime as part of a good dental hygiene program.

and accident prevention. Schools must include these topics in the curriculum also because many families are not well informed enough to cover the topics adequately. Some schools offer health classes at each grade level taught by a health educator. In other schools, health and sex education are integrated into the curriculum and taught by each classroom teacher. Nurses should become active in their community to ensure that these kinds of programs are available to children.

SEX EDUCATION

Children learn about femininity and masculinity from the time they are born. Behaviors, attitudes, and actions of the men and women in the child's life, toward the child and toward each other, form impressions in the child that last a lifetime. There has been much controversy about the proper time and place for formal sex education. Part of the problem seems to stem from the fact that many people automatically think that sex education means adult sexuality and reproduction. However, sex education includes helping children develop positive attitudes toward their own bodies, their own sex, and their own sexual role to achieve optimum satisfaction in being a boy or a girl.

In some schools, sex education is limited to one class, usually in the fifth grade, in which children are shown films about menstruation and their developing bodies. Often these are taught in separate classes for boys and girls. Some health educators strongly recommend that sex education should be started in kindergarten and developed gradually over the successive grades. Learning about reproduction of plants and animals, about birth and nurturing in other animals, and about the roles of the male and the female in family units can lead to the natural introduction of human reproduction, male and female roles, families, and nurturing. If all children grew up in secure, loving, ideal families, much of this could be learned at home. However, many children do not have this type of home, so they need healthy, positive information to help them develop healthy attitudes about their own sexuality. Feelings of self-worth also are woven into these lessons, helping children feel good about themselves and who they are.

Caregivers who feel uncomfortable discussing sex with their children may find it helpful to use books or pamphlets available for various age groups. Generally, a female caregiver finds it easier to discuss sex with a girl, and a male caregiver feels more comfortable with a boy. This can pose special problems for the single caregiver with a child of the opposite sex. Again, printed materials may be helpful. Nurses may be called on to help a caregiver provide information and must be comfortable with their own sexuality to handle these discussions well.

At a young age, children are exposed to a great amount of sexually provocative information through the media. Children who do not get accurate information at home or at school will learn what they want to know from their

A Personal Glimpse

When we had the program on drugs at school, I learned some things. Like when you take drugs you can get sick or even die. In one part of the lesson, we watched a video where a kid took drugs and almost died and during the other part the school nurse showed us samples of drugs. Even though I learned about drugs from the program, I think that all children should be taught this subject by their parent or guardian.

Stephen, age 11

peers, but this information is often inaccurate, making sex education even more urgent. In addition, the Centers for Disease Control currently recommends that elementary school children should be taught about acquired immunodeficiency syndrome and how it is spread. Many school districts are working hard to integrate this information into the health curriculum at all grade levels in a sensitive, age-appropriate manner.

SUBSTANCE ABUSE

In addition to nutrition, health practices, safety, and sex education, school-age children also need substance abuse education. Programs that teach children to "just say no"

Family Teaching
Guidelines to Prevent Substance Abuse

1. Openly communicate values by talking about the importance of honesty, responsibility, and self-reliance. Encourage decision making. Help children see how each decision builds on previous decisions.
2. Provide a good role model for the child to copy. Children tend to copy parents' habits of smoking and drinking alcohol and accept attitudes about drug use, whether they are over-the-counter, prescription, or illicit drugs.
3. Avoid conflicts between what you say and what you do. For example, don't ask the child to lie that you are not home when you are or encourage the child to lie about age when trying to get a lower admission price at amusement centers.
4. Talk about values during family times. Give the child "what if" examples, and discuss the best responses when faced with a difficult situation. For example, "What would you do if you found money that someone dropped?"
5. Set strong rules about using alcohol and other drugs. Make specific rules with specific punishments. Discuss these rules and the reason for them.
6. Be consistent in applying the rules that you set.
7. Be reasonable; don't make wild threats. Respond calmly, carrying out the expected punishment.
8. Get the facts about alcohol and other drugs, and provide children with current, correct information. This helps you in discussions with children and also helps you recognize symptoms if a child has been using them.

(From Growing up drug free: A parent's guide to prevention. Washington DC: U.S. Department of Education, 1990.)

Box 16-1. *Common Products Inhaled as Deliriants*

Model glue
Rubber cement
Cleaning fluids
Kerosene vapors
Gasoline vapors
Butane lighter fluid
Paint sprays
Paint thinner
Varnish
Shellac
Nail polish remover
Liquid typing correction fluid
Propellant in whipped-cream spray cans
Aerosol paint cans
Upholstery-fabric-protection spray cans
Solvents

are one way children can learn they are in control. Teaching children the unhealthy aspects of tobacco and alcohol use and drug abuse should be started in elementary school as a good foundation for more advanced information in adolescence.

Despite the stereotype that children who abuse substances are children of the ghetto, age, race, and socioeconomic status are not limiting factors in this problem. The use of alcohol and other substances to provide mind-altering excitement occurs in children as young as 8 or 9 years of age. Many children, even those as young as elementary school age, from every level of society smoke cigarettes. The risk for starting to smoke is greatest in the sixth and seventh grades. Forty percent of children try cigarettes before they enter high school, with the total reaching 70% before the end of high school. Twelve percent of boys have chewed tobacco or snuff, which is just as addictive and harmful as smoking.

Children may experiment with **inhalants** (substances

Figure 16-7
Helmets are an important aspect of bike safety.

whose volatile vapors can be abused) because they are readily available and may seem no more threatening than an innocent prank. Inhalants classified as **deliriants** contain chemicals that give off fumes that can produce symptoms of confusion, disorientation, excitement, and hallucinations. Many inhalants are commonly found in the home (Box 16-1). The fumes are mind-altering when inhaled. The child initially may experience a temporary high, giddiness, nausea, coughing, nosebleed, fatigue, lack of coordination, or loss of appetite. Overdose can cause loss of consciousness and possible death from suffocation by replacing oxygen in the lungs or depressing the central nervous system, causing respiratory arrest. Permanent damage to the lungs, the nervous system, or the liver can result. Children who experiment with inhalants may proceed to abuse other drugs in an attempt to get similar effects. Addiction occurs in younger children more rapidly than in adults.

Family caregivers must work to develop a strong, loving relationship with the children in the family, teach the children the family's values and the difference between right and wrong, set and enforce rules for acceptable behavior of family members, learn facts about drugs and alcohol, and actively listen to the children in the family (see Family Teaching box: Guidelines to Prevent Substance Abuse). An excellent reference for family caregivers is "How to Raise Drug Free Kids," which is published by the United States Department of Education and can be ordered free by calling

the Department of Education's toll-free number, (800) 624-0100 or via the Internet at http://www.ed.gov/offices/OESE/SDFS/.

Accident Prevention

As stated earlier, accidents continue to be a leading cause of death during this period. Even though school-age children do not require constant supervision, they must be taught certain safety rules and practice them until they are routine (Fig. 16-7). They should understand the function of traffic lights, which family members should obey as a matter of course. Example is the best teacher for any child. Children should know their full name, their caregivers' names, and their own home address and telephone number. Children should be taught the appropriate way to call for emergency help in their community (911 in a community that has such a system). Many communities have safe-home programs that designate homes where children can go if they have a problem on the way home from school. These homes are clearly marked in a way that children are taught to recognize. In many communities, local police officers or firefighters are interested in coming into the classroom to help teach safety. Children gain from meeting police officers and understanding that they have a duty to

Family Teaching
Safety Topics for Elementary School-Age Children

1. Traffic signals and safe pedestrian practices
2. Safety belt use for car passengers
3. Bicycle safety
   a. Wear a helmet
   b. Use hand signals
   c. Ride with traffic
   d. Be sure others see you
4. Skateboard and skating safety
   a. Wear a helmet
   b. Wear elbow and knee pads
   c. Skate only in safe skating areas
5. Swimming safety
   a. Learn to swim
   b. Never swim alone
   c. Always know the water depth
   d. Don't dive head first
   e. No running or horseplay at a pool
6. Danger of projectile toys
7. Danger of all-terrain vehicles
8. Use of life jacket when boating
9. Stranger safety
   a. Who is a stranger
   b. Never accept a ride from someone you don't know
   c. Never accept food or gifts from someone you don't know
   d. Check the license number and try to remember it
10. Good touch and bad touch

TABLE 16-3.   Children's Concept of Biology

Concept	6 to 8 Years	8 to 10 Years	*Implications for Nursing*
Birth	Gradually see babies as the result of three factors—social and sexual intercourse and biogenetic fusion Tend to see baby as emerging from female only; many still see baby as manufactured by outside force—created whole Boys less knowledgeable about baby formation than girls	Begin to put three components together; recognize that sperm and egg come together but may not be sure why Fewer discrepancies in knowledge based on sex differences	Cultural and educational factors play a part in development of where babies come from. Nurse should assess children's ideas about birth and whether they can understand where babies come from and how before teaching. Explanations about role of both parents can begin, but the idea of sperm and egg union may not be understood until 8 or 9 years of age.
Death	May be viewed as reversible Animism (attribution of life) may be seen in some children—death viewed as result of outside force Experiences with death facilitate concept development	Considered irreversible Ideas about what happens after death unclear—related to concreteness of thinking and socio-religious upbringing	Change from vague view of death as reversible and caused by external forces to awareness of irreversibility and bodily causes Fears about death more common at 8—adults should be alert to this Explanations about death, the fact that their thoughts will not cause a death, and they will not die (if illness is not fatal) are needed.
Human body	Know body holds everything inside Use outside world to explain inside Aware of major organs Interested in visible functions of body	Can understand physiology; use general principles to explain body functions; interested in invisible functions of body	Cultural factors may play a part in ability and willingness to discuss bodily functions. Educational programs can be very effective because of natural interest. Assess knowledge of body by using diagrams before teaching.
Health	See health as doing desired activities List concrete practices as components of health Many do not see sickness as related to health; may not consider cause and effect	See health as doing desired activities Understand cause and effect Believe it is possible to be part healthy and part not at the same time; can reverse from health to sickness and back to health	Need assistance in seeing cause and effect Capitalize on positiveness of concept—health lets you do what you really want to do. Young children who are sick may feel they will never get well again.
Illness	Sick children may see illness as punishment; evidence suggests that healthy children do not see illness as punishment Highly anxious children more likely to view illness as disruptive Sickness is a diffuse state; rely on others to tell them when they are ill	Same as 6–8 years of age; can identify illness states, report bodily discomfort, recognize illness is caused by specific factors	Social factors play a part in illness concept. Recognize that some see illness as punishment. Encourage self-care and self-help behavior, especially in older children.

Wieczorek RR, Natapoff J. A conceptual approach to the nursing of children: Health care from birth through adolescence. Philadelphia: JB Lippincott, 1981.

help children, not to punish them. Safety rules should be stressed at home and at school. The Family Teaching box summarizes important safety considerations for school-age children.

THE SCHOOL-AGE CHILD IN THE HEALTH CARE FACILITY

Increased understanding of their bodies, continuing curiosity about how things work, and development of concrete thinking all contribute to helping school-age children understand and accept a health care experience better than younger children. They can communicate better with health care providers, understand cause and effect, and tolerate longer separations from the family.

Nurses who care for school-age children should understand how concepts about birth, death, the body, health, and illness change between the ages of 6 and 10 years (Table 16-3). All procedures must be explained to children and their families, showing the equipment and materials to be used (or pictures of them) and outlining realistic expectations of procedures and treatments. Children's questions should be answered truthfully, including those about pain. Children of this age have anxieties about looking different from other children. An opportunity to verbalize these anxieties will help a child deal with them. School-age children need privacy more than younger children and may not want to have physical contact with adults, a wish that should be respected. Boys may be uncomfortable having a female nurse bathe them, and girls may feel uncomfortable with a male nurse. These attitudes should be recognized and

handled in a way that will ensure as much privacy as possible.

Family caregivers may feel guilty about the child's need for hospitalization and, as a result, may overindulge the child. The child may regress in response to this, but this regression should not be encouraged. Sometimes the family needs as much reassurance as the child.

Discipline and rules have a place on a pediatric unit. Families and children must be informed about the rules as part of the admission routine. Opportunity for interaction with peers, learning experiences, crafts, and projects can help make the child's experience more tolerable (Fig. 16-8).

■ KEY POINTS

- Growth and development during the school-age years is steady at all levels—emotional, social, intellectual, and physical.

- According to Erikson, the developmental task of school-age children is industry versus inferiority. The child engages in many activities using motor, cognitive, and social skills. Success in these activities is necessary for the child to develop a sense of competency.

- A child's success or failures during this period can have a lifelong impact on attitudes and performance.

- The school-age child gains a real sense of self, with individualized moral standards and conscience.

- The family is still the major sustaining force, even

A   B

Figure 16-8
(A) Eight-year-olds still like to listen to stories. (B) Young artist in the hospital playroom.

though much time is spent with peers in activities outside the home.

■ Substance abuse is an ever-increasing concern during this age. Family caregivers must make every effort to be alert to children's use of inhalants, deliriants, alcohol, or tobacco.

■ School-age children need privacy, and this must be respected when planning their care.

■ The changes in a school-age child's understanding of biology influence the child's view of his or her own health care. The nurse needs to understand these concepts to plan nursing care for the school-age child.

CRITICAL THINKING

1. Delsey is upset that 6-year-old Jasmine is a picky eater and often does not want to eat what Delsey has prepared. Explain the advice or reassurance you can give her.

2. Make a safety poster or teaching aid to use in an elementary school classroom. Perhaps you can make this a class project and donate the posters to your pediatric unit or nearby school.

3. Steve, the primary family caregiver of 8-year-old Carolyn, feels that he should offer her sex education and asks your advice. Describe how you will respond.

4. Substance abuse education, including alcohol and tobacco, should be included in the school health program. Discuss effective methods that you believe should be used to present these programs to children.

5. Survey your home and make a list of all the products available that a child could use as an inhalant for a deliriant effect.

6. Seven-year-old Jake is hospitalized with a broken femur. He is shy about having a female nurse care for him. (For female students) What are the characteristics of school-age children that affect how you will care for him? Develop a plan of care for him. (For male students) Use the same situation, but your child is 7-year-old Kimberly.

BIBLIOGRAPHY

Brooks RB. Self-esteem during the school years: Its normal development and hazardous decline. Pediatr Clin North Am 39(3): 537–550, 1992.

Brown J. Be headstrong! Start a bicycle helmet campaign! Contemp Pediatr 9(7):54–73, 1992.

Eschleman MM. Introductory nutrition and diet therapy, 2d ed. Philadelphia: JB Lippincott, 1991.

Jackson DB, Saunders RB. Child health nursing. Philadelphia: JB Lippincott, 1993.

Pillitteri A: Maternal and child health nursing, 2d ed. Philadelphia: JB Lippincott, 1995.

Schuster CS, Ashburn SS. The process of human development, 3d ed. Philadelphia: JB Lippincott, 1992.

Spock B, Rothenberg MB. Dr. Spock's baby and child care. New York: Pocket Books, 1992.

Winkelstein ML. Fostering positive self-concept in the school-age child. Pediatr Nurs 15(3):229–233, 1989.

Wong DL. Whaley and Wong's nursing care of infants and children, 5th ed. St. Louis: Mosby, 1995.

Health Problems of the School-Age Child

BEHAVIORAL PROBLEMS
School Phobia
CENTRAL NERVOUS SYSTEM DISORDERS
Attention Deficit Hyperactivity Disorder
Convulsive Disorders
ALLERGIC REACTIONS
Allergic Rhinitis (Hay Fever)
Asthma
Nursing Process for the Child with Asthma
GASTROINTESTINAL SYSTEM DISORDERS
Appendicitis
Nursing Process for the Child with Appendicitis
Intestinal Parasites
DISORDERS OF ELIMINATION
Enuresis
Encopresis
CARDIOVASCULAR SYSTEM DISORDERS
Rheumatic Fever
Nursing Process for the Child with Rheumatic Fever

ENDOCRINE SYSTEM DISORDERS
Juvenile Diabetes Mellitus (Insulin-Dependent Diabetes Mellitus)
Nursing Process for the Child with Diabetes Mellitus
MUSCULOSKELETAL SYSTEM DISORDERS
Scoliosis
Nursing Process for the Child with Scoliosis
Legg-Calvé-Perthes Disease (Coxa Plana)
Osteomyelitis
Muscular Dystrophy
Juvenile Rheumatoid Arthritis
Fractures
SKIN DISORDERS
Fungal Infections
Parasitic Infections
Skin Allergies
Bites

STUDENT OBJECTIVES

On completion of this chapter, the student will be able to:

1. Identify 10 characteristics that may be seen in a child with attention deficit hyperactivity disorder.
2. Describe a) a grand mal (tonic-clonic) seizure and b) an absence (petit mal) seizure.
3. List factors that can trigger an asthmatic attack, and describe the physiologic response that occurs in the respiratory tract.
4. List the symptoms of appendicitis; differentiate symptoms of the older and the younger child.
5. Identify three intestinal parasites common to children, and state the route of entry for each.
6. Develop a teaching plan for an 8-year-old child with diabetes mellitus; include skin care, insulin administration, and exercise.
7. Describe scoliosis, and identify four methods of correction.
8. Identify the most common form of muscular dystrophy; describe its characteristics.
9. Name the drug of choice in the treatment of juvenile rheumatoid arthritis, and state its primary purpose.
10. List and define the five P's necessary to observe, record, and report when caring for a child in a cast.
11. Describe the treatment for pediculosis of the scalp, and state the protection the nurse must use when treating a child with this condition in the hospital.

KEY TERMS

allergen	lordosis
ankylosis	metered-dose inhaler
anthelmintic	nebulizer
arthralgia	polyarthritis
aura	polydipsia
carditis	polyphagia
chorea	polyuria
diabetic acidosis	school phobia
encopresis	seizure
enuresis	skeletal traction
halo traction	skin traction
hirsutism	soft neurologic signs
hyposensitization	synovitis
insulin reaction	tinea
Kussmaul breathing	traction
kyphoscoliosis	wheezing

Entering school is a stressful time for every child, but especially so for the child with a chronic health problem. Imitation of peers is important during this time, but sometimes this is impossible for the child with a learning disorder, severe allergies, or a problem that limits physical mobility or makes the child feel different from peers. These children must cope with all the normal developmental stresses and the additional stress the health problem causes.

School-age children can learn to manage their health problems. Given enough information and guidance, children can understand and cope with problems such as diabetes and asthma. Nurses and caregivers who care for these children should foster maximum independence and a life as normal as possible.

BEHAVIORAL PROBLEMS

A number of behavioral problems are common in the school-age group. These problems can interfere with socialization, education, and development of the child. Some of these have definite organic causes; in others, the causes are not clearly defined.

School Phobia

School absenteeism is a national problem. Children are absent from school for a variety of reasons, one of which may be **school phobia.** Children who develop school phobia may be good students; more girls than boys are affected. Teachers and nurses can help detect school phobia by paying close attention to absence patterns. School-phobic children may have a strong attachment to one parent, usually the mother, and they fear separation from that parent, perhaps because of anxiety about losing her or him while away from home. School phobia may be the child's unconscious reaction to a seemingly overwhelming problem at school. The parent can unwittingly reinforce school phobia by permitting the child to stay home. The symptoms—vomiting, diarrhea, abdominal or other pain, and even a low-grade fever—are genuine and are caused by anxiety that may approach panic. They disappear with relief of the immediate anxiety after the child has been given permission to stay home.

Treatment includes a complete medical examination to rule out any organic cause for the symptoms and school–family conferences to help the child return to school. Those working with these children must recognize that they really do want to go to school, but for whatever reason cannot make themselves go; these children are not delinquents. The school nurse, the teacher, and other professionals, such as a social worker, a psychologist, and a psychiatrist, all may contribute to resolving the problem. If the child fears a specific factor at school, such as an overly critical teacher, the child may need to be moved to another class or school.

CENTRAL NERVOUS SYSTEM DISORDERS

Although the health problems discussed in this section—attention deficit hyperactivity disorder and convulsive disorders—may not be classified simply as central nervous system disorders, the central nervous system plays an important part in each of them. Both of the conditions have a great impact on the child's success in school and throughout life. Continuing research will help identify the causes and improve treatment. The future holds great promise for children with these conditions.

Attention Deficit Hyperactivity Disorder

Attention deficit hyperactivity disorder (ADHD), or attention deficit disorder, is a syndrome characterized by certain behavioral and perceptual problems. About 3% to 5% of all American children have such a disorder; boys are more commonly affected than girls. The cause of the disorder is unclear: developmental lag, biochemical disorder, and food sensitivities are all theories under consideration. The disorder affects every part of the child's life. The child with ADHD may have these characteristics:

- Impulsive
- Easily distracted
- Often fidgets or squirms
- Has difficulty sitting still
- Has problems following through on instructions despite being able to understand them

- Inattentive when spoken to
- Often loses things
- Goes from one uncompleted activity to another
- Has difficulty taking turns
- Often talks excessively
- Often engages in dangerous activities without considering the consequences.

These children also often demonstrate **soft neurologic signs** (signs of clumsiness or poor coordination that may be appropriate for a younger child). No one child has all of these symptoms. Although it was believed to be resolved by late adolescence, it is now apparent that, at least for some, it continues into adulthood.

Although these children have poor success in the classroom because of their inability to attend, they are not intellectually impaired. The child's poor impulse control also contributes to disciplinary problems in the classroom. Some children with ADHD may have learning disorders, such as dyslexia and perceptual deficits. The child's self-confidence can suffer from feeling inferior to the other children in the class. Special arrangements can be made to provide an educational atmosphere that is supportive for the child without the need for the child to leave the classroom.

DIAGNOSIS

Diagnosis can be made after the child is 3 years old but often is not made until the child reaches school and has trouble settling into the routine. Diagnosis can be difficult and also may be controversial. Many of the symptoms are subjective and rely on the assessment of caregivers and teachers. Some authorities have expressed concern that children are incorrectly labeled as hyperactive by teachers. The symptoms may be a result of environmental factors, which can include broken homes, stress, and unsupportive caregivers.

The most effective approach to diagnosis is a multidisciplinary one involving pediatric specialists, education specialists, a psychologist, the classroom teacher, and others. A careful, detailed history, including school and social functioning, psychological testing, and physical and neurologic examinations can help make the diagnosis.

TREATMENT AND NURSING CARE

Treatment is also multidisciplinary. Learning situations should be structured so that the child has minimal distractions and a supportive teacher. Home support is necessary, requiring structured, consistent guidance from the caregivers. Medication is used for some children. Stimulant medications, such as methylphenidate (Ritalin) and dextroamphetamine (Dexedrine), have often been used. When given in large amounts, these medications may suppress the appetite and affect the child's growth. Pemoline (Cylert) has been used but generally with less success than

A Personal Glimpse

I don't really mind it. When I don't take my meds, I go crazy or bonkers (sometimes). I'm on my pills cause of my behavior [sic] and anger. And also to control my anger and ways I talk (like so I won't say bad words or other bad luagnage [sic]). I was taught about to control your anger, don't let your anger control you.

Eddie, a 9-year-old who takes medication for behavior problems

methylphenidate and dextroamphetamine. Using stimulants for a hyperactive child seems paradoxical, but these drugs apparently stimulate the area of the child's brain that aids in concentration, thus enabling the child to have better control.

In the health care setting, the nurse should maintain a calm, patient attitude toward the child with ADHD. The child should be given only one simple instruction at a time. Limiting distractions, using consistency, and offering praise for accomplishments are invaluable methods of working with these children. The families of children with ADHD need a great deal of support. Primary family caregivers in particular can become frustrated and upset by the constant challenge of dealing with a child with ADHD. Building the child's self-esteem, confidence, and academic success must be the primary goal of all who work with these children.

Convulsive Disorders

Convulsive disorders are not uncommon in children and may result from a variety of causes. A common form of seizure is the acute febrile convulsion that occurs with fevers and acute infections (see Chap. 11). Epilepsy, on the other hand, is a recurrent and chronic convulsive disorder. Epilepsy can be classified as primary (idiopathic), with no known cause, or secondary, resulting from infection, head trauma, hemorrhage, tumor, or other organic or degenerative factor. Primary epilepsy is the most common; its onset generally is between ages 4 and 8 years.

CLINICAL MANIFESTATIONS

Seizures are the characteristic clinical manifestation of both types of epilepsy and may be either partial (focal) or generalized. Partial seizures are limited to a particular area of the brain; generalized seizures involve both hemispheres of the brain.

Partial Seizures Manifestations of partial seizures vary depending on the area of the brain from which they arise. There may be no loss of consciousness or awareness; localized motor activity may be limited to one side of the body and may then spread to other parts. Sensory symptoms may include an **aura** (a sensation that signals an impending attack) involving sight, sound, taste, smell, touch, or emotions (a feeling of fear, for example). Partial seizures are classified as simple, complex, or partial seizures secondarily generalized. In this last type, the partial seizure is considered the primary seizure and can be identified by a tonic-clonic seizure that was not generalized at the onset.

Generalized Seizures Types of generalized seizures include grand mal (major motor), absence (petit mal), akinetic, myoclonic, and infantile spasms.

Grand mal seizures consist of a sudden loss of consciousness, with generalized tonic and clonic movements. If the seizure is preceded by an aura, it is identified as a generalized seizure secondary to a partial seizure. Young children may have difficulty describing an aura but may cry out in response to it. In a primary generalized seizure, loss of consciousness is the initial manifestation. The initial rigidity of the tonic phase (contraction of extensor and flexor muscles) changes rapidly to generalized jerking movements of the muscles (clonic phase). The child may bite the tongue or lose control of bladder and bowel functions. The contraction of respiratory muscles during the tonic phase may cause the child to become cyanotic, appearing briefly to have respiratory arrest. The jerking movements gradually diminish, then disappear, and the child relaxes. The seizure can be brief, lasting less than 1 minute, or it can last 30 minutes or longer. After the episode, some children return rapidly to an alert state, many have a period of confusion, and others experience a prolonged period of stupor. The period after the tonic-clonic phase is called the postictal period.

Absence seizures rarely last longer than 20 seconds. The child loses awareness and stares straight ahead but does not fall. Immediately after the seizure, the child is alert and continues conversation but does not know what was said or done during the episode. Absence seizures can recur frequently, sometimes as often as 50 to 100 a day. They often decrease significantly or stop entirely at adolescence.

Akinetic seizures cause a momentary loss of consciousness, muscle tone, and postural control and can result in serious facial, head, or shoulder injuries. They may recur frequently, particularly in the morning.

Myoclonic seizures are characterized by a sudden jerking of a muscle or group of muscles without loss of consciousness. Myoclonus occurs during the early stages of falling asleep in people who do not have epilepsy.

Infantile spasms occur between 3 and 12 months of age and almost always indicate a cerebral defect and poor prognosis despite treatment. These seizures occur twice as often in boys as in girls and are preceded or followed by a cry.

Muscle contractions are sudden, brief, and symmetric and are accompanied by rolling eyes. Loss of consciousness does not always occur.

DIAGNOSIS

The types of seizures can be differentiated through the use of electroencephalography, skull radiography, computed tomography, a brain scan, and physical and neurologic assessment.

TREATMENT

The main goal of treatment, complete control of seizures, can be achieved for most people through the use of anticonvulsant drug therapy. A number of anticonvulsant drugs are available (Table 17-1). The choice of drug is made based on its effectiveness in controlling seizures and on its degree of toxicity. The oldest and most popular drug is phenytoin (Dilantin). It can cause hypertrophy of the gums after prolonged use.

A few children may be candidates for surgical intervention when the focal point of the seizures is in an area of the brain that is accessible surgically and that is not an area critical to functioning.

Ketogenic diets (high in fat and low in carbohydrates and protein) have been prescribed, but because they are difficult to follow and unappealing to the child, long-term maintenance is difficult.

NURSING CARE

Education and counseling of the child and the family caregivers are important parts of nursing care. They need complete, accurate information about the disorder and the results that can be realistically expected from treatment. Epilepsy does not lead inevitably to mental retardation, but continued and uncontrolled seizures increase the possibility of mental retardation. This emphasizes the importance of early diagnosis and control of seizures.

Although the outlook for a normal, well-adjusted life is favorable, the nurse should inform the child and family about restrictions that may be encountered. Children with epilepsy should be encouraged to participate in physical activities but should not participate in sports in which a fall could cause serious injury, such as rope climbing, and they may have to be careful in contact sports. Unsupervised swimming or underwater swimming should not be permitted. In many states a person with uncontrolled epilepsy is legally forbidden to drive a motor vehicle; this could limit choice of vocation and lifestyle. Despite attempts at educating the general public about epilepsy, many people remain prejudiced about this disorder, and this can limit the epileptic person's social and vocational acceptance.

TABLE 17-1. Antiepileptic–Anticonvulsive Therapeutic Agents

Drug	Indication	Side Effects	Nursing Implications
Carbamazepine (Tegretol)	Generalized grand mal, complex partial, focal motor seizures, mixed seizures	Drowsiness, dry mouth, vomiting, double vision, leukopenia, GI upset, thrombocytopenia	There may be dizziness and drowsiness with initial doses. This should subside within 3–14 days.
Ethosuximide (Zarontin)	Absence seizures, myoclonic (petit mal)	Dry mouth, anorexia, dizziness, headache, nausea, vomiting, GI upset, lethargy, bone marrow depression	Use with caution in hepatic or renal disease.
Clonazepam (Klonopin)	Absence seizures, myoclonic (petit mal)	Double vision, drowsiness, increased salivation, changes in behavior, bone marrow depression	Obtain periodic liver function tests and complete blood count. Monitor for oversedation.
Phenobarbital (Luminol)	Tonic-clonic generalized	Drowsiness, alteration in sleep patterns, irritability, respiratory and cardiac depression, restlessness, headache	Alcohol can enhance the effects of phenobarbital. Blood studies and liver tests are necessary with prolonged use.
Primidone (Mysoline)	Tonic-clonic generalized, complex and simple partial seizures	Behavior changes, drowsiness, hyperactivity, ataxia, bone marrow depression	Adverse effects are the same as for phenobarbital. Sedation and dizziness may be severe during initial therapy—dosage may need to be adjusted by the physician.
Valproic acid (Depakene)	Tonic-clonic, myoclonic absence seizures, mixed seizures	Nausea, vomiting, or increased appetite, tremors, elevated liver enzymes, constipation, headaches, depression, lymphocytosis, leukopenia, increased prothrombin time	Physical dependency may result when used for prolonged period. Tablets and capsules should be taken whole. Elixir should be taken alone, not mixed with carbonated beverages. Increased toxicity may occur with administration of salicylates (aspirin).
Phenytoin (Dilantin)	Tonic-clonic generalized, complex and simple partial	Double vision, blurred vision, slurred speech, nystagmus, ataxia, gingival hyperplasia, hirsutism, cardiac arrhythmias, bone marrow depression	Alcohol, antacids, and folic acid decrease the effect of phenytoin. Instruct the child or caregiver to notify the dentist that he or she is taking phenytoin to monitor hyperplasia of the gums. Inform the child or caregiver that the drug may color the urine pink to red-brown.

General Nursing Considerations with Anticonvulsant Therapy

General nursing considerations with anticonvulsant therapy that apply to all or most of drugs given to children include:

1. Warn the patient and family that patients should avoid activities that require alertness and complex psychomotor coordination (eg, climbing).
2. Medication can be given with meals to minimize gastric irritation.
3. The anticonvulsant medications should not be discontinued abruptly, as this can precipitate status epilepticus.
4. Anticonvulsant medications generally have a cumulative effect, both therapeutically and adversely.
5. Alcohol ingestion increases the effects of anticonvulsant drugs, exaggerating the central nervous system depression.
6. Many of the drugs can cause bone marrow depression (leukopenia, thrombocytopenia, neutropenia, megaloblastic anemia). Regular blood counts are necessary to evaluate bone marrow production.
7. The child receives periodic blood tests to monitor therapeutic levels as opposed to toxic levels.

Adapted from Castiglia PT, Harbin RE. Child health care: Process and practice. Philadelphia: JB Lippincott, 1992.

ALLERGIC REACTIONS

Millions of Americans suffer from allergic diseases, most of which begin in childhood. Children with allergies are hampered by poor appetite, poor sleep, and restricted physical activity in play and at school, often resulting in altered physical and personality development. Children whose parents or grandparents have allergies are more likely to become allergic than other children.

An allergic condition is caused by sensitivity to a substance called an **allergen** (antigen that causes an allergy). There are thousands of allergens; some of the most common are pollen, mold, dust, animal dander, insect bites, tobacco smoke, nuts, chocolate, milk, fish, and shellfish. Drugs can be allergens also, particularly aspirin and penicillin. Some plants and chemicals cause allergic reactions on the skin (discussed later in this chapter).

Allergens may enter the body through various routes, the most common being the nose, throat, eyes, bronchial tissues in the lungs, the skin, and the digestive tract. The first time the child comes in contact with an allergen, no reaction may be evident, but an immune response is stimulated—helper lymphocytes stimulate B lymphocytes to make immunoglobulin E (IgE) antibody. The IgE antibody attaches to mast cells and macrophages. When contacted again, the allergen attaches to the IgE receptor sites, and a response occurs in which certain substances, such as histamine, are released; these substances produce the symptoms known as allergy.

Diagnosis of an allergy requires a careful history and physical examination and possibly skin and blood tests, including a complete blood count, serum protein electrophoresis, and immunoelectrophoresis. Skin testing is gen-

Figure 17-2
Typical facies of allergic rhinitis.

erally done when removal of obvious allergens is impossible or has not brought relief. If a food allergy is suspected, an elimination diet may help identify the allergen. When specific allergens have been identified, patients can either avoid them or, if this is impossible, undergo immunization therapy by injection. This process is called **hyposensitization** or immunotherapy.

Hyposensitization is performed for the allergens that produced a positive reaction on skin testing. The allergist sets up a schedule for injections in gradually increasing doses until a maintenance dose is reached. The patient should remain in the physician's office for 20 to 30 minutes after the injection in case any reaction occurs. Reactions are treated with epinephrine. Severe reactions in children are uncommon, and hyposensitization is considered a safe procedure with considerable benefit for some children.

Symptomatic relief in allergic reactions can be gained through antihistamine or steroid therapy, but the best treatment is prevention.

Allergic Rhinitis (Hay Fever)

Allergic rhinitis in children is most often due to sensitization to animal dander, house dust, pollens, and molds. Pollen allergy seldom appears before 4 or 5 years of age.

CLINICAL MANIFESTATIONS

A watery nasal discharge, postnasal drip, sneezing, and allergic conjunctivitis are the usual symptoms of allergic rhinitis. Continued sniffing, itching of the nose and palate, and the "allergic salute" (Fig. 17-1) are common complaints. Dark circles under the eyes are typical (Fig. 17-2).

Figure 17-1
Allergic salute. The allergic child often pushes his or her nose upward and backward to relieve itching and to free edematous turbinates from contact with the septum. This allows for free passage of air.

TREATMENT

When possible, offending allergens are avoided or removed from the environment. Antihistamine–decongestant preparations, such as Dimetapp, Actifed, and others, can be helpful for some patients. Hyposensitization can be implemented, particularly if antihistamines are not helpful or are needed chronically.

Asthma

Asthma is a spasm of the bronchial tubes due to hypersensitivity of the airways in the bronchial system and inflammation that leads to mucosal edema and mucus hypersecretion. This reversible obstructive airway disease affects at least 10 million people in the United States, including 5% to 10% of all children in the United States.

Asthma attacks are often triggered by a hypersensitive response to allergens; in young children, asthma may be the response to certain foods. Asthma is often triggered by exercise, exposure to cold weather, or such irritants as wood-burning stoves, cigarette smoke, dust, pet dander, and foods (such as chocolate, milk, eggs, nuts, and grains). Infections, such as bronchitis and urinary tract infection, can provoke asthma attacks. In children with asthmatic tendencies, emotional stress or anxiety can trigger an attack. Some children with asthma may have no evidence of an immunologic cause for the symptoms.

Asthma can be either intermittent, with extended periods when the child has no symptoms and does not need medication, or chronic, with the need for frequent or continuous therapy. Chronic asthma affects the child's school performance and general activities and may contribute to poor self-confidence and dependency. Asthma is the most common single cause of school absence.[1]

PATHOPHYSIOLOGY

Spasms of the smooth muscles cause the lumina of the bronchi and bronchioles to narrow. Edema of the mucous membranes lining these bronchial branches, and increased production of thick mucus within them, combine with the spasm to cause respiratory obstruction (Fig. 17-3).

CLINICAL MANIFESTATIONS

The onset of an attack may be very abrupt, or it may progress over several days, evidenced by a dry, hacking cough, **wheezing** (the sound of expired air being pushed through obstructed bronchioles), and difficulty breathing. Asthma attacks often occur at night, waking the child from sleep. The child must sit up and is totally preoccupied with efforts to breathe. Attacks may last for only a short time or may continue for several days. Thick, tenacious mucus may be coughed up or vomited after a coughing episode. In some asthmatic patients, coughing is the major symptom and wheezing occurs rarely, if at all. Many children

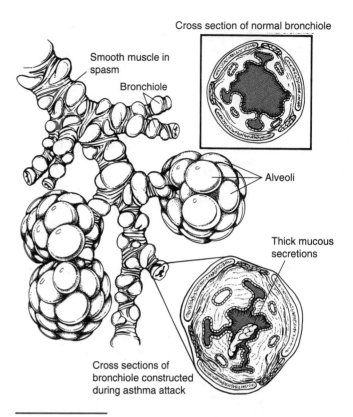

Figure 17-3
Bronchiole airflow obstruction in asthma.

no longer have symptoms after puberty, but this is not predictable. Other allergies may develop in adulthood.

DIAGNOSIS

The history and physical examination are of primary importance in diagnosing asthma. When listening to the child's breathing (auscultation), the examiner hears dyspnea and wheezing, usually generalized over all lung fields. Mucus production may be profuse. Pulmonary function tests are valuable diagnostic tools and indicate the amount of obstruction in the bronchial airways, especially in the smallest airways of the lungs. A definitive diagnosis of asthma is made when the obstruction in the airways is reversed with bronchodilators.

TREATMENT

Prevention is the most important aspect in the treatment of asthma. Children and their families must be taught to recognize the symptoms that lead to an acute attack so that they can be treated as early as possible. These symptoms include increasing cough at night, in the early morning, or on activity; respiratory retractions; and wheezing.[2] Use of a peak flow meter is an objective way to measure airway obstruction, and children as young as 4 or 5 years of age can be taught to use one (see Family Teaching: How to Use a Peak Flow Meter). A peak flow diary should be

Family Teaching

How to Use a Peak Flow Meter

Introduction

Early changes in the airway cannot be felt by your child. By the time the child feels tightness in the chest or starts to wheeze, he or she is already far into an asthma episode. The most reliable early sign of an asthma episode is a drop in the child's peak expiratory flow rate, or the ability to breathe out quickly, which can be measured by a peak flow meter. Almost every asthmatic child over the age of 4 years can and should learn to use a peak flow meter (Figs. A and B.)

Figure A. The Assess peak flow meter.

Figure B. The Mini-Wright peak flow meter.

Figure A.
The Assess peak flow meter.

Figure B.
The Mini-Wright peak flow meter.

Steps to Accurate Measurements

1. Remove gum or food from the mouth.
2. Move the pointer on the meter to zero.
3. Stand up and hold the meter horizontally, with fingers away from the vent holes and marker.
4. With mouth wide open, slowly breathe in as much air as possible.
5. Put the mouthpiece on the tongue and place lips around it.
6. Blow out as hard and fast as you can. Give a short, sharp blast, not a slow blow. The meter measures the fastest puff, not the longest.
7. Repeat steps 1–6 three times. Wait at least 10 seconds between puffs. Move the pointer to zero after each puff.
8. Record the best reading.

Guidelines for Treatment

Each child has a unique pattern of asthma episodes. Most episodes begin gradually, and a drop in peak flow can alert you to start medications before the actual symptoms appear. This early treatment can prevent a flare from getting out of hand. One way to look at peak flow scores is to match the scores with three colors:

Green	Yellow	Red
80%–100% personal best	50%–80% personal best	Below 50% personal best
No symptoms	Mild to moderate symptoms	Serious distress
Full breathing reserve	Diminished reserve	Pulmonary function is significantly impaired
Mild trigger may not cause symptoms	A minor trigger produces noticeable symptoms	Any trigger may lead to severe distress
Continue current management	Augment present treatment regimen	Contact physician

Remember, treatment should be adjusted to fit the individual's needs. Your physician will develop a home management plan with you. When in doubt, consult your physician.

maintained and can also include symptoms, exacerbations, actions taken, and outcomes. Families also must make every effort to eliminate any possible allergens from the home.

Drug Treatment   Bronchodilators are the drugs of choice for treatment of asthma. These drugs are classified into two major groups: 1) theophylline preparations and 2) adrenergic or sympathomimetic drugs. Corticosteroid drugs and cromolyn sodium, a mast cell stabilizer, also are used in addition to the bronchodilators. Epinephrine may be administered subcutaneously in an acute attack.

Theophylline preparations are available in short-acting and long-acting forms. The short-acting forms, such as Theon and Elixicon liquids and aminophylline rectal suppositories, are given about every 6 hours. They are most effective when used only as needed for intermittent episodes of asthma, because they enter the bloodstream quickly. Side effects are nervousness, insomnia, muscular spasms, irritability, palpitations, upset stomach, anorexia, perspiration, and frequent urination.

Long-acting preparations of theophylline, such as Theo-Dur tablets and Theophyl SR capsules, are given every 8 to 12 hours. They are helpful in patients who continually need medication, because these drugs sustain more consistent theophylline levels in the blood than do the short-acting forms. Patients hospitalized for status asthmaticus receive theophylline intravenously (IV).

The beta-adrenergic or sympathomimetic drugs are being used with cromolyn sodium (Intal) often replacing the use of theophylline. Commonly used beta-adrenergic drugs are metaproterenol sulfate (Alupent, Metaprel) and terbutaline sulfate (Brethine). They are short-acting and available in liquid, inhalant, or pill form. These drugs are administered every 6 to 8 hours if breathing difficulty continues despite theophylline administration. In severe attacks, epinephrine by subcutaneous injection often affords quick relief of symptoms. Metaproterenol or isoetharine hydrochloride (Bronkosol) are administered in inhalant form only. Terbutaline can cause tremors in skeletal muscles and increased awareness of the heartbeat. These are normal side effects and not a cause for alarm. Often these effects diminish with continued use of the medication or a decrease in dosage.

Cromolyn sodium prevents mast cells from releasing the chemical mediators that cause bronchospasm and mucous membrane inflammation. It is used to decrease daily wheezing and exercise-induced asthma attacks. A beta-adrenergic drug that functions to open the airways is administered with cromolyn sodium. The beta-adrenergic drug is administered first to maximize the effectiveness of the cromolyn sodium. The child may dislike the taste, which can be minimized by taking sips of water before and after administration. Cromolyn sodium is not useful in severe asthma attacks and can actually worsen an attack, but it is effective as a preventive drug. Side effects are minimal.

Steroids are used in severe or very chronic cases of asthma, but they must be used with great care. They are often prescribed only after other medications have failed to produce the desired effects. Steroids may be given in inhaled form, such as beclomethasone dipropionate (Beclovent), to decrease the systemic effects that accompany oral steroid administration.

Many of these drugs can be given either by a **nebulizer** (tube attached to a wall unit or cylinder that delivers moist air via a face mask) or a **metered-dose inhaler** (hand-held plastic device that delivers a premeasured dose) (Fig. 17-4).

Chest Physiotherapy   Because asthma has multiple causes, treatment and continuing management of the disease require more than medication. Chest physiotherapy includes breathing exercises, physical training, and inhalation therapy. Studies have shown that breathing exercises to improve respiratory function and help control asthma attacks can be an important adjunct to treatment. These exercises teach children how to help control their own symptoms and thereby build self-confidence, which is sometimes lacking in asthmatic children. If the exercises can be taught as part of play activities, children are more likely to find them fun and to practice them more often.

⬆❐ *Nursing Process for the Child With* ⬆❐ *Asthma*

ASSESSMENT

Obtain information from the caregiver about the asthma history, the medications the child takes, and the medications taken within the last 24 hours. Ask if the child has vomited, because vomiting would prevent absorption of oral medications. Ask about any history of respiratory infections; possible allergens in the household, such as pets; type of furniture and toys; whether there is a damp basement (mold spores); and a history of breathing problems after exercise. In the physical examination, include vital signs, observation for diaphoresis and cyanosis, position, type of breathing, alertness, chest movement, intercostal retractions, and breath sounds. Note any wheezing.

If the child is old enough and alert enough to cooperate, involve him or her in gathering the history, and encourage him or her to add information. Ask questions that can be answered "yes" or "no" to decrease tiring the distressed child.

NURSING DIAGNOSES

Work with the child and the child's caregiver to formulate nursing diagnoses. Consider the apprehensions of both the child and the family. Nursing diagnoses may include:

Figure 17-4
(A) Nine-year-old child using a nebulizer. (B) Ten-year-old child using a metered-dose inhaler with spacer.

- Ineffective Airway Clearance related to bronchospasm and increased pulmonary secretions
- Risk for Fluid Volume Deficit related to insensible water loss from tachypnea, diaphoresis, and reduced oral intake
- Fatigue related to dyspnea
- Fear related to sudden attacks of breathlessness
- Health Seeking Behaviors by the family caregivers related to management of home care, disease process, treatment, and control

OUTCOME IDENTIFICATION AND PLANNING

The initial major goals for the child include easing breathing, maintaining adequate fluid intake, and relieving apprehension and fatigue. The family's goals are relieving the child's symptoms and learning how to manage the child's life with asthma. Base the nursing plan of care on these goals.

IMPLEMENTATION

MONITORING RESPIRATORY FUNCTION. Continuously monitor the child while he or she is in acute distress from an asthma attack using pulse oximetry and a cardiopulmonary monitor. If this equipment is unavailable, take the child's respirations every 15 minutes during an acute attack and every 1 or 2 hours after the crisis is over. Observe for nasal flaring and chest retractions; observe the skin for color and diaphoresis. Elevate the child's head. An older child may be more comfortable resting forward on a pillow placed on an overbed table. Monitor the child for response to medications and their side effects, such as restlessness, gastrointestinal (GI) upset, and seizures. Use humidified oxygen and suction as needed during periods of acute distress.

MONITORING AND IMPROVING FLUID INTAKE. During an acute attack, the child may lose a lot of fluid through the respiratory tract and may have a poor oral intake because of coughing and vomiting. Theophylline administration also has a diuretic effect, which compounds the problem. Monitor intake and output. Encourage oral fluids that the child likes. Administer IV fluids as ordered. Monitor IV fluid intake and follow all precautions for parenteral administration. Assess skin turgor and mucous membranes at least every 8 hours. Weigh the child daily to help determine fluid losses.

PROMOTING ENERGY CONSERVATION. The child may become extremely tired from the exertion of trying to breathe. Space activities to provide maximum periods of uninterrupted rest. Provide quiet activities when the child needs diversion. Keep visitors to a minimum and maintain a quiet environment.

REDUCING CHILD AND PARENT ANXIETY. The sudden onset of an asthma attack can be frightening to the child and the family caregivers. Respond quickly when the child has an attack. Reassure the child and the family during an episode of dyspnea. The child's fear of attacks can be increased by the behavior of the caregiver. Teach the child and the caregiver the symptoms of an impending attack and the immediate response needed to decrease the threat of an attack. This knowledge will help them in coping with impending attacks and planning how to handle the attacks. When they are prepared with information, the child and family may be less fearful. Give the child examples of sports figures who have asthma—for example, Olympic track and field athlete Jackie Joyner Kersee and swimmers Amy VanDyken and Tom Dolan.

PROVIDING FAMILY TEACHING. Child and family caregiver teaching is of primary importance in the care of asthmatic children. Family caregivers may overprotect the child because of the fear that an attack will occur when the child is with a babysitter, at school, or anywhere away from the caregiver. Asthma attacks can be prevented or decreased by prompt and adequate intervention. Teach the caregiver and child (within the scope of the child's ability to understand) about the disease process, recognition of symptoms of an impending attack, environmental control, avoidance of infection, exercise, drug therapy, and chest physiotherapy.

Teach the caregiver and the child how to use metered-dose inhaler medications and have them demonstrate correct usage (see Family Teaching: How to Use a Metered Dose Inhaler). Give instructions on home use of a peak flow meter. Urge them to maintain a diary to record the peak flow as well as asthma symptoms, onset of attacks, action taken, and results. Include instructions about administering premedication before the child is exposed to situations in which an attack may occur.

Inform caregivers of allergens that may be in the child's environment, and encourage them to eliminate or control the allergens as needed. Stress the importance of quick response when the child has a respiratory infection. Give instructions for exercise and chest physiotherapy.

Stress to the caregivers the importance of informing the child's classroom teacher, physical education teacher,

school nurse, babysitter, and others who are responsible for the child about the child's condition. With a physician's order, including directions for use, the child should be permitted to bring medications to school and keep them so they can be used when needed.

Provide information on support groups available in the area. The American Lung Association has many materials available to families and can provide information about support groups, camps, and workshops. *Superstuff*, an excellent booklet geared to the elementary- and middle school-age child, is available from the American Lung Association. The Asthma and Allergy Foundation of America and the National Asthma Education Program are also excellent resources.

EVALUATION: GOALS AND OUTCOME CRITERIA

- *Goal*: The child will breathe without distress.
  Criteria: The child's breath sounds are clear, with no wheezing, retractions, or nasal flaring; the skin color is good; the pulse rate is within normal limits.

- *Goal*: The child will not have a fluid deficit.
  Criteria: The child's hourly urine output is 50 mL/kg; mucous membranes are moist; skin turgor is good; weight remains stable.

- *Goal*: The child will have adequate rest.
  Criteria: The child has extended periods of rest; activities are well spaced to avoid tiring the child.

- *Goal*: The child's and caregiver's fear related to impending attacks will be minimized.
  Criteria: The child and the caregiver state the symptoms of an impending attack and appropriate responses and display confidence in their ability to handle an attack.

- *Goal*: The child and the caregiver will gain understanding of how to live with asthma.
  Criteria: The child and the caregiver demonstrate understanding and knowledge of the disease process, treatment, and control through interaction with health care personnel, asking and answering relevant questions and demonstrating techniques as appropriate. The caregiver obtains information to make contact with support groups.

Family Teaching
How to Use a Metered-Dose Inhaler

1. When ready to use, shake the inhaler well with the cap still on. The child should stand, if possible.
2. Remove the cap.
3. Hold the inhaler with the mouthpiece down, facing the child.
4. Be sure the child's mouth is empty.
5. Hold the mouthpiece 1″ to 2″ from the lips.
6. Breathe out normally. Open mouth wide and begin to breathe in.
7. Press top of medication canister firmly while inhaling deeply. Hold breath as long as possible (at least 10 seconds—teach child to count slowly to 10).
8. Breathe out *slowly* through nose or pursed lips.
9. Relax 2–5 minutes, and repeat as directed by physician.

GASTROINTESTINAL SYSTEM DISORDERS

The school-age child may have periodic complaints about a stomach ache or abdominal pain. Usually these complaints are minor, benign, and self-limiting. However, the child's complaints should not be dismissed without being assessed, especially if they seem to be acute, have a regular pattern, or are accompanied by other symptoms.

Appendicitis

Most cases of appendicitis (inflammation of the appendix) in childhood occur in the school-age child. In young children, the symptoms may be difficult to evaluate.

The appendix is a blind pouch located in the cecum near the ileocecal junction. Obstruction of the lumen of the appendix is the primary cause of appendicitis. The obstruction is usually caused by hardened fecal matter or a foreign body. This obstruction causes circulation to be slowed or interrupted, resulting in pain and necrosis of the appendix. The necrotic area can rupture, causing escape of fecal matter and bacteria into the peritoneal cavity and resulting in the complication of peritonitis.

CLINICAL MANIFESTATIONS

Symptoms in the older child may be the same as in an adult: pain and tenderness in the right lower quadrant of the abdomen, nausea and vomiting, fever, and constipation. These symptoms are uncommon in young children, however, because many children already have a ruptured appendix when first seen by the physician. The young child has difficulty localizing the pain, may act restless and irritable, and may have a slight fever, a flushed face, and a rapid pulse. Usually the white blood cell count is slightly elevated. It may take several hours to rule out other conditions and make a positive diagnosis. When appendicitis is suspected, laxatives and enemas are contraindicated because they increase peristalsis and thereby increase the possibility of rupturing an inflamed appendix.

TREATMENT

Surgical removal of the appendix is necessary and should be performed as soon as possible after diagnosis. If the appendix has not ruptured before surgery, the operative risk is nearly negligible. Even after perforation has occurred, the mortality rate is less than 1%.

Food and fluids by mouth are withheld before surgery. If the child is dehydrated, IV fluids are ordered. If fever is present, the temperature should be reduced to below 102°F (38.9°C).

Recovery is rapid and usually uneventful. The child is ambulated early and can leave the hospital a few days after surgery. If peritonitis or a localized abscess occurs, gastric suction, parenteral fluids, and antibiotics may be ordered.

✽⚘ *Nursing Process for the Child*
↩➤ *With Appendicitis*

ASSESSMENT

When a child is admitted with a diagnosis of possible appendicitis, an emergency situation exists. The family caregiver who brings the child to the hospital is often upset and anxious. The admission assessment must be performed quickly and skillfully. Obtain information about the child's condition for the last several days to formulate a picture of how the condition has developed. Emphasize GI complaints, appetite, bowel movements for the last few days, and general activity level. During the physical assessment, include vital signs, especially noting any elevation of temperature, presence of bowel sounds, abdominal guarding, and nausea or vomiting. Report immediately diminished or absent bowel sounds. Provide the child and caregiver with careful explanations about all procedures that are to be performed. Use special empathy and understanding to alleviate the child's and family's anxieties.

NURSING DIAGNOSES

As soon as the medical diagnosis of appendicitis has been confirmed, the child is prepared for surgery. Some nursing diagnoses might include:

- Fear of child and family caregiver related to emergency surgery

- Pain related to necrosis of appendix and surgical procedure

- Risk for Fluid Volume Deficit related to decreased intake

- Ineffective Family Coping: Compromised related to knowledge deficit

OUTCOME IDENTIFICATION AND PLANNING

Because of the urgent nature of the child's admission and preparation for surgery, great efforts must be taken to provide calm, reassuring care, both to the child and the caregiver. A major goal for both the child and caregiver is relieving fear. Additional goals for the child are relieving pain and maintaining fluid intake. Another goal for the family is coping with the child's condition.

REDUCING FEAR. Although procedures must be performed quickly, consider both the child's and the family's fear. The child may be extremely frightened by the sudden change of events and also may be in considerable pain. The family caregiver may be apprehensive about impending surgery. Introduce various health care team members by name and title as they come into the child's room to perform procedures. Explain to the child and the family what is happening and why. Explain the postanesthesia care unit (recovery room) to the child and the family. Encourage the family and child to verbalize fears, and try to allay these fears as much as possible. Let family members know where to wait during surgery, how long the surgery will last, where dining facilities are located, and where the surgeon will expect to find them after surgery. If possible, demonstrate deep breathing, coughing, and abdominal splinting to the child and have him or her practice it. Throughout the preoperative care, be sensitive to fears, whether verbalized or not, and provide understanding care.

REDUCING PAIN. Preoperatively, analgesics are not given because they may conceal signs of tenderness that are important for diagnosis. Provide comfort through positioning and gentle care while performing preoperative procedures. Heat to the abdomen is contraindicated because of the danger of rupture of the appendix. Postoperatively, assess the child hourly for pain and administer analgesics as ordered. Provide quiet activities to help divert the child's attention from the pain. The child may fear ambulation postoperatively because of pain. Many children (and adults, too) are worried that the stitches will pull out. Reassure the child that this worry is understood but that the sutures (or staples) are intended to withstand the strain of walking and moving about. Activity is essential to the child's recovery but should be as pain-free as possible. Help the child understand that as activity increases, the pain will decrease. The child whose appendix ruptured before surgery may also have pain related to the nasogastric tube, abdominal distention, or constipation.

MONITORING FLUID INTAKE. Dehydration can be a concern, especially if the child had bouts of nausea and vomiting preoperatively. On admission to the hospital, the child is maintained NPO until after surgery. Measure and record intake and output. Administer IV fluids as ordered and using appropriate nursing measures. Postoperatively, check dressings to detect evidence of excessive drainage or bleeding, indicating loss of fluids. Clear oral fluids are usually ordered soon after surgery; after the child takes and retains fluids successfully, a progressive diet is ordered. Assess, record, and report bowel sounds at least every 4 hours because the physician may use this as a gauge to determine when the child can have solid food.

PROVIDING FAMILY TEACHING. The child who has had an uncomplicated appendectomy usually convalesces quickly and can return to school within 1 or 2 weeks. Teach the caregiver to keep the incision clean and dry. Activities are limited according to the recommendations of the physician. The child who has had a ruptured appendix is hospitalized for a week or more and is more limited in activities postoperatively. Instruct the family to observe for signs and symptoms of complications postoperatively, including fever, abdominal distention, and pain. Emphasize the need for making and keeping follow-up appointments.

EVALUATION: GOALS AND OUTCOME CRITERIA

■ *Goal:* Fears of the child and family will be alleviated.
Criteria: The child and family verbalize fears and ask questions preoperatively; the child cooperates with health care personnel.

■ *Goal:* The child's pain will be controlled.

Criteria: The child's pain is at an acceptable level, as evidenced by the child's verbalization of pain according to a pain scale (see Chap. 4).

■ *Goal:* The child will have adequate fluid intake.
Criteria: The child's skin turgor is good, vital signs are within normal limits, weight remains stable, and hourly urine output is at least 50 mL/kg.

■ *Goal:* Caregivers will cope effectively and provide appropriate care for the child.
Criteria: Caregivers discuss recovery expectations, demonstrate wound care as needed, and review signs and symptoms to report.

Intestinal Parasites

A few intestinal parasites are common in the United States. They are especially common in young and school-age children. Hand-to-mouth practices contribute to infestations.

ENTEROBIASIS (PINWORM INFECTION)

The pinworm (*Enterobius vermicularis*) is a white, threadlike worm that invades the cecum and may enter the appendix. Pinworms are spread from person to person by articles contaminated with pinworm eggs. The infestation is common in children and occurs when the pinworm eggs are swallowed. The eggs hatch in the intestinal tract and grow to maturity in the cecum. The female worm, when ready to lay her eggs, crawls out of the anus and lays the eggs on the perineum.

Itching around the anus causes the child to scratch and trap new eggs under the fingernails, which often causes reinfection when the child's fingers go into the mouth. Clothing, bedding, food, toilet seats, and other articles become infected, and the infestation spreads to other members of the family. Pinworm eggs can also float in the air and be inhaled.

The life cycle of these worms is 6 to 8 weeks, after which reinfestation commonly occurs unless treated. The incidence is highest in school-age children and next highest in preschoolers. All members of the family are susceptible.

Clinical Manifestation and Diagnosis Intense perianal itching is the primary symptom of pinworms. Young children who cannot clearly verbalize their feelings may be restless, sleep poorly, or have episodes of bedwetting.

The usual method of diagnosis is to capture the eggs from around the anus, using cellophane tape, and examine them under a microscope. Adult worms also may be seen as they emerge from the anus when the child is lying quietly or sleeping. The cellophane tape test for identifying worms is performed in the early morning just before, or as soon as, the child wakens:

1. Wind clear cellophane tape around the end of a tongue blade, sticky side outward.

2. Spread the child's buttocks and press the tape against the anus, rolling from side to side.
3. Transfer the tape to a microscope slide and cover with a clean slide to send to the laboratory. The tongue blade can be placed in a plastic bag if the caregiver does not have slides or a commercially prepared kit.
4. The tape is examined microscopically in the laboratory for eggs.

Treatment and Nursing Care   Treatment consists of the use of an **anthelmintic** (a medication that expels intestinal worms [vermifuge]). Mebendazole (Vermox) is the most commonly used product. The medication should be repeated in 2 or 3 weeks to eliminate any parasites that hatch after the initial treatment. Because pinworms are easily transmitted, the nurse should encourage all family members to be treated as well.

Children and caregivers may be especially disturbed by having worms. They may need reassurance from the nurse that pinworm infestation is as common as an infection or a cold. This support is important when caring for a child with any type of intestinal parasite.

As a preventive measure, the nurse should teach the child to wash the hands after bowel movements and before eating. The child should also be encouraged to observe other hygiene measures, such as regular bathing and daily change of underclothing. The nurse must teach caregivers to keep the child's fingernails short and clean. Caregivers also need to know that bedding should be changed frequently to avoid reinfestation. All bedding and clothing, especially underclothing, should be washed in hot water.

ROUNDWORMS

Ascaris lumbricoides is a large intestinal worm found only in humans. Infestation is from the feces of infested people. It is usually found in areas where sanitary facilities are lacking and human excreta is deposited on the ground.

The adult worm is pink and 9″ to 12″ long. The eggs hatch in the intestinal tract, and the larvae migrate to the liver and lungs. The larvae reaching the lungs ascend up through the bronchi, are swallowed, and reach the intestine, where they grow to maturity and mate. Eggs are then discharged into the feces. Full development requires about 2 months. In tropical countries, where infestation may be heavy, bowel obstructions may present serious problems. Generally, however, no symptoms are present in ordinary infestations. Identification is made by means of microscopic examination of feces for eggs. Pyrantel pamoate (Antiminth) is the medication commonly used. The nurse must teach caregivers that improved hygiene practices, with sanitary disposal of feces, including diapers, are necessary to prevent infestation.

HOOKWORMS

The hookworm lives in the human intestinal tract, where it attaches itself to the wall of the small intestine. Eggs are discharged in the feces of the host. These parasites are prevalent in areas where infected human excreta is deposited on the ground and where the soil, moisture, and temperature are favorable for the development of infective larvae of the worm. In the southeastern United States and tropical West Africa, the prevailing species is *Necator americanus*.

Clinical Manifestation and Diagnosis   After feces containing eggs are deposited on the ground, larvae hatch. They can survive there as long as 6 weeks and usually penetrate the skin of barefoot people. They produce an itching dermatitis on the feet (ground itch). The larvae pass through the bloodstream to the lungs and into the pharynx, where they are swallowed and reach the small intestine. In the small intestine, they attach themselves to the intestinal wall, where they feed on blood. Heavy infestation may cause anemia through loss of blood. Chronic infestation produces listlessness, fatigue, and malnutrition. Identification is made by examination of the stool under the microscope.

Treatment and Nursing Care   Pyrantel pamoate or mebendazole may be used in the treatment of hookworms. The nurse must stress the need for the affected child to receive a well-balanced diet with additional protein and iron. Transfusions are rarely necessary. To prevent hookworm infestation, the nurse should instruct caregivers to keep children from running barefoot where there is any possibility of ground contamination with feces.

GIARDIASIS

Giardiasis is not caused by a worm but by a protozoan parasite, *Giardia lamblia*. It is a common cause of diarrhea in world travelers and is also prevalent in children who attend day care centers and other types of residential facilities; it may be found in contaminated mountain streams or pools frequented by diapered infants. The child ingests the cyst containing the protozoa. The cyst is activated by stomach acid and passes into the duodenum, where it matures, causing diarrhea, weight loss, and abdominal cramps. Identification and diagnosis are made through examination of stool under the microscope.

Metronidazole (Flagyl) or quinacrine (Atabrine) is effective in treating the infestation. The nurse should alert the caregiver that quinacrine causes a yellow discoloration of the skin. To prevent infestations, the nurse should stress to caregivers the importance of careful handling of soiled diapers, especially in a child care facility. Handwashing, avoiding pools and streams used by diapered infants, and avoiding contact with infected persons are also important.

DISORDERS OF ELIMINATION

Although difficulties with diarrhea or constipation are common in school-age children, the most common cause for stress in the child and the caregiver is a problem with continence. Enuresis or encopresis can cause many days of frustration and discouragement for both the child and the caregiver.

Enuresis

Enuresis, or bedwetting, is involuntary urination beyond the age when control of urination commonly is acquired. Many children do not acquire complete nighttime control before 5 to 7 years of age, and occasional bedwetting may be seen in children as late as 9 or 10 years of age. Boys have more difficulty than girls, and in some instances enuresis may persist into the adult years.

Enuresis may have a physiologic or psychological cause and may indicate a need for further exploration and treatment. Physiologic causes may include a small bladder capacity, urinary tract infection, and lack of awareness of the signal to empty the bladder because of sleeping too soundly. Persistent bedwetting in a 5- or 6-year-old child may be a result of rigorous toilet training before the child was physically or psychologically ready. Enuresis in the older child may express resentment toward family caregivers or a desire to regress to an earlier level to receive more care and attention. Emotional stress also can be a precipitating factor. The health care team also needs to consider the possibility that enuresis can be a symptom of sexual abuse.

If a physiologic cause has been ruled out, efforts should be made to discover possible causes, including emotional stress. If the child is interested in achieving control—for instance, to go to camp or visit friends overnight—waking the child during the night to go to the toilet or limiting fluids before retiring may be helpful. However, these measures should not be used as a replacement for searching for the cause. Help from a pediatric mental health professional may be needed.

The family caregiver may become extremely frustrated about having to deal with smelly, wet bedding every morning. The child may go to great efforts to hide the fact that the bed is wet. Health care personnel must take a supportive, understanding attitude toward the problems of the caregiver and the child, allowing each of them to ventilate feelings and providing a place where emotions can be freely expressed.

Encopresis

Encopresis is chronic involuntary fecal soiling beyond the age when control is expected (about 3 years of age). Speech and learning disabilities may accompany this problem. If

there are no organic causes (eg, worms, megacolon), encopresis indicates a serious emotional problem and the need for counseling for the child and the family caregivers. It is thought that overcontrol or undercontrol by a caregiver can cause encopresis. Recommendations for treatment differ; the most important aspect, however, is recognition of the problem and referral for treatment and counseling.

CARDIOVASCULAR SYSTEM DISORDERS

The child's cardiovascular system experiences a period of slow growth with few problems through the school-age years. The primary threat to the cardiovascular system during this age is rheumatic heart disease as a complication of rheumatic fever.

Rheumatic Fever

Rheumatic fever is a chronic disease of childhood, affecting the connective tissue of the heart, joints, lungs, and brain. An autoimmune reaction to group A beta-hemolytic streptococcal infections, rheumatic fever occurs throughout the world, particularly in the temperate zones. Rheumatic fever has become less common in developed countries, but there have been recent indications of increased occurrences in some areas of the United States.

Rheumatic fever is precipitated by a streptococcal infection such as strep throat, tonsillitis, scarlet fever, or pharyngitis, which may be undiagnosed or untreated. The resultant rheumatic fever manifestation may be the first indication of trouble. An elevation of antistreptococcal antibodies, indicative of recent streptococcal infection, however, can be demonstrated in about 95% of the rheumatic fever patients tested within the first 2 months of onset. An antistreptolysin-O titer measures these antibodies.

CLINICAL MANIFESTATIONS

A latent period of 1 to 5 weeks follows the initial infection. The onset is often slow and subtle. The child may be listless, anorectic, and pale. He or she may lose weight and complain of vague muscle, joint, or abdominal pains. Often there is a low-grade late afternoon fever. None of these is diagnostic by itself, but if such signs persist, the child should have a medical examination.

Major manifestations of rheumatic fever are **polyarthritis** (migratory arthritis), **chorea** (disorder characterized by emotional instability, purposeless movements, and muscular weakness), and **carditis** (inflammation of the heart). The onset may be acute rather than insidious, with severe carditis or arthritis as the presenting symptom. Chorea generally has an insidious onset.

Polyarthritis Polyarthritis moves from one major joint to another (ankles, knees, hips, wrists, elbows, shoulders). The joint becomes painful to either touch or movement (**arthralgia**) and hot and swollen. Body temperature is moderately elevated; the erythrocyte sedimentation rate (ESR) is increased. Although extremely painful, this type of arthritis does not lead to the disabling deformities that occur in rheumatoid arthritis.

Chorea The onset of chorea is gradual, with increasing incoordination, facial grimaces, and repetitive involuntary movements. Movements may be mild and remain so, or they may become increasingly violent. Active arthritis is rarely present when chorea is the major manifestation. Carditis occurs, although less commonly than when polyarthritis is the major condition. Attacks tend to be recurrent and prolonged but are rare after puberty. It is seldom possible to demonstrate an increase in the antistreptococcal antibody level because of the generally prolonged latency period.

Corticosteroids and salicylates are of little value in the treatment of uncomplicated chorea. The child may be sedated with phenobarbital, chlorpromazine (Thorazine), haloperidol (Haldol), or diazepam (Valium). Bed rest is necessary, with protection such as padding the bed sides if the movements are severe.

Carditis Carditis is the major cause of permanent heart damage and disability among children with rheumatic fever. Carditis may occur alone or as a complication of either arthritis or chorea. Presenting symptoms may be vague enough to be missed. The child may have a poor appetite or pallor, perhaps a low-grade fever, listlessness, and moderate anemia. Careful observation may reveal slight dyspnea on exertion. Physical examination shows a soft systolic murmur over the apex of the heart. Unfortunately, such a child may have been in poor physical health for some time before the murmur is discovered.

Acute carditis may be the presenting symptom, particularly in young children. An abrupt onset of high fever, perhaps as high as 104°F (40°C), tachycardia, pallor, poor pulse quality, and a rapid decrease in hemoglobin are characteristic. Weakness, prostration, cyanosis, and intense precordial pain are common. Cardiac dilatation usually occurs. The pericardium, myocardium, or endocardium may be affected.

DIAGNOSIS

Rheumatic fever is difficult to diagnose and sometimes impossible to differentiate from other diseases. The possible serious effect of the disease demands early and conscientious medical treatment. However, avoid causing apprehension and disrupting the child's life, because the condition could prove to be something less serious. The nurse should not attempt a diagnosis but should understand the criteria on which a presumptive diagnosis is based.

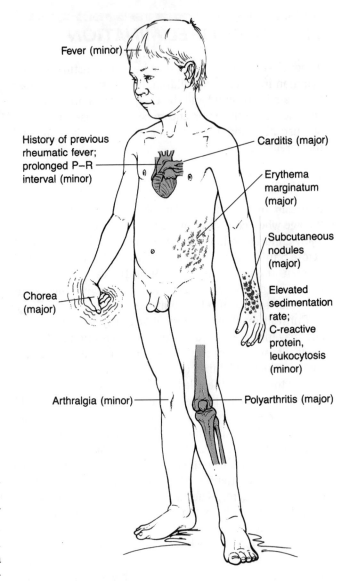

Figure 17-5
Major and minor manifestations of rheumatic fever.

The modified Jones criteria (Fig. 17-5) are generally accepted as a useful rule for guidance when deciding whether to treat the patient for rheumatic fever. The criteria are divided into major and minor categories. The presence of two major, or one major and two minor, criteria indicates a high probability of rheumatic fever if supported by evidence of a preceding streptococcal infection. This system is not infallible, however, because no one criterion is specific for the disease, and additional manifestations can help confirm the diagnosis.

TREATMENT

The chief concern in caring for a child with rheumatic fever is the prevention of residual heart disease. As long as the rheumatic process is active, progressive heart damage is possible. Bed rest, therefore, is essential to reduce the workload of the heart. The length of the period of bed rest cannot be arbitrarily stated; guidelines are given in Table 17-2.

Residual heart disease is treated in accordance with its severity and its type with digitalis, restricted activities, diuretics, and a low-sodium diet as indicated.

Laboratory tests, although nonspecific, provide an evaluation of the disease activity to guide treatment. Two commonly used indicators are the ESR and the presence of C-reactive protein. The ESR is elevated in the presence of an inflammatory process and is nearly always increased in the polyarthritis or carditis manifestation of rheumatic fever. It remains elevated until clinical manifestations have ceased and any subclinical activity has subsided. It seldom increases in uncomplicated chorea. Therefore, ESR elevation in a choreic patient may indicate cardiac involvement.

C-reactive protein is not normally present in the blood of healthy people, but it appears in the serum of acutely ill people, including those ill with rheumatic fever. As the patient improves, C-reactive protein disappears.

Leukocytosis is also an indication of an inflammatory process. Until the leukocyte count returns to a normal level, the disease probably is still active.

Drug Therapy Medications used in the treatment of rheumatic fever include penicillin, salicylates, and corticosteroids. Penicillin is administered to eliminate the hemolytic streptococci. If the child is allergic to penicillin, erythromycin is used. Penicillin administration continues after the acute phase of the illness to prevent the recurrence of rheumatic fever.

Salicylates are given in the form of acetylsalicylic acid (aspirin) to children, with the daily dosage calculated according to the child's weight. Aspirin relieves pain and reduces the inflammation of polyarteritis. It is also used for its antipyretic effect. The continued administration of a relatively large dosage may cause toxic effects; individual tolerance differs greatly.

For mild or severe carditis, corticosteroids appear to be the drug of choice because of their prompt, dramatic action.

Administration of salicylates or corticosteroids is not expected to alter the course of the disease, but the control of the toxic manifestations enhances the child's comfort and sense of well-being and helps reduce the burden on the heart. This is of particular importance in acute carditis with congestive heart failure. Diuretics may be administered when needed in severe carditis.

PREVENTION

Because the peak of onset of rheumatic fever occurs in school-age children, health services for this age group take on added importance. The overall approach is to promote continuous health supervision for all children, including the school-age child. The use of well-child conferences or clinics needs to increase to provide continuity of care for school-age children. The nurse who has contact in any way with school-age children must be aware of the importance of teaching the public about the need to have upper respiratory infections evaluated for group A beta-hemolytic streptococcus and the need for treatment with penicillin. The nurse also should stress that the child must take the complete prescription of penicillin (usually 10 days' supply), even though the symptoms disappear and the child feels well.

TABLE 17-2. Bed Rest Guidelines in Children with Acute Rheumatic Fever

Cardiac Status	Management
No carditis	Bed rest for 2 weeks and gradual ambulation for 2 weeks even if on salicylates
Carditis, no heart enlargement	Bed rest for 4 weeks and gradual ambulation for 4 weeks
Carditis, with enlargement	Bed rest for 6 weeks and gradual ambulation for 6 weeks
Carditis, with heart failure	Strict bed rest for as long a heart failure is present and gradual ambulation for 3 months

Behrman RE, Vaughan VC, eds. Nelson's textbook of pediatrics, 13th ed. Philadelphia: WB Saunders, 1987.

◤◥ *Nursing Process for the Child With* ◣◢ *Rheumatic Fever*

ASSESSMENT

Conduct a thorough evaluation of the child's physical condition, beginning with a careful review of all systems. Note any signs that may be classified as major or minor manifestations. Include in the physical assessment observation for elevated temperature and pulse and careful examination for erythema marginatum, subcutaneous nodules, swollen or painful joints, or signs of chorea. A throat culture determines if there is an active infection. Obtain a complete, up-to-date history from the child and the caregiver. Ask about a recent sore throat or upper respiratory infection. Find out when the symptoms began, the extent of the illness, and what, if any, treatment was obtained. Include the school-age child in the nursing interview to help contribute to the history.

NURSING DIAGNOSES

The nursing diagnoses vary depending on the manifestations displayed. Use the nursing assessment to determine the appropriate diagnoses, such as:

- Pain related to arthralgia

- Diversional Activity Deficit related to prescribed bed rest

- Activity Intolerance related to carditis or arthralgia

- Risk for Injury related to chorea

- Risk for Noncompliance with prophylactic drug therapy related to financial or emotional burden of lifelong therapy

- Risk for Altered Health Maintenance related to knowledge deficit about the condition, need for long-term therapy, and risk factors

OUTCOME IDENTIFICATION AND PLANNING

The goals for nursing care are determined in cooperation with the child and the caregiver. Goals for the child include reducing pain, providing diversional activities, conserving energy, and preventing injury. Goals for the caregiver include complying with drug therapy and increasing knowledge about the long-term care of the child. Throughout planning and implementation, bear in mind the child's developmental stage.

IMPLEMENTATION

PROVIDING COMFORT MEASURES AND REDUCING PAIN. Position the child to relieve joint pain. Large joints usually are involved, including the knees, ankles, wrists, and elbows. Carefully handle the joints when moving the child to help minimize pain. Even the weight of blankets may cause pain; be alert to this possibility and improvise covering as needed. Try warm baths and gentle range-of-motion exercises to help alleviate some of the joint discomfort. Give the child a pain scale indicator to express the level of pain (see Fig. 4-5 in Chap. 4).

Salicylates are administered in the form of aspirin to reduce fever and relieve joint inflammation and pain. Because of the risks of long-term administration of salicylates, note any signs of toxicity and record and report them promptly. Tinnitus, nausea, vomiting, and headache are all important signs of toxicity. Administer aspirin after meals or with a glass of milk to lessen GI irritation. Enteric-coated aspirin is also available for patients who are sensitive to its effects. Large doses may alter the prothrombin time and thus interfere with the clotting mechanism. Salicylate therapy is usually continued until all laboratory findings are normal.

The child whose pain is not controlled with salicylates may be administered corticosteroids. Side effects such as **hirsutism** (abnormal hair growth) and "moon face" may be upsetting to the child and family. Toxic reactions such as euphoria, insomnia, gastric irritation, and growth suppression must be watched for and reported. Because premature withdrawal of a steroid drug is likely to cause a relapse, it is important to discontinue the drug gradually by decreasing dosages.

PROVIDING DIVERSIONAL ACTIVITIES. Children vary greatly in how ill they feel during the acute phase of rheumatic fever. For those who do not feel very ill, bed rest can cause distress or resentment. Be creative in finding diversional activities that allow bed rest but prevent restlessness and boredom. Do not use the television as an all-day babysitter. Quiet games can provide some entertainment. Use of a computer can be beneficial because both entertaining and educational games are available, and most children enjoy working with a computer. Simple needlework or model building are other useful diversional activities. During the school year, make efforts (or encourage the caregiver) to provide the child with a tutor and work from school; this helps relieve boredom and also maintains contact with peers. Plan all activities with the child's developmental age in mind.

PROVIDING SENSORY STIMULATION AND PROMOTING ENERGY CONSERVATION. The pain of arthralgia may be so great that the child will not want to be involved in any kind of activity. Administer analgesics as ordered to help decrease the inflammation of the joints and decrease the pain. Provide rest periods between activities to help pace the child's energies and provide for maximum comfort. During times of increased cardiac involvement or exacerbations of joint pain, the child may want to rest and perhaps have someone read a story. This may be a good time to choose a book that involves the child's imagination and that has enough excitement to create ongoing interest. Peers may be encouraged to visit, but these visits must be monitored so that the child is not overly tired. The child's classroom could be encouraged to write to the child to provide contact with everyday school activities and keep the child in touch. If the child has chorea, inform visitors that the child cannot control these movements and that they are as upsetting to the child as to others.

PREVENTING INJURY. The child with chorea may be frustrated with his or her inability to control the movements. Provide an opportunity for the child to express feelings. Protect the child from injury by keeping the side rails up and padding them. Do not leave a child with chorea unattended in a wheelchair. Use all appropriate safety measures.

PROMOTING COMPLIANCE WITH DRUG THERAPY. A child does not become immune from future attacks of rheumatic fever after the first illness. Rheumatic fever can recur whenever the child has a group A beta-hemolytic streptococcal infection if the child is not properly treated. For this reason, the child who has had rheumatic fever must be maintained on prophylactic doses of penicillin for 5 years or longer. Whenever the child is to have oral surgery, including dental work, extra prophylactic precautions should be taken, even into adulthood. Because of this long-term therapy, noncompliance can become a problem for both financial and emotional reasons. Oral penicillin is usually prescribed, but if compliance is poor, monthly injections can be substituted. Encourage the family to contact the local chapter of the American Heart Association for help in finding economical sources of penicillin. Become informed about other resources that may be available in your community. Stress to the child and the family the need to prevent recurrence of the disease with the danger of heart damage. Follow-up care must be ongoing, even into adulthood.

PROVIDING FAMILY TEACHING. Inform the family and child about the importance of having all upper respiratory infections checked by a health care provider to prevent another bout of a streptococcal infection. Be certain that they understand that the child can have recurrences and that a future recurrence could have much more serious effects. If the child has had carditis and heart damage has occurred, instruct the caregiver that the child must be regularly followed to evaluate the damage. The child may need to be maintained on cardiac medications. Instruct the family about these medications. Mitral valve dysfunction is a common aftereffect of severe carditis. A girl who has had mitral valve damage from cardiac involvement may have problems in adulthood during pregnancy. Inform the caregiver that heart failure for such a girl is a possibility during pregnancy, and she should be given the option to have a mitral valve replacement if needed.

Teaching time is an excellent opportunity to stress the importance of preventing rheumatic fever. Other children in the family may benefit if caregivers are given this information.

EVALUATION: GOALS AND OUTCOME CRITERIA

- *Goal*: The child's joint pain will be minimal.
Criteria: The child voices that the pain level is decreased, using a pain scale to express degree of pain.

- *Goal*: The child on bed rest will become engaged in activities.
Criteria: The child displays interest and is actively involved in age-appropriate activities.

- *Goal*: The child will learn when and how to conserve energy.
Criteria: The child rests quietly during rest periods, identifies when he or she needs rest, and engages in quiet diversional therapy.

- *Goal*: The child is not injured from chorea movements.
Criteria: The child remains free of injury.

- *Goal*: The child and family will follow through on prophylactic medication.
Criteria: The child and family voice understanding of the importance of prophylactic medication and identify means for obtaining it.

- *Goal*: The family will learn about follow-up care.
Criteria: The caregivers voice understanding of the need for follow-up care and indicate how they will obtain it.

ENDOCRINE SYSTEM DISORDERS

Diabetes mellitus is the most significant endocrine disorder that affects children of school age. Other conditions that may affect schoolchildren are disorders of the pituitary gland that alter growth and diabetes insipidus. The incidence of these latter conditions is low.

Juvenile Diabetes Mellitus (Insulin-Dependent Diabetes Mellitus)

At least 10 to 12 million Americans have been diagnosed with diabetes. A significant number of them are children: it is estimated that diabetes mellitus affects about one in 600 children between the ages of 5 and 15 years. The incidence of this condition continues to increase.

Diabetes is often considered an adult disease, but at least 5% of cases begin in childhood, usually at about 6 years of age or around the time of puberty. Management of diabetes in children is different from adults and requires conscientious care geared to the child's developmental stage.

Diabetes is classified into two major types: type 1, insulin-dependent diabetes mellitus (IDDM), and type 2, non–insulin-dependent diabetes mellitus. As noted in Table 17-3, diabetes in children is type 1.

PATHOGENESIS

The exact pathophysiology of diabetes is not completely understood; however, it is known to result from dysfunction of the beta (insulin-secreting) cells of the islets of Langerhans in the pancreas. It is believed that the presence of an acute infection during childhood may trigger a mechanism in genetically susceptible children, activating beta-cell dysfunction and disrupting insulin secretion. Other conditions that may contribute to IDDM are pancreatic tumors, pancreatitis, and long-term corticosteroid use. Normally, the sugar derived from digestion and assimilation of foods is burned to provide energy for the body's activities. Excess sugar is converted into fat or glycogen and stored in the body tissues. Insulin, a hormone secreted by the pancreas, is responsible for the burning and storage

TABLE 17-3.   **Comparison of Type 1 and Type 2 Diabetes**

Assessment	Type 1 (Insulin-Dependent)	Type 2 (Non–insulin-Dependent)
Age of onset	5–7 y or at puberty	40–65 y
Type of onset	Abrupt	Gradual
Weight changes	Marked weight loss is often initial sign	Associated with obesity
Other symptoms	Polydipsia	Polydipsia
	Polyuria (often begins as bed-wetting)	Polyuria
	Fatigue (marks fall in school)	Fatigue
	Blurred vision (marks fall in school)	Blurred vision
	Glycosuria	Glycosuria
	Polyphagia	
	Pruritus	Pruritus
	Mood changes (may cause behavior problems in school)	Mood changes
Therapy	Hypoglycemic agents never effective; insulin needed	Managed by insulin injection or diet alone; oral hypoglycemic agents a possibility
	Diet only moderately restricted; no dietary foods used	Diet tends to be strict
	Common-sense foot care for growing children	Good skin and foot care necessary
Period of remission	Period of remission for 1–12 mo generally follows initial diagnosis	Not demonstrable

Adapted from Pillitteri A. Maternal and child health nursing, 2d ed. Philadelphia: JB Lippincott, 1995.

of sugar. In diabetes, the secretion of insulin is inadequate or nonexistent, allowing sugar to accumulate in the bloodstream and spill over into the urine. In children, diabetes causes an abrupt, pronounced decrease in insulin production, resulting in decreased ability to derive energy from the food eaten. Large amounts of protein and fat are used to supply the child's energy needs, causing loss of weight and slowed growth. This combination of failure to gain weight and lack of energy may be the initial reason the child is brought to the attention of the health care provider. However, the child may not be seen by a health care provider until symptoms of acidosis are evident.

CLINICAL MANIFESTATIONS

Classic symptoms of diabetes mellitus are **polyuria** (dramatic increase in urinary output, probably with enuresis), **polydipsia** (abnormal thirst), and **polyphagia** (increased food consumption). These symptoms are usually accompanied by weight loss or failure to gain weight and lack of energy. Symptoms of diabetes in children often have an abrupt onset.

If the child's symptoms are not noted and referred for diagnosis, the disorder is likely to progress to **diabetic acidosis.** Because of inadequate insulin production, carbohydrates are not converted into fuel for energy production. Fats are then mobilized for energy but in the absence of glucose are incompletely oxidized. Ketone bodies (acetone,

diacetic acid, and oxybutyric acid) accumulate. They are readily excreted in the urine, but in this excretion the acid–base balance of body fluids is upset, resulting in acidosis. Diabetic acidosis is characterized by drowsiness, dry skin, flushed cheeks and cherry-red lips, acetone breath with a fruity smell, and **Kussmaul breathing** (abnormal increase in the depth and rate of the respiratory movements). Nausea and vomiting may occur. If untreated, the child lapses into coma and exhibits dehydration, electrolyte imbalance, rapid pulse, and subnormal temperature and blood pressure.

Treatment for acidosis includes keeping the patient warm. The child needs skilled nursing care and may be admitted to a pediatric intensive care unit, if available. Blood and urine are tested to evaluate the degree of acidosis. If the child cannot urinate, a catheter is inserted. Gastric lavage may be performed to relieve abdominal distention and eliminate the danger of aspiration. Regular insulin is given IV, along with IV electrolyte fluids.

DIAGNOSIS

Early detection and control are critical in postponing or minimizing later complications of diabetes. The nurse should observe carefully for any signs or symptoms in all members of a family that has a history of diabetes. The family also should be taught to observe the children for frequent thirst, urination, and weight loss. All relatives of diabetics are considered a high-risk group and should have periodic testing.

At each visit to a health care provider, children who have a family history of diabetes should be monitored by finger stick glucose monitoring or dipstick testing for glycosuria. If the blood glucose level is elevated or glycosuria is present, a fasting blood sugar (FBS) is performed. An FBS of 200 mg/dL or higher almost certainly is diagnostic for diabetes when other signs such as polyuria and weight loss despite polyphagia are present.

Although glucose tolerance tests are performed in adults to confirm diabetes, they are not commonly used in children. The traditional oral glucose tolerance test is often unsuccessful in children because they may vomit the concentrated glucose that must be swallowed.

TREATMENT

Management of diabetes in children includes insulin therapy, a meal plan, and an exercise plan. Treatment of the diabetic child involves the family and child and a number of health team members, such as the nurse, the pediatrician, the nutritionist, and the diabetic nurse educator. After diabetes is diagnosed, the child may be hospitalized for a period. This allows the condition to be stabilized under supervision. This is a trying time, and the nurse must plan care with an understanding of the emotional impact of the diagnosis. The child's teacher, the school nurse, and others who supervise the child during daily activities must be informed of the diagnosis.

Insulin Insulin therapy is an essential part of the treatment of diabetes in children. The dosage of insulin is adjusted according to blood glucose levels so that the levels are maintained near normal. Two kinds of insulin are often combined for the best results. Insulin can be grouped into rapid-acting, intermediate-acting, and long-acting (Table 17-4). An intermediate-acting and a rapid-acting insulin

often are given together. Some preparations come in a premixed proportion of 70% intermediate-acting and 30% rapid-acting insulins, eliminating the need for mixing.

Insulin reaction (insulin shock, hypoglycemia) is caused by insulin overload, resulting in too rapid metabolism of the body's glucose. This may be due to a change in the body's requirement, carelessness in diet (such as failure to eat proper amounts of food), an error in insulin measurement, or excessive exercise. Because diabetes in children is very labile (unstable, fluctuating), the child is subject to insulin reactions. Some of the symptoms of impending insulin shock in children are any type of odd, unusual, or antisocial behavior, headache and malaise, blurred vision and faintness, and undue fatigue or hunger. Children often have hypoglycemic reactions in the early morning. The nurse must observe the child at least every 2 hours during the night. Note tossed bedding, which would indicate restlessness, and any excessive perspiration. If necessary, try to arouse the child. As the child becomes regulated and observes a careful diet at home, parents need not watch so closely but should have a thorough understanding of all aspects of this condition. Blood glucose monitoring is often scheduled for this early morning time, especially while the child is hospitalized.

Treatment of an insulin reaction should be *immediate*. Give the child sugar, candy, orange juice, or one of the commercial products designed for this emergency. Repeated or impending reactions require consultation with the physician.

If the child cannot take a sugar source orally, glucagon should be administered subcutaneously to bring about a prompt increase in the blood glucose level. Every adult responsible for a diabetic child should clearly understand the procedure for administering this drug and should have easy access to it. Glucagon is a hormone produced by alpha

TABLE 17-4. Types of Insulin: Onset, Peak, and Duration

Action	Preparation	Onset (h)	Peak (h)	Duration (h)
Rapid-acting	Regular iletin [Pork, beef]	½–1	2–4	6–8
	Humulin R [Human (Lilley)]	½–1	2–4	6–8
	Novolin [Human (Squibb)]	½	2½–5	8
	Semilente	½–1	5–10	12–16
Intermediate-acting	NPH [Pork, beef]	1½–2	6–12	24
	Humulin N [Human (Lilley)]	1–2	6–12	18–24
	Novolin N [Human (Squibb)]	1½	4–12	24
	Lente [Beef, pork]	2–4	6–12	18–26
	Humulin 70/30 [70% N, 30% R]	½	4–8	24
	Novolin 70/30 [70% N, 30% R]	½	4–8	24
Long-acting	Protamine zinc [Beef, pork]	4–8	14–24	28–36
	Ultralente [Beef, pork]	4–8	14–24	28–36

cells of the pancreatic islets. An elevation in the blood glucose level results in insulin release (in a normal person), but a decrease in the blood glucose level stimulates glucagon release. The released glucagon in the bloodstream acts on the liver to promote glycogen breakdown and glucose release.

Glucagon is available as a pharmaceutical product, packaged as a powder in individual dose units. To prepare the dose, add the diluent, which comes with the powdered drug, with a sterile syringe and needle. The solution is then drawn up into the syringe and administered in the same manner as insulin.

Glucagon acts within minutes to restore consciousness, after which the child can take candy or sugar. This treatment prevents the long delay in waiting for a physician to administer glucose IV or for an ambulance to reach the facility. It is, however, not a substitute for proper medical supervision.

Insulin Regimen   Most newly diagnosed diabetic children show a decreased need for insulin during the first weeks or months after control is established. This is often referred to as the "honeymoon period," and it should be explained to the family in advance to avoid false hope. As the child grows, the need for insulin increases and continues to do so until the child reaches full growth. Again, family caregivers need to know that this is normal and that the child's condition is not getting worse.

Methods of Giving Insulin.   The child may not be able to take over the management of the insulin dose as early as blood glucose monitoring, but he or she can watch the preparation of the syringe and learn the technique for drawing up the dosage. Encouraging the child to watch until it becomes routine may be helpful. By 8 or 9 years of age, the child should be thinking out the dose and getting the feel of the syringe. The child also may draw up the dose and prepare for self-administration. The age at which this is possible cannot be stated arbitrarily. No two children mature at the same rate; some may be able to do this much earlier than others. Automatic injection devices can help the child self-administer insulin at a younger age. The child should be encouraged to take over the management of the therapy when ready. If included in decision making, the child can learn the importance of the routine and accept the restrictions the disease imposes.

Insulin Pumps.   An insulin pump is a method of continuous insulin administration that is useful for some diabetics. The pump is about the size of a transistor radio and can be worn strapped to the waist or on a shoulder strap. It delivers a steady low dose of insulin through a syringe housed in the pump and connected by polyethylene tubing to a small-gauge subcutaneous needle implanted in the abdomen. Extra insulin is released at mealtimes and other times when needed by pressing a button. The pump does not sense the blood glucose level; therefore, careful blood

glucose monitoring (at least four times a day) is necessary to adjust the dosage as needed. The pump must be removed to bathe, swim, or shower. The child may want to wear loose clothing that will hide the pump. The needle site must be regularly observed for redness and irritation. The site is changed every 24 to 48 hours using aseptic technique.

Unique Needs of the Adolescent   Adolescence is an extremely trying period for many diabetics, as it is for other young people. Diabetics, like normal adolescents, must work from dependence to independence. Even when an adolescent has accepted responsibility for self-care, it is not unusual for him or her to rebel against the control that this condition demands, become impatient, and appear to ignore future health. The adolescent may skip meals, drop diet controls, or neglect glucose monitoring. Going barefoot and neglecting proper foot care also can cause problems for the diabetic adolescent. It can be a difficult time for both the family and the adolescent. The caregivers naturally become concerned and are apt to give the adolescent more controls to rebel against. Special care should be taken by the family, teachers, nurses, and physicians to see that these young people find enough maturing satisfaction in other areas and do not need to rebel in this vital area.

The adolescent who completely understands all aspects of the condition (especially if allowed to assume control of treatment previously) should be allowed to continue. Should the adolescent run into difficulty, an adolescent clinic can be of great value. Here the adolescent can discuss problems with understanding people who respond with care, providing dignity and attentive listening.

◥◤ Nursing Process for the Child With
◣◢ Diabetes Mellitus

ASSESSMENT

Ask the caregiver about the child's symptoms leading up to the present illness. Ask about the child's appetite, weight loss or gain, evidence of polyuria or enuresis in a previously toilet-trained child, polydipsia, dehydration (which may include constipation), irritability, and fatigue. Include the child in the interview and encourage him or her to contribute information. Assess the child's developmental stage to determine appropriate nursing diagnoses and plan effective care (Table 17-5). If the child is first seen in diabetic coma, adjust the initial nursing assessment accordingly.

In the physical assessment, measure the height and weight and examine the skin for evidence of dryness or slowly healing sores. Note signs of hyperglycemia, record vital signs, and collect a urine specimen. Perform a blood glucose level determination using a bedside glucose monitor.

TABLE 17-5. Developmental Guidelines for Diabetic Child Responsibilities*

Issue	Age (yr)					
	Under 4	4–5	6–7	8–10	11–13	14+
Food	Teaching focuses on parents	Knows likes and dislikes	Can begin to tell sugar content of food and know foods he or she should *not* have	Has more ability to select foods according to criteria—like exchange lists	Knows if foods fit own diet plan	Helps plan meals and snacks
Insulin	Parents take responsibility for care	Can tell where injection should be. Can pinch the skin.	Can begin to help with aspects of injections	Gives own injections with supervision	Can learn to measure insulin	Can mix two insulins
Testing		Can choose finger for finger stick. Can wash finger with soap and water. Collects urine; should watch caregiver do testing; helps with recording.	Can do own finger stick using automatic puncture device. Can help with some aspects of the blood test. Can do own urine test and record results.	Can do blood tests with supervision	Can see test results forming a pattern	Can begin to use test results to adjust insulin
Psychological		Identifies with being "bad" or "good"—these words should be avoided. A child this age may think he or se is bad if the test is said to be "bad."	Needs many reminders and supervision	Needs reminders and supervision. Understands only immediate consequences, not long-term consequences, of diabetes control. "Scientific" mind developing—intrigued by tests.	May be somewhat rebellious Concerned with being "different"	Understands long-term consequences of actions, including diabetes control Independence and self-image are important Rebellion continues and some supervision and continued support is still needed

* These are only guidelines. Each child is an individual. Talk to your health care provider about any concerns you may have.
Adapted from Hess V. Diabetes: Stuff and more stuff. Lincoln, NE: HERC Publishing, 1989.

NURSING DIAGNOSES

Base nursing diagnoses on the nursing assessment, with adjustments for the child's developmental stage. In addition to "Noncompliance related to long-term treatment," nursing diagnoses may include:

- Risk for Injury related to insulin deficiency

- Ineffective Family Coping: Compromised related to home management of hypoglycemia and hyperglycemia

- Fear of child and caregiver related to insulin administration

- Altered Nutrition: Less than Body Requirements related to decrease in insulin production

- Risk for Infection related to circulatory or sensory impairment
- Anxiety of child and caregiver related to diagnosis of diabetes and complications
- Self-Esteem Disturbance related to chronic illness and insulin dependency

OUTCOME IDENTIFICATION AND PLANNING

The major goals for the child include preventing injury and infection, relieving fear about insulin administration, maintaining adequate nutrition, and preserving independence and self-concept. Goals for the family include managing hypo- and hyperglycemia, insulin administration, and nutrition for the child. Additional goals for the child and caregivers include learning about diabetes, its management, and possible complications.

PREVENTING INJURY. The child who is seen in the health care facility with diabetes may be newly diagnosed or may be experiencing an unstable episode as a result of illness or changing needs. The child's blood glucose level must be monitored to maintain it within normal limits. Assess the blood glucose level at least twice a day, before breakfast and before the evening meal, by means of bedside glucose monitoring.

On initial diagnosis of diabetes, until some stability is achieved, the blood glucose level may be assessed as often as every 4 hours. Because this procedure involves a finger stick, the child may object and resist this testing. Offer encouragement and support, helping the child to express fears and acknowledging that the finger stick does hurt and it is acceptable to dislike it. Consider the child's developmental stage when performing the testing. School-age children can be involved in much of the process. Encourage the child to choose the finger to be used and clean it with soap and water. Automatic-release instruments make it easier for the child to do the finger stick. Teach the child to read the results and learn the desired level. School-age children are in the stage of industry versus inferiority and usually are interested in learning new information. Appeal to this developmental characteristic to gain the child's cooperation.

Monitor the child at least every 4 hours for signs of hyper- or hypoglycemia (see Family Teaching: Signs of Hyperglycemia and Hypoglycemia). If the blood glucose level is higher than 240 mg/dL, the urine may be tested for ketones. Be aware of the most likely times for an increase or decrease in the blood glucose level in relation to the insulin the child is receiving.

PROMOTING FAMILY COPING IN THE MANAGEMENT OF HYPOGLYCEMIA AND HYPERGLYCEMIA. Since regular monitoring of the blood glucose level is necessary, teach the child and the caregiver how to perform monitoring. Teach them the signs of both hyperglycemia and hypo-

glycemia and how to be prepared to take the appropriate action, if necessary. They must be alert to signs of hypoglycemia, especially when insulin is at peak action (see Table 17-4). Teach them to treat blood glucose levels lower than 60 mg/dL with juice, sugar, or nondiet soda. If the blood glucose level cannot be checked promptly, the child should still consume a simple carbohydrate if there are any signs of hypoglycemia.

If the child cannot swallow, glucagon or dextrose should be administered following the physician's orders. Glucagon is commercially available and can be administered intramuscularly. Teach the caregiver how to mix and administer glucagon.

Instruct the child to get help immediately when signs of hypoglycemia occur and to carry and take sugar cubes, Lifesavers, gumdrops, or a small tube of cake frosting. The reaction should be followed with a snack of a complex carbohydrate, such as crackers, and a protein, such as cheese, peanut butter, or half of a meat sandwich. The snack is needed to maintain the increase in blood glucose level created by the simple carbohydrates and to prevent another hypoglycemic reaction.

Reassure the caregiver and the child that hypoglycemia is much more likely to occur than hyperglycemia. If there is any doubt as to whether the child is having a hypoglycemic or a hyperglycemic reaction, treat it like hypoglycemia. Instruct them to keep a record of the hypoglycemic reactions to determine if there is a pattern and if the insulin schedule or food plan needs adjustment.

Exercise decreases the blood glucose level because carbohydrates are being burned for energy. The therapeutic program should be adjusted to allow for this increase in energy requirements to avoid hypoglycemia. Adjustments

Family Teaching
Signs of Hyperglycemia and Hypoglycemia

Signs of Hyperglycemia
- Polyphagia (excessive hunger)
- Polyuria (excessive urination)
- Dry mucous membranes
- Poor skin turgor
- Lethargy
- Change in level of consciousness

Signs of Hypoglycemia
- Shaking
- Irritability
- Hunger
- Diaphoresis
- Dizziness
- Drowsiness
- Pallor
- Changed level of consciousness
- Feeling "strange"

Nursing Care Plan
for the Child with Diabetes Mellitus

Tessie is a 9-year-old girl who has been hospitalized after recently being diagnosed with diabetes mellitus. Her blood sugar levels have been fluctuating greatly, and she has had an episode of diabetic acidosis. Her physician plans to monitor her condition to determine her insulin and food needs and to stabilize her condition.

NURSING DIAGNOSIS

Altered Nutrition, Less than Body Requirements related to decreased insulin production

GOAL: *Tessie's nutrition requirements will be met.*

OUTCOME CRITERIA:

- Tessie eats food at meals and snack times.
- Tessie's caregivers demonstrate understanding of the food plan by making appropriate menu selections.

Nursing Interventions	Rationale
Stress the need to follow a nutritional plan that includes well-balanced meals eaten at regular times; teach caregivers how to supplement with complex carbohydrates and protein snack when meals are delayed.	Understanding the relationship of blood glucose and food in diabetes will prepare the child and family to make informed decisions about Tessie's diet in different situations.
Teach Tessie and her family how to adjust her meal plan for home, school, and restaurant settings.	Planning for meals in various settings enables the family to encourage a normal active life for Tessie. Including Tessie in the planning helps her feel that she has some control and prepares her for independent decision-making about food choices when away from her family.

NURSING DIAGNOSIS

Risk for Infection related to circulatory or sensory impairment

GOAL: *Tessie will not contract any infections.*

OUTCOME CRITERIA:

- Tessie's skin is clear and intact with no signs or symptoms of infection.
- Tessie and her family demonstrate skin inspection and skin care.
- Tessie and her family describe the importance of promptly reporting infections.

Nursing Interventions	Rationale
Teach Tessie and her caregiver to inspect her skin daily and promptly treat small skin breaks.	Infections occur more frequently in the diabetic child due to decreased circulation. Prompt treatment prevents further complications.
Teach Tessie and her caregiver skin hygiene with emphasis on foot care.	Good hygiene with emphasis on good foot care is the first line of defense for lifelong health habits for the diabetic.
Teach Tessie and her family to be alert for signs of respiratory or urinary infections to report promptly.	Bacterial and fungal infections can become serious if not treated promptly.

(continued)

Nursing Care Plan (Continued)
for the Child with Diabetes Mellitus

NURSING DIAGNOSIS

Ineffective Family Coping: Compromised related to home management of hypoglycemia and hyperglycemia

GOAL: *Tessie and her family will learn to cope with diabetes.*

OUTCOME CRITERIA:

- Tessie and her family discuss diabetes, its physiology, and treatment.
- Tessie and her family list signs and symptoms of hyper- and hypoglycemia and how to handle each.
- Tessie is able to administer insulin with family supervision.

Nursing Interventions	Rationale
Use every opportunity to provide information in small doses. Provide written backup for oral presentations. Have Tessie and caregiver repeat the information or ask them questions to determine they have understood what was taught.	Although information is presented, often the learner's anxiety level may be high and information is not absorbed. Small doses of learning at a time are easier to digest. Feedback is necessary to determine what was learned.
Teach Tessie and her family the signs of hyper- and hypoglycemia and appropriate responses for each. Discuss how exercise and routine childhood illness may effect Tessie's blood sugar and adjustments that might need to be made.	Episodes of hyper- and hypoglycemia can be life threatening. The child and family need to know how to respond quickly to either event. They also need to know how exercise can be wisely handled in Tessie's daily life and how to respond when she is ill.
Teach Tessie and her caregiver the correct way to give insulin, including site rotation. Supervise return demonstrations by Tessie and her caregiver. Set up a site rotation chart to use.	Giving injections may be the most threatening part of the illness to the child and family. Patience while providing ample practice will help them gain confidence.
Stress the importance of Tessie's wearing a Medic Alert identification medal or bracelet.	This identification can be lifesaving in an emergency.

NURSING DIAGNOSIS

Self Esteem Disturbance related to chronic illness, insulin dependency

GOAL: *Tessie's self esteem will improve.*

OUTCOME CRITERIA:

- Tessie discusses necessary adjustments to her daily activities and schedule.
- Tessie names several people to inform about her diabetic condition.

Nursing Interventions	Rationale
Encourage Tessie to become active in self care.	Provides Tessie with a feeling of control over her illness.
Teach Tessie she can engage in normal activities, including sleepovers, as long as she confides in a responsible adult who is able to identify hypo- and hyperglycemia and respond appropriately.	The child is assured that she can take part in normal activities. Stresses the need for someone else to be responsible for Tessie's condition in the case of an emergency.

also may be needed in the child's school schedule. For instance, physical education should never be scheduled right before lunch for a diabetic child. Also, the diabetic child should not be scheduled for a late lunch period.

Many children are subject to minor infections and illnesses during the school years with little long-term effect. However, the diabetic child is more susceptible to long-term complications. When the diabetic child has an infection and fever, the temperature and metabolic rate increase and the body needs more sugar and therefore more insulin to make the sugar available to the body. Although the child may not be eating due to vomiting or anorexia, the body still needs insulin. Insulin should never be skipped during illness. Blood glucose levels should be checked every 2 to 4 hours during this time. Fluids need to be increased. Instruct the caregivers to contact the physician when the child becomes ill, especially if the child is vomiting, cannot eat, or has diarrhea, so that close supervision can be maintained. Give the caregiver guidelines for care of an ill child with the initial diabetic instructions.

It is extremely important for the child to wear a Medic Alert identification medal or a bracelet, with information about diabetic status. Identification cards, such as those carried by many adult diabetics, are seldom practical for a child.

PROVIDING FAMILY TEACHING ON INSULIN ADMINISTRATION. Teach the family caregiver and the child the correct way to give insulin. Disposable syringes make caring for equipment relatively easy. A doll may be used to practice the actual administration until the caregiver (and child, if old enough) is comfortable and confident. Provide direct supervision until proficiency is demonstrated.

This part of the treatment is probably the most threatening aspect of the illness. Remember your feelings when you gave your first injection in nursing school. A great deal of empathy and warm support are needed by the child and family.

Give clear instructions concerning the importance of rotating injection sites (Fig. 17-6). If used too frequently, a site is apt to become indurated and eventually fibrosed, hindering proper insulin absorption. The atrophic hollows in the skin, or the lumps of hypertrophied tissue, are unsightly as well. Some people appear to have a greater skin sensitivity than others. Areas on both the upper arms, upper thighs, abdomen, and buttocks can be used. Use of a careful plan allows several weeks to elapse before a site is used again. Starting from the inner, upper corner of the area, each injection is given 1/2" below the preceding one, going down in a vertical line, with the next series starting 1/2" outward at the upper level. If there is any sign of induration, the local site should be avoided for weeks after all signs of irritation have disappeared. A chart recording the sites used and the rotation schedule is recommended.

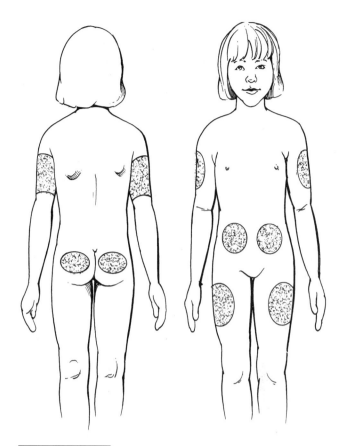

Figure 17-6
Subcutaneous injection sites.

ENSURING ADEQUATE AND APPROPRIATE NUTRITION. The child with diabetes needs a sound nutritional program that provides adequate nutrition for normal growth while it maintains the blood glucose at near-normal levels. The food plan should be well balanced, with foods that take into consideration the child's food preferences, cultural customs, and lifestyle (see Parent Teaching: Child's Diabetic Food Plan). Help the child and caregiver to understand the importance of eating regularly scheduled meals. Special occasions can be planned so that the child does not feel left out of celebrations. If a particular meal is going to be late, the child should have a complex carbohydrate and protein snack. Children should be included in meal planning when possible so that they learn what is permissible and what is not. In this way they will be able to handle eating when they are on their own in school and in social situations.

PREVENTING INFECTION AND SKIN BREAKDOWN. Skin breakdowns, such as blisters and minor cuts, can become major problems for the diabetic child. Teach the caregiver and child to inspect the skin daily and promptly treat even small breaks in the skin. Encourage daily bathing. Teach the child and caregiver to dry the skin well after bathing, and give careful attention to any area where skin touches skin, such as the groin, axilla, or other skin folds. Emphasize good foot care. This includes wearing well-fitting shoes, inspecting between toes for cracks, trimming nails straight across, wearing clean socks, and not going barefoot. Establishing these habits early will help the child prepare for lifelong care of diabetes.

Diabetic children may be more susceptible to urinary tract and upper respiratory infections. Teach the child and caregiver to be alert for signs of urinary tract infection, such as itching and burning on urination. Instruct them to report signs of urinary tract or upper respiratory infections to the physician promptly.

REDUCING CHILD AND FAMILY ANXIETY. When the diagnosis of diabetes is confirmed, the family caregiver may feel devastated. A young child will not understand the implications, but the school-age or adolescent child will experience a great amount of fear and anxiety. The caregiver may have feelings of guilt, resentment, or denial. Other family members also may experience strong feelings about the illness. All of these feelings and concerns must be recognized and resolved to work successfully with the diabetic child. Encourage the family to express these feelings and fears. Involve the caregiver in caring for the child during hospitalization as a means of helping him or her deal with feelings. Carefully listen to questions and answer them completely and honestly. Many materials are available to give to the caregiver to read, but be sure the caregiver can read and understand them. Videos are also available that are helpful in educating the diabetic and the family. Recommend available community support groups. Cover home care in detail. Provide the family caregiver with a support person to contact when questions arise after discharge.

Because so much information must be absorbed in a brief time, the caregivers may seem forgetful or confused. Careful, patient repetition of all aspects of diabetes and the child's care is necessary. When anxiety levels are high, information is often heard but not digested. Provide written material in a form they can easily understand. Have them repeat information, and ask them questions to confirm that they understand. Demonstrate warmth and caring throughout the teaching to increase the family's comfort and confidence in the response they can expect to their questions and apprehensions.

PROMOTING SELF-CARE AND POSITIVE SELF-ESTEEM. The school-age or older child may experience some strong feelings of inadequacy or being "sick." These feelings must be expressed and handled. To help allay fear, teach the child as much as is appropriate for his or her age. Tell the child about athletes and other famous people who are diabetic. When possible, another child who is diabetic may visit so that the child does not feel so alone. Encourage the child to become active in helping with self-care. Answer questions about how diabetes will affect the child's activities. Summer camps for children with diabetes are available in many areas and can help develop the child's self-assurance.

The diabetic child can participate in normal activities. However, at least one friend should be told about the diabetic condition, and the child should not go swimming or hiking without a responsible person nearby who knows what to look for and what to do if the child should have a reaction.

Some older children are sensitive about their condition and fear that they seem different from their friends. Even with the best instruction and preparation, they may feel this way and wish to keep their condition secret. They must understand that a teacher or some other adult in their environment must be acquainted with their condition. Classroom teachers need to know which of their students have such a condition and should understand the signs of an impending reaction.

Diabetic children under good control need not be kept from such activities as campouts, overnight trips with the school band, or other similar activities away from home. Of course, these children must be capable of measuring their insulin and giving their own injections. Some young people may find that a desire to participate in such an activity can be the factor that helps them overcome reluctance to measure and administer their own insulin.

EVALUATION: GOALS AND OUTCOME CRITERIA

■ *Goal:* The child will not experience injury related to abnormal blood glucose levels.

Family Teaching
Child's Diabetic Food Plan

1. Plan well-balanced meals that are appealing to child.
2. Be positive with child when talking about foods that child can eat; downplay the negatives.
3. Space three meals and three snacks throughout the day. Daily caloric intake is divided to provide 20% at breakfast, 20% at lunch, 30% at dinner, and 10% at each of the snacks.
4. Calories should be made up of 50%–60% carbohydrates, 15%–20% protein, and no more than 30% fat.
5. Avoid concentrated sweets such as jelly, syrup, pie, candy bars, and soda pop.
6. Artificial sweeteners may be used.
7. Child must not skip meals. Make every effort to plan meals with foods that child likes.
8. Include foods that contain dietary fiber, such as whole grains, cereals, fruits and vegetables, nuts, seeds, and legumes. Fiber helps prevent hyperglycemia.
9. Dietetic food is expensive and unnecessary.
10. Teach child day by day about the food plan to encourage independence in food selections when at school or away from home.

Criteria: The child's blood glucose level is 60 to 100 mg/dL; the urine is negative for acetone; there are no signs of hyperglycemia or hypoglycemia.

■ *Goal*: The child and caregiver will demonstrate coping mechanisms for management of hypo- and hyperglycemia.
Criteria: The child and caregiver list the signs of hyper- and hypoglycemia and how to handle each; they ask questions to clarify information.

■ *Goal*: The child and caregiver will evidence reassurance about insulin administration.
Criteria: The child and caregiver demonstrate insulin injection, describe various types of insulin and their reaction and peak times, and develop a site rotation schedule.

■ *Goal*: The child and caregiver will demonstrate understanding of nutritional needs.
Criteria: The child eats food at meals and snack times; the child and caregiver demonstrate understanding of meal planning by making appropriate menu selections.

■ *Goal*: The child will experience no skin breakdown or infection.
Criteria: There are no signs of infection; the skin is clear and intact; the child and caregiver demonstrate skin inspection and care and discuss the importance of promptly reporting infections.

■ *Goal*: The child and caregiver will express anxieties.
Criteria: The child and caregiver express fears and anxieties and participate in hospital care and planning for home care.

■ *Goal*: The child and caregiver will demonstrate understanding of long-term home care.
Criteria: As appropriate for age, the child discusses necessary adjustments to the daily schedule and activities and names several people to inform about the diabetic condition. The caregiver demonstrates support of the child in managing daily and long-term care of diabetes.

■ *Goal*: The child demonstrates a positive attitude about the condition.
Criteria: The child expresses feelings about having diabetes and demonstrates appropriate participation in activities and realistic goal planning.

MUSCULOSKELETAL SYSTEM DISORDERS

The long bones of the extremities grow rapidly during the school-age period. "Growing pains" are a frequent complaint but rarely indicate serious disease. School age is a time of increasing physical activity, including team sports. Peer approval and group or team participation at school and in after-school activities are important to the school-age child. Minor skeletal injuries, such as sprains and minor fractures, may make the child a temporary celebrity. However, a serious skeletal defect or injury may influence the child's ability to cope with peer relationships and create social adjustment problems.

Scoliosis

Scoliosis, a lateral curvature of the spine, occurs in two forms, structural and nonstructural (functional). The latter is more common. Structural scoliosis is caused by rotated and malformed vertebrae. Nonstructural scoliosis can have several causes: poor posture, muscle spasm due to trauma, or unequal length of legs. When the primary problem is corrected, elimination of the functional scoliosis has begun.

Most cases of structural scoliosis are idiopathic (no known cause); a few are caused by congenital deformities or infection. Idiopathic scoliosis is seen in older school-age children at 10 years of age and older. Although mild curves occur as often in boys as in girls, idiopathic scoliosis requiring treatment occurs eight times more frequently in girls than in boys.[3]

DIAGNOSIS

Nurses play an important role in screening for scoliosis. School nurses and others who contact children in a health care setting at age 10 and beyond should conduct or assist with screening programs. Many states require regular examination of students for scoliosis beginning in the fifth or sixth grade. Scoliosis screening should last through at least eighth grade. A school nurse often does the initial screening. Nurses in the health care setting are also responsible for screening these children during regular well-child visits.

During examination, the undressed child is observed from the back, noting any lateral curvature of the spinal column, asymmetry of the shoulders, shoulder blades, or hips, and an unequal distance between the arms and waist (Fig. 17-7). The examiner then asks the child to bend at the hips (touch the toes) and observes for prominence of the scapula on one side and curvature of the spinal column.

TREATMENT

Treatment is by application of electrical stimulation, braces, traction, casts, and spinal fusion, which may include internal fixation with rods. Curvatures of less than 25° are observed closely but not treated. Curvatures between 25° and 40° are corrected with electrical stimulation or a Milwaukee brace, and those more than 40° are usually corrected surgically. Treatment is long term and usually lasts through the rest of the child's growth cycle.

Figure 17-7
(A) Posterior view of child's back with lateral curvature. (B) View of child bending over with prominence of scapular area and asymmetry of flank demonstrated.

Electrical Stimulation   Electrical stimulation may be used as an alternative to bracing for the child with a mild to moderate curvature. Electrodes are applied to the skin or surgically implanted. Treatment occurs at night while the child is asleep. The leads are placed to stimulate muscles on the convex side of the curvature to contract as impulses are transmitted. This causes the spine to straighten. If external electrodes are used, the skin under the leads must be checked regularly for irritation. This treatment is the least disruptive to the child's life, but there is some controversy about its effectiveness.

Braces   The brace most commonly used is the Milwaukee brace, which exerts pressure on certain areas to maintain correct posture or immobilization (Fig. 17-8). The Milwaukee brace is considered the most effective spinal brace for the treatment of scoliosis. It exerts lateral pressure and longitudinal traction, thus achieving vertical

alignment. The brace does not correct the existing curvature but prevents further progression of the curve.

The brace should be worn constantly, except during bathing or swimming. It should be worn over a T-shirt or undershirt to protect the skin and the leather of the brace. The throat mold of the brace can be covered with soft cloth if sweating or irritation occurs.

Wearing the Milwaukee brace creates a distinct change in body image, usually in adolescence, a time when body consciousness is at an all-time high. The need to wear the brace and deal with the limitations it involves may cause anger; the change in body image can cause a grief reaction. Handling these feelings successfully requires understanding support from the nurse, family, and peers. Sometimes it is helpful for the patient in a Milwaukee brace to talk with other scoliosis patients and learn how they have coped. Understanding the disorder itself and the important benefits of treatment also can ease the adjustment.

Casts and Traction   Some orthopedic surgeons continue to use casts, with varying success. Before the cast is applied, the child should be given an explanation of the procedure and what the treatment is intended to accomplish. The adolescent girl needs reassurance that the cast will not interfere with breast development.

Care of this child is similar to the care of a child in any kind of cast: regular observation and recording of color, temperature, presence or absence of edema, sensation, and motion; proper positioning; meticulous skin care; and patient teaching. When ready for discharge, the child needs

Figure 17-8
Milwaukee brace.

an understanding of cast care, a firm mattress (and probably a bed board), and family support. If return to school is impossible, arrangements need to be made for a tutor at home or a communication hookup with the school. Casts need to be changed periodically to continue the correction as the child grows.

In a severe curvature, the cast is sometimes combined with **halo traction** (Fig. 17-9). Halo traction may be added to the body cast using stainless steel pins inserted into the skull and into the femurs. Weights are increased gradually to promote correction. When the curvature has been corrected, spinal fusion is performed.

The strange appearance of the halo traction apparatus magnifies the problems of body image; in addition, the head may need to be shaved. The child needs a thorough explanation of what will occur during the procedure and, if possible, should have the opportunity to talk with a child who has had this kind of traction. The nurse can help the child ventilate any feelings of fear, anger, depression, and embarrassment. Family members also need support in managing their own feelings about the child in halo traction.

Frequent shampooing, cleansing of the pin sites, and observation for signs of complications are critical in the care of children in halo traction. Any sign of infection, cyanosis, respiratory distress, diplopia (double vision), pupil irregularity, numbness, paralysis, or inability to void should be documented and reported at once. Particular care should be taken to prevent bumping the halo, because it magnifies sounds. Turning the child at least every 2 hours and performing skin care with alcohol every 4 hours help prevent tissue breakdown. Breathing exercises and range-of-motion activities reduce the possibility of other complications.

Rod Implantation   Rigid stainless steel rods may be implanted along the spinal column to maintain reduction of the curvature, combined with spinal fusion. This procedure, done only in severe curvatures, is frightening to the child and family. This is major surgery, and the child and family must be well prepared for it. The child can expect to have postoperative pain and will have to endure days of remaining flat in bed, being turned only in a log-rolling fashion. Because this is an elective procedure, thorough preoperative teaching can be carried out for the child and the family. The child may be given a patient-controlled analgesia pump to control pain. A Foley catheter is usually inserted because of the need to remain flat. The rods remain in place permanently. About 6 months after surgery, the child will be able to take part in most activities except contact sports (such as tackle football, gymnastics, and wrestling). Because the bones are fused and rods are implanted, this procedure arrests the child's growth in height, which contributes to the emotional adjustment that the child and family must make.

Nursing Process for the Child With Scoliosis

ASSESSMENT

The child with scoliosis must be reassessed every 6 to 9 months. Document the degree of curvature and related impairments. This is a sensitive age for children, when privacy and the importance of being like everyone else are top priorities. Keep this in mind when assessing the child. Provide privacy and protect the child's modesty.

The child who is admitted to a health care facility for application of a Milwaukee brace or other instrumentation may be carrying a lot of unseen emotional baggage. Be sensitive to this emotional state. The family caregivers also may be upset but may be trying to hide it for the child's sake. In addition to routine assessment, look for clues to the emotional state of both the child and family caregivers.

NURSING DIAGNOSES

Assess the emotional state of the child and caregiver to help determine effective nursing diagnoses. The type of treatment involved also affects the selection of nursing diagnoses. Some diagnoses for application of a Milwaukee brace are:

■ Impaired Physical Mobility related to restricted movement

Figure 17-9
Halo traction applied to a body cast. Although this appears top heavy, the child can ambulate with traction in place.

- Risk for Impaired Skin Integrity related to mechanical irritation of brace
- Risk for Noncompliance related to long-term treatment
- Risk for Body Image Disturbance related to wearing a brace continuously

OUTCOME IDENTIFICATION AND PLANNING

Consult the child and caregiver when establishing nursing goals. Be especially sensitive to the child's needs. Goals for the child may include minimizing the disruption of activities and maintaining skin integrity and self-image. Goals for the child and caregiver include complying with long-term care.

IMPLEMENTATION

PROMOTING MOBILITY. Prescribed exercises must be practiced and performed as directed. Encourage and support the child during these exercises. The child may need to be in traction for 1 or 2 weeks before the brace is applied. This can be emotionally traumatic.

Evaluate the child's environment after the brace has been applied and take precautions to prevent injury. Help the child practice moving about safely: going up and down stairs, getting in and out of vehicles, chairs, or desks, and getting out of bed. Teach the child to avoid hazardous surfaces. Listen carefully to the child and the family caregiver to determine any other hazards in the home or school environment. Advise the family caregiver to contact school personnel to ensure that the child has comfortable, supportive seating at school and that adjustments are made in the physical education program.

PREVENTING SKIN IRRITATION. When the brace is first applied, check the child regularly to confirm proper fit. Assess any areas of rubbing, discomfort, or skin irritation and adjust the brace as necessary. Teach the child how to inspect all areas under the brace daily. Instruct the child and caregiver that reddened areas should be reported to the physician so that adjustments can be made. Skin under the pads should be massaged daily. Daily bathing is essential, and clean cotton underwear or a T-shirt should be worn under the brace to provide protection.

PROMOTING COMPLIANCE WITH THERAPY. The child must wear the brace for years, until the spinal growth is completed, and needs to be weaned from it gradually for another 1 or 2 years, wearing it only at night. During this period, the caregivers and the child need emotional support from the nursing staff. Be certain that the child and caregivers have a complete understanding of the importance of wearing the brace continually. To encourage compliance, teach them about the complications that may occur if correction is unsuccessful. Inform the caregiver about the need to monitor the child for compliance. Help the caregiver understand the importance of being empathetic to the child's need to be like others during this period of development. Offer ways in which the caregiver can help the child deal with adjustment to the therapy.

PROMOTING POSITIVE BODY IMAGE. The child should be involved in all aspects of care planning. Self-image and the need to be like others is so important at this age. Learning to be confident enough to handle the comments of peers can be difficult for the child. Give the child frequent opportunities to ventilate feelings about being different. Help the child select clothing that blends with current styles but is loose enough to hide the brace. Encourage the child to find extracurricular activities with which the brace will not interfere. Active sports are not permitted, but many other activities are available. Help the child focus and enhance a positive attribute, such as hair or complexion. Encourage the child and caregiver to discuss accommodations with school personnel together.

EVALUATION: GOALS AND OUTCOME CRITERIA

- *Goal*: The child will move effectively within the limits of the brace.
  Criteria: The child ambulates without injury.

- *Goal*: The child's skin will remain intact.
  Criteria: The child uses methods to reduce skin irritation and bathes regularly. Skin remains free from irritation and breakdown.

- *Goal*: The child will comply with therapy.
  Criteria: The child wears the brace as directed. Caregivers report compliance, and the child's condition also evidences compliance.

- *Goal*: The child will exhibit positive coping behaviors.
  Criteria: The child is self-confident and has an attractive, well-groomed appearance; the child verbalizes feelings about the need to wear the brace.

Legg-Calvé-Perthes Disease (Coxa Plana)

Legg-Calvé-Perthes disease is an aseptic necrosis of the head of the femur. It occurs four to five times more often in boys than in girls and 10 times more often in whites than in African-Americans. It can be caused by trauma to the hip, but generally the cause is unknown. Symptoms first noticed are pain in the hip or groin and a limp, accompanied by muscle spasms and limitation of motion. These symptoms mimic **synovitis** (inflammation of a joint, most commonly the hip in children), which makes immediate diagnosis difficult. Radiographic examination may need to be repeated several weeks after the initial visit to demonstrate vascular necrosis for a definitive diagnosis.

There are three stages of the disease, each lasting 9

months to 1 year. In the first stage, radiographic studies show opacity of the epiphysis. In the second stage, the epiphysis becomes mottled and fragmented, and during the third stage, reossification occurs.

In the past, immobilization of the hip through the use of braces and crutches, bed rest with traction, or casting was considered essential for recovery without deformity. However, restricting a child's activity for 2 years or more was extremely difficult. Current treatment focuses on containing the femoral head within the acetabulum during the revascularization process so that the new femoral head will form to make a smoothly functioning joint. The method of containment varies with the portion of the head affected. Use of a brace that holds the necrotic portions of the head in place during healing is considered an effective method of containment. Reconstructive surgery is now possible, enabling the child to return to normal activities within 3 to 4 months.

The prognosis for complete recovery without difficulty later in life depends on the child's age at the time of onset, the amount of involvement, and the cooperation of the child and the family caregivers. Nursing care focuses on helping the child and caregivers to manage the corrective device and the importance of compliance to promote healing and avoid long-term disability.

Osteomyelitis

Osteomyelitis is an infection of the bone usually caused by *Staphylococcus aureus*. Acute osteomyelitis is twice as common in boys and results from a primary infection such as a staphylococcal skin infection (impetigo), burns, a furuncle (boil), a penetrating wound, or a fracture. The bacteria enter the bloodstream and are carried to the metaphysis of a bone, where an abscess forms, ruptures, and spreads the infection along the bone under the periosteum.

Symptoms usually begin abruptly with fever, malaise, and pain and localized tenderness over the metaphysis of the affected bone. There is limitation of joint motion. Diagnosis is based on laboratory findings of leukocytosis (15,000–25,000 cells or more), an increased ESR, and positive blood cultures. Radiographic examination does not reveal the process until 5 to 10 days after the onset.

Treatment for acute osteomyelitis must be immediate. Intravenous antibiotic therapy is started at once and is continued for at least 6 weeks. Depending on the physician and the compliance of the child and family, a short course of IV antibiotics may be followed by administration of oral antibiotics to complete treatment. Surgical drainage of the involved metaphysis may be performed. If the abscess has ruptured into the subperiosteal space, chronic osteomyelitis follows.

If prompt, specific antibiotic treatment is vigorously employed, acute osteomyelitis may be brought under control rapidly and extensive bone destruction of chronic osteomyelitis is prevented. If extensive destruction of bone

has occurred before treatment, surgical removal of necrotic bone becomes necessary.

During the acute stage, nursing care includes reducing pain by positioning the affected limb, minimizing movement of the limb, and administering medication. Transmission-based precautions may be required if the wound is open and draining. Follow the usual procedure for IV antibiotic therapy, including careful observance of the venipuncture site and monitoring the rate, dosage, and time of antibiotic. An intermittent infusion device or peripherally inserted central catheter may be used for long-term IV therapy.

Monitor oral nutrition and fluids, as the child's appetite may be poor during the acute phase (it improves in later stages). Weight-bearing on the affected limb must be avoided until healing has occurred, as pathologic fractures occur very easily in the weakened stage. Physical therapy helps restore the function of the limb.

Muscular Dystrophy

Muscular dystrophy is a hereditary, progressive, degenerative disease of the muscles. The most common form of muscular dystrophy is Duchenne (pseudohypertrophic) muscular dystrophy. Duchenne muscular dystrophy, an X-linked recessive hereditary disease, occurs almost exclusively in males and is carried by females. When muscular dystrophy has been diagnosed in a child, the mother and the siblings should be tested to see if they have the disease or are carriers.

The first signs are noted in infancy or childhood, when the child finds it difficult to stand or walk, usually at about 3 years of age; later, trunk muscle weakness develops. Mild mental retardation often accompanies this disease. The child cannot rise easily to an upright position from a sitting position on the floor; instead, he or she rises by climbing up the lower extremities with the hands (Fig. 17-10). Weakness of leg, arm, and shoulder muscles progresses gradually. Increasing abnormalities in gait and posture appear by school age with **lordosis** (forward curvature of the lumbar spine, or swayback), pelvic waddling, and frequent falling (Fig. 17-11). The child becomes progressively weaker, usually becoming wheelchair-bound by 10 to 12 years of age (middle school or junior high school age). The disease continues into adolescence and young adulthood, when the patient usually succumbs to respiratory failure.

In addition to symptoms in the first 2 years of life, the diagnosis can be confirmed by highly increased serum creatinine phosphokinase, aldolase, and serum glutamic oxaloacetic transaminase levels, as well as a decrease in muscle fibers seen in a muscle biopsy.

No effective treatment for the disease has been found, but research is rapidly closing in on genetic identification, which promises exciting changes in treatment in the future. The child is encouraged to be as active as possible to delay muscle atrophy and contractures. Physiotherapy, diet

Figure 17-10
Child "climbing up" lower extremities.

Figure 17-11
Characteristic posture of a child with Duchenne muscular dystrophy. Along with the typical toe gait, the child develops a lordotic posture as Duchenne dystrophy causes further deterioration.

to avoid obesity, and parental encouragement help keep the child active.

Once a child becomes wheelchair-bound, **kyphoscoliosis** (hunchback) develops, causing a decrease in respiratory function and an increase in the incidence of infections. Breathing exercises are a daily necessity for these children.

The nurse should advise the family to keep the child's life as normal as possible, which may be difficult. This disease can drain the emotional and financial reserves of the entire family. The nurse might suggest assistance through the Muscular Dystrophy Association of America (810 7th Avenue, New York, NY 10019), through local chapters of this organization, and by talking with other parents who face the same problem.

Juvenile Rheumatoid Arthritis

Juvenile rheumatoid arthritis (JRA) is the most common connective tissue disease of childhood. (Connective tissues are those that provide a supportive framework and protective covering for the body, such as the musculoskeletal system and skin and mucous membranes.) Joint inflammation occurs first and if untreated leads to irreversible changes in joint cartilage, ligaments, and menisci (the crescent-shaped fibrocartilage in the knee joints), eventually causing complete immobility. The occurrence of JRA appears to peak at two age levels: 1 to 3 years and 8 to

12 years. It can be subdivided into three different types: systemic, polyarticular (involving five or more joints), and pauciarticular (involving four or fewer joints, most often the knees and the ankles) (Table 17-6). This disease has a long duration, but 80% to 90% of children with JRA reach adulthood without serious disability.[4]

The goal of treatment is to maintain mobility and preserve joint function. Treatment can include drugs, physical therapy, and surgery. Early diagnosis and drug therapy to control inflammation and other systemic changes can reduce the need for other types of treatment.

Enteric-coated aspirin is the drug of choice for JRA; an effective antiinflammatory drug, it is inexpensive, is easily administered, and has few side effects when carefully regulated. Administering aspirin with food or milk is important to decrease GI irritation and bleeding. Acetaminophen is not an appropriate substitute because it lacks antiinflammatory properties. Teach family caregivers the importance of regular administration of aspirin, even when the child is not experiencing pain. The primary purpose of aspirin is not to relieve pain but to decrease inflammation of the joints.

When aspirin is no longer effective, nonsteroidal antiinflammatory drugs, indomethacin, gold preparations, antimalarials, steroids, penicillamine, or immunosuppressives may be used. All of these are toxic and must be closely monitored.

Physical therapy includes exercise, application of splints, and heat. Implementing this program at home requires the cooperation of the nurse, physical therapist, and physician. Joints must be immobilized by splinting during active disease, but gentle daily exercise is necessary to prevent **ankylosis** (immobility of a joint). Stress to the caregivers the importance of encouraging the child to perform independent activities of daily living to maintain function and independence. The family caregiver must be patient, allowing the child time to accomplish necessary tasks.

Depending on the degree of disease activity, range-of-motion exercises, isometric exercises, swimming, and riding a tricycle or bicycle may be part of the treatment plan. Inform caregivers that these exercises should not increase pain; if exercise does trigger increased pain, the amount of exercise should be decreased.

Fractures

A fracture is a break in a bone, usually accompanied by vascular and soft-tissue damage, and is characterized by pain, swelling, and tenderness. Children's fractures differ from those of adults in that generally they are less complicated, heal more quickly, and usually occur from different causes. The child has an urge to explore the environment but lacks the experience and judgment to recognize possible hazards. In some instances, caregivers may be negligent in their supervision, but often the child uses immature judgment or is simply too fast for them.

The bones most commonly fractured in childhood are the clavicle, femur, tibia, humerus, wrist, and fingers. The classification of a fracture reflects the kind of bone injury sustained (Fig. 17-12). If the fragments of fractured bone are separated, the fracture is said to be complete. If fragments remain partially joined, the fracture is termed in-

---

TABLE 17-6.   **Characteristics of Different Types of Juvenile Rheumatoid Arthritis**

Characteristic	Polyarthritis	Pauciarticular	Systemic
Frequency of occurrence	40%–50%	40%–50%	10%–20%
Number of joints involved	5 or more	4 or fewer	Variable
Sex ratio (F:M)	3:1	5:1	1:1
Systemic involvement	Moderate	Not present	Prominent
Uveitis*	5%	20%	Rare
Fever	Rare	Rare	Common
Sensitivity			
Rheumatoid factors	10%	Rare	Rare
Antinuclear bodies	40%–50%	75%–85%	10%
Course	Systemic disease is generally mild; articular involvement may be unremitting	Systemic disease is absent; major cause of morbidity is uveitis	Systemic disease is often self-limited; arthritis is chronic and destructive in 50%
Prognosis	Guarded to moderately good	Excellent except for eyesight	Moderate to poor

* Uveitis—an inflammation of the middle (vascular) tunic of the eye; includes the iris, ciliary body, and choroid.
Adapted from Cassidy JT. Connective tissue diseases and amyloidosis. In FA Oski, et al., eds. Principles and practice of pediatrics. Philadelphia: JB Lippincott, 1990.

Simple/closed   Compound/open   Spiral   Greenstick

Figure 17-12
Types of fractures. All are examples of complete fractures except **D**, which is an incomplete fracture.

complete. Greenstick fractures are one kind of incomplete fracture common in children due to incomplete ossification. When a broken bone penetrates the skin, the fracture is called compound, or open. A simple, or closed, fracture is a single break in the bone without penetration of the skin. Spiral fractures, which twist around the bone, are frequently associated with child abuse and are caused by a wrenching force. Fractures in the area of the epiphyseal plate (growth plate) can cause permanent damage and severely impair growth (Fig. 17-13).

TREATMENT

Most childhood fractures are treated by realignment and immobilization, using either traction or closed manipulation and casting. A few patients with severe fractures or additional injuries, such as burns and other soft-tissue damage, may require surgical reduction, internal or external fixation, or both. Internal fixation devices include rods, pins, screws, and plates made of inert materials that will not trigger an immune reaction. They allow early mobilization of the child to a wheelchair, crutches, or a walker.

External fixation devices are used primarily in complex fractures, often with other injuries or complications. These devices are applied under sterile conditions in the operating room and may be augmented by soft dressings and

Figure 17-13
One form of epiphyseal injury; a crushing injury (as might occur in a fall from a height) can destory the layer of germinal cells of the epiphysis, resulting in disturbance of growth.

elevation by means of an overhead traction rope. External fixation devices rarely are used on young children.

Casts The kind of cast used is determined by the age of the child, the severity of the fracture, the type of bone involved, and the amount of weight-bearing. Most casts are formed from gauze strips impregnated with plaster of Paris or other synthetic material, such as fiberglass or polyurethane resin, that is pliable when wet but hardens when dry. Synthetic materials are lighter in weight and present a cleaner appearance because they can be sponged with water when soiled; they even come in colors. Synthetic casts dry more rapidly than plaster of Paris. The lightweight casts tend to be used as arm casts and hip spicas for infants and small children.

The child and the family should be taught what to expect after the cast is applied and how to care for the casted area. A stockinette is applied over the area to be casted, and the bony prominences are padded before the wet plaster rolls

are applied. Although the wet plaster of Paris feels cool on the skin when it is applied, evaporation soon causes a temporary sensation of warmth. The cast will feel heavy and cumbersome.

While the cast is wet, it should be handled only with open palms, because fingertips can cause indentations and result in pressure points. If the cast has no protective edge, it should be petaled (see Fig. 9-22 in Chap. 9) with adhesive tape strips. If the cast is close to the genital area, plastic should be taped around the edge to prevent wetting and soiling of the cast.

After the fracture has been immobilized, any complaints of pain signal complications and should be recorded and reported immediately. Observing, documenting, and reporting the five P's is essential to good nursing care:

- *Pain*—Any sign of pain should be noted and the exact area determined.
- *Pulse*—If an upper extremity is involved, brachial, radial, ulnar, and digital pulses should be checked.

COMMUNICATIONS BOX

Seven-year-old Jimmy is in skeletal traction for a severely fractured femur.
As the nurse enters his room, he turns his head away from the door.

INEFFECTIVE COMMUNICATION

Nurse: Hey, Jimmy. What's the trouble?
Jimmy: Nothin'.
Nurse: What do you mean, "nothin?"
Jimmy: (Just shrugs)
Nurse: What's the matter . . . Cat got your tongue?
Jimmy: (Shrugs again)
Nurse: Jimmy, I can't help you if you won't talk to me.
Jimmy: (Turns away from the nurse)
Nurse: OK, Sport. When you decide to talk, let me know. (Leaves the room)

The nurse treats Jimmy as a "pal," but isn't skilled at using open-ended questions. The response "cat got your tongue?" is almost a sure turn-off to a youngster. The nurse ends up leaving the room without finding out what Jimmy's problem was. He will continue to have pain until it builds to a point where he can't stand it any more, and then it will take longer for the pain medication to bring comfort.

EFFECTIVE COMMUNICATION

Nurse: Hi, Jimmy. You look like you are having some pain. Tell me where it hurts.
Jimmy: (Points to thigh)
Nurse: Can you tell me how it feels?
Jimmy: It feels kind of burny.
Nurse: Kind of burny? Show me exactly where the burny feeling is.
Jimmy: Right here (pointing). And it kind of feels jabby.
Nurse: OK, Jimmy. You did a good job of showing me exactly how it feels. I'll get some medicine to make it feel better. After I give you the medicine I'll read a story to you if you like.

The nurse recognized Jimmy had some kind of problem. Pain was the most likely choice. If it had not been pain, Jimmy would have most likely responded verbally to set her straight. By asking open-ended questions that couldn't be answered with just "yes" or "no," the nurse got more definite responses from Jimmy. After telling Jimmy he/she would get him medicine for the pain, the nurse offered the special treat of a story.

If a lower extremity is involved, femoral, popliteal, posterior tibial, and dorsalis pedis pulses should be assessed.

- *Paresthesia*—Check for any diminished or absent sensation, or for numbness or tingling.
- *Paralysis*—Check hand function by having the child try to hyperextend the thumb or wrist, oppose the thumb and little finger, and adduct all fingers. Check function of the foot by having the child try to dorsiflex and plantarflex the ankles and flex and extend the toes.
- *Pallor*—Check the color of the extremity and the nail beds distal to the site of the fracture. Pallor, discoloration, and coldness indicate circulatory impairment.

In addition to the five P's, any foul odor or drainage on or under the cast, "hot spots" on the cast (warm to touch), looseness or tightness, or any elevation of temperature must be noted, documented, and reported. Family caregivers should be instructed to watch carefully for these same danger signals.

Children and caregivers should be cautioned not to put anything down inside the cast, no matter how much the casted area itches. Small toys and sticks or sticklike objects should be kept out of reach until the cast has been removed.

When the fracture has healed, the cast is removed with a cast cutter. This can be frightening for the child unless the person using the cast cutter explains and demonstrates that the device will not cut flesh but only the hard surface of the cast. The child should be told that there will be vibration from the cast cutter, but it will not burn.

After cast removal, the area that was casted should be soaked in warm water to help remove the crusty layer of skin that has accumulated. Application of oil or lotion may prove comforting. Family caregivers and the child must be cautioned against scrubbing or scraping this area because the tender layer of new skin underneath the crust may bleed.

Traction Traction is a pulling force applied to an extremity or other part of the body. A system of weights, ropes, and pulleys is used to realign and immobilize fractures, reduce or eliminate muscle spasm, and prevent fracture deformity and joint contractures.

There are two basic types of traction: skin traction and skeletal traction. **Skin traction** pulls on tape, rubber, or plastic materials attached to the skin and indirectly exerts pull on the musculoskeletal system. Examples of skin traction are Bryant's traction, Buck extension traction, Russell traction, and sidearm traction. **Skeletal traction** exerts pull directly on skeletal structures by means of a pin, wire, tongs, or other device surgically inserted through a bone.

Bryant's traction is often used for the treatment of a fractured femur in children younger than 2 years of age. These fractures are often transverse or spiral fractures. The use of Bryant's traction entails some risk of compromised

circulation and may result in contracture of the foot and lower leg, particularly in an older child. The child's legs are wrapped with elastic bandages that should be removed at least daily for skin assessment and then rewrapped. Skin temperature and the color of the legs and feet must be checked frequently to detect any circulatory impairment. Severe pain may indicate circulatory difficulty and should be reported immediately. When a child is in Bryant's traction, the hips should not rest on the bed—the nurse should be able to pass a hand between the child's buttocks and the sheet.

Buck extension traction is used for short-term immobilization. The child's body provides the countertraction to the weights. It is used to correct contractures and bone deformities such as Legg-Calvé-Perthes disease. Russell traction (Fig. 17-14) seems to be more effective for older

Figure 17-14
Types of traction. **(A)** Buck extension, a form of skin traction. **(B)** Russell traction, a type of skin traction. Two lines of traction (one horizontal and one vertical) allow for good bone alignment for healing. **(C)** 90 degree–90 degree (skeletal) traction. The lower leg is in a boot cast, and a wire pin is inserted into the distal femur.

children. A child in either type of traction, however, tends to slide down until the weights rest on the bed or the floor. The child should be pulled up to keep the weights free, the ropes must be in alignment with the pulleys, and the alignment should be checked frequently. An older child may coax a roommate to remove the weights or the sandbags used as weights.

Sidearm traction (Fig. 17-15) is sometimes used for fractures of the humerus or the elbow. It can be applied as skin traction or, when a pin is inserted into the bone, as skeletal traction.

Children in any kind of traction must be carefully monitored to detect any signs of neurovascular complications. Skin temperature and color, presence or absence of edema, peripheral pulse, sensation, and motion must be assessed every hour for the first 24 hours after traction has been applied and every 4 hours unless ordered otherwise. Skin care must be meticulous. Skin preparation (Skin-Prep) should be used to toughen the skin rather than lotions or oils, which soften the skin and contribute to tissue breakdown.

Children in skeletal traction require special attention to pin sites. Pin care should be performed every 8 hours with povidone-iodine or hydrogen peroxide solution. Sterile gloves are worn and sterile applicators used (Fig. 17-16). Any sign of infection (odor, local inflammation, or elevated temperature) must be recorded and reported at once.

External Fixation Devices Children whose fractures are severe enough to require the use of external fixation also need special skin care at pin sites. The sites are left open to the air and should be inspected and cleansed every 8 hours. The appearance of the pins puncturing the

Figure 17-16
Pin sites with povidone-iodine and sterile gauze applied.

skin and the unusual appearance of the device can be upsetting to the child, so be sensitive to any anxiety the child expresses.

As early as possible, the child (if old enough) or family caregivers should be taught to care for the pin sites. External fixation devices are sometimes left in place for as long as 1 year; therefore, it is important that the child accepts this temporary change in body image and learns to care for the affected site. Children with these devices will probably work with a physical therapist during the rehabilitation period and will have specific exercises to perform. Before discharge from the hospital, the child should feel comfortable in moving about and should be able to recognize the signs of pin infection.

Crutches Children with fractures of the lower extremities and other lower leg injuries often must learn to use crutches to avoid weight-bearing on the injured area. Several types of crutches are available, the most common being axillary crutches, principally used for temporary situations. Forearm, or Canadian, crutches usually are recommended for children who need crutches permanently, such as paraplegic children with braces. Trough, or platform, crutches are more suitable for children with limited strength or function in the arms and hands.

The use of crutches is generally taught by a physical therapist, but it can be the responsibility of nurses. The type of crutch gait to be taught is determined by the amount of weight-bearing permitted, the child's degree of stability, whether or not the knees can be flexed, and the specific goal of treatment.

SKIN DISORDERS

School-age children often have minor bruises, abrasions, or rashes that generally cause few problems. There are, however, common fungal and parasitic disorders that can

Figure 17-15
Dunlop traction, a variation of sidearm traction.

become serious if not controlled and cured. Allergic skin reactions are not uncommon. Because a large part of the school-age child's time is spent away from home, the child is exposed to poisonous plants that cause allergic reactions or to bites from insects, animals, or snakes; these need attention.

Fungal Infections

Fungal infections of the skin are superficial infections caused by fungi that live in the outer (dead) layers of the skin, the hair, and nails. **Tinea** (ringworm) is the term commonly applied to these infections, which are further differentiated by the part of the body infected.

TINEA CAPITIS (RINGWORM OF THE SCALP)

Ringworm of the scalp is called *tinea capitis* or *tinea tonsurans*. The most common cause is *Microsporum audouinii*, transmitted from person to person through combs, towels, hats, barber scissors, or direct contact. A less common type, *Microsporum canis*, is transmitted from animal to child. Tinea capitis begins as a small papule on the scalp and spreads, leaving scaly patches of baldness. The hairs become brittle and break off easily. Griseofulvin, an oral antifungal antibiotic, is the medication of choice. Because treatment may be prolonged (3 months or more), compliance must be reinforced. Children who are being properly treated may attend school. Hair loss is not permanent.

TINEA CORPORIS (RINGWORM OF THE BODY)

Tinea corporis is ringworm of the body that affects the epidermal layer of the skin. The lesions appear as a scaly ring with clearing in the center and may occur on any part of the body. They resemble the lesions of scalp ringworm. The child usually contracts tinea corporis from contact with an infected dog or cat. Topical antifungal agents, such as clotrimazole, econazole nitrate, tolnaftate, and miconazole, are effective. Griseofulvin also is used in this condition.

TINEA PEDIS (RINGWORM OF THE FEET; ATHLETE'S FOOT)

Tinea pedis (athlete's foot) is the scaling or cracking of the skin between the toes. Examination under a microscope of scrapings from the lesions is necessary for definite diagnosis. Transmission is by direct or indirect contact with skin lesions from infected people. Contaminated sidewalks, floors, pool decks, and shower stalls spread the condition to those who walk barefoot. Tinea pedis, usually found in adolescents and adults, is becoming more prevalent among school-age children due to the popularity of plastic shoes.

Care includes washing the feet with soap and water, then gently removing scabs and crusts and applying a topical agent such as tolnaftate. Griseofulvin by mouth is also useful. During the chronic phase, the use of ointment, scrupulous foot hygiene, frequent changing of white cotton socks, and avoidance of plastic footwear are helpful. Continuing application of a topical agent for up to 6 weeks is recommended.

TINEA CRURIS (RINGWORM OF THE INNER THIGHS AND INGUINAL AREA)

Tinea cruris (jock itch) is caused by the same organisms that cause tinea corporis. It is more common in athletes and is uncommon in preadolescent children. Tinea cruris is pruritic and localized to the area. Treatment is the same as for tinea corporis. Sitz baths also may be soothing.

Parasitic Infections

Parasites are organisms that live on or within another living organism, from which they obtain their food supply. Lice and the scabies mite both live by sucking the blood of the host.

PEDICULOSIS

Pediculosis (lice infestation) may be caused by *Pediculus humanus capitis* (head lice), *Pediculus humanus corporis* (body lice), or *Phthirus pubis* (pubic lice). Head lice are the most common infestation in children. Animal lice are not transferred to humans.

Head lice are passed from child to child by direct contact or indirectly by contact with combs, headgear, or bed linen. Lice, which are rarely seen, lay their eggs, called nits, on the head, attaching them to strands of hair. The nits can be seen as tiny pearly white flecks attached to the hair shafts. They look much like dandruff, but dandruff flakes can be flicked off easily, whereas the nits are tightly attached and not easily removed. The nits hatch in about 1 week, and the lice become sexually mature in about 2 weeks. Severe itching of the scalp is the most obvious symptom.

Use of lindane (Kwell) shampoo, which is prescribed by a physician, gives the most satisfactory results. After wetting the hair with warm water, the Kwell is applied like any ordinary shampoo; about 1 oz is used. The head should be lathered for 4 minutes, then rinsed thoroughly and dried. After the hair is dry, it should be combed with a fine-toothed comb dipped in warm white vinegar to remove remaining nits and nit shells. Shampooing may be repeated in 2 weeks to remove any lice that may have been missed as nits and since hatched. Avoid getting Kwell into the eyes or on mucous membranes. When treating a child in the hospital for pediculosis, wear a disposable gown, gloves, and head cover for protection.

Family caregivers are often embarrassed when the school nurse sends word that the child has head lice. They can be reassured that lice infestation is common and can happen to any child; it is not a reflection on the caregiver's

Family Teaching
Eliminating Pediculi Infestations

1. Wash all child's bedding and clothing in hot water and dry in hot dryer.
2. Vacuum carpets, car seats, mattresses, and upholstered furniture very thoroughly. Discard vacuum dust bag.
3. Wash pillows, stuffed animals, and other washable items the same way clothing is washed.
4. Dry-clean unwashable items.
5. If items cannot be washed or dry-cleaned, seal in plastic bag for 2 weeks to break reproductive cycle of lice.
6. Wash combs, brushes, and other hair items (rollers, curlers, barrettes, etc.) in shampoo, soaking for 1 hour.
7. If you discover the infestation yourself, report to child's school or day care.
8. School should disinfect headphones.

housekeeping. All family members should be inspected and treated as needed. See Family Teaching: Eliminating Pediculi Infestations for other useful information.

SCABIES

Scabies is a skin infestation caused by the scabies mite, *Sarcoptes scabiei*. The female mite burrows in areas between the fingers and toes and in warm folds of the body, such as the axilla and groin, to lay eggs. Burrows are visible as dark lines, and the mite is seen as a black dot at the end of the burrow. Severe itching occurs, causing scratching with resulting secondary infection.

The areas are treated with lindane lotion or crotamiton (Eurax). The body is first scrubbed with soap and water, and then the lotion is applied on all areas of the body except the face. With lindane, a second coat can be applied, then all washed off in 24 hours. For crotamiton, a second coat is applied in 24 hours, and the patient then waits an additional 48 hours to wash it off. Caregivers should follow the tips recommended for pediculosis. All who had close contact with the child within a 30- to 60-day period should be treated. The rash and itch may continue for several weeks, even though the mites have been successfully eliminated.

Skin Allergies

One of the most common allergic skin reactions is eczema (atopic dermatitis), which is discussed in Chapter 11. Other skin disorders of allergic origin include hives (urticaria) and giant swellings (angioedema) and rashes caused by poison ivy, poison oak, and other plants or drug reactions. Skin rashes are common in school-age children. Some are caused by infectious diseases and others by allergy. Whatever the cause, rashes are usually treated with topical preparations, such as lotions, ointments, and greases, plus

cool soaks. The itching must be relieved as much as possible because scratching can introduce additional pathogens to the affected area.

HIVES (URTICARIA) AND GIANT SWELLINGS (ANGIOEDEMA)

Hives appear in different sizes and on many different parts of the body and are usually caused by foods or drugs. They are bright red and itchy and can occur on the eyelids, tongue, mouth, hands, or feet, or in the brain or stomach. When affecting the mouth or tongue, hives can cause difficulty in breathing; in the stomach, the swelling can produce pain, nausea, and vomiting. Swelling in brain tissue causes headache and other neurologic symptoms.

Foods such as chocolate, nuts, shellfish, berries or other raw fruit, fish, and highly seasoned foods are likely to cause hives. Possible drug allergens include aspirin and related drugs, laxatives, antiinflammatory drugs, tranquilizers, and antibiotics (penicillin is the most common allergen of this group). Sometimes it is impossible to identify the cause.

Treatment is aimed at reducing the swelling and relieving the itching. If the allergen can be identified, it can be removed from the child's environment and hyposensitization can be performed. If the allergen is a certain food, that food must be eliminated from the child's diet. Antihistamines (topical or systemic) are used to relieve itching and reduce swelling. Cool soaks also help relieve itching. Fingernails should be kept short and clean. In severe cases, corticosteroids may be necessary.

PLANT ALLERGIES

Poison ivy, oak, and sumac are common causes of contact dermatitis. Of these, poison ivy is the worst offender, particularly during the summer (Fig. 17-17). The cause of the

Figure 17-17
The lesions of poison ivy. Note the linear distribution. (Courtesy of the Centers for Disease Control and Prevention, Atlanta, GA.)

allergy is an extremely potent oil, urushiol, that is present in all parts of these plants. Its effects vary from slight inflammation and itching to severe, extensive swelling that can virtually immobilize the child. This disorder causes intense itching (pruritus) and forms tiny blisters that weep and continue to spread the inflammation.

Antihistamines or oral steroids help relieve itching and prevent scratching. Cool soaks, Aveeno baths, calamine lotion, or topical steroids help minimize discomfort. The child should be taught to recognize and avoid the poisonous plants. The plants also should be removed from the environment when possible.

Bites

Because school-age children are active, inquisitive, and not completely inhibited in their actions, they commonly suffer bites, both animal and human, as well as insect stings and bites. Many of these are minor, particularly if the skin is not broken. Some, however, can have life-threatening implications if proper care is not given.

ANIMAL BITES

Children enjoy pets, but often they are not alert to possibly dangerous encounters with pets or wild animals. Dog bites are common. Fortunately, because of rabies vaccination programs for dogs, few dog bites cause rabies; in fact, cats are the domestic animal most likely to carry rabies. Any pet who bites should be held until it can be determined whether the animal has been vaccinated against rabies. If not, the child must undergo a series of injections to prevent this potentially fatal disease. The series consists of both active and passive immunizations. Active immunity is established with five injections of human diploid cell vaccine beginning on the day of the bite and on days 3, 7, 14, and 28. Human rabies immune globulin is given on the first day along with the diploid cell vaccine.

All animal and human bites should be thoroughly washed with soap and water. An antiseptic such as 70% alcohol or povidone-iodine should be applied after the wound has been thoroughly rinsed. The wound must be observed for signs of infection until well healed. Animal bites should be promptly reported to the proper authorities.

Children should be taught at an early age about the danger of animal bites, particularly of strange or wild animals, such as skunks, raccoons, bats, and squirrels.

SPIDER BITES

Spider bites can cause serious illness if untreated. Bites of black widow and brown recluse spiders and scorpions demand medical attention. Absorption of their poison can be slowed by applying ice to the affected area until medical care is obtained.

TICK BITES

Wood ticks carried by chipmunks, ground squirrels, weasels, and wood rats can cause Rocky Mountain spotted fever. Most cases are found in the South Atlantic, South Central, and Southeastern United States. Dogs are often the carriers to humans. People living in areas where ticks are common can be immunized against this disease.

Deer ticks, carried by white-footed mice and white-tailed deer found in the Northeast, Midwest, and West, can carry the organism that causes Lyme disease. The first stage of the disease begins with a lesion at the site of the bite. The lesion appears as a macule with a clear center. The second stage occurs several weeks to months later if the patient is not treated. The symptoms of this stage may affect the central nervous system and the heart. If untreated, the third stage may occur months to years later, causing arthritis, neurologic disorders, and bone and joint disease.

Children and adults should wear long pants, long-sleeved shirts, and insect repellent when walking in the woods. Pant legs should be tucked into socks. If a tick is found on the body, alcohol may be applied and the tick carefully removed with tweezers. Care should be taken not to crush the tick, to prevent the release of pathogenic organisms. A health care provider must be consulted if there is any suspicion that a child or an adult has been bitten by a deer tick.

SNAKE BITES

Snake bites demand immediate medical intervention. The wound should be washed, ice applied, and the body part involved immobilized. Prompt transport to the nearest medical facility is essential.

INSECT STINGS OR BITES

Insect stings or bites can prove fatal to children who are sensitized. Swelling may be localized or may include an entire extremity. Circulatory collapse, airway obstruction, and anaphylactic shock can cause death within 30 minutes if the child is untreated. Immediate treatment is necessary and may include injection of epinephrine, antihistamines, or steroids. These children should wear a Medic Alert bracelet and carry an anaphylaxis kit that includes a plastic syringe of epinephrine and an antihistamine. The teacher, school nurse, and anyone who cares for the child should be alerted to the child's allergy and should know where the anaphylaxis kit is and how to use it if needed.

■ KEY POINTS

■ Most illnesses during the school-age years are short term and minor, but for some children this is a time of visits to a health care facility and many trips to the health care provider.

- Children with long-term or chronic diseases such as scoliosis, asthma, rheumatic fever, or diabetes may be self-conscious about being different from their classmates.

- Children need to have positive self-esteem. Illness may threaten the child's self-confidence and can contribute to self-doubt.

- Children's interest in science creates a fascination with their bodies and how they work.

- School-age children can be involved in their health care, learning how the illness is affecting their bodies, how to help care for themselves, and what the future may hold.

- An important aspect of teaching the asthmatic child and family is helping them learn to anticipate an impending episode and respond appropriately. Exercise and activity are an essential part of therapy for the child with asthma.

- The diabetes of childhood is insulin-dependent diabetes mellitus, which is managed by insulin replacement, diet, and exercise.

- The diabetic child and family members must be included when teaching about all aspects of caring for the child's diabetes.

- Nurses who care for school-age children have a responsibility to be observant for scoliosis.

- Goals in caring for a child with juvenile rheumatoid arthritis include preserving joint function and preventing physical deformities.

- The adventurous school-age child often explores new horizons and because of immature judgment may be exposed to the dangers of fractures, poison ivy, and animal bites, particularly when in hazardous or wooded areas.

CRITICAL THINKING

1. A coworker says to you, "That Jeff in room 204 is bouncing off the walls." You are assigned to him. Using behavior techniques for the ADHD child, tell how you will plan his care.

2. You are in the grocery store and see a child having a grand mal seizure. No other adult is around. Explain what you will do.

3. Five-year-old Malcolm has been sent home from kindergarten with a note advising of an outbreak of pinworms. There are five children between 2 and 8 years of age in the household where he lives, including cousins. Ex-

plain to his aunt, who cares for the children, what she should do to handle the problem.

4. Describe the guidance you would give 8-year-old Raoul, a diabetic who plans to play Little League baseball.

5. Ten-year-old Carrie must wear a Milwaukee brace. She says she thinks it's really ugly. Identify the nursing diagnosis appropriate for this problem. Indicate planning, implementation, and evaluation for this diagnosis.

6. Describe the signs to observe for to detect neurovascular complications in a child in traction.

REFERENCES

1. Eggleston PA. Asthma. In Oski FA, ed. Principle and practices of pediatrics. Philadelphia: JB Lippincott, 1990.
2. Kattan M. Managing and preventing asthma emergencies. Contemp Pediatr 5(11):22, 1988.
3. Sponseller PD, Toto VT. Bone, joint, and muscle problems. In Oski FA, ed. Principle and practices of pediatrics. Philadelphia: JB Lippincott, 1990.
4. Cassidy JT. Connective tissue diseases and amyloidosis. In Oski FA, ed. Principle and practices of pediatrics. Philadelphia: JB Lippincott, 1990.

BIBLIOGRAPHY

Bechler-Karsch A. Assessment and management of status asthmaticus. Pediatr Nurs 20(3):217–223, 1994.
Capen CL, Dedlow ER, Robillard RH, Fuller BM, Fuller CP. The team approach to pediatric asthma education. Pediatr Nurs 20(3):231–237, 1994.
DeWitt S. Nursing assessment of the skin and dermatologic lesions. Nurs Clin North Am 25(1):235–245, 1990.
Eden-Kilgour S, Gibson DE. Nursing management of children with scoliosis. J Pract Nurs 40(2):34–38, 1990.
Ellett ML. Constipation/encopresis: A nursing perspective. J Pediatr Health Care 4(3):141–146, 1990.
Hess V. Diabetes: Stuff and more stuff. Lincoln, NE: HERC, 1989.
Jackson DB, Saunders RB. Child health nursing. Philadelphia: JB Lippincott, 1993.
Kropfelder L, Winkelstein M. A case management approach to pediatric asthma. Pediatr Nurs 22(4):291–295, 1996.
Kuster PA. Reducing risk of house dust mite and cockroach allergen exposure in inner-city children with asthma. Pediatr Nurs 22(4):297–303, 1996.
Pillitteri A. Maternal and child health nursing, 2d ed. Philadelphia: JB Lippincott, 1995.
Ryan-Wenger NM, Walsh M. Children's perspective on coping with asthma. Pediatr Nurs 20(3):224–228, 1994.
Savinetti-Rose B. Developmental issues in managing children with diabetes. Pediatr Nurs 20(1):11–15, 1994.
Scoloveno MA, Yarcheski A, Mahon NE. Scoliosis treatment effects on selected variables among adolescents. West J Nurs Res 12(5):601–618, 1990.
Sharts-Hopko NC. Ritodrine, reexamined. MCN 18(1):56, 1993.
Willis J. Common pests. Commun Outlook 24–25, 1990.
Wong DL. Whaley and Wong's nursing care of infants and children, 5th ed. St. Louis: Mosby, 1995.

Chapter 18

Growth and Development of the Adolescent: 11 to 18 Years

STUDENT OBJECTIVES

On completion of this chapter, the student will be able to:

1. Define key terms.
2. State the age of a) the preadolescent and b) the adolescent.
3. Describe the psychosocial development of the preadolescent.
4. Name the physical changes that make the child appear uncoordinated in early adolescence.
5. List the secondary sexual characteristics that appear in a) adolescent boys and b) in adolescent girls.
6. Name the nutrients that are commonly deficient in the diets of adolescents.
7. State a) the major cognitive task of the adolescent according to Piaget and b) the psychosocial task according to Erikson.
8. Discuss the adolescent's need to conform with peers.
9. Explain some of the problems that adolescents face when making career choices today.
10. Discuss the influence of peer pressure on psychosocial development.
11. Discuss the necessity for orderly psychosocial development of identity and trust before adolescents are ready for intimate relationships.
12. Discuss adolescent body image and associated problems.

KEY TERMS

early adolescence	menarche
heterosexual	orthodontia
homosexual	puberty
malocclusion	

Adolescence comes from the Latin word meaning "to come to maturity," a fitting description of this stage of life. The adolescent is maturing physically and emotionally, growing from childhood toward adulthood and seeking to understand what it means to be grown up.

Early adolescence (preadolescence, pubescence) begins at about age 10 in girls and about age 12 in boys with a dramatic growth spurt that signals the advent of **puberty** (reproductive maturity). During this stage, the child's body begins to take on adultlike contours, the primary sex organs enlarge, secondary sexual characteristics appear, and hormonal activity increases. This early period ends with the onset of menstruation in the female and production of sperm in the male.

The bone growth that began during intrauterine life continues through adolescence and is usually completed by the end of this period. Other growth during this time includes maturing of reproductive organs and tremendous psychosocial growth.

Adolescents are fascinated, and sometimes fearful and confused, by the changes occurring in their bodies and their thinking processes. They begin to look grown up, but they do not have the judgment or independence to participate in society as an adult. These young people are strongly influenced by their peer group and often resent parental authority. Roller-coaster emotions characterize this age group, as does intense interest in romantic relationships (Fig. 18-1).

The adolescent years can be a time of turmoil and uncertainty that creates conflict between family caregivers and children. If these conflicts are resolved, normal development can continue. Unresolved, the conflicts can foster delays in development and prevent the young person from maturing into a fully functioning adult.

Body image is critical to adolescents. Health problems that threaten body image, such as acne, obesity, dental or vision problems, and trauma, can seriously interfere with development.

PREADOLESCENT DEVELOPMENT

During the period between 10 and 12 years of age, there is a great variation in the rate of growth between boys and girls. This variability in growth and maturation can be a

Figure 18-1
Intense interest in the opposite sex characterizes adolescence.

concern to the child who develops rapidly or the one who develops more slowly than his or her peers. Children of this age do not want to be different from their friends. There is much overlapping of developmental characteristics in the preadolescent child between the stages of late school age and early adolescence, but nevertheless there are unique characteristics to set it apart (Table 18-1).

Physical Development

Preadolescence begins in the female between the ages of 9 and 11 years and is marked by a growth spurt that lasts about 18 months. Girls grow about 3" each year until **menarche** (the beginning of menstruation), after which growth slows considerably. Early in adolescence, girls begin to develop a figure, the pelvis broadens, and axillary and pubic hair begins to appear, along with many changes in hormone levels. The variation between girls is great and often is a cause for much concern by the "early bloomer" or the "late bloomer." Young girls who begin to develop physically as early as 9 years of age are often embarrassed by these physical changes. In girls, the onset of menarche marks the end of the preadolescent period.

Boys enter preadolescence a little later, usually between 11 and 13 years of age, and grow generally at a slower, steadier rate than do girls. During this time, the scrotum and testes begin to enlarge, and the skin of the scrotum begins to change in coloring and texture with sparse hair at the base of the penis. Boys who start their growth spurt later often are concerned about being shorter than their peers. In boys, the appearance of nocturnal emissions is often used as the indication that the preadolescent period has ended.

TABLE 18-1. Growth and Development of the Preadolescent: 10–13 Years

Physical	Motor	Personal–Social	Language	Perceptual	Cognitive
Average height 56¾″–59″ (144–150 cm) Average weight 77–88 lb (35–40 kg) Pubescence may begin Girls may surpass boys in height Remaining permanent teeth erupt	Refines gross and fine motor skills May have difficulty with some fine motor coordination due to growth of large muscles before that of small muscles; hands and feet are first structures to increase in size; thus, actions may appear uncoordinated during early preadolescence Can do crafts Uses tools increasingly well	Attends school primarily for peer association Peer relationships of greatest importance Intolerant of violation of group norms Can follow rules of group and adapt to another point of view Can use stored knowledge to make independent judgments	Fluent in spoken language Vocabulary 50,000 words for reading; oral vocabulary of 7,200 words Uses slang words and terms, vulgarities, jeers, jokes, and sayings	Can catch or intercept ball thrown from a distance Possible growth spurts may cause myopia	Begins abstract thinking Conservation of volume Understands relation among time, speed, and distance Ability to sympathize, love, and reason are all evolving Right and wrong become logically clear

Preparation for Adolescence

Preadolescents need information about their changing bodies and feelings. Sex education that includes information about the hormonal changes that are occurring, or will be occurring, is necessary to help them through this developmental stage.

Girls need information that will help them handle their early menstrual periods with minimal apprehension. Most girls have irregular periods for the first year or so; they need to know that this is not a cause for worry. They have many questions about protection during the menstrual period and the advisability of using sanitary pads or tampons. They may fear that "everybody will know" when they have their first period, and must be allowed to express this fear and be reassured.

Boys also need information about their bodies. Erections and nocturnal emissions are topics they need to discuss, as well as the development of other male secondary sex characteristics.

Both boys and girls need information about changes in the opposite sex, including discussions that address their questions. This kind of information helps them increase their understanding of human sexuality. School programs may provide a good foundation for sex education, but each preadolescent needs an adult to turn to with particular questions. Even a well-planned program does not address all the needs of the preadolescent. The best school program

begins early and builds from year to year as the child's needs progress (see Chap. 16).

Preadolescence is an appropriate time for discussions that will help the young teen resist pressures to become sexually active too early. Family caregivers may turn to a nurse acquaintance for guidance in preparing their child. Perhaps the most important aspect of discussions about sexuality is that honest, straightforward answers must be given in an atmosphere of caring concern. Children whose need for information is not met through family, school, or community programs will get their information—often inaccurate—from peers, movies, television, or other media.

ADOLESCENT DEVELOPMENT

Adolescence spans the ages of about 13 to 18 years. Some males do not complete adolescence until they are 20 years old. The rate of development during adolescence varies greatly from one teen to another. It is a time of many physical, emotional, and social changes. During this period, the adolescent is engaged in a struggle to master the developmental tasks that lead to successful completion of this stage of development (Table 18-2). A prerequisite for the completion of these tasks is completion of the developmental tasks of earlier stages of development.

TABLE 18-2. Developmental Tasks of Adolescence

Basic Task	Associated Tasks
Appreciate own uniqueness*	Identify interests, skills, and talents Identify differences from peers Accept strengths and limitations Challenge own skill levels
Develop independent internal identity*	Value self as a person Separate physical self from psychological self Differentiate personal worth from cultural stereotypes Separate internal value from societal feedback
Determine own value system*	Identify options Establish priorities Commit self to decisions made Translate values into behaviors Resist peer and cultural pressure to conform to their value system Find comfortable balance between own and peer/cultural standards, behaviors, and needs
Develop self-evaluation skills*	Develop basis for self-evaluation and monitoring Evaluate quality of products Assess approach to tasks and responsibilities Develop sensitivity to intrapersonal relationships Evaluate dynamics of interpersonal relationships
Assume increasing responsibility for own behavior*	Quality of work, chores Emotional tone Money management Time management Decision making Personal habits Social behaviors
Find meaning in life	Accept and integrate meaning of death Develop philosophy of life Begin to identify life or career goals
Acquire skills essential for adult living	Acquire skills essential to independent living Develop social and emotional abilities and temperament Refine sociocultural amenities Identify and experiment with alternatives for facing life Acquire employment skills Seek growth-inducing activities
Seek affiliations outside of family	Seek companionship with compatible peers Affiliate with organizations that support uniqueness Actively seek models or mentors Identify potential emotional support systems Differentiate between acquaintances and friends Identify ways to express sexuality
Adapt to adult body functioning	Adapt to somatic (body) changes Refine balance and coordination Develop physical strength Consider sexuality and reproduction issues

* Tasks deemed crucial to continued maturation
Adapted from Schuster CS, Ashburn SS. The process of human development: A holistic life-span approach, 3rd ed. Philadelphia: JB Lippincott, 1992.

Physical Development

Rapid growth occurs during adolescence. Girls begin growing during the preadolescent period and achieve 98% of their adult height by the age of 16. Boys start growing around 13 years of age and may continue to grow until 20 years of age. The rapid growth of the skeletal system, which outpaces the muscular system, causes the long, lanky appearance of many teens and contributes to the clumsiness often seen during this age.

During the first menstrual cycles, ovulation does not usually occur because increased estrogen levels are needed to produce an ovum mature enough to be released. However, at 13 to 15 years of age, the cycle becomes ovulatory, and pregnancy is possible. The girl's breasts take on an adult appearance by age 16, and pubic hair is curly and abundant.

By the age of 16 years, the penis, testes, and scrotum are adult in size and shape, and mature spermatozoa are being produced. Male pubic hair also is adult in appearance and amount. After age 13, muscle strength and coordination develop rapidly. The larynx and vocal cords enlarge, and the voice deepens. The "change of voice" makes the teenage male's voice vary unexpectedly, which occasionally causes embarrassment for the teen.

Psychosocial Development

Adolescence is a time of transition from childhood to adulthood. Between the ages of 10 and 18 years, adolescents move from Freud's latency to the genital stage, from Erikson's industry versus inferiority to identity versus role confusion, and from Piaget's concrete operational thinking to formal operational thought. They develop a sense of moral judgment and a system of values and beliefs that will affect their entire life. The foundation provided by family, school, and community experiences is still a strong influence, but tremendous power is exerted by the peer group. Trends and fads among adolescents dictate clothing choices, hair styles, music, and other recreational choices (Fig. 18-2). The adolescent whose family caregivers make it difficult to conform are adding another stress to an already emotion-laden period. Peer pressure to experiment with potentially dangerous practices such as drugs, alcohol, and reckless driving also can be strong, and adolescents may need careful guidance and understanding support to help resist this peer influence.

Personality Development

Erikson considered the central task of adolescence to be the establishment of identity. Adolescents spend a lot of time asking themselves, "Who am I as a person? What will I do with my life? Marry? Have children? Will I go to college? If so, where? If not, why not? What kind of career should I choose?"

Figure 18-2
For many teens, hanging out with friends is an important way to share common interests and to gain a sense of belonging.

Adolescents are confronted with a greater variety of choices than ever before. Sex role stereotypes have been shattered in most careers and professions. More women are becoming lawyers, physicians, plumbers, and carpenters; more men are entering nursing or choosing to become house-husbands while their wives earn the primary family income. Transportation has made greater geographic mobility possible, so that many youngsters can spend summers or a full school year in a foreign country, plan to attend college thousands of miles from home, and begin a career in an even more remote location. Making decisions and choices is never simple and, with such a tremendous variety of options, it is understandable that adolescents often are preoccupied with their own concerns.

When identity has been established, generally between the ages of 16 and 18 years, adolescents seek intimate relationships, usually with members of the opposite sex. *Intimacy*—mutual sharing of one's deepest feelings with another person—is impossible unless both persons have established a sense of trust and a sense of identity. Intimate relationships are a preparation for long-term relationships, and people who fail to achieve intimacy may develop feelings of isolation and experience chronic difficulty in communicating with others.

Most intimate relationships during adolescence are **heterosexual**, or between members of the opposite sex. Sometimes, however, young people form intimate attachments with members of the same sex, or **homosexual** relationships. Because our culture is predominately heterosexual and is still struggling with trying to understand homosexual relationships, these relationships can cause great anxiety for family caregivers and children. Although some parts of American society are beginning to accept homosexual relationships as no more than another lifestyle, prejudice still exists. So great a stigma has been attached to homosexuality that many adolescents fear they are homosexual if they are uncomfortable about heterosexual intimacy. However, this is a normal problem that occurs as adolescents move from same-sex peer group activities to dating peers of the opposite sex.

Body Image

Body image is closely related to self-esteem. Seeing one's body as attractive and functional contributes to a positive sense of self-esteem. During adolescence, the desire not to be different can extend to feelings about one's body and can cause adolescents to feel that their bodies are inadequate, even though they are really healthy and attractive.

American culture tends to equate a slender figure with feminine beauty and acceptability and a lean, tall, muscular figure with masculine virility and strength. Adolescents who feel that they are underdeveloped suffer great anxiety, particularly males. Adolescent girls have even undergone plastic surgery to augment their breasts to relieve this anxiety. Girls in this age group often feel that they are too fat and try strange, nutritionally unsound diets to reduce their weight. Some literally starve themselves, and even after their bodies have become emaciated, truly believe that they are still fat and therefore unattractive. This condition is called *anorexia nervosa* and is discussed further in Chapter 19.

It is important for adolescents to establish a positive body image by the end of their developmental stage. Because bone growth is completed during adolescence, a person's height will remain basically the same throughout adult life, even though weight can fluctuate greatly. Tall girls who long to be petite and boys who would like to be 6 feet tall may need guidance and support to bring their expectations in line with reality and learn to have positive feelings about their bodies and accept them the way they are.

NUTRITION

Nutritional requirements are greatly increased during periods of rapid growth in adolescence. Adolescent boys need more calories than do girls throughout the growth period.

Appetites increase, and most teens eat frequently. Families with teenage boys often jokingly say that they cannot keep the refrigerator filled. Nutritional needs are related to growth and sexual maturity rather than age.

Even though adolescents understand something about nutrition, they may not relate this understanding to their dietary habits. Their accelerated growth rate and, for some, increased physical activities mean that they need more food to supply their energy requirements. Because adolescents are seeking to establish their independence, their food choices are sometimes not wise and tend to be influenced by peer preference rather than parental advice. Teens frequently skip meals, especially breakfast, snack on foods that provide empty calories, and eat a lot of fast foods. The era of fast-food meals has given adolescents easy access to high-calorie, nutritionally unbalanced meals. Too many fast-food meals and nutritionally empty snacks can result in nutritional deficiencies (Fig. 18-3).

When good nutritional habits have been established in early childhood, adolescent nutrition is likely to be better balanced than when nutritional teaching has been insufficient. Being part of a family that practices sound nutrition helps ensure that occasional lapses into sweets, fast foods, and other peer group food preferences will not create serious deficiencies. Nutrients that are often deficient in the teen's diet include calcium, iron, zinc, vitamins A, D, B_6, and folic acid. Calcium needs increase during skeletal growth. Girls need additional iron because of losses during

Figure 18-3
Teens often choose convenient junk foods, which lack nutritional value.

TABLE 18-3. Food Sources of Nutrients Commonly Deficient in Preadolescent and Adolescent Diets

Common Nutrient Deficiencies	Food Sources
Vitamin A	Liver, whole milk, butter, cheese; sources of carotene such as yellow vegetables, green leafy vegetables, tomatoes, yellow fruits
Vitamin D	Fortified milk, fish liver oils
Vitamin B_6 (pyridoxine)	Liver, kidney, chicken, fish, pork, eggs, whole-grain cereals, legumes
Folacin (folic acid)	Green leafy vegetables, liver, kidney, meats, fish, nuts, legumes, whole grains
Calcium	Milk, hard cheese, yogurt, ice cream, small fish eaten with bones (eg, sardines), dark-green vegetables, tofu, soybeans, calcium-enriched orange juice
Iron	Lean meats, liver, legumes, dried fruits, green leafy vegetables, whole-grain and fortified cereals
Zinc	Oysters, herring, meat, liver, fish, milk, whole grains, nuts, legumes

menstruation. Boys also need additional iron during this growth period (Table 18-3).

In their quest for identity and independence, some adolescents experiment with food fads and diets. Adolescent girls, worried about being fat, fall prey to a variety of fad diets. Athletes also may follow fad diets that may include supplements in the belief that these diets enhance body building. These diets often include increased amounts of protein and amino acids, which cause diuresis and calcium loss. Carbohydrate loading, practiced by some during the week before an athletic event, increases the muscle glycogen level to two to three times normal and may hinder heart function. A meal that is low in fat and high in complex carbohydrates eaten 3 to 4 hours before an event is much more appropriate for the teen athlete.

Adolescents need a balanced diet consisting of three servings from the milk–dairy group, two or three servings (6–7 oz total) from the meat group, three or four servings from the fruit group, four or five servings from the vegetable group, and 9 to 11 servings from the grain group (Fig. 18-4). Adolescents often resist pressure from family members to eat balanced meals; all family caregivers can do is to provide nutritious meals and snacks and regular mealtimes. A good example may be the best teacher at this point.

A refrigerator stocked with ready-to-eat nutritious snacks can be a good weapon against snacking on empty calories.

Families with low incomes may have difficulty providing the kind of foods that meet the requirements for a growing teen. These families need help to learn how to make low-cost, nutritious food selections and plan adequate meals and snacks. The nurse can be instrumental in helping them plan appropriate food purchases. For instance, the nurse might recommend fruit and vegetable stores or farm stands that accept food stamps.

Ethnic and Cultural Influences

Culture also influences adolescent food choices and habits. For example, many Mexican-Americans are accustomed to having their big meal at noon. When school lunches do not provide such a heavy meal, the Mexican-American adolescent may supplement the lunch with sweets or fast foods. In the Asian community, milk is not a popular drink, and this can result in a calcium deficiency. Many Asians are lactose-intolerant; therefore, other products high in calcium, such as tofu (soybean curd), soybeans, and greens, should be recommended to increase calcium intake.

Be alert to cultural dietary influences on the adolescent, and take these into consideration when helping the adolescent and the family devise an adequate food plan.

Certain religions recommend a vegetarian diet, and other persons follow a vegetarian diet for ecologic or philosophic reasons. If planned with care, vegetarian diets can provide needed nutrients. The most common types of vegetarian diets are:

- *Semivegetarian*—includes dairy products, eggs, and fish; excludes red meat and possibly poultry
- *Lacto-ovovegetarian*—includes eggs and dairy products; excludes meat, poultry, and fish
- *Lactovegetarian*—includes dairy products; excludes meat, fish, poultry, and eggs
- *Vegan*—excludes all food of animal origin, including dairy products, eggs, fish, meat, and poultry.

Vegan diets may not provide adequate nutrients without careful planning. All vegetarians should include whole-grain products, legumes, nuts, seeds, and fortified soy substitutes if low-fat dairy products are unacceptable.

HEALTH PROMOTION AND MAINTENANCE

Adolescents have much the same need for regular health checkups, protection against infection, and prevention of accidents as do younger children. They also have special needs that can best be met by health professionals with in-depth knowledge and understanding of adolescent con-

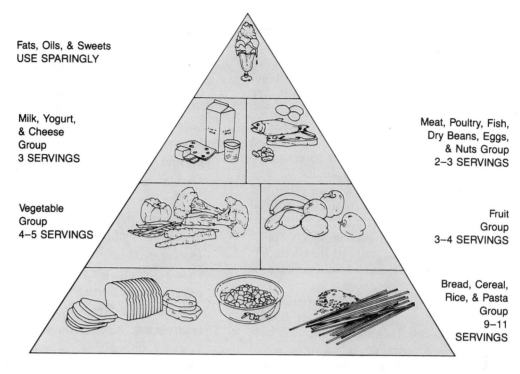

Fats, Oils, & Sweets
USE SPARINGLY

Milk, Yogurt,
& Cheese
Group
3 SERVINGS

Meat, Poultry, Fish,
Dry Beans, Eggs,
& Nuts Group
2–3 SERVINGS

Vegetable
Group
4–5 SERVINGS

Fruit
Group
3–4 SERVINGS

Bread, Cereal,
Rice, & Pasta
Group
9–11
SERVINGS

Smaller number of servings for Teen Girls—Larger number of servings for Teen Boys

What Counts as 1 Serving? ▶

The amount you eat may be more than one serving.
For example, a dinner portion of spaghetti would count as 2 or 3 servings.

Bread, Cereal, Rice & Pasta Group	Vegetable Group	Fruit Group	Milk, Yogurt & Cheese Group	Meat, Poultry, Fish, Dry Beans, Eggs & Nuts Group	Fats & Sweets
1 slice of bread	½ cup of chopped raw or cooked vegetables	1 piece of fruit or melon wedge	1 cup of milk or yogurt	2½ to 3 ounces of cooked lean meat, poultry, or fish	LIMIT CALORIES FROM THESE especially if you need to lose weight
½ cup of cooked rice or pasta	1 cup of leafy raw vegetables	¾ cup of juice	1½ ounces of natural cheese	Count ½ cup of cooked beans, or 1 egg, or 2 tablespoons of peanut butter as 1 ounce of lean meat	
½ cup of cooked cereal		½ cup of canned fruit	2 ounces of processed cheese		
1 ounce of ready-to-eat cereal		¼ cup of dried fruit			

Figure 18-4
Food guide pyramid adapted for adolescent girls and boys. (From United States Department of Agriculture.)

cerns. The number of adolescent clinics and health centers has increased, along with innovative health services such as school-based clinics, crisis hotlines, homes for runaways, and rehabilitation centers for adolescents who have been involved with alcohol or other drugs or with prostitution. Staff members in these programs provide teens with services needed for healthy growth.

Routine Checkups

A routine physical examination is recommended at least twice during the teen years, although annual physical examinations are encouraged. At this time, a complete his-

tory of developmental milestones, school problems, behavioral problems, family relationships, and immunizations should be completed. Immunization for measles, mumps, and rubella (MMR) is given if the second dose of the MMR vaccine was not administered during the late school age; however, a urine pregnancy screening is advisable before the rubella vaccine is administered to a girl of childbearing age. A booster of diphtheria and tetanus toxoid (dT) is given around 14 to 16 years of age (about 10 years after the last booster). If the teen has not been immunized with hepatitis B vaccine, immunization also is recommended at this time. Any other immunizations that are incomplete should be updated. Tuberculin testing is included at one visit at least and, depending on the community, may be recommended at both visits if there is an interval of several years between visits.

Height, weight, and blood pressure are measured and recorded. Vision and hearing screening are done if they have not been part of a regular school screening program. Up to the age of 16 years, adolescents need to be screened for scoliosis. Thyroid enlargement should be checked through age 14. Sexually active girls must have a pelvic examination, screening for sexually transmitted diseases (STDs), and a Pap smear (Fig. 18-5). Urinalysis is performed on all female adolescents, and a urine culture is performed if the girl has any symptoms of a urinary tract infection, such as urgency or burning and pain on urination. This is an excellent time for the nurse to counsel the adolescent girl about sexual activity, STDs, and human immunodeficiency virus (HIV) infection.

Adolescents must be given privacy, individualized attention, confidentiality, and the right to participate in decisions about their health care. They may feel uncomfortable and out of place in a pediatrician's waiting room, where most of the patients are 3 feet tall, or in a waiting room filled with adults. There are adolescent clinics and physicians who specialize in adolescent health care, but many adolescents do not have these facilities available to them.

Continuity of care helps build the adolescent's confidence in the service and the caregivers. Professionals dealing with teens should recognize that the physical symptoms offered as the reason for seeking care are often not the most significant problem about which the adolescent is concerned. An attitude of nonjudgmental accep-

Figure 18-5
The adolescent is usually nervous about her first pelvic examination and pap smear. Careful explanation by the nurse regarding these procedures may ease some of these fears.

A Personal Glimpse

Every year, around our birthdays, my little brother and I always go to our pediatrician's office. After being called by the nurse, we both go down to a tiny room with bright walls, baby pictures, and the kind of mobiles that are hung over a crib, the same kind of decorations that cover the entire office. I suppose the room itself is comforting, but then I have to strip down to my underwear right in front of my 6-year-old brother. To make matters worse, I have to put on a skimpy little gown that hardly covers my underwear and wait in a room with huge windows and blinds that don't close, overlooking the next building's parking lot. It's so embarrassing, having to climb up onto the examining table, with a gown falling down underneath me. Why can't the gowns be longer? It isn't just 6-year-olds who have to wear them!

Jessica, age 12

tance on the part of health care personnel can often encourage the adolescent to ask questions and share feelings and concerns about a troubling matter. Adolescents may be accompanied to the health care facility by a family caregiver, but they need to have an opportunity to be interviewed alone. Questions must be asked in a way that is concrete and specific so that the adolescent will give direct answers. The interviewer must be alert to verbal and nonverbal clues.

DENTAL CHECKUPS

Adolescents need continued regular dental checkups every 6 months. Dental **malocclusion** (improper alignment of the teeth) is a common condition that affects the way the teeth and jaws function. Correction of the malocclusion with dental braces improves chewing ability and appearance. The treatment of the malocclusion with dental braces is called **orthodontia**. Braces have become very common among adolescents since about half of them have malocclusions that can be corrected. Orthodontic treatment is usually started in early adolescence or late school age. Since braces have become so widespread among teens, they are readily accepted.

Family Teaching

The adolescent years are difficult for the maturing young person and often are just as difficult for the caregiver. Caregivers must allow the independent teen to flourish while continuing to safeguard him or her from risky and immature behavior. Caregivers and adolescents struggle with issues related to sexuality, substance abuse, accidents, discipline, poor nutrition, and volatile emotions.

Learning about adolescent physical and psychosocial development can help caregivers struggling to understand their teen. Caregivers will find information on sexuality and substance abuse enlightening and useful. The caregiver's communication skills may be enhanced by attending workshops or consulting counselors, teachers, religious leaders, or health care workers. Good communication between adolescents and their caregivers is essential to fostering healthy relationships between them. Caregivers may need both guidance in preparing their teen for adulthood and emotional support to feel successful in this difficult period. Take every opportunity to provide the family caregiver with information and support.

Health Education and Counseling

Before adolescents can take an active role in their own health care, they need information and guidance on the need for health care and how to meet that need most effectively. Education and counseling about sexuality, STDs, contraception, substance abuse, and mental health are a vital part of adolescent health care. Some of this teaching should, and sometimes does, come from family caregivers, but often the caregivers' lack of information, or their discomfort in discussing these topics, means that the job will have to be done by health professionals.

SEXUALITY

A good foundation in sex education can help the adolescent take pride in having reached sexual maturity; otherwise, puberty can be a frightening, shameful experience. Girls who have not been taught about menstruation until it occurs are understandably alarmed. Those who have been taught to regard it as "the curse" rather than an entrance into womanhood will not have positive feelings about this part of their sexuality.

Boys who are unprepared for nocturnal emissions may feel guilty, believing that they have caused these "wet dreams" by sexual fantasies or masturbation. They need to understand that this is a normal occurrence and simply the body's method of getting rid of surplus semen.

Assuming that adolescents are adequately prepared for the events of puberty, sex education during adolescence can deal with the important issues of responsible sexuality, contraception, and venereal disease. More adolescents today are sexually active than ever, resulting in an alarmingly rapid increase in teenage pregnancies and STDs. The

incidence of HIV infection, in particular, is increasing among adolescents.

Girls need to learn the importance of regular pelvic examinations and Pap smears and the technique for breast self-examination, a monthly self-care procedure (Fig. 18-6). Boys need to learn that testicular cancer is one of the most common cancers in young men between the ages of 15 and 34 and must be taught how and when to perform testicular self-examination (see Family Teaching: Testicular Self-Examination) (Fig. 18-7).

Masturbation   Adolescents' growing awareness of their sexuality, sexually provocative material in the media, and lack of acceptable means to gratify sexual desires make masturbation a common practice during adolescence. Unlike young children's genital exploration, adolescent masturbation can produce orgasm in the female and ejaculation in the male. Generally, it is a private, solitary activity, but occasionally it occurs with other members of the peer group. Health professionals recognize masturbation as a positive way to release sexual tension and increase one's knowledge of body sensations. The nurse can reassure adolescents that masturbation is common in both males and females and is a normal outlet for sexual urges.

SEXUAL RESPONSIBILITY

Not all adolescents are sexually active, but the numbers increase with each year of age. Although abstinence is the only completely successful protection, all adolescents need to have information concerning safe sex practices to be prepared for the occasion when they wish to be sexually intimate with someone. Adolescents do not have a good record of using contraceptives to prevent pregnancy. Many teens give excuses such as "sex shouldn't be planned," because if it is planned, it is wrong or they feel guilty. They need to feel that it "just happened" in the heat of the moment, not because they really wanted or planned it. Many adolescents are beginning to realize that much more than pregnancy may be at risk, but their attitude of "it won't happen to me," typical of their developmental age, continues to contribute to their increasing sexual activity.

Some adults continue to resist providing contraceptive information to adolescents in school, believing that such information encourages teens to become sexually active. However, as HIV infection becomes a greater threat to every sexually active person, this argument becomes harder to defend. Adolescents need contraceptive information to prevent pregnancy, but, more importantly, they need straightforward information about using condoms to protect themselves against HIV infection. Both male and female adolescents need this information, and girls must be advised to carry their own condoms if they believe there is any possibility that they may have sexual intercourse.

Condoms have been claimed to have an 85% effectiveness rate. Condoms with spermicidal foam have an effective

Breast Self-Examination (BSE)

Here is one way to do BSE:

1 Stand before a mirror. Inspect both breasts for anything unusual, such as any discharge from the nipples, puckering, dimpling, or scaling of the skin.

The next two steps are designed to emphasize any change in the shape or contour of your breasts. As you do them you should be able to feel your chest muscles tighten.

2 Watching closely in the mirror, clasp hands behind your head and press hands forward.

Breast self-examination should be done once a month so you become familiar with the usual appearance and feel of your breasts. Familiarity makes it easier to notice any changes in the breast from one month to another. Early discovery of a change from what is "normal" is the main idea behind BSE.

If you menstruate, the best time to do BSE is 2 or 3 days after your period ends, when your breasts are least likely to be tender or swollen. If you no longer menstruate, pick a day, such as the first day of the month, to remind yourself it is time to do BSE.

4 Raise your left arm. Use three or four fingers of your right hand to explore your left breast firmly, carefully, and thoroughly. Beginning at the outer edge, press the flat part of your fingers in small circles, moving the circles slowly around the breast. Gradually work toward the nipple. Be sure to cover the entire breast. Pay special attention to the area between the breast and the armpit, including the armpit itself. Feel for any unusual lump or mass under the skin.

5 Gently squeeze the nipple and look for a discharge. (If there is a discharge, see your doctor.) Repeat the exam on your right breast.

3 Next, press hands firmly on hips and bow slightly toward your mirror as you pull your shoulders and elbows forward.

Some women do the next part of the exam in the shower. Fingers glide over soapy skin, making it easy to concentrate on the texture underneath.

6 Steps 4 and 5 should be repeated lying down. Lie flat on your back, left arm over your head and a pillow or folded towel under your left shoulder. This position flattens the breast and makes it easier to examine. Use the same circular motion described earlier.
Repeat on your right breast.

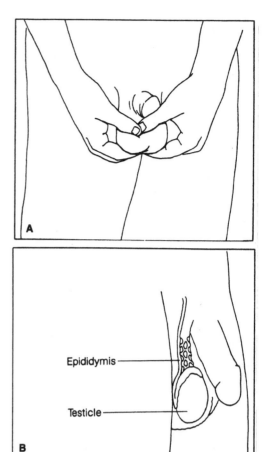

Family Teaching
Testicular Self-Examination

1. Perform the examination once a month after a warm bath or shower. The scrotum is relaxed from the warmth. Select a day that is easy to remember, such as the first or last day of the month.
2. Stand in front of a mirror, if possible, and look for any swelling on the skin of the scrotum.
3. Examine each testicle, one at a time, using both hands.
4. Place the index and middle fingers under the testicle and the thumbs on top. Roll each testicle gently between the thumbs and fingers. One testicle is normally larger than the other (see Fig. 15A).
5. The epididymis is the soft, tubelike structure located at the back of the testicle that collects and carries sperm. This must not be mistaken for an abnormal lump (see Fig. 5B).
6. Most lumps are found on the sides of the testicle, although they may appear on the front. Report any lump to your health care provider at once.
7. Testicular cancer is highly curable when treated promptly.

Figure 18-7
Drawings from the National Cancer Institute pamphlet, "What You Need to Know About Testicular Cancer," NIH Publication 88-1565, Revised June 1988. (A) Examine each testicle with index and middle fingers under testicle and thumbs on top; (B) Cross section of scrotum showing position of the epididymis and the testicle.

rate of 95%, but when users are taught how to use them correctly, the rate of effectiveness increases to 99%. The effectiveness of protection from HIV and other STDs should follow the same percentages. The safest condom is one made of latex with a prelubricated tip or reservoir and pretreated with nonoxynol-9 spermicide. Family Teaching: Safe Condom Use and Figure 18-8 provide guidelines for use.

Other STDs that sexually active adolescents need to know about are syphilis, gonorrhea, genital herpes, genital warts, and chlamydial and trichomonal infections. Prevention of STDs is the primary aim of education for adolescents. However, if prevention proves ineffective, the most important factor is referral for treatment. Many adolescents are reluctant to seek treatment, fearing that their family caregivers will discover their activity. Crisis hotlines are valuable resources to assure adolescents that treatment is vital for them and their partners, and confidentiality is ensured.

Health care personnel who work with adolescents seeking treatment for an STD must be nonjudgmental, supportive, and understanding. The adolescents need treatment and information about preventing spread of the STD to others, as well as how to prevent contracting another STD. See Chapter 19 for a thorough discussion of STDs and related nursing care.

SUBSTANCE ABUSE

As adolescents search for identity and independence, they are susceptible to many pressures from society and their peers. Adolescents may experiment with substances that may be habit-forming or addictive and ultimately will harm them. This may be done "just for kicks," to "go along with the crowd" (peer group), or to rebel against the authority of family caregivers or other adults. Some substances that are abused by adolescents also are abused by many adults, and to some adolescents, using these substances may appear sophisticated.

Alcohol and certain other drugs provide an escape, how-

Figure 18-6
Breast self-examination as presented by the National Cancer Institute. (NIH Publication No. 88-1556, 1988.)

Family Teaching
Safe Condom Use

1. Use a new condom each time.
2. The safest type of condom is prelubricated latex with a tip or reservoir that has been pretreated with nonoxynol-9 spermicide.
3. If the condom is not pretreated, you may lubricate it with water or water-based lubricant, such as K-Y Jelly *and* a spermicidal jelly or foam containing nonoxynol-9.
4. Do not use oil-based products such as mineral oil, cold cream, or petroleum jelly for lubrication; they may weaken the latex.
5. Put the condom on as soon as the penis is erect. Retract the foreskin if not circumcised, and unroll the condom over the entire length of the penis.
6. Leave a ½" space at the end. Press out the tip of the condom to remove air bubbles.
7. The outside of the condom may be lubricated as much as desired with a water-soluble lubricant.
8. If the condom starts to slip during intercourse, hold it on. Do not let it slip off. Condoms come in sizes, so if you have a problem with slipping, look for a smaller size.
9. After ejaculation, hold the rim of the condom at the base of the penis, and withdraw before losing the erection.
10. Remove the condom and tie a knot in the open end. Dispose of it so that no one can come in contact with semen.
11. Heat can damage condoms. Store them in a cool, dry place.
12. Immediately after intercourse, both partners should wash off any semen or vaginal secretions with soap and water.

ever brief, from the pressures that the adolescent may feel. Alcohol is the mind-altering substance most commonly abused by adolescents. Other substances that adolescents may abuse are tobacco (including smokeless tobacco), alcohol, marijuana, cocaine or "crack," heroin, other street drugs, and prescription drugs. Adolescents can often obtain tobacco products despite recent federal legislation to enforce strict age limitations on their sale.

Programs developed to educate students about substance abuse meet with varying success. Health care personnel must stress to adolescents that abuse of mind-altering drugs is often accompanied by irresponsible sexual behavior, further complicating their lives. Chapter 19 discusses these problems in more detail.

MENTAL HEALTH

The turmoil that adolescents experience while searching for self-esteem and self-confidence can cause stress that may lead to depression, suicide, and conduct disorders. Academic and social pressures add to that stress. The family also may be under stress due to unemployment or economic difficulties, separation, divorce, or death of one of the caregivers. Health care personnel must be sensitive to signs that the adolescent is having problems. Adolescents need the opportunity to ventilate their fears, concerns, and frustrations. The rapport between family caregivers and teens may not be such that the adolescent can express these feelings to them. Many schools have mental health personnel on staff who can provide counseling when it is needed. Adolescents need counseling to work through troublesome situations and to avoid chronic mental health problems. Mental health assessment is an important part of the total health assessment of the adolescent.

Figure 18-8
Putting on a condom: (A) Press the air out ½ inch at the tip of the condom; (B) holding the tip of the condom, carefully roll it down the shaft of the erect penis; (C) be certain that the condom covers the full length of the penis with the rim of the condom at the base of the penis.

Accident Prevention

In every part of society, increasing numbers of adolescents are dying as a result of violence; this includes motor vehicle accidents, homicide, suicide, and other causes. The homicide rate is about seven times higher for African-American adolescents than for whites (Fig. 18-9), and the overall number of violent deaths is much greater for males than for females in every age group between 10 and 19 years (Fig. 18-10). White males between 15 and 19 years are killed in motor vehicle accidents twice as frequently as African-American males in this age group. Alcohol and other drugs are often involved in fatal accidents. Death is not the only negative outcome of violence: many adolescents are injured and hospitalized or treated in emergency departments, and many suffer psychological injury from being the victim of violence.

Violence is on the rise in schools, and not just inner-city schools. Weapons are being detected on students in schools all over the country. Guns and knives are the weapons most often found. The problem has become so serious that some schools have installed metal detectors to protect students.

Adolescents also are victims of violence in their own homes in greater numbers than any other age group of children. Date rape and other violence in a dating relationship has become common.

Students have formed groups such as Students Against Drunk Driving to promote safety in driving. Many schools provide support groups that help students work through their grief after schoolmates have met with violent death.

Much work needs to be done to understand the reason for this increasing violence. One factor may be that adolescents act recklessly without benefit of mature judgment. Adolescents have relatively ready access to guns and often use them as a means to solve problems. Efforts to control gun sales have met with little success in the United States Congress.

Nurses who have any contact with adolescents must make every effort to help them work through their problems in a nonviolent way. The nurse can become involved at the school or community level, becoming an advocate for adolescents and an educator to promote safe driving as well as helmet wear and safety practices when using a motorcycle, all-terrain vehicle, bicycle, skateboard, or in-line skates. Nurses also can work with support groups that offer counseling to adolescents involved in date violence. The nurse can provide a positive role model for adolescents as a community member and a health care worker.

THE ADOLESCENT IN THE HEALTH CARE FACILITY

When adolescents are hospitalized, it is usually because of a major health problem such as an injury from violence or from a motor vehicle accident, substance abuse, attempted suicide, or a chronic health problem intensified by the physiologic changes of adolescence. Adolescents must cope with the stress of hospitalization, possibly dramatic alterations in body image, partial or total inability to conform with peer group norms, and an interrupted search for identity.

Adolescents fear loss of control and loss of privacy. Pro-

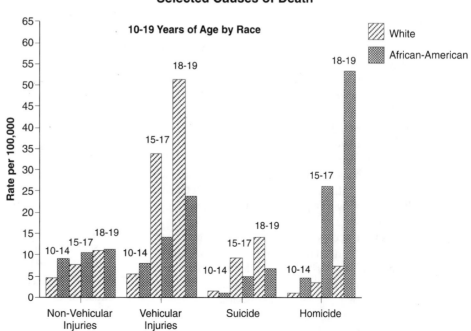

Figure 18-9
Selected causes of death for adolescents by race. These statistics are from Child Health USA '90. United States Department of Health and Human Services, HRS-M-CH 90-1, October, 1990. They are updated every 10 years.

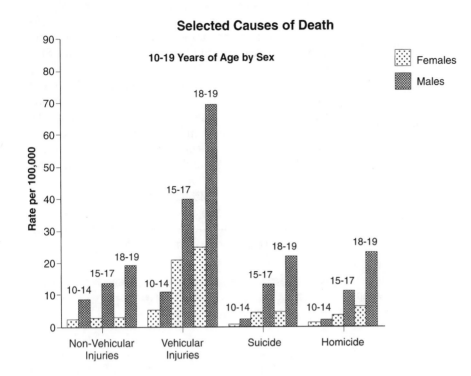

Figure 18-10
Selected causes of death by sex. These statistics are from Child Health USA '90. United States Department of Health and Human Services, HRS-M-CH 90-1, October, 1990. They are updated every 10 years.

vide opportunities for the adolescent to make choices whenever possible. Protect the adolescent's privacy by providing screening and adequate covering during procedures.

Adolescents may react with anger and refuse to cooperate when they feel threatened. Be aware of this possible reaction, and avoid labeling such an adolescent as a difficult patient.

The admission interview for an adolescent may be more successful if the family caregiver and the adolescent are interviewed separately. This provides the opportunity to gain information that the adolescent may not want to reveal in the presence of the family caregiver. Thoroughly assess the adolescent's developmental level, listen carefully with empathy to his or her concerns, encourage maximum participation in self-care, and provide sufficient information to make this participation possible. As with all patients, clear, honest explanations about treatments and procedures are essential.

During the admission interview, advise the adolescent of the unit's rules. Adolescents need to know what limits are set for their behavior while hospitalized. To share feelings and gain information, many find it helpful to discuss their health problem with a peer who has had the same or a related problem.

Adolescents need access to a telephone to contact peers and keep up social contacts. Recreation areas are important. In settings specifically designed for adolescents, recreation rooms can provide an area where teens can gather to do schoolwork, play games and cards, and socialize. In many hospitals with adolescent units, video games as well as television are provided in each patient room. Teens are encouraged to wear their own clothes. Girls can be encour-

aged to shampoo and style their hair and wear their usual makeup.

The adolescent's health problem may require a lengthy hospitalization and intense rehabilitation efforts. Adequate preparation and guidance can help make that difficult experience easier and less damaging to normal growth and development.

■ KEY POINTS

■ Adolescence is a turbulent time during which adolescents often feel confused.

■ Children go through many physical and emotional changes on their way to adulthood, beginning in the preadolescent years.

■ Adolescents have many struggles in their search for identity and independence.

■ Adolescents face many pressures and temptations that often are difficult to resist.

■ A warm, accepting family environment, positive school experiences, and good health give the adolescent the best chance of reaching adulthood with a positive sense of self, the ability to form close relationships, and the capacity to make sound decisions about life.

■ Nutritional needs are increased during adolescence because of the rapid physical growth that occurs during this period.

■ Many factors influence an adolescent's nutritional needs and food intake. Caregivers must be alert to nutritional deficiencies and make an effort to provide sound nutritional guidance.

■ Adolescents are trying to identify their career options and determine what they want to do with their lives. Many more career opportunities are available to them than at any previous time. This abundance of choices can place more pressure on the teen when making decisions.

■ Adolescents need a strong support system to help them through this stressful stage of development.

■ Only after adolescents complete the task of establishing their identity are they ready to establish an intimate relationship, the next task of development according to Erikson. Developing intimate relationships brings an additional set of problems.

■ Adolescents need a program of health maintenance in a setting that meets their needs for privacy, individualized attention, confidentiality, and the right to participate in decisions about their health care.

■ Substance abuse, sexual activity, sexual and physical abuse, and accidents can further complicate an adolescent's life. Peer pressure may be extremely influential in affecting the adolescent's attitudes and behaviors related to these issues.

■ Adolescents may need to deal with violence in school, a widespread problem.

■ In the health care facility, the adolescent fears loss of control and loss of privacy. The nurse caring for the hospitalized adolescent must be sensitive to the adolescent's needs and provide care that is supportive and provides for as much participation by the adolescent as possible. Health problems that threaten the adolescent's body image may threaten the satisfactory completion of developmental tasks.

? CRITICAL THINKING

1. Mr. Krasas is the custodial parent of Gina, age 11. He is concerned about providing her with appropriate sex education information. Describe the guidance you will give him.
2. Mattie is the mother of 13-year-old Chantal. Chantal has decided she will not eat meat or poultry because animals had to be killed to obtain it. Mattie is concerned about Chantal's nutrition. Design a teaching plan for Mattie that helps her provide the nutrients that are often deficient in adolescents.
3. Jamal is an adolescent athlete. He has told you he is planning to use a carbohydrate-loading diet before a big track meet. Using your knowledge about carbohydrate loading, detail the guidance you will give him.
4. You have the opportunity to talk with a group of 15-year-old girls. Describe the guidance you will give them about breast self-examination and Pap smears.
5. Caitlin is 15 years old. She scornfully tells you that girls don't need to know anything about condoms. State your answer to her, and design a teaching plan to use with adolescent boys and girls covering guidelines for condom use.
6. You are working in an adolescent clinic. Identify and describe all aspects of a complete physical for a) a 15-year-old girl and b) a 15-year-old boy.

BIBLIOGRAPHY

Castiglia PT, Harbin RE. Child health care: Process and practice. Philadelphia: JB Lippincott, 1992.

Cohall AT, Mayer R, Cohall K, et al. Teen violence: The new morality. Contemp Pediatr 8(9):76–86, 1991.

Cohen MI. Adolescents: Left behind by our health care system. Contemp Pediatr 9(7):33–44, 1992.

Dimond DA. Let's talk about sex. Contemp Pediatr 9(7):19–29, 1992.

Eschleman MM. Introductory nutrition and diet therapy, 3d ed. Philadelphia: Lippincott-Raven, 1996.

Jackson DB, Saunders RB. Child health nursing. Philadelphia: JB Lippincott, 1993.

Libbus MK. Condoms as primary prevention in sexually active women. MCN 17(5):256–260, 1992.

Pillitteri A. Maternal and child health nursing, 2d ed. Philadelphia: JB Lippincott, 1995.

Schuster CS, Ashburn SS. The process of human development, 3d ed. Philadelphia: JB Lippincott, 1992.

Starn J, Paperny DM. Computer games to enhance adolescent sex education. MCN 15(4):250–253, 1990.

Wong DL. Whaley and Wong's nursing care of infants and children, 5th ed. St. Louis: Mosby, 1995.

Chapter 19

Health Problems of the Adolescent

EATING DISORDERS
  Obesity
  Anorexia Nervosa
  Bulimia
  Nursing Process for the Adolescent With an Eating Disorder

SKIN DISORDERS
  Acne Vulgaris

MENSTRUAL DISORDERS
  Premenstrual Syndrome
  Dysmenorrhea
  Amenorrhea

INFECTIOUS DISEASES
  Infectious Mononucleosis
  Pulmonary Tuberculosis

THE SEXUALLY ACTIVE ADOLESCENT
  Vaginitis
  Sexually Transmitted Diseases
  Nursing Process for the Adolescent Girl With AIDS
  Adolescent Pregnancy

MALADAPTIVE RESPONSES TO THE STRESSES OF ADOLESCENCE
  Substance Abuse
  Suicide

STUDENT OBJECTIVES

On completion of this chapter, the student will be able to:

1. Define key terms.
2. Discuss the goal of health care professionals who work with obese adolescents.
3. State two goals of treatment for the hospitalized anorexic patient.
4. Discuss alcohol abuse and its impact on adolescents.
5. List nine types of drugs commonly abused by adolescents, and state at least one negative effect of each.
6. State the third leading cause of death in the 10- to 19-year-old age group.
7. Discuss the factors involved in causing acne vulgaris.
8. List the drugs commonly used for a) mild acne, b) inflammatory acne, and c) severe acne.
9. Describe infectious mononucleosis.
10. Identify the only certain way to prevent sexually transmitted diseases.
11. Identify the drug of choice to treat a) gonorrhea and b) syphilis.
12. Identify how the human immunodeficiency virus is transmitted.
13. Discuss how the developmental tasks of adolescence conflict with the developmental tasks of pregnancy.

KEY TERMS

alcohol abuse	menarche
alcoholism	mittelschmerz
amenorrhea	obesity
anorexia nervosa	overweight
bulimia	polyphagia
chancre	premenstrual syndrome
comedones	sebum
dependence	substance abuse
dysmenorrhea	tolerance
gynecomastia	vaginitis
impunity	withdrawal symptoms

Many adolescent health problems result from the rapid physiologic changes that are taking place, the adolescent's reaction to those changes, and the stress, conflict, and confusion that characterize adolescence. As adolescents struggle with questions about identity, independence, career, sexuality, morality, and emotions, alterations in their size and physical appearance make them uncomfortable and unfamiliar even with themselves. Coping with these changes and uncertainties is difficult for every adolescent, but for some it is impossible. Lacking adequate coping mechanisms, many adolescents feel there is no solution but escape and seek that escape through alcohol or drugs, running away, committing suicide, or other self-destructive behavior. Motor vehicle accidents, homicide, and suicide are common causes of death in the adolescent age group.

The complex interrelationship between psychological well-being and physical health, although not completely understood, is evident throughout life but particularly during adolescence. Emotions and attitudes affect nutrition and other health behaviors and can result in general or systemic disorders, which in turn can lead to further psychological stress. The high number of adolescent pregnancies also is believed to be a result of inappropriate responses to the stresses of adolescence.

Nurses are assuming an increasingly important role in helping adolescents understand, manage, and prevent health problems. Fulfillment of this role demands an understanding of adolescent growth and development and the ability to listen and observe carefully and project a sensitive, nonjudgmental attitude.

EATING DISORDERS

Eating disorders are among the most common health problems of adolescents. The most common of these are obesity, anorexia nervosa, and bulimia. Food represents nurturing and security and, as a result, may be consumed inappro-priately to try to solve problems. This misuse can result in health problems that have long-term or permanent effects.

Obesity

Obesity is a national problem in the United States, largely as a result of an overabundance of food and too little exercise. The thin figure, particularly for women, has become so idealized that being fat can handicap a person socially and professionally and severely damage self-esteem. **Obesity** generally is defined as an excessive accumulation of fat that increases body weight by 20% or more over ideal weight (see Appendix B). **Overweight**, although not necessarily signifying obesity, means that a person's weight is more than average for height and body build.

Obesity often begins in childhood and, if not treated successfully, leads to chronic obesity in adult life. The obese adolescent often feels isolated from the peer group, normally a source of support during this period. Because of the obesity, the adolescent often is embarrassed to participate in sports, thus eliminating one method of burning excess calories. Many use food as a means of satisfying emotional needs, establishing a vicious cycle. Adolescents' eating habits include skipping meals, especially breakfast, and indulging in late-night eating. This behavior compounds the problem because the calories they consume before going to bed are not used for energy but are stored as fat. Snacking while watching television also contributes to the overindulgence in caloric intake.

Some adolescents suffer from **polyphagia** (compulsive overeating). They lack control of their food intake, cannot postpone their urge to eat, hide food for later secret consumption, eat when not hungry or to escape from worries, and expend a great deal of energy thinking about securing and eating food. Not all compulsive eaters are overweight, and in some ways this disorder resembles anorexia nervosa.

Many factors, including genetic, social, cultural, metabolic, and psychological, contribute to the development of obesity. Children of obese parents are likely to share this problem not only because of some inherited predisposition toward obesity but also because of family eating patterns and the emotional climate surrounding food. Certain cultures equate obesity with being loved and being prosperous. If these values carry over into a modern family, the adolescent is torn between the standards of the peer group and those of the family.

Obesity is difficult to treat in any age group but especially in adolescence. Much of teenage life centers around food, such as after-school snacks, the ice cream shop, late-night diners, the pizza parlor, and fast-food restaurants serving high-fat, high-calorie foods with little nutritional value. Diets that emphasize nutritionally sound meals and reduced caloric intake produce results too slowly for impatient teenagers. Thus, the many quick-weight-loss programs, diet pills, and diet books find a ready market among adolescents.

Treatment must include a thorough exploration of the obese adolescent's food attitudes. Sometimes, a team approach is necessary, using the skills of a psychiatrist or psychologist, nutritionist, nurse, or other counselor. Summer camps that center on weight reduction with nutritious, calorie-controlled food, exercise, and activity are successful for some adolescents but are too costly for many families. In addition, many teens may fall back into old habits after summer camp is over unless there is a continuing support system.

Caregivers who work with obese adolescents should try to make these youngsters feel like worthwhile persons, stressing that obesity does not automatically make them unacceptable. Finding the support of a caring adult who will help the adolescent gain control of this aspect of his or her life can help give the necessary incentive to lose weight (see Family Teaching: Tips for Caregivers of Obese Teens).

Anorexia Nervosa

Preoccupation with reducing diets and the quest for the "perfect" (ie, thin) figure sometimes leads to **anorexia nervosa**, or self-inflicted starvation. This disorder occurs most commonly in adolescent white females, although there are reported cases among males and among African-American, Hispanic, and Asian adolescents. First described more than 100 years ago, anorexia has increased in incidence in recent years and is currently estimated to affect as many as 1% of adolescent girls. It is found in all the developed countries. Two age ranges are identified as the usual age of onset—11 to 13 years and 19 to 20 years. Although considered a psychiatric problem, it causes severe physiologic damage and even death.

CHARACTERISTICS

These adolescents are often described as successful students who tend to be perfectionists, trying always to please parents, teachers, and other adults. The families of anorexic adolescents characteristically show little emotion and display no evidence of conflict within the family. An adolescent in a controlled family environment, in which the parents do not freely express emotions, may try to establish independence and identity by controlling his or her own appetite and body weight. Depression is common in these adolescents. Anorexic persons deny weight loss and actually see themselves as fat, even when they look obviously skeletal to others. They often adhere to a rigid program of exercise to further their efforts in weight reduction. They also may make demands on themselves for cleanliness and order in their environment or engage in rigid schedules for studying and other ritualistic behavior. These adolescents deny hunger but often suffer from fatigue.

Family Teaching
Tips for Caregivers of Obese Teens

1. Have teen keep a food diary for a week. Include food eaten, time eaten, what teen was doing, and how teen felt before and after eating; identify what stimulates urge to eat.
2. Study diary with teen to look for eating triggers.
3. Set a reasonable goal of no more than 1 or 2 lbs a week or perhaps maintaining weight with no gain.
4. Advise teen to eat only at specific, regular mealtimes.
5. Recommend teen eats only at dining or kitchen table (not in front of TV or on the run).
6. Have teen use small plates to make amount of food look like more.
7. Teach teen to eat slowly—count and chew each bite (25 to 30 is a good goal).
8. Suggest the teen try to leave a little on the plate when done.
9. Have teen survey home and get rid of tempting high-calorie foods.
10. Stock up on low-calorie snacks—carrot sticks, celery sticks, and other raw vegetables.
11. Help teen get involved in an active project that occupies time and also helps burn calories—any active team sport, or bicycling, walking, hiking, swimming, skating.
12. Promote walking instead of riding whenever possible.
13. Establish group or buddy system.
14. Weigh only once a week, on the same scale, at the same time of day, in the same clothing.
15. Make a chart to keep track of teen's weight.
16. Help teen focus on a positive asset and make the most of it to help build self-concept.
17. Encourage good grooming; group could work on putting on a "mini" fashion show, choosing with guidance clothes that help maximize best features. This could be done simply by using magazine illustrations if actual clothing is not available.
18. Reward each small success with positive reinforcement.
19. Enlist cooperation of all family members to support the teen with encouragement and a positive atmosphere.

CLINICAL MANIFESTATIONS AND DIAGNOSIS

Persons with anorexia are visibly emaciated and almost skeletal. They appear sexually immature, have dry skin and brittle nails, and often have lanugo (downy hair) over their backs and extremities. Other symptoms include amenorrhea (absence of menstruation), constipation, hypothermia, bradycardia, low blood pressure, and anemia.

The American Psychiatric Association identifies the following criteria for the diagnosis of anorexia nervosa:[1]

- Weight loss 15% below that expected for age and height; or failure to make expected weight gain during a period of growth, leading to body weight 15% below that expected

- Intense fear of gaining weight or becoming fat, even though underweight
- Disturbance in the way the body is experienced (eg, feeling fat even when emaciated, or perceiving one part of the body to be too fat, even though underweight)
- Amenorrhea, as evidenced by absence of three consecutive menstrual cycles.

TREATMENT

Adolescents diagnosed with anorexia nervosa may be hospitalized to achieve the two goals of treatment: correction of malnutrition and identification and treatment of the psychological cause. An approach involving several disciplines is necessary. Therapy is required to help the adolescent gain insight into the problem. In addition, family therapy, nutritional therapy, and behavior modification are used. Affected adolescents fear they will gain too much weight; therefore, a compromise between what the physician prefers and what the adolescent desires may be necessary.

Adolescents with anorexia have become experts in manipulating others and their environment. Once treatment begins, they may try to avoid gaining weight by ordering only low-calorie foods, by disposing of their meals in plants, trash, toilets, or dirty linen, or by exercising in the hall or jogging in place in their room. In some instances, nasogastric tube feedings or hyperalimentation is necessary to provide nutritional support.

In treatment based on behavior modification, the patient may be deprived of all privileges, such as visitors, television, and telephone, until she begins to gain weight. Privileges are then gradually restored. These techniques are effective only when the patient and the caregivers understand the program and its purpose and have agreed on individualized goals and rewards.

Group therapy may be used, relying on peer support and the opportunity to associate with other patients with the same diagnosis in a nonthreatening setting.

The long-term outlook for the adolescent with anorexia is unclear. Death may occur from suicide, infection, or the effects of starvation. Some adolescents recover completely, others have eating problems into adulthood, and still others have problems with social adjustment that are not related to eating. Predicting the outcome is difficult, and more studies are needed before a definitive answer is available (Fig. 19-1).

Bulimia

Bulimia nervosa (usually referred to simply as bulimia) is characterized by binge eating followed by purging. The typical bulimic person is a white female in late adolescence. Most often, the bulimic person is of normal weight or overweight. Those who are underweight usually fulfill the criteria for anorexia nervosa. Some anorexic persons periodi-

Figure 19-1

This anorexic teen, who is in the later stages of treatment, continues to meet with the counselor to discuss her food choices, exercise program, and overall well-being.

cally practice binging and purging. Bulimia is seen increasingly in young adult women as well.

The binging often occurs late in the day when the adolescent is alone. Secrecy is an important aspect of the process. The adolescent eats large quantities of food within 1 or 2 hours. This binging is followed by guilt, fear, shame, and self-condemnation. To avoid weight gain from the food eaten, the adolescent follows the binging with purging by means of self-induced vomiting, laxatives, diuretics, and excessive exercise.

CLINICAL MANIFESTATIONS AND DIAGNOSIS

The clues to bulimia may be few but may include dental caries and erosion from frequent exposure to stomach acid, throat irritation, and endocrine and electrolyte imbalances that may cause cardiac irregularities and menstrual problems. Calluses or abrasions may be noted on the back of the hand from frequent contact with the teeth while inducing vomiting. Possible complications are esophageal tears and acute gastric dilatation. Hypokalemia also may occur, especially if the adolescent abuses diuretics to prevent weight gain. Other behavior problems seen in many bulimic persons include drug abuse, alcoholism, stealing (especially food), promiscuity, and other impulsive activities.

According to the American Psychiatric Association's *DSM-IV*, the diagnostic criteria for bulimia include:

- Recurrent episodes of binge eating
- A feeling of lack of control over behavior during binges
- Self-induced purging, use of laxatives or diuretics,

and strict dieting, fasting, or vigorous exercise to prevent weight gain

- Average of at least two binge-eating episodes a week over a 3-week period
- Obsessiveness regarding body weight and shape.

TREATMENT

Treatment of bulimia is varied. Many aspects of the treatment are similar to treatment of the adolescent with anorexia. Food diaries often are used as a tool to assess the adolescent's eating patterns. In some instances, antidepressant drugs may be useful. The nurse can refer the adolescent to a support group that may prove helpful.

▶ ◥ Nursing Process for the Adolescent ◤ ◢ With an Eating Disorder

ASSESSMENT

Begin the assessment of the adolescent with an eating disorder with a complete history, including previous illnesses, allergies, a dietary history, and a description of eating habits. The adolescent may not give an accurate dietary history or description of eating habits. Question the family caregiver in a separate interview to gain added information. In the physical assessment include height, weight, blood pressure, temperature, pulse, and respirations. Carefully inspect and evaluate the skin, mucous membranes, state of nutrition, and state of alertness and cooperation. Finish the assessment with complete documentation.

NURSING DIAGNOSES

Nursing diagnoses vary with the specific eating disorder, the physical condition of the adolescent, the length of time the adolescent has had the condition, and other accompanying conditions. The following diagnoses may be useful in planning care:

- Altered Nutrition: Less Than Body Requirements related to self-induced vomiting and use of laxatives or diuretics
- Self Esteem Disturbance related to fear of obesity and potential rejection
- Risk for Activity Intolerance related to fatigue secondary to malnutrition
- Constipation or Diarrhea related to decreased food and fluid intake and use of laxatives
- Risk for Impaired Skin Integrity related to loss of subcutaneous fat and dry skin secondary to malnutrition
- Noncompliance with treatment regimen related to unresolved conflicts over food and eating
- Ineffective Family Coping: Compromised related to eating disorders, treatment regimen, and dangers associated with an eating disorder

OUTCOME IDENTIFICATION AND PLANNING

The major goals for the adolescent with an eating disorder relate to meeting nutritional needs and improving self-concept and self-esteem. Other goals include establishing appropriate activity levels, maintaining normal bowel activity, maintaining skin integrity, preserving social relationships, and complying with the treatment program. The goals for the family include understanding the condition, learning how to manage the condition and its treatment, and reinforcing the adolescent's self-esteem.

IMPLEMENTATION

IMPROVING NUTRITION. The adolescent with anorexia nervosa has a compulsive desire to be thin and an unrealistic body image. The adolescent with bulimia, on the other hand, may consume large amounts of food followed by purging to avoid the excessive weight gain that could result from such consumption. In either instance, the adolescent does not receive the nutrients needed to achieve adequate growth during this period of development.

Supervise food intake. Weigh the adolescent at the same time each day, but do not make an issue of weight fluctuation. Be observant when weighing the patient: the adolescent may try to add weight by putting heavy objects in pockets, shoes, or other hiding places. While being weighed, the patient should wear minimal clothing (preferably a patient gown with no pockets) and bare feet.

The physician and a dietitian work with the adolescent to devise a food plan to meet the adolescent's nutrition requirements. The food plan is not geared to a sudden weight gain but a slow, steady gain with an established goal that has been agreed on by the health care team and the adolescent. Often the adolescent keeps a food diary, which is reviewed daily with the health team.

Patients with eating disorders are often manipulative and deceptive. Observe the patient during and after eating to make certain the teen eats the required food and does not get rid of it after apparently consuming it.

Contract agreements are often recommended for patients with eating disorders. These agreements, usually part of a behavioral modification plan, specify the adolescent's and the staff's responsibilities for the diet, activity expectations for the teen, and other aspects of the adolescent's behavior. The contract also may spell out specific privileges that can be gained by meeting the contract goals. This places the teen in greater control of the outcome.

In addition to daily weights, test urine for ketones and regularly evaluate the skin turgor and mucous membranes to gather further information about nutritional status. Report and document immediately evidence of deteriorating physical condition. If weight loss continues, nasogastric tube feedings may need to be implemented. This possibility also can be included in the contract.

If the adolescent's condition is at a critical stage, with

fluid and electrolyte deficiencies, parenteral fluids are necessary immediately to hydrate the patient before further treatment can be implemented. Observe the adolescent continuously to prevent any attempt to remove intravenous lines or otherwise disrupt the treatment. Closely monitor serum electrolytes, cardiac and respiratory status, and renal complications. During administration of parenteral fluids, continue to encourage the adolescent to maintain an oral intake.

REINFORCING POSITIVE SELF-ESTEEM.   The nurse must function as an active, nonjudgmental listener to the adolescent. Consistent assignment of the same nursing personnel to care for the adolescent helps establish a climate in which the adolescent can relate to the nurse and begin to build a positive self-concept. Report and document without delay any signs of depression. Also report and document any negative feelings expressed by the adolescent. Do not minimize or ignore these feelings. Reinforce positive behavior. Psychotherapy and counseling groups are necessary to help the adolescent work through feelings of negative self-worth. Encourage the adolescent to express fears, anger, and frustrations and help the patient recognize that these are feelings that everyone has from time to time. Never ridicule or belittle these feelings. Encourage the adolescent to explore ways in which destructive feelings may be changed. These are feelings that can be dealt with in counseling sessions; therefore, report and document them carefully.

BALANCING REST AND ACTIVITY.   Exercise and activity are important parts of the contract negotiated with the adolescent. Explain to the adolescent that fatigue is a result of the extreme depletion of energy reserves related to nutritional deficits. Encourage the adolescent to become involved in all activities of daily living. Provide ample rest periods when the adolescent's energy reserves are depleted. Discourage the adolescent from pushing beyond endurance and closely observe for secretive excessive activity.

MONITORING BOWEL HABITS.   Make a careful record of bowel movements. The adolescent may not be reliable as a reporter of bowel habits, so devise methods to prevent the teen from using the bathroom without supervision. Report at once and document constipation or diarrhea. Watch carefully to prevent the teen from obtaining and taking a laxative. These patients are devious and may go to great lengths to obtain a laxative to purge themselves of food. Report immediately any evidence or suspicions of this type of behavior.

MAINTAINING SKIN INTEGRITY.   Good skin care is essential in the care of the adolescent with a severely restricted nutritional intake. The skin may be dry and tend to break down easily because of the lack of a subcutaneous fat cushion. Inspect daily for redness, irritation, or signs of decubitus ulcer formation. Observe specifically the bony prominences. Encourage the adolescent to be out of bed most of the day. When the teen is in bed, encourage regular position changes so that no pressure areas develop.

IMPROVING COMPLIANCE.   The long-term outcome for adolescents with eating disorders is precarious. Adolescents with severe eating disorders often have multiple inpatient admissions. During inpatient treatment, goals should be set and plans made for discharge. Specific consequences must be established for noncompliance. Counseling must continue after discharge. A support group referral may be helpful in encouraging compliance. Family involvement is necessary. The adolescent must recognize that discharge from the health care facility does not mean that he or she is "cured."

IMPROVING FAMILY COPING.   The family of the adolescent needs counseling along with the adolescent. Some families may deny that the teen has a problem or that the problem is as severe as health care team members perceive it to be. Family therapy meets with varied success. Usually, the earlier family therapy is initiated, the better the results. Family members must be able to identify behaviors of their own that contribute to the adolescent's problem. Family members also must learn to cooperate with behavior modification programs and, with guidance, carry them out at home when necessary. Ongoing contact between the family, the adolescent, and consistent health team members is essential. (See Nursing Care Plan for the Adolescent With an Eating Disorder.)

EVALUATION: GOALS AND OUTCOME CRITERIA

The evaluation of an adolescent with an eating disorder is an ongoing process that continues throughout the hospital stay. Goals and outcome criteria include:

- *Goal*: The adolescent will gain a predetermined amount of weight per week.
  Criteria: The adolescent's mucous membranes are moist and skin turgor is good; at least 80% of each meal is eaten; weight gain is 1 to 2 lb (450–900 g) a week.

- *Goal*: The adolescent will evidence improved self-esteem.
  Criteria: The adolescent verbally expresses positive attitudes, maintains peer relationships, and improves grooming.

- *Goal*: The adolescent will pace activity to avoid fatigue.
  Criteria: The adolescent is involved in activity as prescribed in a contract; no excessive activity is detected.

- *Goal*: The adolescent's bowel elimination will be normal.
  Criteria: The adolescent will experience no episodes of diarrhea or constipation. The adolescent will not attempt deceit to obtain laxatives.

Text continues on page 417.

Nursing Care Plan
for the Adolescent with an Eating Disorder

Felicia is a 15-year-old who has had a complete physical examination to determine why she has lost weight. After her examination and testing was completed, a diagnosis of anorexia nervosa was made. Felicia denies that she is underweight. She has been hospitalized to initiate treatment because her weight has dropped to 87 pounds (39.5 kg).

NURSING DIAGNOSIS

Altered Nutrition: Less than Body Requirements related to self-induced vomiting and use of laxatives

GOAL: *Felicia's nutrition will improve, reaching a goal weight of 100 pounds; maintain adequate fluid intake*

OUTCOME CRITERIA

- Felicia gains at least 1.5 pounds (680 grams) per week
- Felicia eats her meals completely
- Felicia is involved in plans to improve her nutrition
- Felicia does not interrupt parenteral fluid administration
- Felicia's mucous membranes are moist, her skin turgor good
- Felicia's electrolytes, cardiac and respiratory status, and renal function are within normal limits

Nursing Interventions	Rationale
Supervise Felicia's intake by observing her during and after meals.	An adolescent with an eating disorder may go to any length to avoid eating.
Weigh Felicia daily at the same time with the same type of clothes on. Make certain nothing can be secreted in pockets or other hiding places that could add to her weight.	An adolescent can be very innovative in finding ways to hide heavy objects on herself to increase her weight gain.
Include Felicia with other health care providers to establish a mutually agreed upon long-term weight goal and food plan that provides her with a slow, steady, weekly weight gain. Make a contract agreement with Felicia to clearly state expectations and privileges that she can gain or lose.	The adolescent is central to the planning process and cannot be made to meet goals set by others. Her participation and agreement to specific plans give her a feeling of more control of the overall outcome, encouraging her to stick to the plan.
Observe Felicia continuously when parenteral fluids are being administered to prevent any attempts to disrupt the IV line. Also encourage her to take oral fluids at the same time.	The anorectic adolescent may deprive herself so much that the fluid and electrolyte deficiencies become life threatening. A balance must be restored before any further treatment can begin.
Test Felicia's urine for ketones and evaluate her skin turgor and mucous membranes regularly.	These tests provide further indication of Felicia's nutritional status.

NURSING DIAGNOSIS

Risk for Self Esteem Disturbance related to fear of obesity and potential rejection

GOAL: *Positive self esteem will be reinforced*

OUTCOME CRITERIA

- Felicia verbally expresses positive attitudes about herself

(continued)

Nursing Care Plan (Continued)
for the Adolescent with an Eating Disorder

Nursing Interventions	Rationale
Be a nonjudgmental, active listener; never minimize or ignore feelings expressed by Felicia. Report any negative feelings or any signs of depression expressed by Felicia.	This is a first step in establishing and maintaining a climate of trust with Felicia. Felicia's negative feelings and expression of depression are important to the therapeutic treatment plan. All health care providers need to know about signs of depression to alert them to take appropriate precautions.

NURSING DIAGNOSIS

Risk for Activity Intolerance related to fatigue secondary to malnutrition

GOAL: *Felicia will balance rest and activity*

OUTCOME CRITERIA

• Felicia follows her contract for activity
• Felicia is not excessively active
• Felicia paces her activity to avoid fatigue

Nursing Interventions	Rationale
Teach Felicia that a nutritional deficit depletes energy reserves and results in fatigue; encourage her to engage in activities of daily living, but provide for rest periods when her energy is low. Discourage Felicia from pushing herself beyond her physical limits, and observe closely for secretive excessive exercise.	Felicia needs to understand that activity and rest are related to her nutritional status and that a healthy balance is crucial to overall health. The adolescent with an eating disorder may attempt to burn off excess calories with exercise.

NURSING DIAGNOSIS

Constipation or diarrhea related to decreased food and fluid intake or use of laxatives.

GOAL: *Felicia will maintain normal bowel habits*

OUTCOME CRITERIA

• Felicia has bowel movements every day or every other day
• Felicia's stools are soft formed

Nursing Interventions	Rationale
Observe Felicia's trips to the bathroom and keep a careful record of Felicia's bowel habits; report and document any occurrence of diarrhea or constipation at once. Observe Felicia carefully to be certain she does not have opportunity for purging or taking a laxative.	Typically, Felicia may not be a reliable reporter of her bowel habits. A nurse observer is necessary to validate her stools. These adolescents can be devious and will go to almost any length to prevent weight gain.

NURSING DIAGNOSIS

Risk for Impaired Skin Integrity related to loss of subcutaneous fat and dry skin secondary to malnutrition

GOAL: *Felicia's skin integrity will be maintained*

OUTCOME CRITERIA

• Felicia's has no areas of red, dry, irritated skin
• Felicia has no decubitus ulcer formations

(continued)

Nursing Care Plan (Continued)
for the Adolescent with an Eating Disorder

Nursing Interventions	Rationale
Inspect Felicia' skin daily for redness, irritation, or dryness. Provide good skin care.	Signs of redness, irritation, and dryness are preliminary signs for skin breakdown and formation of decubitus ulcers.
Protect any bony prominences that may break down. Encourage position changes when Felicia is in bed to prevent decubiti formation.	Protection of pressure on bony surfaces and frequent changes of position improve circulation and prevent formation of decubitus ulcers.

NURSING DIAGNOSIS

Noncompliance With Treatment Regimen related to unresolved conflicts over food and eating

GOAL: *Felicia will improve compliance*

OUTCOME CRITERIA

- Felicia keeps counseling appointments
- Felicia joins a support group
- Felicia continues to gain weight as per her contract agreement

Nursing Interventions	Rationale
Make plans for Felicia's discharge while she is still in the hospital. Include counseling plans in the contract.	Eating disorders are not cured with one hospitalization. Counseling is necessary to continue after discharge.
Encourage Felicia to make and maintain contact with a support group after discharge.	A support group may strengthen Felicia's desire to comply with the treatment regimen.
Make clear to Felicia the established consequences for noncompliance with the program.	Consequences for noncompliance are important to reinforce the need to follow the program
	Consequences set out a disciplinary action which will occur if the adolescent fails to follow the program.

NURSING DIAGNOSIS

Ineffective Family Coping: Compromised related to eating disorders, treatment regimen, and dangers associated with an eating disorder

GOAL: *The family's understanding of illness and treatment goals will improve*

OUTCOME CRITERIA

- The family attends counseling sessions
- The family identifies behaviors that impact negatively on Felicia's behavior

Nursing Interventions	Rationale
Provide for counseling Felicia's family as well as counseling for her.	It is important for the family to understand the dynamics of the problem and to face their possible contribution to the disorder.
Teach Felicia's family members about the behavior modification program she is using. Provide guidance on how to carry out the program at home.	Eating disorders are not cured simply because the adolescent is discharged. Counseling, a continuation of the treatment program, and adherence to the contract agreement Felicia has signed are essential. For these reasons, the family must become involved.

■ *Goal*: The adolescent's skin will show no evidence of breakdown.
Criteria: The adolescent's skin is intact, with no signs of redness, irritation, or excessive pressure.

■ *Goal*: The adolescent will show signs of compliance.
Criteria: The adolescent agrees to, signs, and adheres to a contract agreement, keeps counseling appointments, joins a support group, and continues to gain or maintain weight as per contract agreement.

■ *Goal*: The family will evidence signs of improved coping.
Criteria: The family attends counseling sessions and identifies behaviors that aggravate the adolescent's condition.

SKIN DISORDERS

Acne Vulgaris

Acne, one of the most common health problems of adolescence, may be only a mild case of oily skin and a few blackheads, or it may be a severe type with ropelike cystic lesions that leave deep scars, both physical and emotional. To adolescents who want to be attractive and popular, however, even a mild case of acne (often called "zits") can cause great anxiety, shyness, and social withdrawal.

Characterized by the appearance of **comedones** (blackheads and whiteheads) and papules and pustules on the face and, to some extent, the back and chest, acne is caused by a variety of factors, including:

- Increased hormonal levels, especially androgens
- Hereditary factors
- Irritation and irritating substances, such as vigorous scrubbing and cosmetics with a greasy base
- Growth of anaerobic bacteria.

Each hair follicle has an associated sebaceous gland that, in adolescents, produces increased **sebum** (oily secretion). The sebum is blocked by epithelial cells and becomes trapped in the follicle. When this collection becomes infected by anaerobic organisms, inflammation occurs, causing papules, pustules, and nodules (Fig. 19-2). Several types of acne lesions are often present at one time.

TREATMENT AND NURSING CARE

The topical medications benzoyl peroxide (Clearasil, Benoxyl) and tretinoin (Retin-A) come in a variety of forms, such as topical cleansers, lotions, creams, sticks, pads, gels, and bars. The usual treatment plan for mild acne is topical application of one of these medications once or twice a day. These medications should not be applied to normal skin or allowed to get into the eyes or nose or on other mucous membranes. Antibiotics, such as erythromycin and tetracy-

Figure 19-2
Acne of face and chest.

cline, may be administered for inflammatory acne. Antibiotic therapy requires an extended treatment course of at least 6 to 12 months, followed by tapering of the dosage.

Isotretinoin (Accutane) may be used for severe inflammatory acne. This potent, effective oral medication is used for hard-to-treat cystic acne. Side effects are common but often diminish when the drug dosage is reduced. Warn the adolescent about some of the side effects, including dry lips and skin, eye irritation, temporary worsening of acne, epistaxis (nosebleed), bleeding and inflammation of the gums, itching, photosensitivity (sensitivity to the sun), and joint and muscle pain. Isotretinoin is a pregnancy category X drug: it must not be used at all during pregnancy because of serious risk of fetal abnormalities. Any adolescent girl who is to be treated with isotretinoin must first be given a urine test to rule out pregnancy and must use an effective form of contraception for a month before beginning isotretinoin therapy.

Even though the adolescent's perception of the disfigurement caused by acne may seem out of proportion to the actual severity of the condition, acknowledge and accept his or her feelings. Teach the adolescent and the family caregiver to wash the lesions gently with soap and water; do not scrub vigorously. Comedones should be removed gently, following the recommendations of the physician and using careful aseptic techniques. Careful removal produces no scarring—a goal for every teen.

Understanding and support by the nurse and family caregiver are the most important aspects of caring for the adolescent with acne. Reassure the teen that eating chocolate and fatty foods does not cause acne, but a well-balanced, nutritious diet promotes healing.

MENSTRUAL DISORDERS

The beginning of menstruation, called **menarche**, normally occurs between the ages of 9 and 16 years. For many girls this is a joyous affirmation of their womanhood, but others may have negative feelings about this event, depending on how they have been prepared for menarche and for their roles as women. Irregular menstruation is common during the first year until a regular cycle is established.

Some adolescent girls have dull, aching abdominal pain at the time of ovulation (midcycle, hence the name **mittelschmerz**). The cause is not completely understood, but the discomfort usually lasts only a few hours and is relieved by analgesics, a heating pad, or a warm bath.

Premenstrual Syndrome

Women of all ages are subject to the discomfort of **premenstrual syndrome** (PMS), but the symptoms may be alarming to the adolescent. Symptoms include edema (resulting in weight gain), headache, increased anxiety, mild depression, and mood swings. The major cause of PMS is thought to be water retention following progesterone production after ovulation (Fig. 19-3).

Generally, the discomforts of PMS are minor and can be relieved by reducing salt intake during the week before menstruation, taking mild analgesics, and applying local heat. When symptoms are more severe, the physician may prescribe a mild diuretic to be taken the week before menstruation to relieve edema; occasionally, oral contraceptive pills are prescribed to prevent ovulation.

Dysmenorrhea

Dysmenorrhea (painful menstruation) is classified as primary or secondary. Many adolescent girls experience pain associated with menstruation, including cramping abdominal pain, leg pain, and backache. *Primary dysmenorrhea* occurs as part of the normal menstrual cycle without any associated pelvic disease. The increased secretion of prosta-

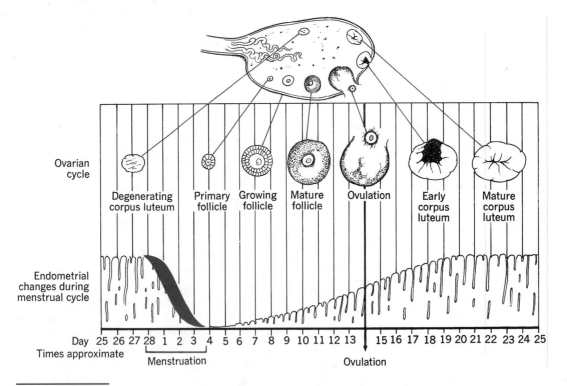

Figure 19-3

Schematic representation of a 28-day ovarian cycle. Menstruation occurs with shedding of the endometrium. The follicular phase is associated with the rapidly growing ovarian follicle and the production of estrogen. Ovulation occurs midcycle, and mittelschmerz may occur. The secretory phase follows in preparation for the fertilized ovum. If fertilization does not occur, the corpus luteum begins to degenerate, estrogen and progesterone levels decline, and menstruation again occurs.

glandins, which occurs in the last few days of the menstrual cycle, is thought to be a contributing factor in primary dysmenorrhea. Nonsteroidal antiinflammatory drugs (NSAIDs), such as ibuprofen (Advil, Motrin), inhibit prostaglandins and are the treatment of choice for primary dysmenorrhea. These drugs are most effective when taken before cramps become too severe. Because NSAIDs are irritating to the gastric mucosa, they always should be taken with food and discontinued if epigastric burning occurs.

Secondary dysmenorrhea is the result of pelvic pathologic changes, most often pelvic inflammatory disease (PID) or endometriosis. The adolescent girl who has severe menstrual pain should be examined by a physician to determine if any pelvic pathologic changes are present. Treatment of the underlying condition helps relieve severe dysmenorrhea.

Amenorrhea

The absence of menstruation, or **amenorrhea**, can be primary (no previous menstruation) or secondary (missing three or more periods after menstrual flow has begun). Primary amenorrhea after 16 years of age warrants a diagnostic survey for genetic abnormalities, tumors, or other problems. Secondary amenorrhea can be the result of discontinuing contraceptives, a sign of pregnancy, the result of physical or emotional stressors, or a symptom of an underlying medical condition. A complete physical examination, including gynecologic screening, is necessary to help determine the cause.

INFECTIOUS DISEASES

Infectious Mononucleosis

Sometimes called the "kissing disease," infectious mononucleosis ("mono") is caused by the Epstein-Barr virus, one of the herpesvirus group. The organism is transmitted through saliva. There is no immunization available, and treatment is symptomatic. Adolescents and young adults seem to be most susceptible to this disorder, although sometimes it also is seen in younger children.

CLINICAL MANIFESTATIONS

Infectious mononucleosis can present a variety of symptoms, ranging from mild to severe and including symptoms that mimic hepatitis. Symptoms include sore throat with enlarged tonsils, fever, palatine petechiae (red spots on the soft palate), swollen lymph nodes, and enlargement of the spleen, accompanied by extreme fatigue and lack of energy. In some instances, headache, abdominal pain, and epistaxis are also present.

DIAGNOSIS

Diagnosis of infectious mononucleosis is based on clinical symptoms, laboratory evidence of lymphocytes in the peripheral blood (with 10% or more abnormal lymphocytes present in a peripheral blood smear), and a positive heterophil agglutination test. Monospot is a valuable diagnostic test; rapid, sensitive, inexpensive, and simple to perform, it can detect significant agglutinins at lower levels, thus allowing earlier diagnosis. Infectious mononucleosis often is confused with streptococcal infections because of the fever and the appearance of the throat and tonsils.

TREATMENT AND NURSING CARE

No cure exists for infectious mononucleosis; treatment is based on symptoms. An analgesic–antipyretic, such as acetaminophen, usually is recommended for the fever and headaches. Fluids and a soft, bland diet are encouraged to reduce throat irritation. Corticosteroids sometimes are used to relieve the severe sore throat and fever. Bed rest is suggested to relieve fatigue but is not imposed for a specific amount of time. If the spleen is enlarged, the adolescent is cautioned to avoid contact sports, which might cause a ruptured spleen. Because the immune system is weakened, the adolescent must take precautions to avoid secondary infections.

The course of mononucleosis is usually uncomplicated. Fever and sore throat last from 1 week to 10 days. Fatigue generally disappears 2 to 4 weeks after the appearance of acute symptoms but may last as long as 1 year. The limitations that this disorder impose on the teenager's school and social life may cause depression. In most instances, however, the adolescent can resume normal activities within 1 month after symptoms present. Nursing care includes encouraging the adolescent to express feelings about the interruptions the illness is causing in school, social, and work plans. Long-term effects rarely are seen.

Pulmonary Tuberculosis

Tuberculosis is present in all parts of the world and is the most important chronic infectious disease in terms of illness, death, and cost.[2] In the United States, the incidence of tuberculosis declined until the late 1980s, when an increasing number of cases were identified. Tuberculosis in patients infected with the human immunodeficiency virus (HIV) has been credited with causing this increase.

Tuberculosis is caused by *Mycobacterium tuberculosis*, a bacillus that is spread by droplets of infected mucus that become airborne when the infected person sneezes, coughs, or laughs. The bacilli, when airborne, are inhaled into the respiratory tract of the unsuspecting person and become implanted in lung tissue. This process is the beginning of a primary lesion.

CLINICAL MANIFESTATIONS

Primary tuberculosis is the original infection that goes through various stages and ends with calcification. Primary lesions in children generally are unrecognized. The most common site of a primary lesion is the alveoli of the respiratory tract. Most cases arrest with the calcification of the primary infection. However, in children with poor nutrition or health, the primary infection may invade other tissues of the body, including the bones, joints, kidneys, lymph nodes, and meninges. This is called miliary tuberculosis. In the small number of children with miliary tuberculosis, there may be general symptoms of chronic infection, such as fatigue, loss of weight, and low-grade fever accompanied by night sweats.

Secondary tuberculosis is a reactivation of a healed primary lesion. This often occurs in adults and contributes to the exposure of children to the organism. Although secondary lesions are more common in adults, they may occur in adolescents. Symptoms resemble those in an adult, including cough with expectoration, fever, loss of weight, malaise, and night sweats.

DIAGNOSIS

The tuberculin skin test is the primary means by which tuberculosis is detected. A skin test can be performed using a multipuncture device that deposits purified protein derivative (PPD) intradermally (tine test) or by intradermal injection of 0.1 mL of PPD. Either of these tests is administered on the inner aspect of the forearm. The site is marked and read at 48 and 72 hours. Redness, swelling, induration, and itching of the site indicate a positive reaction. Persons with a positive reaction are further examined by radiographic evaluation. Sputum tests of young children are rarely helpful because children do not produce a good specimen. Screening by means of skin testing is recommended for all children at 12 months, before entering school, in adolescence, and annually for children in high-risk situations or communities, including children in whose family there is an active case, Native Americans, and children who recently immigrated from Central or South America, the Caribbean, Africa, Asia, or the Middle East. Other high-risk children are those infected with HIV, those who are homeless or live in overcrowded conditions, and those immunosuppressed from any cause.

TREATMENT

Drug therapy for tuberculosis includes administration of isoniazid (INH), often in combination with rifampin. Although INH has been known to cause peripheral neuritis in children with poor nutrition, few problems occur in children whose diets are well balanced. Rifampin is tolerated well by children, but it causes body fluids such as urine, sweat, tears, and feces to turn orange-red. A possible disadvantage for adolescents is that it may permanently stain contact lenses. Rifamate is a combination of rifampin and INH. Other drugs that may be used are ethambutol, streptomycin, and pyrazinamide.

Drug therapy is continued for 9 to 18 months. After chemotherapy has begun, the child or adolescent may return to school and normal activities unless clinical symptoms are evident. An annual chest radiograph is necessary from that time on.

PREVENTION

Prevention requires improvements in social conditions such as overcrowding, poverty, and poor health care. Also needed are health education, medical, laboratory, and radiographic facilities for examination, and control of contacts and persons suspected of infection.

A vaccine called bacille Calmette-Guérin (BCG) is used in countries with a high incidence of tuberculosis. It is given to tuberculin-negative persons and is said to be effective for 12 years or longer. Mass vaccination is not considered necessary in parts of the world where the incidence of tuberculosis is low. After administration of BCG vaccine, the skin test will be positive, so screening is no longer an effective tool. The use of BCG vaccine remains controversial.

THE SEXUALLY ACTIVE ADOLESCENT

The age at which adolescents become sexually active has been decreasing in recent years, and with that decrease has come an increase in the complications resulting from sexual activity. Problems that result from sexual activity of adolescents include sexually transmitted diseases (STDs), genital infections, and adolescent pregnancy.

Vaginitis

Vaginitis (inflammation of the vagina) can result from a number of causes, such as diaphragms or tampons left in place too long, irritating douches or sprays, estrogen changes caused by birth-control pills, and antibiotic therapy. Actually, these causes are precursors, providing an opportunity for the organisms to become active. The most common causes of vaginitis are *Candida albicans*, bacterial vaginosis (caused by *Gardnerella vaginalis* and other organisms), and *Trichomonas*. *Trichomonas* is the only one of these organisms transmitted solely by sexual contact (Table 19-1).

Sexually Transmitted Diseases

The incidence of STDs is highest in adolescents. The diseases range from infections that can be easily treated to life-threatening diseases such as HIV infection (Table 19-

TABLE 19-1. Infectious Causes of Vaginitis

Organism/Incidence	Symptoms	Sexual Transmission	Treatment
Candida albicans First episodes occur in adolescence, especially in sexually active girls	Severe itching, exacerbated just before menstruation Odor not present Milky "cottage cheese"–like discharge may be noted on examination	Normally present in vagina, most often results from glycosuria, antibiotic therapy, birth-control pills, steroid therapy, or other factor that alters normal pH of vagina May result from oral–genital sex	Nystatin, miconazole (Monistat), or clotrimazole (Gyne-Lo-trimin) vaginal suppositories or creams
Bacterial Vaginosis (multiple organisms) Common among adolescent girls; sexual partner will probably also be infected	About half of patients have no symptoms Fishy odor after intercourse Discharge, if present, grayish and thin	Sexually transmitted	Metronidazole (Flagyl)* or ampicillin; sexual partners may be treated
Trichomonas Most frequently diagnosed STD	Itching with severe infection, especially after menstruation Discharge has foul odor and may be frothy, gray or green	Sexually transmitted	Metronidazole (Flagyl)*; sexual partners also should be treated

* Flagyl is not ordered for the pregnant patient due to possible danger to fetus.

2). Infants infected with STDs usually are infected prenatally or during birth. Children infected after the neonatal period must be considered victims of sexual abuse until disproved. Severe or repeated cases of PID or severe genital warts are warning signs that the girl should be tested for HIV.

Prevention is the most important aspect in the campaign against STDs. The only certain way to avoid contracting an STD is sexual abstinence. However, sexual activity in adolescents indicates that this is often not a practical solution. Condoms with spermicide, discussed in Chapter 18, provide protection, although they are not fail-safe. Adolescents must be educated about all aspects of the consequences of sexual activity.

GONORRHEA

More than 1 million cases of gonorrhea are reported annually, and an equal number of cases are believed to be undiagnosed. It is one of the most commonly reported communicable diseases in the United States. Also called "the clap," "the drips," or "the dose," gonorrhea has mild primary symptoms, particularly in females, and often goes undetected and thus untreated until it progresses to serious pelvic disorders. This disease can cause sterility in males.

There are several drugs that may be used to treat gonorrhea, but the current drug of choice is ceftriaxone (Rocephin) followed by a week of oral doxycycline (Vibramycin)

to prevent an accompanying chlamydial infection. Adolescents are asked to name their sexual contacts so that they also may be treated. Penicillin-resistant strains of the organism have developed, so penicillin is no longer an effective method of treatment. Adolescents must learn that their bodies will not develop immunity to the organism and they might become infected again if they continue to expose themselves to the risk.

CHLAMYDIAL INFECTION

Chlamydial infections have replaced gonorrhea as *the* most common STD in the United States. Symptoms may be mild, causing a delay in diagnosis and treatment until serious complications and transmission to others have occurred.

Adolescents must be made aware of the seriousness of PID, a common result of a chlamydial infection. Pelvic inflammatory disease can cause sterility in the female, primarily by causing scarring in the fallopian tubes, which prohibits the passage of the fertilized ovum into the uterus. A tubal pregnancy may be the consequence of a chlamydial infection. In the male, sterility may result from epididymitis caused by a chlamydial infection.

Tetracycline or doxycycline is used to treat chlamydial infection. In the pregnant adolescent, erythromycin can be used to avoid the teratogenic effects of these drugs. All sexual partners must be treated.

TABLE 19-2. Major Sexually Transmitted Diseases

Infection and Agent	Transmission	Symptoms	Possible Complications	Prevention
Gonorrhea—gonococcus: *Neisseria gonorrhoeae*	Sexual contact; mother to fetus during vaginal delivery	Yellow mucopurulent discharge of the genital area, painful or frequent urination, pain in the genital area; may be asymptomatic. Frequent cause of pelvic inflammatory disease	Sterility, cystitis, arthritis, endocarditis	Public should be educated on safe sex practices; mother should be tested before delivery. Newborn's eyes should be treated with tetracycline ointment, erythromycin ointment, or silver nitrate. All contacts should be treated with antibiotics
Chlamydia—bacteria: *Chlamydia trachomatis*	Sexual contact; mother to fetus during vaginal delivery	Mucopurulent genital discharge, genital pain, dysuria. Frequent cause of pelvic inflammatory disease, often in combination with gonorrhea	Sterility	Public should be educated about safe sex practices. Sexual contact should be avoided when lesions are present. Infected mothers should have a cesarean delivery
Genital herpes virus: herpes simplex type 2	Sexual contact; mother to fetus during vaginal delivery	Genital soreness, pruritus, and erythema; vesicles appear that usually last for about 10 days; during which time transmission of virus is likely		Public should be educated about safe sex practices. Sexual contact should be avoided when lesions are present. Infected mothers should have a cesarean delivery
Syphilis—spirochete: *Treponema pallidum*	Sexual contact; mother to fetus via placenta; blood transfusions if donor is in early stage of disease and undiagnosed	Primary stage: genital lesion, enlarged lymph nodes. Secondary stage (6 weeks later): lesions of skin and mucous membrane, with generalized symptoms of headache and fever	Tertiary stage: central nervous system and cardiovascular damage, paralysis, psychosis	Public should be educated about safe sex practices. Screen blood donors; do serologic testing before and during pregnancy. Avoid contact with body secretions from infected patients
Acquired immunodeficiency syndrome (AIDS)—virus: human immunodeficiency virus	Sexual contact; exposure to blood or blood products; mother to fetus	Active phase: rash, cough, malaise, night sweats, lymphadenopathy. Asymptomatic phase: no symptoms, but test is positive for HIV antigens. AIDS-related complex: lymphadenopathy, diarrhea, oral candidiasis, weight loss, fatigue, skin rash, recurrent infections, fever. AIDS: rare infections such as *Pneumocystis carinii* pneumonia or rare cancers such as Kaposi sarcoma or B-cell lymphomas	Neurologic impairment	Public should be educated about safe sex practices, especially high-risk groups. Blood or blood products used for transfusion should be carefully screened. Intravenous drug abusers should not share needles. Universal precautions should be used consistently in all health care settings. Institute measures to avoid needlesticks among health care workers

Adapted from Craven RF, Hirnle CJ. Fundamentals of nursing: Human health and function. Philadelphia: JB Lippincott, 1992.

GENITAL HERPES

Genital herpes has reached epidemic proportions in the United States. The disease begins as a vesicle that ruptures to form a painful ulcer on the genitalia. The initial ulcer lasts 10 to 12 days. Recurrent episodes occur intermittently and last 4 to 5 days. No cure is available, but acyclovir (Zovirax) is useful in relieving or suppressing the symptoms. Genital herpes is associated with a much higher than average risk for cervical cancer; therefore, the female who has genital herpes should have an annual Pap smear. Genital herpes is not transmitted to the fetus in utero, but if there is an active case of genital herpes at the time of delivery, the infant should be delivered by cesarean birth to avoid infection during passage through the vagina. In newborns, the infection can become systemic and cause death.

SYPHILIS

Caused by the spirochete *Treponema pallidum*, syphilis is a destructive disease that can involve every part of the body. Untreated, it can have devastating long-term effects. Infected mothers are highly likely to transmit the infection to their unborn infants.

Syphilis is spread primarily by sexual contact. Symptoms of the primary stage usually appear about 3 weeks after exposure. If allowed to progress without treatment, syphilis has a secondary stage, a latent stage, and a tertiary stage.

The cardinal sign of the primary stage is the **chancre**, a hard, red, painless lesion at the point of entry of the spirochete. This can appear on the penis, the vulva, or the cervix. It also can appear on the mouth, the lips, or the rectal area as a result of oral–genital or anal–genital contact. The secondary stage, marked by rash, sore throat, and fever, appears 2 to 6 months after the original infection. Signs of both the first and second stages disappear without treatment, but the spirochete remains in the body. The latent period can persist for as long as 20 years without symptoms; however, blood tests are still positive. In the tertiary stage, syphilis causes severe neurologic and cardiovascular damage, mental illness, and gastrointestinal disorders.

Syphilis responds to one intramuscular injection of benzathine penicillin; if the adolescent is sensitive to penicillin, oral tetracycline can be administered for a 15-day course of treatment. If treatment is not obtained before the tertiary stage, the neurologic and cardiovascular complications can lead to death.

ACQUIRED IMMUNODEFICIENCY SYNDROME

Acquired immunodeficiency syndrome (AIDS) is caused by HIV, which attacks and destroys the T-helper lymphocytes (CD4 +). The T-helper lymphocytes are the cells that direct the immune response to viral, bacterial, and fungal infections and remove some malignant cells from the body. There are four distinct stages in AIDS:

1. Early stage: the patient has symptoms similar to those of influenza; there is rapid reproduction of the virus
2. Middle period: may last for years, with few symptoms; there is slow reproduction of the virus and loss of T4 cells
3. Period of transition with symptoms
4. Crisis period: may last months or years.

Transmission of HIV is by contact with infected blood or sexual contact with an infected person. The virus cannot be transmitted through casual contact. The diagnosis of any STD increases the statistical risk of HIV infection by 300%.

Because not all persons who test positive for HIV develop AIDS immediately, the Centers for Disease Control and Prevention have established criteria that places patients under AIDS surveillance. The most significant of these criteria for adolescents and adults is a CD4 + T-lymphocyte count of fewer than 200 cells/μL (the normal count is 600–1,200 cells/μL), or less than 14% of total lymphocytes, and, for women, the addition of invasive cervical cancer.[3]

Infants usually are infected through the placenta during prenatal life, in the birth process when contaminated by the mother's blood, or through breast-feeding. Children and teens also can be infected through sexual abuse. Adolescents are most often infected through intimate heterosexual or homosexual relations and through intravenous drug use. Some hemophiliacs who received blood products before 1985 were infected, but safeguards are now in place and the blood supply has become much safer.

Although most children with AIDS are between the ages of 1 and 4 years, an alarming increase has occurred among adolescents since 1990, causing great concern in those who work with adolescents. African-American adolescents have a disproportionately high rate of AIDS. In April 1992, the House Select Committee on Children, Youth, and Families completed a study entitled "A Decade of Denial; Teens and AIDS in America," stating that HIV "is spreading unchecked among the nation's adolescents, regardless of where they live or their economic status." Exactly how many teens are HIV positive is unknown; however, the number of those diagnosed increased more than six times between 1989 and 1992 and is currently continuing to rise. Reporting methods were changed in 1993 to include any person reported to have a CD4 + cell count of less than 200/μL, greatly increasing the numbers reported.

Teenagers' attitude of **impunity** (the belief that nothing can hurt them) and the increasing rate of sexual activity in this age group, often involving multiple partners, contribute to the fear that this group will experience widespread illness from HIV. The incubation period for HIV can vary from 3 to 8 years; thus, many who contract the disease in adolescence will not have symptoms until they are in their 20s, when they are at their reproductive peak. The proper use of a condom with spermicide (see Chap. 18) during any type of sexual contact is a must to prevent the spread of HIV. Adolescent girls may have sexual experiences with older men who have had many previous sexual partners. This increases the risk for the girl and, in turn, can increase the risk for any adolescent boy with whom she is sexually intimate. Adolescent boys are also at increased risk if they engage in unprotected homosexual relations, use intravenous drugs, have multiple partners, or have sex with a prostitute.

Cultural influences may play an important role. The adolescent girl often finds it difficult to insist that her partner use a condom. If the partner refuses and claims to be "safe" (uninfected) or protests that the condom decreases his pleasure, she might give in for fear of breaking up the relationship. In addition, in some cultures, the more sexual conquests a boy has, the more manly he is considered.

About 20% to 30% of the infants born to HIV-infected mothers develop AIDS. Although the infants may test positive in the first year of life, testing is not reliable until 15 months of age because the infant may retain antibodies from the mother for this length of time. However, for affected infants younger than 1 year of age, the disease can move rapidly to AIDS and serious complications. Failure to thrive, *Pneumocystis carinii* pneumonia, recurrent bacterial infections, progressive encephalopathy, and malignancy often develop in affected infants. Some of these children progress quickly to terminal illness and death, but with aggressive chemotherapy some of them are living long enough to enter school.

Adolescents manifest the symptoms of HIV much the same as do adults. Females rarely have Kaposi sarcoma, a cancer often seen in homosexual men. Many women, including adolescents, present with a chronic infection of vaginitis caused by *C albicans* that has not responded to local antifungal treatments. These infections may be controlled by oral systemic medications. The female who tests positive for HIV should have a pelvic examination every 6 months to detect early STDs and institute vigorous treatment.

🔖🔖 *Nursing Process for the Adolescent*
🔖🔖 *With AIDS*

ASSESSMENT

When assessing the adolescent with AIDS, gather a complete history, including chief complaint, presenting symptoms, past medical history, immunization status, family history, and social history. Interview the family caregiver if present, but be certain to provide the adolescent with a private interview. The teen may be extremely reluctant to reveal either social or sexual history, especially in the presence of a family member. Review carefully the teen girl's

history of vaginal candidiasis, PID, and sexual activity. Review the teen boy's sexual activity, including partners who are of the same sex or who are drug users. The adolescent may have various emotions, including anger, denial, guilt, and rebelliousness. It is important to accept all these emotions as legitimate reactions to the illness.

During the physical assessment, maintain strict universal precautions. Include vital signs, especially observing for fever, which may indicate infection, and perform a thorough survey of all body systems. Observe for poor skin turgor, rashes or lesions, alopecia, mucous membrane lesions or thrush, weight loss, mental or neurologic changes, respiratory infections or signs of tuberculosis, diarrhea or abdominal pain, vaginal discharge, perineal lesions, or genital warts. Help prepare the adolescent for diagnostic tests that must be performed.

NURSING DIAGNOSES

Following careful assessment of the adolescent, develop nursing diagnoses by thoroughly reviewing the assessment data and identifying the actual or potential problems. Nursing diagnoses may include:

- Risk for Infection related to increased susceptibility secondary to a compromised immune system

- Risk for Infection Transmission related to the infectious nature of the virus (not an approved NANDA diagnosis)

- Risk for Impaired Skin Integrity related to perineal and anal tissue excoriation secondary to genital candidiasis or genital warts

- Pain related to symptoms of the disease

- Altered Nutrition: Less Than Body Requirements, related to anorexia, oral or esophageal lesions, or diarrhea

- Social Isolation related to rejection by others secondary to the diagnosis of AIDS

- Hopelessness related to the diagnosis and prognosis

- Ineffective Family Coping: Compromised related to the diagnosis of AIDS

OUTCOME IDENTIFICATION AND PLANNING

Planning the nursing care of an adolescent with AIDS can be challenging. The adolescent needs much support to accept the diagnosis and move in a positive direction to follow the treatment plan to the best of his or her ability. The nurse can play a critical role in helping the teen understand the treatment and prognosis and their impact on his or her life. Major goals for the adolescent include maintaining the highest level of wellness possible by preventing infection and the spread of the infection, maintaining skin integrity, minimizing pain, improving nutrition, alleviating social isolation, and diminishing a feeling of hopelessness. The primary goal for the family is improving coping skills and helping the teen cope with the illness.

PREVENTING INFECTION. In the health care facility, strict adherence to appropriate infection control measures is extremely important. A primary goal is to teach the adolescent to prevent infections. Teach good handwashing technique; the patient should take care to wash between the fingers and under rings and should use a pump-type soap. He or she should keep nails trimmed to avoid harboring microorganisms under the nails. Teach the teen that skin care includes showering (not a tub bath) with a mild soap (no strong, perfumed soaps), using an emollient cream, and patting the skin dry, avoiding vigorous rubbing.

Raw fruits and vegetables should be washed and peeled or cooked to avoid the danger of bacteria, and meats must be well cooked. The teen must avoid unpasteurized dairy products and foods grown in organic fertilizer.

Instruct the teen to brush the teeth at least three times a day, using a soft toothbrush and a nonabrasive toothpaste. Routine dental care is vital.

The household where the adolescent lives must be cleaned carefully and regularly. A household bleach solution of one part bleach to 10 parts of water is a good solution to use. Particular attention should be paid to the refrigerator, the stove, the oven, and the microwave to prevent contamination of foods during preparation or storage. Household items that may be contaminated should be discarded in double plastic bags to prevent spread to others. Laundry bleach should be used when washing the adolescent's clothing, especially underwear.[4]

Teach the adolescent that pets should be cared for by someone else. Cleaning an aquarium or bird cage or emptying a cat's litter box can expose the adolescent to opportunistic organisms that will attack the compromised immune system. Help the adolescent learn to avoid persons who have any infectious disease. Advise him or her that prompt attention to an apparently minor infection helps avoid more serious illness. The adolescent with AIDS should not receive any live vaccine immunizations but should continue to receive other immunizations, as indicated.

PREVENTING TRANSMISSION. The good hygienic practices necessary to protect the teen from an acquired or opportunistic infection also help prevent transmission of the virus to others. The adolescent needs counseling about sexual practices. One of the most emotionally difficult tasks for the adolescent may be to list sexual contacts. This is a delicate matter that must be approached in a nonjudgmental, sympathetic manner, but the teen needs to understand that anyone with whom he or she has been sexually intimate may be infected and must be identified. In reviewing sexual contacts, the teen may find that the sexual partner from whom he or she contracted the virus already knew that he or she was infected. Infection with HIV does not necessarily mean that the teen was promiscuous. The adolescent may have been sexually intimate with only one person, and that person may have assured the teen that he or she was not infected. The adolescent may be extremely angry about exposure by a trusted person.

Teach the adolescent safe sex practices. The adolescent needs to understand that he or she is protecting not only future sexual partners from contracting the disease but also himself or herself from contracting other strains of the virus. Both boys and girls need to have complete instructions on the use of condoms and spermicide (see Chap. 18). The adolescent must not be sexually intimate with anyone without using a condom, no matter what kind of argument the other person uses. Also, the teen needs to learn that HIV is transmitted through vaginal intercourse, oral–genital contact, anal intercourse, or any contact with blood or body fluids, including menstrual discharge. The teen who practices oral–genital sex must learn to use a dental dam (a square of latex worn in the mouth to prevent contact of body fluids with mucous membranes of the mouth).

The adolescent girl needs counseling about pregnancy. The probability of transmitting the virus to her unborn child may be as high as 30%, and there is currently no way to determine if she will pass the virus to her child. She must consider that even if her infant is not infected, she will probably not live to see the child reach adulthood. All of these considerations are overwhelming, and the adolescent needs continuous support to understand, accept, and deal with them.

A discussion of the teen's use of illicit, injectable drugs is important. Counsel the adolescent about the importance of stopping drug use. However, the reality is that he or she may not quit, so explain how to sterilize needles using chlorine bleach. A mixture of one part bleach to five parts water should be drawn through the needle into the syringe, flushing two or three times and finally rinsing with water. Remember that the adolescent has the right to decide how to conduct his or her life, and remain nonjudgmental through all contacts with the teen.

PROTECTING SKIN INTEGRITY. Skin lesions are common symptoms of many STDs. The adolescent must report any new skin lesion to the health care provider for diagnosis and immediate treatment. The best preventive measure is to follow careful infection control measures, including careful handwashing, and to protect skin integrity by using skin emollients to guard against dryness, avoiding harsh, perfumed soaps, and guarding against injury to the skin. In advanced disease, nursing measures are implemented to protect and pad pressure points and improve peripheral circulation.

RELIEVING PAIN. Pain is caused by several manifestations of AIDS. Skin and mucous membrane lesions may be very painful. Topical anesthetic solutions, such as viscous lidocaine, and meticulous mouth care can relieve pain caused by oral mucous membrane infections. Smoking, alcohol, and spicy or acidic foods irritate the oral mucous membranes and often cause additional pain. Pelvic inflammatory disease, a common complication of STDs, is usually accompanied by abdominal pain. The adolescent with respiratory complications also has bouts of chest pain. Administer analgesics to relieve pain and use all appropriate nursing measures to help the adolescent be more comfortable. As the disease develops, the pain may be greater, and every effort must be made to provide comfort.

IMPROVING NUTRITION. Anorexia, or a poor appetite, is a common problem of the patient with AIDS. Dehydration, diarrhea, infection, malabsorption, oral candidiasis, and some drugs also can contribute to the adolescent's poor state of nutrition. Malnutrition can cause additional problems with increased and more serious infections. The adolescent's diet must be more nutritious and higher in calories than normal. Several small meals supplemented by high-calorie, high-protein snacks may be desirable. Dietary supplements, such as Ensure and Isocal, also may be useful. Explore the adolescent's food likes and dislikes and develop a meal plan using this information. If malnutrition becomes severe, the adolescent may need tube feedings or parenteral nutrition.

EASING SOCIAL ISOLATION AND HOPELESS-NESS. The adolescent may fear having others know about the illness because he or she anticipates a negative reaction from peers and family. Provide the teen with supportive counseling and guidance to help him or her deal with these fears. The teen may not feel that he or she can tell the family for fear of rejection. In fact, many families have rejected their children who have AIDS, but many others have risen to the challenge; although they may tell the teenager they do not like his or her behavior, they continue to offer love and support. The adolescent may need support to help tell social acquaintances as well. If there is an adolescent HIV support group available through the hospital or community, the teen should be referred to it. Adolescents often find that adult support groups are not as helpful because the adults' needs are different from those of adolescents. The adolescent is actually facing death before having a chance to experience adulthood.

The fact that the adolescent is facing an early death may give him or her a special sense of purpose to "spread the word" to others. The adolescent needs support and guidance to set priorities and must have help to accomplish these goals. School officials may need to be told, and the family can be helpful during this time. If the family is not supportive, the adolescent needs even more support from health care providers.

HELPING THE FAMILY TO COPE. The adolescent must be involved in telling the family about the diagnosis if they do not already know. The sexual activity of adolescent children is a topic many families have a difficult time dealing with, especially if the activity is homosexual or promiscuous. The family caregivers usually need support as much as the adolescent does. They often are devastated by the prospect of their child's illness and early death. If the adolescent is pregnant or has a child, the family also must con-

sider the future of that child. For the family who plays a supportive role in the adolescent's life, the period after diagnosis is a difficult one. Teach the family as much about the disease as possible. They must learn how to prevent the spread of the virus among family members and opportunistic infections and must be taught about treatments and medications, nutrition guidelines, and the signs and symptoms to be alert for. Stress the importance of reporting even minor complications to the health care provider, and suggest ways to help support the adolescent (Table 19-3).

Although teaching the adolescent and the family all of this information is necessary, remember that a person can absorb only so much information at one time. To teach them successfully—and to be sure they understand the information—do not present too much information at one time. Give the family and the adolescent written materials that repeat the information, and review it verbally with them, asking questions and clarifying information until they show evidence of clear understanding of the concepts they need to know. While teaching, be sensitive to unspoken feelings and questions and carefully bring them into the discussion to provide the entire family with the best possible support and information.

EVALUATION: GOALS AND OUTCOME CRITERIA

- *Goal*: The adolescent will experience minimal risk of infection.
  Criteria: The adolescent practices good hygiene measures and identifies ways to prevent infection and ways to protect his or her health at home.

- *Goal*: The adolescent will not spread the disease to others.
  Criteria: The adolescent practices infection control measures and identifies sexual partners and safer sexual practices.

- *Goal*: The adolescent's skin integrity will remain intact.
  Criteria: The adolescent protects the skin and mucous membranes and promptly reports skin lesions or infections.

- *Goal*: The adolescent will experience minimal pain from complications of the disease.
  Criteria: The adolescent learns to manage pain and rests comfortably with minimal discomfort.

- *Goal*: The adolescent's food intake will meet his or her nutritional needs.
  Criteria: The adolescent eats nutritionally sound meals, includes frequent small meals in the food plan, and maintains his or her weight.

- *Goal*: The adolescent will not experience social isolation.
  Criteria: The adolescent voices fears about social isolation and makes and carries out plans to maintain relationships.

TABLE 19-3. Counseling Patients at Different Stages of HIV Infection

Stage	Focus
Immediately after learning of positive HIV test (regardless of disease stage)	Assist patient in accepting diagnosis and encourage him or her to verbalize feelings (anger, fear, hopelessness, etc.) Explain the difference between being HIV positive and having AIDS Explain how HIV is spread (by direct contact with infected body fluids—usually through sex, sharing needles, or blood transfusion) Counsel the patient on how to avoid transmitting the virus to others or contracting yet another strain Teach the patient some safer sex strategies, such as using condoms, dental dams; use role-playing to demonstrate how to negotiate the use of these barriers Explain the pros and cons of contraceptives, such as intrauterine devices, oral contraceptives, and nonoxynol-9 in women with HIV Discuss why and how to notify sex partners of infection; explain that partners need counseling, testing, and, if HIV positive, referral for treatment; offer to help with the notification process, if necessary Discuss pregnancy and childbearing, as appropriate; explain rates of transmission from mother to newborn; suggest early prenatal care if patient is or becomes pregnant If patient uses illicit, injectable drugs, explain how to sterilize needles with chlorine bleach: use a 5-to-1 ratio of water to bleach, draw the mixture up into the syringe two or three times, then flush with plain water Discuss the importance of primary health care, and provide appropriate referrals Provide educational literature on HIV, and refer patient to local support services and rehabilitation programs
Asymptomatic, CD4 cells >500 cells/μL blood	Review health maintenance activities: the need for regular gynecologic examinations and Pap smears, adequate diet, regular exercise, 8 to 10 hours sleep/night, cutting back on alcohol, tobacco, and use of recreational drugs (if not ready to stop use) Stress the importance of health care follow-up Assess the patient's support systems: Does he or she have friends or relatives who can help out when symptoms develop? Does he or she have physical and economic access to health care? Refer to support groups, financial assistance programs
Asymptomatic, CD4 cells >500 cells/μL blood, on antiretroviral medicines	Discuss prescribed drugs: indications, schedules doses, how to recognize and manage side effects Discuss long-term family plans, especially arrangements for child (or children) at the parent's incapacity or death
Visible symptoms: weight loss, thinning hair, darkening nails, skin rashes	Encourage small, frequent meals, or suggest nutritional supplements, such as Ensure, to prevent weight loss Offer strategies for masking signs of illness, such as bright nail polish and attractive scarves or wigs Explore ways for the patient to initiate age-appropriate discussion of HIV status with family Counsel patient to specify guardianship for any child he or she has in a legal will Discuss advanced directive alternatives available in your state, such as do-not-resuscitate status and health care proxy options
After hospitalization for opportunistic infection	Reassess home support—the need to call in a visiting nurse or volunteer buddy Counsel patient to finalize do-not-resuscitate status or health care proxy arrangements per state
End stage	Provide physical comfort through frequent turning on an air mattress, hydration therapy, lubricating skin massages Acknowledge the anticipatory grief of family members and friends

Kelly PJ, Holman S. The new face of AIDS. AJN 93(3)26–34, 1993. Used with permission. All rights reserved.

■ *Goal*: The adolescent will make adjustments to his or her future expectations.

Criteria: The adolescent expresses feelings about his or her future, seeks support from others, and begins to make realistic future plans.

■ *Goal*: The family will show evidence of coping with the illness and supporting the teen.

Criteria: The family expresses anxieties, voices understanding of the illness, and supports the adolescent in future plans.

Adolescent Pregnancy

The rate of adolescent pregnancy is about one in 10 girls, resulting in 1 million adolescent pregnancies each year. About half of these result in live births; the remainder are aborted spontaneously or electively. The rate of adolescent pregnancy is higher in the United States than in any other country that keeps accurate statistics. In 1989, more than two thirds of the infants born to teenagers were born to single mothers,[5] and this statistic remains unchanged more than seven years later. When this statistic is coupled with the fact that single-parent children are more likely to live in poverty, the magnitude of the problem becomes clear.

Many factors may contribute to the high rate of teen sexual activity and pregnancy. Adolescents are continuously bombarded with sex-oriented media. Teenagers have easy access to cars. They have less parental supervision, including after school, when many parents are still at work. Society is mobile, and few people know their neighbors or feel responsible for them, so neighbors do not report a teen's activity as they might in closely knit neighborhoods. Many teenagers have sex with no concern about the potential outcome. On the other hand, a girl may want to become pregnant to prove she is "grown up," to prove her femininity, to show self-assertion or hostility toward her family, or to fulfill a desire to have a baby who will love her and whom she can love. Adolescents from low socioeconomic groups may see motherhood as a form of economic survival with allotments of money, food stamps, and medical and dental care. They may see this as a way to escape economic oppression. Unfortunately, they believe this will provide economic and personal independence. More than one of these reasons, or others, may be involved in any teenage pregnancy.

The pregnant adolescent may have a poor record of success in school, a low self-image, poor family relationships, and inadequate financial means. She commonly receives inadequate prenatal care. These factors place her future and the future of her unborn infant in jeopardy.

Pregnancy is associated with its own developmental tasks, and these collide with the normal developmental tasks of adolescence, often with unsatisfactory results. As an adolescent, she is seeking independence; as an expectant mother with inadequate resources, she remains dependent. She is seeking identity, but the only identity she gains is that of a young, confused, at-risk mother-to-be. Her acute awareness of body image must accept the silhouette of pregnancy, certainly not in keeping with the slim figure desired by most adolescent girls. Pregnancy brings about many hormonal changes, on top of those that occur during adolescence. The adolescent's lack of knowledge about pregnancy and parenthood may cause her to have increased, unrealistic fears about herself and her pregnancy. As an adolescent, she is still trying to clarify her values and develop a positive self-concept, but the pregnancy will have a negative impact on her self-concept, especially if the father of the infant or her parents reject her or her pregnancy.

Once pregnancy has been confirmed, the adolescent must decide whether to terminate the pregnancy by elective abortion or to carry it to term. If she chooses to have the baby, she must then decide whether to keep it or relinquish it for adoption. These are difficult choices, particularly for a frightened, often unsupported, immature girl. Health professionals must provide the facts and guidance that will enable the girl to make an informed choice. School nurses, social workers, teachers, and counselors may be her only resources. Most pregnant adolescents choose to keep their babies, whether they marry the father or not. In many instances, the grandmother or grandparents of the newborn help raise the infant.

In most schools, the pregnant adolescent is encouraged to stay in school rather than drop out (Fig. 19-4). If this is not the case, the girl should be encouraged to continue her education elsewhere, even if it means relocation. Some urban schools sponsor prenatal classes and child care programs intended to encourage, support, and provide assistance to the girl in continuing her education throughout her pregnancy and parenthood.

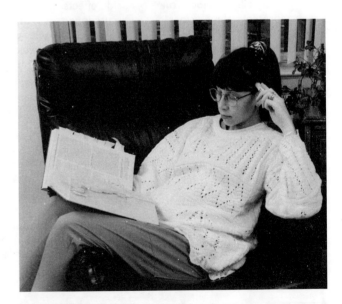

Figure 19-4
Although many adolescent mothers do not complete high school, some are able to continue and complete their education.

A Personal Glimpse

Easter vacation of my junior year, I told my mom that I hadn't gotten my period for a long time. She asked me if there was any chance of me being pregnant. I said, "I don't know. Maybe." So we went to the store to get a pregnancy test. I took it and it turned dark pink immediately. When Mom told me I was pregnant, an immediate fear went through me and I started to cry. She gave me a hug and told me that I had to tell Brian (the father).

When I told him, I began to cry, because I thought for sure he was going to leave me. We sat down to talk about what we were going to do. I don't believe in abortion, but I just thought to myself, "I'm only 16! I didn't even get a chance to run around!"

But I decided to have the baby and not give it up for adoption. I kept thinking about getting fat and whether I'd be heavy after I had the baby. I cut way back on what I was eating so I wouldn't gain any weight. But when I went for a checkup they told me I had to start eating because the baby wouldn't develop right if I didn't.

I was too scared to tell my dad, so I got Mom to call and tell him. He was so mad at me, and he just wanted to grab hold of Brian and put him in jail, since he was 18. He didn't want me around him and said I was just following in my mother's footsteps and that I'd probably quit school. But then, after a couple of months, Dad talked to Brian and me and he was excited about the baby. I told my dad I wasn't quitting school and that I was planning to go to nursing school.

My mom and grandparents were happy but they wished it wouldn't have happened to me, being so young. They all got pregnant young, too, so they knew what it was like.

I didn't want anyone at school to know because I thought everyone would just look down on me or just talk about me and call me a slut. I hid it the rest of my junior year, but by senior year needless to say I couldn't hide it anymore. The teachers were great. They didn't treat me any differently. I felt funny, though, because I was the only pregnant girl in school.

My girlfriends didn't care. In fact, they were excited and made bets on whether it would be a boy or a girl. Some of the guys didn't really care and still talked to me, but most of them just ignored me. I think that bugged me the most, because before I got pregnant the guys would be around me all the time. One guy who had been like a brother to me didn't even talk to me—maybe a "hi" now and then, but that was it.

Before I had my baby, I was scared of the unknown, but everything went great. Brian was even with me in the delivery room. And after I had her, I was so excited because I could still fit into my old jeans and I didn't even get stretch marks. Must have been the cocoa butter I rubbed on my stomach and butt all the time.

Sarah, age 19

Adolescent clinics are beginning to play a particularly important role in the management of teenage pregnancy. Many of these clinics use a team approach to work with the girl, perhaps the young father, and the girl's parents; the physician, nurse practitioner or nurse midwife, nutritionist, and social worker offer understanding, supportive care, teaching, and counseling during the prenatal period and follow-up care after delivery. These clinics help reduce some of the risk factors common in a teen pregnancy by providing prenatal care in a comfortable, nonthreatening atmosphere. If the adolescent has chosen abortion, these clinics also can provide follow-up care and contraceptive counseling. Adolescent clinics offer care for STDs, HIV, substance abuse, and other adolescent health problems.

The adolescent has a higher incidence of pregnancy-induced hypertension, which places the infant at risk for inadequate circulation and the mother at risk for convulsions and death. The infant is more likely to be of low birth

COMMUNICATIONS BOX

Jenna, a 14-year-old, has come to the family planning clinic. She is in the exam room. Minimal information has been collected. She is picking at her clothes and seems very nervous.

INEFFECTIVE COMMUNICATION

Nurse: Hello, Jenna. I need to get some more information from you.

Jenna: (Becoming somewhat defiant) Why do you have to ask so many questions?

Nurse: You have to give us background information so we can take care of you.

Jenna: Well, I don't want my family to know that I was here.

Nurse: Oh, but we have to contact your parent or caregiver.

Jenna: (Loudly, with determination) Oh, no, you won't. I'll just not stay here if that's what happens.

Nurse: You'll have to cooperate with us, Jenna.

Jenna: (Very loud) Oh, no, I don't! I'm getting out of here.

The nurse has lost in this episode. Jenna will not be cooperative with him/her. Jenna gave many clues to her level of anxiety at the beginning by picking at her clothes and showing general signs of nervousness. The nurse did not read or at least did not respond to the signals. As Jenna showed more signs of anxiety by openly becoming defiant, the nurse simply dug in and plodded on. By not being sensitive to Jenna's signals, the nurse never even found out what the teen wanted.

EFFECTIVE COMMUNICATION

Nurse: Hello, Jenna. My name is Mrs. Kelley. Can you tell me how I can help you today?

Jenna: (Hesitantly) Well, I think I might be pregnant.

Nurse: Tell me what makes you suspect that.

Jenna: I haven't had my period for two months.

Nurse: Can you remember when you had your first period?

Jenna: I was 10 years old, I think.

Nurse: (Warmly) Good, you do remember. Jenna, can you tell me how sexually active you've been? I mean, how many sexual partners, and how often.

Jenna: I only have had one boyfriend. We maybe have sex a couple times a month.

Nurse: How does thinking that you may be pregnant make you feel?

Jenna: Scared. And excited, too.

Nurse: I can understand that. I would like to do an examination and take some tests, so we know just whether you are pregnant, or if there is some other reason for your delayed period. We can deal with it one step at a time.

Jenna: OK.

Throughout this interview, the nurse treated Jenna with respect and concern, starting by simply telling Jenna her name. This gives Jenna the feeling of value. Because Mrs. Kelley read Jenna's nervousness and showed her concern with gentle, open-ended questions, Jenna responded, giving the information and cooperation that were needed. Mrs. Kelley in no way was accusing Jenna of anything, and carefully stated her questions to convey that message.

weight, with possibly fatal complications. Nutrition of the mother and the fetus may be severely compromised, and there may be social problems that will affect the mother and the infant for their entire lives.

Nurses who work with pregnant adolescents must resolve their own feelings to maintain a helpful, nonjudgmental attitude. These teenagers are fragile emotionally and mentally during this crisis. The nurse must develop a trusting relationship with the adolescent. Knowledge and understanding of adolescent psychosocial development are essential. Never fall into the habit of stereotyping adolescent mothers. As nurses work with the adolescent and develop a trusting relationship, they can help the girl look to the future and guide her in making realistic plans. The pregnant adolescent has many problems to face and needs strong support, but with good prenatal and postnatal care and planning, the experience can become an opportunity for growth.

ADOLESCENT FATHERHOOD

Adolescent fathers are often overlooked in discussions about adolescent pregnancy. However, more emphasis recently has been placed on the adolescent father's role. Several factors affect the father's role in the pregnancy. The adolescent girl who has had multiple partners may not be sure who the father is, or she may not care enough for the father to want to involve him in her pregnancy and her future. Many boys deny their role in the pregnancy or lose interest in the girl when she announces her pregnancy. All these factors help determine the degree of responsibility that the teenage father takes. When a cooperative, interested father is involved in education about the pregnancy, parenthood, and future contraception, a better outlook for the couple can be expected. The adolescent couple commonly has serious financial problems, often has unrealistic expectations, and may look forward to years of struggle. Support from the families of both adolescents can help improve the couple's future. The newborn who has two well-informed parents with a good support system clearly has a greater advantage than one who does not.

MALADAPTIVE RESPONSES TO THE STRESSES OF ADOLESCENCE

Substance Abuse

Substance abuse is the misuse of an addictive substance that changes the mental state of the user. The addictive substances commonly abused are tobacco, alcohol, and controlled or illicit drugs. Adolescents, influenced by peers and, in some instances, family adults, use drugs and alcohol to avoid facing their problems, escape and forget the pain of life as they see it, add excitement to social events, or bow to peer pressure. Throughout history, people have

used alcohol and other mood-altering drugs as a means of relieving the tensions and pressures of their lives. Many cultures still sanction use of some of these substances but object to their *abuse* (excessive use, or use in a way that is medically, socially, or culturally unacceptable).

The unfortunate fact is that frequent use or abuse of these substances can lead to addiction or **dependence** (a compulsive need to use a substance for its satisfying or pleasurable effects). Dependence may be psychological, physical, or both. Psychological dependence means that the substance is desired for the effects or sensations it produces—alertness, euphoria, relaxation, a sense of well-being, and a false sense of control over problems. Physical dependence results from drug-induced changes in body tissue function that require the drug for normal activity. The magnitude of physical dependence determines the severity of **withdrawal symptoms** (physical and psychological symptoms that occur when the drug is no longer being used), such as vomiting, chills, tremors, and hallucinations. The symptoms vary with the amount, type, frequency, and duration of drug use. Continued use of an addictive substance can result in **tolerance** (the ability of body tissues to endure and adapt to continued or increased use of a substance), requiring larger doses of the drug to produce the desired effect.

Four stages of use have been identified that help describe the progression of substance abuse (Table 19-4). Using the clues from these stages, the nurse who works in any capacity with adolescents can be more alert to signs of possible substance abuse.

The adolescents at greatest risk of becoming substance abusers are those who:

- Have families in which alcohol or drug abuse is or has been present
- Suffer from abuse, neglect, or loss or have no close relationships as a result of a dysfunctional family
- Have behavior problems, such as aggressiveness, or are excessively rebellious
- Are slow learners or have learning disabilities or attention deficit disorder
- Have problems with depression and low self-esteem.

In some instances, early identification of these factors by family, teachers, counselors, or other caregivers and prompt referral for treatment can help avoid the potential tragedy of substance abuse.

The most effective and least expensive treatment for substance abuse is prevention, beginning with education in the early school years. Information about drugs and about coping with problems without drugs should be provided. "Scare" techniques are completely ineffective because they arouse disbelief and often add the tempting thrill of danger. The impact of educational programs may be diluted if children come from a home where alcohol or other drugs are used by family caregivers.

TABLE 19-4. Progression of Substance Abuse in Adolescents

Stage	Predisposition	Behavior	Family Reaction
Stage 1. Experimentation, Learning the Mood Swing			
Infrequent use of alcohol/ marijuana	Curiosity	Learning the mood	Often unaware
No consequences	Peer pressure	Feels good	Denial
Some fear of use	Attempt to assume adult role	Positive reinforcement	
Low tolerance		Can return to normal	
Stage 2. Seeking the Mood Swing			
Increasing frequency in use of various drugs	Impress others	Using to get high	Attempts at elimination
Minimal defensiveness	Social function	Pride in amount consumed	Blaming others
Tolerance	Modeling adult behavior	Used to relieve feelings (ie, anxieties of dating)	
		Denial of problem	
Stage 3. Preoccupation with the Mood Swing			
Peer group activities revolve around use	Using to get loaded, not just high	Begins to violate values and rules	Conspiracy of silence
Steady supply		Use before and during school	Confrontation
Possible dealing		Use despite consequences	Reorganization with or without affected person
Few or no straight friends		Solitary use	
Consequences frequent		Trouble with school	
		Overdoses, "bad trips," blackouts	
		Promises to cut down or attempts to quit	
		Protection of supply, hides use from peers	
		Deterioration in physical condition	
Stage 4. Using to Feel Normal			
Continue to use despite adverse outcomes	Use to feel normal	Daily use	Frustration
Loss of control		Failure to meet expectations	Anger
Inability to stop		Loss of control	May give up
Compulsion		Paranoia	
		Suicide gestures, self-hate	
		Physical deterioration (poor eating and sleep habits)	

Adgar H. Adolescent drug abuse. In Oski FA, ed. Principles and practice of pediatrics 2nd ed. Philadelphia: JB Lippincott, 1994.

ALCOHOL ABUSE

In many parts of American culture, drinking alcoholic beverages is considered acceptable and desirable social behavior. Although the purchase of alcohol is legally restricted to adults older than 21 years of age in all states and the District of Columbia, it is available in many homes and, consequently, is the first drug most adolescents try. Alcohol is the most commonly abused drug among adolescents. **Alcohol abuse** occurs when a person ingests a quantity sufficient to cause intoxication (drunkenness). **Alcoholism** (chronic alcohol abuse or dependence) has reached epidemic proportions in America—an estimated 4.6 million teenagers have a drinking problem.[6]

Drinking often begins in the late school-age years and increases in frequency throughout adolescence. Some adolescents use alcohol in combination with marijuana and other drugs, potentiating the effects of both substances and increasing the probability of intoxication.

Alcoholism is costly in dollars and in damage to the lives of alcohol abusers and their families. During adolescence, alcohol abuse is closely linked to automobile accidents. A car is another symbol of adult status and a means to escape adult supervision. Drinking with friends before or while driving often has tragic results. Most states have a standard of blood alcohol content of 0.1% as the level to determine charges of driving under the influence, but 12 states have lowered the limit to 0.08%. The point that many adolescents miss is that fine motor control and judgment are affected at even lower levels, and driving ability may be decreased. The number of fatal alcohol-related accidents involving adolescents has decreased since all states have set 21 years as the legal age for drinking, but it still remains high.

Adolescents who receive treatment and counseling for problem drinking are more likely to recover than adults who have been problem drinkers over a long period. However, adolescents are difficult to treat due to their feelings of immortality and the rapid progression of the disease in adolescents.

Treatment   Alcoholism is not a weakness of character but a major, chronic, progressive, and potentially fatal disease process that affects every organ of the body, mental health, and social competence. Alcoholism is thought to be inherited, so children with a family history of alcoholism may be prone to alcohol problems. Treatment is lengthy and expensive and has no chance of success until the alcoholic acknowledges the problem and his or her helplessness to deal with it.

Treatment begins with detoxification ("drying out") and management of withdrawal symptoms. After that, a well-balanced diet, high-potency vitamins (especially vitamin B), and plenty of rest help eliminate harmful side effects of the disease.

Counseling to identify and address the problems that led to compulsive drinking is an essential part of treatment. Many counselors who work with alcoholic patients are people who are recovering from a drinking problem themselves. This experience gives the counselor additional insight and empathy for the problem and the victim and adds credibility to the counseling offered.

Alcoholics Anonymous (AA), the best known of all self-help groups, offers fellowship and understanding to the compulsive drinker. There are chapters in every sizable community, and many have special programs for adolescents as well as for families of alcoholics (Alateen, Al-Anon). Anyone who has a desire to stop drinking is welcomed into AA and is helped to stay sober by taking it "one day at a time." Recovery from alcoholism is a lifetime matter. The earlier the problem is diagnosed, the better the person's chances to respond to treatment. Ongoing support from health professionals, peers, family, and community is essential to successful treatment.

TOBACCO ABUSE

Tobacco is the second most commonly abused drug among adolescents. *Any* use of tobacco is abuse. More than 70% of young people try tobacco, by either smoking or chewing.[7] Many adolescents smoke because it gives them a feeling of maturity. Threats of long-term physical illnesses are far enough in the future that adolescents tend to ignore

them. Many elementary and secondary schools have developed programs that warn children of the dangers of smoking, but the danger seems distant, and children believe that they can quit any time they want to. The more immediate result of smoking that may stir interest in adolescents is the fact that their hair, breath, and clothes smell bad. Adolescents also have strong feelings of fairness and justice, so they may respond to the fact that children who are around persons who smoke are at increased risk for respiratory illness and cancer.

The use of "smokeless tobacco" (snuff or chewing tobacco) has increased steadily among adolescent males in the last 10 years. These teenagers believe that they are not damaging their lungs, but this type of tobacco use can cause mouth, lip, and throat cancers that are disfiguring and life-threatening.

Adolescents whose family caregivers smoke are especially prone to become smokers, and they have difficulty accepting the fact that they are seriously endangering themselves by smoking. Most hospitals, schools, and public buildings have adopted no-smoking policies. Perhaps the pressure of society will help deter smoking in the future. There is an effort at the federal level to discourage adolescents from beginning to smoke, but adolescents do not seem to be responding to the warnings. This may be due in part to the above-mentioned attitude among adolescents that nothing can hurt them.

MARIJUANA ABUSE

The third most commonly abused drug among adolescents is marijuana. In 1995, 21.2% of high school seniors used marijuana currently, up from the 14% of seniors who claimed they were current users of marijuana and hashish in 1992. Although marijuana use is lower than in the peak year of 1979, the rate of adolescent smokers has been increasing since 1992. More than 40% have tried the drug at some time.[7] Many adolescents believe that marijuana smoking is not risky.

The effects of marijuana are mostly behavioral. It affects judgment, sense of time, and motivation. These effects make driving hazardous and may even cause hallucinations at higher doses. In addition, marijuana smoke is three to five times more carcinogenic than cigarette smoke. The marijuana available today may be three to five times more potent than that smoked in the 1960s.[8] Because marijuana is illegal, there is no manufacturing control over it, and the user has no idea where it came from or the additives that may have been used. Nurses must make every effort to inform adolescents about the dangers of marijuana and to discourage them from using it.

COCAINE ABUSE

Although cocaine does not rank among the first three drugs most commonly used by adolescents, it is an extremely dangerous drug. Use of cocaine and its derivative, "crack," had decreased among adolescents after the peak in 1985, but statistics since 1992 indicate that cocaine use is no longer decreasing. Cocaine and crack use can be found everywhere, from inner cities to rural neighborhoods.

Cocaine, a fine, white, powdery substance, directly affects the brain cells, causing a physical and psychological effect. It usually is inhaled or smoked and is absorbed through the mucous membranes into the bloodstream. The physical results are an increase in pulse, respirations, blood pressure, and temperature. The psychological effect is a feeling of euphoria and increased sociability. The high is reached in about 20 minutes and lasts 20 to 30 minutes. In contrast, crack enters the bloodstream in about 30 seconds, with a fast, powerful, but short high that lasts only about 5 minutes. As a result of the rapid, short high from crack, users tend to seek repeated highs over a short period, decreasing the time it takes to become addicted. Because of the rapid absorption of crack, immediate cardiac arrest can occur from its use. After smoking crack, the user may experience a "crash" that causes depression. To relieve this depression, crack users turn to alcohol and marijuana. This multiple use further complicates the effects of the drug. Some cocaine users inject cocaine to obtain a faster high and thus add to their risk of contracting HIV from contaminated needles.

Nurses must stress to adolescents the danger of using cocaine and crack. School education programs should start at the elementary level. Nurses can perform a community service by volunteering to present programs to local schoolchildren. Children and adolescents must be alerted to the dangers of these drugs and taught ways to refuse the offer of drugs. A complete drug-education program also should include activities that help the students increase their feeling of self-worth.

NARCOTICS

The most commonly abused narcotics are morphine and heroin. These drugs decrease anger, sex drive, and hunger by producing a dreamlike, euphoric state. Highly addictive and extremely expensive, narcotics result in teenage prostitution, pushing (selling) drugs, and robbery as a means to support the drug habit. As mentioned earlier, any of the drugs that are injected subject adolescents to the added risk of contracting HIV from using contaminated needles.

Although heroin use, in actual numbers, is lower than that of other illicit drugs, adolescents' use of heroin has increased, due to several factors. In general, there is a decrease among teens in the perceived danger of drug use. This trend seems to be evident across the entire scope of illicit drug use. Since heroin is now available in a form that can be smoked, the threat of HIV infection is no longer a deterrent.

OTHER ABUSED DRUGS

Other mood-altering drugs commonly abused by adolescents include psychotomimetic (psychedelic) drugs, hypnotics, amphetamines, and analgesics.

Psychedelic drugs, although not addictive in a physical sense, can create a psychological dependence from the hallucinations that result. This category of drugs includes LSD, PCP ("angel dust"), psilocybin (derived from mushrooms), mescaline, DMT (derived from plants), and airplane glue. Effects can include intoxication, "bad trips," and overdosage.

Hypnotics are as addictive as narcotics, and withdrawal from them must be carefully controlled to prevent delirium, seizures, or death. Barbiturates, glutethimide (Doriden), ethchlorvynol (Placidyl), and methaqualone (Quaalude) are the most commonly abused drugs in this group and are sometimes used with alcohol, increasing the intoxicating effects such as sleepiness, slurred speech, and impaired cognitive and motor function.

Amphetamines ("uppers") produce increased alertness, wakefulness, reduced awareness of fatigue, and increased confidence and energy. Although not physically addicting, they encourage psychological dependence and are abused by millions of Americans, many of whom become trapped in a destructive cycle of uppers and "downers" (barbiturates).

Analgesics, particularly those combining phenacetin, caffeine, and a hypnotic, often are abused by adolescents. Empirin and Fiorinal are two examples. Chronic abuse can result in blood and kidney disorders.

Anabolic steroids are not mood-altering drugs, but their abuse among athletes is a cause for great concern. Adolescent athletes take the anabolic steroids to build up muscle mass in the belief that the drug will increase their athletic ability. These athletes take megadoses of illegally obtained drugs. Other adolescents may take them to build muscles and to achieve a "manly" appearance they believe will make them more attractive. The side effects of euphoria and decreased fatigue make these drugs even more inviting to adolescents. Some use also has been reported in high school female athletes.

The use of excessively large doses of steroids may cause **gynecomastia** (excessive development of mammary glands in the male) or premature fusion of the long bones, stunting growth in the adolescent who has not yet completed growth. Liver damage, predisposition to atherosclerosis, acne, hypertension, aggressiveness, and psychotic and manic symptoms also may result.[9] School programs about drug abuse should include the topic of anabolic steroid abuse.

Treatment   The best treatment for the abuse of all of these drugs is prevention. When prevention is ineffective, emergency care and long-term treatment become necessary. An overdose or a "bad trip" may force the adolescent to seek treatment. Emergency measures may even require artificial ventilation and oxygenation to restore normal respiration.

Long-term treatment involves many health professionals, such as psychiatric nurses, psychologists or psychiatrists, social workers, drug rehabilitation counselors, and community health nurses. The teen is an important member of the treatment team and must admit the problem and the need for help and be willing to take an active part in treatment. Both outpatient and inpatient treatment programs are available. Many of these programs are geared specifically to adolescents. The human services section of the local telephone directory provides specific listings.

Suicide

Suicide is the third leading cause of death in adolescents 10 to 19 years of age, falling just short of the homicide rate (see Fig. 18-9 in Chap. 18). Because some deaths reported as accidents, particularly one-car accidents, are thought to be suicides, the rate actually may be higher. Adolescent males commit suicide four times more often than girls, but girls attempt suicide five times more often than boys. Boys use more violent means of committing suicide than girls and therefore are more often successful. Suicide is twice as common among Native American adolescents as among whites and twice as common among white adolescents as among African-Americans.[10]

Adolescents who have attempted suicide once have a high risk of attempting it again, perhaps more effectively. Attempted suicide rarely occurs without warning and usually is preceded by a long history of emotional problems, difficulty in forming relationships, feelings of rejection, and low self-esteem. Loss of one or both parents through death or divorce, a family history that includes suicide of one or more members, and lack of success in academic or athletic performance are other common contributing factors. To this history is added one or more of the normal developmental crises of adolescence: difficulty in establishing independence, identity crisis, lack of intimate relationships, breakdown in family communication, a sense of alienation, and a conflict that interferes with problem solving. The adolescent's situation may be further complicated by an unwanted or unplanned pregnancy, drug addiction, or physical or sexual abuse, leading to depression and a feeling of total hopelessness.

Health professionals involved with adolescents and family caregivers must be aware of the factors that place a teen at risk for suicide, as well as the hints that signal an impending suicide attempt (see Family Teaching: Adolescent Suicide Warning Signs for Caregivers). Some of these desperate youngsters will verbalize their hopelessness with statements such as, "I won't be around much longer" or "After Monday, it won't matter anyhow." They may begin giving away prized possessions or appear suddenly elated after a long period of acting dejected. Never ignore these behaviors, and make an effort to ensure the teen's safety until counseling and treatment resources are in place. Strive to help the teen understand that although suicide is an option in problem solving, it is a final option, and there are other options that are not so final. Be aware of the community resources, such as hotlines and counselors,

Family Teaching
Adolescent Suicide Warning Signs for Caregivers

Warning Signs in Teen's Behavior

1. Previous suicide attempt
2. Thoughts of wishing to kill self
3. Plans for self-destructive acts
4. Feeling "down in the dumps"
5. Withdrawal from social activities
6. Loss of pleasure in daily activities
7. Change in activity—increase or decrease
8. Poor concentration
9. Complaints of headaches, upset stomach, joint pains, frequent colds
10. Change in eating or sleeping patterns
11. Strong feelings of guilt, inadequacy, hopelessness
12. Preoccupation with thoughts of people dying, getting sick, or being injured
13. Substance abuse
14. Violence, truancy, stealing, or lying
15. Lack of judgment
16. Poor impulse control
17. Rapid swing in appropriateness of expressed emotions
18. Pessimistic view of self and world

Changes in Teen's Interpersonal Relationships

1. Conflicts with peers
2. Loss of boyfriend or girlfriend
3. School problems—behavioral or academic
4. Feelings of great frustration, being misunderstood, or not being part of the group
5. Lack of positive support from family, peers, or others
7. Earlier suicide of family member, friend, or classmate
8. Separations, deaths, births, moves, or serious illnesses in the family

Pfeffer CR. Spotting the red flags for adolescent suicide. Contemp Pediatr 6(2):65, 1989.

that specialize in working with persons who are contemplating or have attempted suicide.

During the initial interview with the adolescent, include questions that draw out feelings of alienation, depression, and hopelessness. If any of these indications are present, report and document these findings immediately. Question the family caregiver about any such signs and follow through with seeking additional help for the adolescent.

■ KEY POINTS

■ Adolescence for many teens is filled with a multitude of problems. Minor problems can seem major and major ones insurmountable.

- Teens with a positive self-esteem and a supportive family environment are more likely to weather this turbulent time with fewer problems than those with a poor self-image, fewer successes, and an unfavorable home environment.

- The choices adolescents make related to nutrition, friends and associates, alcohol and other drugs, sexuality, and school and career plans can affect their entire adult life.

- The primary objective in adolescent health care is prevention of health problems. Providing competent, compassionate care for adolescents with physiologic and psychological problems is the second objective, and the third is to restore health as quickly and completely as possible.

- Motor vehicle accidents, homicide, and suicide are the leading causes of death among adolescents. Nurses play an important part in promoting adolescent safety.

- Health problems of adolescents include poor nutrition, sexually transmitted diseases, substance abuse, and suicide. Nurses must identify these problems and refer the adolescent and family for help.

? CRITICAL THINKING

1. Tanya, 16 years old, is 65" (165 cm) tall and weighs 98 lb (44.5 kg). She moans about how fat her thighs are. You believe she is anorexic. List the symptoms you will observe for, in addition to her weight loss.

2. Tanya's diagnosis of anorexia nervosa is confirmed, and she is hospitalized for treatment. Develop a nursing care plan for her.

3. Explore the options available in your community for a pregnant 10th-grade girl. Can she continue school? What sources for maternity care are available if she has no health insurance? Will child care be available to her after she has the baby so she can return to school?

4. Brian is HIV positive and lives with his family. The family is frightened that other members may get the virus. Describe how you can reassure the family and help prevent spread of the virus in the home. Identify the guidelines you will give the family caregivers to help them protect Brian from infectious or opportunistic diseases.

5. Identify factors that put adolescents at greatest risk of becoming substance abusers.

6. Explain the most likely reasons why alcohol is the most commonly abused drug among adolescents.

REFERENCES

1. American Psychiatric Association. Diagnostic and statistical manual of mental disorders—revised, 4th ed. Washington, DC: American Psychiatric Association, 1994.
2. Starke JR. Tuberculosis. In Oski F. Principles and practices of pediatrics, 2d ed. Philadelphia: JB Lippincott, 1994.
3. Centers for Disease Control and Prevention. 1993 revised classification system for HIV infection and expanded surveillance case definition for AIDS among adolescents and adults. MMWR 41(No. RR-17:2), 1992.
4. Kelly PJ, Holman S. The new face of AIDS. Am J Nurs 93(3): 26–34, 1993.
5. Lewit EM. Teenage childbearing. Future of Children 2(2): 186–191, 1992.
6. Adger H. Adolescent drug abuse. In Oski F. Principles and practices of pediatrics, 2d ed. Philadelphia: JB Lippincott, 1994.
7. NIDA Capsule Series C-83-07. Facts about teenagers and drug abuse, 1995.
8. Goldenring JM. 20 questions: A drug talk they'll remember. Contemp Pediatr 9(1):56–79, 1992.
9. Engel NS. Anabolic steroid use among high school athletes. MCN 14(6):417, 1989.
10. Cohall AT, Mayer R, Cohall K, et al. Teen violence: The new morality. Contemp Pediatr 8(9):81, 1991.

BIBLIOGRAPHY

Boland MG, Czarniecki L. Starting life with HIV. RN 54(1):54–58, 1991.

Clarke PF, Byrne MW. A step up from home care: Enhanced care for medically complex HIV-infected children. MCN 18(3): 94–98, 1993.

Ferraro AR. Bulimia: A look from within. Pediatr Nurs 16(2): 187–191, 1990.

Fleming BW, Munton MT, Clarke BA, et al. Assessing and promoting positive parenting in adolescent mothers. MCN 18(1): 32–37, 1993.

Jackson DB, Saunders RB. Child health nursing. Philadelphia: JB Lippincott, 1993.

Jackson MM. Tuberculosis in infants, children, and adolescents: New dilemmas with an old disease. Pediatr Nurs 19(5): 437–443, 1993.

Jaffe ES. Working with troubled teens. RN 54(2):58–62, 1991.

Morgan IS. Recognizing depression in the adolescent. MCN 19(3): 148–155, 1994.

Nelson JA. HIV in adolescents. MCN 20(1):34–37, 1995.

Novotny J. Adolescents, acne, and the side effects of Accutane. Pediatr Nurs 15(3):247–248, 1989.

Pfeffer CR. Spotting the red flags for adolescent suicide. Contemp Pediatr 6(2):59, 1989.

Pillitteri A. Maternal and child health nursing, 2d ed. Philadelphia: JB Lippincott, 1995.

Ridel J, Moon MW. Children with HIV becoming adolescents: Caring for long-term survivors. Pediatr Nurs 22(3):220, 1996.

Roller CG. Drawing out young mothers. MCN 17(5):254–255, 1992.

Washburn P. Identification, assessment, and referral of adolescent drug abusers. Pediatr Nurs 17(2):137–140, 1991.

Whatley JH. Effects of health locus of control and social network on adolescent risk taking. Pediatr Nurs 17(2):145–148, 1991.

Wong DL. Whaley and Wong's nursing care of infants and children, 5th ed. St. Louis: Mosby, 1995.

A Child in Crisis

The Child in a Stressed Family

STUDENT OBJECTIVES

On completion of this chapter, the student will be able to:

1. Identify the behaviors of the pregnant drug abuser that put her fetus in danger.
2. Describe the effects that cocaine abuse during pregnancy may have on the fetus.
3. Identify nursing care that may be helpful when caring for crack cocaine infants.
4. Describe characteristics of the infant with fetal alcohol syndrome.
5. Describe the unpredictable behavior of an addicted parent and its effect on the child.
6. List six behaviors that suggest there is an addiction problem in the child's family.
7. Identify how poor parenting skills may lead to child abuse.
8. State the amount of time that a health care facility can hold a child while investigating for possible child abuse.
9. Identify the circumstances under which physical punishment can be classified as abusive.
10. Describe the differences between bruises that occur accidentally to a young child and those that have been inflicted in an abusive manner.
11. Define Munchausen syndrome by proxy.
12. Identify ways that a child may be emotionally abused.
13. List the services offered by the National Runaway Hot Line.
14. Describe emotional reactions a child may have to divorce.
15. Describe the effects of homelessness on the health care of children.

KEY TERMS

child neglect
co-dependent parent
dysfunctional family
fetal alcohol syndrome
incest
latchkey child
microcephaly

micrognathia
neonatal abstinence
   syndrome
palpebral fissures
philtrum
sexual abuse
sexual assault

Substance abuse is a family problem. If one member of the family abuses cigarettes, alcohol, or drugs, every member of that family is affected. The problem has grown to alarming proportions since the early 1980s. The number of infants born to substance-abusing mothers has grown consistently during this time, resulting in a large number of babies who face great physical and emotional challenges with few or limited family resources (see Fig. 6-10 in Chap. 6). In addition, children who have at least one parent who is a substance abuser are at risk for a variety of problems that researchers relate to substance abuse in the family. Behavior problems, school failures, and child abuse are just a few of the negative results that can occur.

THE INFANT OF A SUBSTANCE-ABUSING MOTHER

Maternal substance abuse takes an enormous toll on the unborn child. Most illicit drugs cross the placenta easily, and it is estimated that the concentration of these drugs in the fetus can be as high as 50% of that in the mother. Use of more than one drug at a time (polydrug use), including alcohol and cigarettes, is common among women. The compounded effects of these drugs further compromises the well-being of the fetus. Cigarette smoking impairs fetal development as severely as illicit drugs and alcohol. Cigarettes are the most commonly abused substance. According to some research, at least 25% of pregnant women use nicotine, and 5% to 8% are at risk for alcohol-related prenatal problems.[1]

Although substance abuse occurs among women of all economic and social backgrounds, the pregnant substance abuser may have no prenatal care or may receive irregular care. Substance abuse is very difficult to overcome even for well-motivated pregnant women. Drug treatment programs tailored for pregnant and parenting women are cost-effective and have been proven to help them overcome their addiction problems and greatly improve birth outcomes. Unfortunately, programs of this type are very difficult to find and when found are often overburdened.

The first trimester is the most dangerous time for fetal exposure to teratogens. In some cases the pregnant woman who is dependent on illicit drugs may be more interested in getting her next supply of drugs than in keeping an appointment. If the woman's financial status does not provide enough money for food, health care, and drugs, she may use her limited resources to get more drugs. As a result, the unborn child suffers not only from the effects of the drugs but from nutritional deprivation and inadequate care. In addition, the illicit drug abuser may be sexually promiscuous, perhaps practicing prostitution to obtain money to support her habit. Thus, she puts herself and her unborn child in jeopardy for sexually transmitted diseases. If she injects drugs, she also may be at great risk for HIV infection or hepatitis. Many women with a substance abuse problem deny or try to hide their drug dependence, avoiding contact with health care workers for fear of detection.

The Effect of Cocaine on the Neonate

During pregnancy, cocaine (often used in the form of "crack" because it is cheaper) causes vasoconstriction of the placental blood vessels, resulting in a variety of problems. Spontaneous abortion, premature birth, and premature separation of the placenta are common. The decrease in circulation to the fetus can cause intrauterine growth retardation. In addition, disorganized behavioral states may be detected both prenatally and postnatally. Serious congenital anomalies, which may include permanent neurologic damage, can occur as a result of polydrug use. Many cocaine users also use other drugs, specifically alcohol, marijuana, and cigarettes, and these further endanger the health of the fetus.

At birth, newborns who have been exposed to cocaine often are irritable, quivery, and easily startled and cry at any sound or even the softest touch. Most newborns of drug-dependent women show signs of **neonatal abstinence syndrome** (NAS), characterized by central nervous system hyperirritability, gastrointestinal dysfunction, respiratory distress, and vague autonomic symptoms, including yawning, sneezing, sweating, stuffy nose, mottling, increased tearing, and fever.[2] At birth, these infants commonly have a low birth weight and poor Apgar scores. The infant may not be able to take nutrition normally and may need gavage feeding. Breast-feeding is not attempted because cocaine can stay in breast milk for 60 hours after drug use.

Many of these newborns are admitted to the neonatal intensive care unit because of prematurity, very low birth weight, and other birth problems. At times, the mother may abandon the infant in the hospital, so the infant must be sent to a foster home when ready for discharge.

NURSING CARE OF THE COCAINE-EXPOSED INFANT

Caring for cocaine-exposed infants is challenging. They often suffer from poor sleep patterns, diarrhea, and dehydration. They commonly do not respond to the usual means of quieting infants, such as swaddling, offering pacifiers, and rocking; it may help to wrap the infant securely with arms brought to the midline and hold him or her snugly against the body in an upright position. When the infant is rocked, the movement should be vertical (up and down) rather than the usual back-and-forth method. Reducing stimuli, such as noise, bright lights, and sudden movements, helps quiet the infant. Soft music also may help. These infants seem to take nourishment better when held upright and fed slowly. They may need to have smaller, more frequent feedings because they tire so quickly.

If the mother plans to take the baby home, intensive teaching is required. The mother should be drug-free and enrolled in a program to support her resolve to quit using drugs. The mother needs to learn basic parenting skills. In addition, the infant may show many signs that can be interpreted as rejection of the caregiver; the caregiver must understand that these behaviors are general reactions and not specifically directed at him or her. Provide caregivers with complete instructions, including written materials. Be certain that the teaching materials are presented at a level and in language the caregiver can understand.

Close home contact should be planned to follow up on the infant after discharge. The Brazelton Neonatal Assessment Scale (see Fig. 7-13 in Chap. 7) can be used to determine the progress of the infant's development. Encourage the caregiver to phone for help if there is a problem with the infant. Ongoing support for these families is essential.

The Effect of Heroin and Other Opiates on the Neonate

Crack cocaine has become the most commonly abused illicit drug since its appearance in the 1980s. However, heroin and other opiates continue to be used, and in some parts of the country heroin use is increasing. The death rate for neonates of heroin-addicted mothers is greater than that for babies of nonaddicted mothers.

The effects of maternal abuse of these drugs are similar to those of crack cocaine. Hypoxia during labor may cause meconium staining and aspiration pneumonia in the newborn, contributing to increased illness and possible death. These infants often have jaundice, aspiration pneumonia, transient tachypnea, respiratory distress syndrome, and congenital malformations. Prenatal care is commonly poor. The infant may have a high-pitched cry and increased muscle tone and may be irritable. Infants of mothers who have been taking methadone have much the same withdrawal symptoms. However, these infants may have a higher birth weight because the mother had more consistent prenatal care.

Withdrawal symptoms apparently are related to the mother's drug habit. Newborns whose mothers took large doses over a long period have the most severe withdrawal. Timing of withdrawal symptoms is related to how close to delivery the mother took heroin. The closer to delivery the last dose occurred, the later the withdrawal symptoms appear. These symptoms may continue for 2 months or more.

Nursing care of the infant of a heroin or opiate abuser is similar to the care of the infant of a cocaine-addicted mother. Paregoric is used to treat infants with opiate-induced NAS to manage the symptoms. Phenobarbital is used in infants with nonopiate NAS. Some physicians may prescribe the two drugs in combination.

The Neonate With Fetal Alcohol Syndrome

Alcohol is second only to nicotine as the substance most commonly abused by pregnant women. Any ingestion of alcohol during pregnancy is considered unwise. Moderate maternal drinking has been demonstrated to produce infants with poor intrauterine growth and congenital anomalies, and heavy maternal drinking produces even greater abnormalities. The abnormalities characteristically seen in the infant whose mother consumed alcohol during pregnancy are commonly referred to as fetal alcohol effects (FAE) or **fetal alcohol syndrome** (FAS). Infants with FAS are shorter, weigh less, and may have **microcephaly** (small head), facial deformities, hearing disorders, poor coordination, minor joint and limb abnormalities, heart defects, delayed development, and mental retardation. The facial deformities are characteristic and include short **palpebral fissures** (opening between the eyes), a flat **philtrum** (vertical groove in the middle of the upper lip), a thin upper lip, a short, upturned nose, and **micrognathia** (a small lower jaw) (Fig. 20-1). Infants may have a few or many of these abnormalities. Neonates are jittery and may evidence failure to thrive.

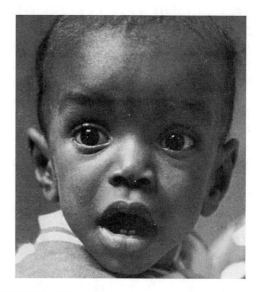

Figure 20-1

A 15-month-old child with fetal alcohol syndrome.

The fetus may be affected by a number of factors related to the mother's drinking. The alcoholic mother may be malnourished. She may have an alcohol-induced illness, such as gastric hemorrhage or cirrhosis of the liver. Alcohol crosses the placenta easily, directly affecting the fetus as well as being present in the amniotic fluid that the fetus ingests.

At birth, the infant may be hypoglycemic from the effect of the alcohol. All infants at risk should be screened with a reagent strip in the nursery within the first few hours after birth. Symptoms of neonatal hypoglycemia for which the nurse should be alert include tremors, lethargy, seizures, irregular respirations, and apnea. These neonates also may have respiratory distress syndrome.

Newborns with FAS need a quiet, nonstimulating environment. Intravenous fluids are administered as needed to avoid dehydration, and anticonvulsant drugs are administered if the infant is having seizures.

The number of infants believed to have FAE may be twice the number of those with FAS. Many of these infants are not clearly identified. The effects of FAE include alcohol-related physical features, growth retardation, and various cognitive deficits. They are believed to be, at least in part, the result of the mother's consuming lower levels of alcohol, as well as possible genetic differences in susceptibility.

Infants and toddlers with FAS often have difficulty with feedings. They also may be hyperactive or have attention deficit disorders, intellectual slowness, poor fine-motor control, and developmental delay of gross motor skills. Children with FAS and FAE need a supportive educational environment throughout their school years.

PARENTS ADDICTED TO DRUGS OR ALCOHOL

More than 10% of children come from a home that is affected by the alcoholism of one or both parents. Alcoholism exacts a terrible toll on the functioning of the family. Children of alcoholics are four times more likely to become alcoholics themselves. When other substances are included in the statistics, the number of affected homes increases substantially. Many women who abuse drugs and alcohol were themselves victims of physical, emotional, or sexual abuse as children.[3]

The Effect of Parental Substance Abuse on the Family

Developmental delays occur in young children of substance abusers. Infants of cocaine abusers avoid the caregiver's gaze, contributing further to bonding delays. The parent who is addicted may be so involved in procuring the drug that any pretense of good parenting is forgotten. The parent, caught up in the ups and downs of addiction, is not dependable and cannot provide any stability for the child. The parent may waver between overindulgence—smothering the child with attention, leniency, and gifts—and the opposite behavior of irritability, unreasonable accusations, threats, and anger. This unpredictable behavior has a severe impact on the relationships in the family. Children of substance-abusing parents often become loners, avoiding relationships with others for fear that the substance-abusing parent might do or say something to embarrass them in front of their peers.

As the parent's substance abuse worsens, there is an increase in the dysfunction and social isolation of the family. The **co-dependent parent** supports, directly or indirectly, the addictive behavior of the other parent. This behavior usually involves making excuses for the addict's actions and expecting others (ie, the children) to overlook the parent's moodiness, erratic behavior, and consumption of alcohol or drugs. Co-dependency may add to the dilemma of children living with an addicted parent.

Children Coping With Parental Addiction

Children rarely talk about the parent's problem, even to the other parent. These children often suffer from guilt, anxiety, confusion, anger, depression, and addictive behavior. Children react in a variety of ways. An older child, often a girl, may take on the responsibility of running the household, taking care of the younger children, making meals, and performing the tasks that the parent normally should do. These children may become overachievers in school but remain isolated emotionally from their peers and teachers. Another child in the family may try to deflect the embarrassment and anger of the other siblings, trying to make everyone feel good. As these children become adolescents or young adults, they may have problems such as substance abuse or eating disorders. The child in the family who "acts out" and engages in delinquent behavior is most likely to come to the attention of social services and be identified as a child who needs help.

Behaviors that may alert nurses and other health care personnel to an addiction problem in the family are:

- The loner child who avoids interaction with classmates
- The child who is failing in school or has numerous episodes of unexcused absences or truancy
- The child with frequent minor physical complaints, such as headaches or stomach aches
- The child who steals or commits acts of violence
- The aggressive child
- The child who abuses drugs or alcohol.

Box 20-1. *Resources for Information and Help with Drug and Alcohol Problems*

If you suspect your child may be using alcohol or drugs, you've got to confront the situation directly. Your doctor, local hospital, school social worker, or county mental health society may be able to refer you to a treatment facility.

A number of helpful national organizations are just a phone call away. if you have a computer and access to the Internet, several also offer valuable information at their World Wide Web sites.

Center for Substance Abuse Treatment: For drug and alcohol information and referral, call 1-800-662-HELP.

The National Clearinghouse for Alcohol and Drug Information: For pamphlets, publications, and materials for schools, call 1-800-SAY-NOTO. Web site: www.health.org

American Council for Drug Education: Call 1-800-488-DRUG.

National Helplines: For referrals to local treatment facilities, self-help and family-support groups, and crisis centers, call 1-800-HELP-111.

National Families in Action: Call 770-934-6364. Web site: www.emory.edu/NFIA

National Family Partnership: Call 314-845-1933.

PRIDE (Parents' Resource Institute for Drug Education): Call 770-458-9900. Web site: www.prideusa.org

Community Anti-Drug Coalitions of America: For information on current issues or legislation, call 1-800-DRUGS-50.

Al-Anon/Alateen Family Group Headquarters, Inc.: Call 1-800-356-9996.

Alcoholics Anonymous World Services: Check the phone directory for your local AA chapter or call 212-870-3400.

Nar-Anon Family Group Headquarters, Inc.: Call 310-547-5800.

Cocaine Helpline: Call 1-800-COCAINE.

Partnership for a Drug-Free America: Web site: www.drugfreeamerica.org

U.S. Department of Education: Web site: www.ed.gov

U.S. Department of Justice Clearinghouse: Web site: www.ncjrs.org

Reader's Digest and Parent Soup: Co-hosted web site: www.drugfreekids.com

From Ola, P. & D'Aulaire, E. How to raise drug free kids. Washington, D.C.: U.S. Department of Education, 1997.

Nurses and others who work with children must be alert to these signals for help. Children can benefit from programs that support them and help them understand what is happening in the home. Such a program may include group therapy sessions at school, in which the child learns that others have the same problems, reducing his or her feelings of isolation. Other programs may include the whole family, perhaps as part of the program for the addicted parent who is trying to break the addiction. Professional help is necessary to prevent the child from developing more serious problems. The earlier the child can be identified and treatment begun, the better the prognosis. Box 20-1 provides a list of resources for drug and alcohol problems.

CHILD ABUSE

Every family faces many types of stress at one time or another. In addition to substance abuse, events that create stress for a family include illness, job loss, economic crisis or poverty, relocation, birth, death, and trauma. How the family handles these stresses affects greatly the emotional, social, and physical health of each member of the family. A **dysfunctional family** is one that cannot resolve these

stresses and work through them in a positive, socially acceptable manner. The atmosphere in such a family creates additional stress for all family members. Because of the lack of support within the family for individual members, these members respond negatively to real or perceived problems. This may set the stage for child abuse, runaway children, substance abuse, and other unhealthy coping behaviors. Single-parent families often face multiple pressures at the same time, creating additional stress and adding to the risk of dysfunctional coping.

Although child abuse has occurred throughout history, the evolution of cultural practices in the United States during the last few decades of the 20th century has emphasized the rights of children. Thus, any sort of mistreatment and abuse of children is regarded as unacceptable. The term *child abuse* has come to mean any intentional act of physical, emotional, or sexual abuse, including acts of negligence, committed by a person responsible for the care of the child.

Each year, increasing numbers of child abuse cases are brought to the attention of authorities. Estimates of the number of children treated in emergency departments range from 500,000 to 1 million annually. However, this may be only the tip of the iceberg, because many more cases may go undetected.

Child abuse is not limited to one age group and can

be detected at any age. The courts have even viewed fetal exposure to drugs and alcohol as child abuse. Surprisingly, adolescents have the greatest incidence of abuse. In children younger than 2 years of age, the rate is estimated at six per 1,000; the rate in children 15 to 17 years of age escalates to more than 14 per 1,000.[4]

Child abuse has long-term effects. The abused child may be hyperactive, may exhibit angry, antisocial behavior, or may be especially withdrawn. Abusive parents often were abused themselves as children; thus, the problem of child abuse continues in a cyclical fashion from generation to generation. Abusive parents can be found at all socioeconomic levels, but families with greater financial means may be able to evade detection more easily. Low-income families show greater evidence of violence, neglect, and sexual abuse, according to some studies. Commonly, abusive parents have inadequate parenting skills; therefore, they have unrealistic expectations of the child and do not respond to the child's behavior appropriately.

State laws require health care personnel to report suspected child abuse. This requirement overrides the concern for confidentiality. Loss of nursing license is the usual penalty for the nurse who does not report suspected child abuse. These laws were enacted to protect the nurse from reprisal for accusing a caregiver (eg, being sued for slander). Usually, the health care facility can hold the child for 72 hours after suspected abuse has been reported so that a caseworker can investigate the charge. After this 72-hour period, a hearing is held to determine if the charges are true and to decide where the child should be placed.

The demand for foster care has risen with the increased use of crack cocaine. The children of families in which alcohol and other substances are abused tend to enter foster care at a younger age than those from the general population.[5]

Physical Abuse

Physical abuse often occurs when the caregiver is unfamiliar with normal child behavior. Inexperienced caregivers do not know what is normal behavior for a child and become frustrated when the child does not respond to them in the way they expect. Some young women become pregnant to have a child to love, expecting that love to be returned in full measure. When the child resists the mother's control or seems to do the opposite of what she expects, she takes it as a personal affront and becomes angry, possibly responding with physical punishment. Some cultures support physical punishment for children, citing the old principle "Spare the rod, spoil the child." Despite evidence that physical punishment often results in negative behavior and other forms of punishment are more effective, corporal punishment continues to be approved, even in some schools. However, physical punishment that leaves marks, causes injury, or threatens the child's physical or emotional well-being is considered abusive.

When a child is brought to a physician or hospital because of physical injuries, family caregivers may attribute the injury to some action of the child that is not in keeping with the child's age or level of development. The caregiver may also attribute the injury to an action of a sibling. Whenever the child's symptoms do not match the injury the caregiver describes, be alert for possible abuse. However, do not accuse the caregiver before a complete investigation takes place.

Young, active children often have a number of bruises that occur from their usual activities. Most of these bruises occur over bony areas such as the knees, elbows, shins, and forehead. Bruises that occur in areas of soft tissue, such as the abdomen, buttocks, genitalia, thighs, and mouth, may be suspect. Bruises in the inner aspect of the upper arms may indicate that the child raised the arms to protect the face and head from blows. Bruises may be distinctive in outline, clearly indicating the instrument that was used. Hangers, belt buckles, electrical cords, hand prints, teeth (from biting), and sticks all leave identifiable marks. Bruises may be in varying stages of healing, indicating that not all the injuries occurred during one episode (Fig. 20-2).

On a radiograph, bone fractures in various stages of healing may be noted. Spiral fractures of the long bones of a young child are considered a cardinal sign of abuse. Infants who have been harshly shaken may not show a clear picture of abuse, but computed tomography scanning may demonstrate cerebral edema or cerebral hemorrhage.

Burns are another common type of injury seen in the abused child (Fig. 20-3). Although burns may be accidental in young children, certain types of burns are highly suspi-

Figure 20-2
The child who has been physically abused usually has old and fresh bruises about the head, face, and body and may either look sad and forlorn or be actively seeking to please, sometimes even particularly involved with and attentive to the abusing parent.

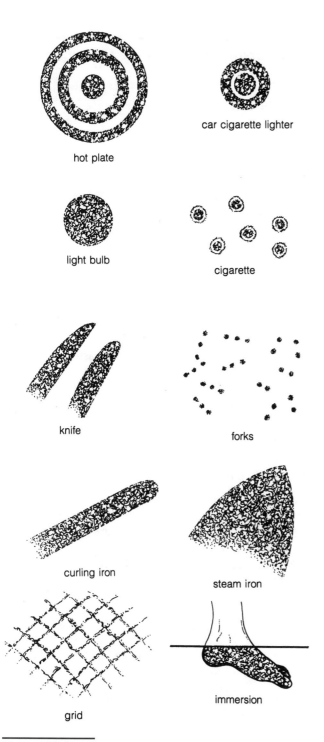

Figure 20-3
Burn patterns from objects used for inflicting burns in child abuse.

cious. Cigarette burns are common abuse injuries. Burns from immersion of a hand in hot liquid, a hot register (as evidenced by the grid pattern), a steam iron, or a curling iron are not uncommon. Caregivers have been known to immerse the buttocks of a child in hot water if they thought the child was uncooperative in toilet training. Caregivers

are often unaware of how quickly a child can be seriously burned. A burn that is neglected or not reported immediately must be considered suspicious until all the facts can be gathered and examined.

Munchausen by Proxy Syndrome

In Munchausen by proxy syndrome, one person either fabricates or induces illness in another to get attention. When injury to a child is involved, the mother is most often the person who has the syndrome. Often, the mother injures the child to get the attention of medical personnel. She may slowly poison the child with prescription drugs, alcohol, or other drugs, or she may suffocate the child to cause apnea. The mother appears very attentive to the child and often is familiar with medical terminology. This situation is frustrating for health care personnel because it is difficult to catch the suspect in the act of endangering the child. Close observation of the caregiver's interactions with the child is necessary. For instance, if episodes of apnea occur only in the presence of the caregiver, be alert for this syndrome. The caregiver who suffers from this syndrome must receive psychiatric help.

Emotional Abuse and Neglect

Injury from emotional abuse can be just as serious and lasting as physical abuse, but it is much more difficult to identify. Several types of emotional abuse can occur, including:

- Verbal abuse, such as humiliation, scapegoating, unrealistic expectations with belittling, and erratic discipline
- Emotional unavailability, when caregivers are absorbed in their own problems
- Insufficient or poor nurturing or threatening to leave the child or otherwise end the relationship
- Role reversal, in which the child must take on the role of parenting the parent and is blamed for the parent's problems.

Children may show evidence of emotional abuse by appearing worried or fearful or having vague complaints of illness or nightmares. Caregivers may display signs of inappropriate expectations of the child when in the health care facility, sometimes mocking or belittling the child for age-appropriate behavior. In young children, failure to thrive may be a sign of emotional abuse. In the older child, poor school performance and attendance, poor self-esteem, and poor peer relationships may be clues.

Child neglect is failure to provide adequate hygiene, health care, nutrition, love, nurturing, and supervision that is needed for growth and development. If a child is not given adequate care for a serious medical condition, the caregivers are considered neglectful. For example, if a child is seriously burned (even though it is accidental) and the caregivers do not take the child for evaluation and treatment until several days later, the caregiver may be judged to be neglectful. Often, the child with failure to thrive as a result of being underfed, deprived of love, or constantly criticized can be classified as neglected; however, be careful not to make an unsubstantiated accusation of neglect.

Sexual Abuse

Sexual abuse of children has existed in all ages and cultures, but seldom has it been admitted when it is perpetrated by parents or other relatives in the home. **Incest** (sexually arousing physical contact between family members not married to each other) occurs in an estimated 240,000 to 1 million American families annually, and that number is growing each year. As with other types of child abuse, sexual abuse knows no socioeconomic, racial, religious, or ethnic boundaries. However, substance abuse, job loss, and poverty are contributing factors. Like other forms of child abuse, sexual abuse is being recognized and reported more often. The National Center for Child Abuse and Neglect defines **sexual abuse** as contacts or interactions between a child and an adult when the child is being used for sexual stimulation of the perpetrator or other person. Sexual abuse also may be committed by someone younger than 18 years of age if that person is in a position of power or control over the other.[6]

Several terms are commonly used when sexual abuse is discussed. From a legal viewpoint, sexual contacts between a child and another person in a caretaking position, such as a parent, babysitter, or teacher, is classified as sexual abuse. Sexual contacts made by someone who is not functioning in a caretaker role is classified as **sexual assault**. Incest includes fondling of breasts, genitalia, intercourse (vaginal or anal), oral–genital contact, exhibitionism, and voyeurism.

Regardless of the relationship of the perpetrator to the child, the outcome of the abuse is devastating. Episodes of sexual abuse that involve a person the child trusts seem to be the most damaging. Incest often goes unreported because the person committing the act uses intimidation by means of threats, appealing to the child's desire to be loved and to please, convincing the child of the importance of keeping the act secret.

When a child is sexually assaulted by a stranger, the caregivers usually become aware of the incident, promptly report it, and take the child for a physical examination. However, in the case of incest, the child rarely tells another person what is happening. The child may exhibit physical complaints, such as various aches and pains, gastrointestinal upsets, changes in bowel and bladder habits (including enuresis), nightmares, and acts of aggression or hostility. Some of these complaints or behaviors may be the presenting problem when the child is seen by a health care provider.

▶ ⌐ Nursing Process in the Care of an ◀ ⌐ Abused Child

ASSESSMENT

When assessing a child who may have been abused or neglected, be thorough and complete in observation and documentation. The child should have a complete physical assessment, and all bruises, blemishes, lacerations, areas of redness and irritation, and marks of any kind on the child's body must be carefully described and accurately documented. It may be necessary to request that photographs be taken. Observe the interaction between the child and the caregiver, and carefully document your observations using nonjudgmental terms. The child's body language may be revealing, so be alert for significant information. For example, if the child shrinks away from contact by the caregiver or health care practitioner or, on the other hand, is especially clinging to the caregiver, watch for other signs of inappropriate behavior. These assessments vary with the child's age (Table 20-1).

Perhaps the most difficult part may be to maintain a nonjudgmental attitude throughout the assessment and examination. Be calm and reassuring with the child, letting the child lead the way, when possible.

NURSING DIAGNOSES

The nursing diagnoses vary with the type of abuse or neglect that the child may have experienced. Appropriate nursing diagnoses for a child with a fracture, for example, include care before and after the fracture has been set and casted. Various nursing diagnoses are appropriate for the care of a child with burns, based on the care needed for the burns. A child who is nutritionally deprived needs diagnoses that address nutritional needs. Nursing diagnoses that may be of use are:

- Anxiety by child related to history of abuse and fear of abuse from others

- Ineffective Individual Coping by the nonabusive parent related to fear of violence from abusive partner or feelings of powerlessness

- Ineffective Family Coping: Disabling related to unknown cause

- Ineffective Family Coping: Disabling related to unrealistic expectations of child by parent

OUTCOME IDENTIFICATION AND PLANNING

Major goals for the abused child include relieving anxiety and alleviating injuries. An important family goal is to improve coping skills of the caregiver or family.

TABLE 20-1.   Nursing Assessments: Signs of Abuse in Children

Physical Signs	Behavioral Signs
Physical Abuse	
Bruises and welts: may be on multiple body surfaces or soft tissue; may form regular pattern (eg, belt buckle)	Less compliant than average
Burns: cigar or cigarette, immersion (stocking/glovelike on extremities or doughnut-shaped on buttocks or genitals), or patterned as an electrical appliance (eg, iron)	Signs of negativism, unhappiness
	Anger, isolation
	Destructive
	Abusive toward others
Fractures: single or multiple; may be in various stages of healing	Difficulty developing relationships
Lacerations or abrasions: rope burns; tears in and around mouth, eyes, ears, or genitalia	Either excessive or absent separation anxiety
	Inappropriate caretaking concern for parent
Abdominal injuries: ruptured or injured internal organs	Constantly in search of attention, favors, food, etc.
Central nervous system injuries: subdural hematoma, retinal or subarachnoid hemorrhage	Various developmental delays (cognitive, language, motor)
Physical Neglect	
Malnutrition	Lack of appropriate adult supervision
Repeated episodes of pica	Repeated ingestions of harmful substances
Constant fatigue or listlessness	Poor school attendance
Poor hygiene	Exploitation (forced to beg or steal; excessive household work)
Inadequate clothing for circumstances	Role reversal with parent
Inadequate medical or dental care	Drug or alcohol use
Sexual Abuse	
Difficulty walking or sitting	Direct or indirect disclosure to relative, friend, or teacher
Thickening or hyperpigmentation of labial skin	Withdrawal with excessive dependency
Vaginal opening measures >4 mm horizontally in preadolescence	Poor peer relationships
	Poor self-esteem
Torn, stained, or bloody underclothing	Frightened or phobic of adults
Bruises or bleeding of genitalia or perianal area	Sudden decline in academic performance
Lax rectal tone	Pseudomature personality development
Vaginal discharge	Suicide attempts
Recurrent urinary tract infections	Regressive behavior
Nonspecific vaginitis	Enuresis or encopresis
Venereal disease	Excessive masturbation
Sperm or acid phosphatase on body or clothes	Highly sexualized play
Pregnancy	Sexual promiscuity
Emotional Abuse	
Delays in physical development	Distinct emotional symptoms or functional limitations
Failure to thrive	Deteriorating conduct
	Increased anxiety
	Apathy or depression
	Developmental lags

Jackson DB, Saunders RB. Child health nursing. Philadelphia: JB Lippincott, 1993. Data from Council on Scientific Affairs. AMA diagnostic and treatment guidelines concerning child abuse and neglect. JAMA 254(6):796–800, 1985.

IMPLEMENTATION

RELIEVING THE CHILD'S ANXIETY.   Observe the child for behavior that indicates anxiety, such as withdrawal, ducking or shying away from the nurse or caregivers, guarding, and avoiding eye contact. Assign one nurse to care for the child so that the child can relate to one person consis-

tently. Provide physical contact such as hugging, rocking, and caressing only if the child accepts it. Identify nursing actions that seem to comfort the child, and use them consistently. Use a calm, reassuring, and kind manner, and provide a safe atmosphere in which the child has an opportunity to express feelings and fears. Use play to help the child express some of these emotions. Be careful not to do anything that might alarm or upset the child. Psychological support is provided through social services or an abuse team.

SUPPORTING THE NONABUSIVE CAREGIVER. One caregiver in the family may be the abuser, and the other is not. The nonabusive caregiver is a victim as well as the child. Give the nonabusive caregiver an opportunity to express fears and anxieties. He or she may feel powerless in the situation. Help the passive caregiver decide whether to continue the relationship or leave it. Try to preserve the caregiver's self-esteem, as this is not an easy decision to make. Remember that confidentiality is essential when discussing such problems.

OBSERVING INTERACTION BETWEEN THE CARE-GIVER AND CHILD. While caring for the abused child when the caregiver is present, use the opportunity to observe how the caregiver relates to the child and how the child reacts to the caregiver. Give the caregiver the same courtesy extended to all caregivers. Offer a compliment when the caregiver does something well in caring for the child. Give the caregiver an opportunity to discuss in private any concerns; during this time, you may be able to gain his or her confidence.

PROMOTING PARENTING SKILLS. Often, abuse occurs when a caregiver is unfamiliar with normal growth and development and the behaviors common to a particular stage of development. Help the caregiver develop realistic expectations of the child; to help accomplish this goal, design a teaching plan and include the caregiver in caring for the child. Teach the caregiver expected responses from the child, and help him or her learn about normal development. Praise the caregiver for displaying positive behaviors. Point out specific behaviors of the child and explain them to the caregiver. Explore the reasons for the caregiver's absence when he or she does not visit regularly. Discuss specific behaviors of the child that are upsetting to the caregiver and explain that these are common for the child's age.

The caregiver may be facing temporary or permanent placement of the child in another home. Help the caregiver and the child accept this change. Emotions that a caregiver has had over a long period cannot be easily switched off. The assistance of social services and a child life specialist is beneficial in these situations. Act as a member of the team to aid in the transition. The foster parents may need support from the nursing staff to help ease the child's transition to the new home. Abused children must be followed carefully after discharge from the health care facility to ensure that their well-being is protected.

EVALUATION: GOALS AND OUTCOME CRITERIA

- *Goal*: The child will exhibit decreased signs of anxiety.
  Criteria: The child's play, facial expressions, and posture are relaxed; the child displays no withdrawal or guarding during contacts with the nursing staff.

- *Goal*: The nonabusive caregiver will begin to cope with fears and feelings of powerlessness.
  Criteria: The nonabusive caregiver expresses fears and concerns and makes plans to resolve problems.

- *Goal*: The caregiver will exhibit positive interaction with the child.
  Criteria: The caregiver talks with the child, is sensitive to his or her needs, and refrains from making unreasonable demands on the child.

- *Goal*: The caregiver will be involved in the child's care and will demonstrate knowledge of growth and development and ways to handle the child's misbehavior.
  Criteria: The caregiver states age-appropriate behavior for the child, discusses ways to handle the child's irritating behavior, and is involved in counseling or other discharge plans.

THE RUNAWAY CHILD

In the United States, as many as 750,000 to 2 million adolescents run away from home each year. A child can be considered a runaway after being absent from home overnight or longer without permission from a family caregiver. Most children who run away from home are 10 to 17 years of age.

A child may run away from home in response to circumstances that he or she views as too difficult to tolerate. Physical abuse, incest, alcohol or drug abuse, divorce, stepfamilies, pregnancy, school failure, and truancy may contribute to the child's desire to escape. However, some adolescents are not runaways but rather "throwaways" who have been forced to leave home and are not wanted by the adults in the home. Often, the throwaways have been forced out of the home because their behavior is unacceptable to family caregivers or because of other family stresses such as divorce, remarriage, and job loss.

Runaway or throwaway adolescents often turn to stealing, drug dealing, and prostitution to provide money for alcohol, drugs, food, and possibly shelter. Many of these adolescents live on the streets because they cannot pay for shelter and avoid going to public shelters for fear of being found by police. They may become victims of pimps or drug dealers who use the adolescents for their own gain.

There are numerous programs to help runaways, especially in urban areas. A 24-hour National Runaway Hot Line (1-800-231-6946) is available to give runaways information and referral. This service may help the runaway find a safe place to stay and may provide counseling, shelter, health care, legal aid, message relay to the family, and transportation home, if desired. Runaways are not forced to go home but may be encouraged to let their family know they are alright. Other free hotline numbers are also available.

A sexually transmitted disease, pregnancy, AIDS, or drug overdose are the usual reasons that runaways are seen at a health care facility. When caring for such a child, be nonjudgmental. Any indication of being disturbed or disgusted by the adolescent's lifestyle may end any chance of cooperation and cause the adolescent to refuse to give any additional information. Try to build a trusting relationship with the child. Remember that the runaway viewed his or her problems as so great that escaping was the only way to resolve them. Counseling is necessary to begin to resolve the problems.

Health teaching for the runaway must be suited to his or her lifestyle and must be at a level the child can understand. Without prying excessively, try to find out the runaway's living circumstances and adjust the teaching plans accordingly. Remember that the child's problems did not come about overnight, nor will they be resolved quickly. Caring for a runaway can be frustrating, challenging, and sometimes rewarding for the health care staff.

THE LATCHKEY CHILD

As a result of the increased number of families in which both parents work and the increase in single-parent families in which the parent must work, many children need after-school care and supervision; unfortunately, adequate or appropriate child care may not be readily available. A **latchkey child** is one who comes home to an empty house after school each day because the family caregivers are at work. The term was coined because these children often wear the house key around their neck. These children usually spend several hours alone before an adult comes home from work (Fig. 20-4). The number of latchkey children may be as high as 10 million in the United States.

Latchkey children often have fears about being at home alone. When there is more than one child and the older child is responsible for the younger one, conflicts can arise. The older child may have to assume responsibility that is beyond the normal expectations for the child's age. This can be a difficult situation for the caregivers and the children. The caregivers must carefully outline permissible activities and safety rules. There should be a plan in place to help the older child solve any problem that may arise that involves both children. The older child should not feel that the complete responsibility is on his or her shoulders, but rather that it is a shared responsibility with the caregiver. Some schools have after-school latchkey programs that provide safe activities for children. In addition, some communities have programs in which an adult telephones the child regularly every day after school or there is a telephone

Figure 20-4
A 12-year-old boy and his 9-year-old sister come home to an empty house to await arrival of their caregiver.

hotline the child can call (see Family Teaching: Tips for Latchkey Children).

Despite concerns that latchkey children are more likely to become involved with smoking, stealing, or taking drugs, researchers have not found sufficient data to support this fear. Children who are given responsibility of this kind and who are recognized for their dependability usually live up to the expectations of the adults in their social environment.

Nurses must recognize the need for after-school services for these children and take an active role in the community to plan and support such services. Maintain a list of the facilities available to support families with latchkey children. The nurse can give caregivers guidance in planning children's after-school activities and offer support to the caregivers in their attempts to provide for their children.

DIVORCE AND THE CHILD

Divorce has increased to the point where one in two marriages ends in divorce. About 50% of the children experience the separation or divorce of their parents before they complete high school. Some children may experience more than one divorce, because 40% of those who remarry divorce for the second time.[3] Divorce can be traumatic for

Family Teaching
Tips for Latchkey Children

1. Teach the child to keep the key hidden and not show it to anyone.
2. Plan with the child the routine to follow when arriving home; plan something special each day.
3. Plan a telephone contact on the child's arrival home—either have the child call you or you call the child.
4. Always let the child know if you are going to be delayed.
5. Review safety rules with the child. Post them on the refrigerator as a reminder.
6. Use a refrigerator chart to spell out daily responsibilities, and have the child check them off as they are completed.
7. Let the child know how much you appreciate his or her responsible behavior.
8. Have a trusted neighbor for backup if the child needs help; be sure the child knows the telephone number, and post it by the phone.
9. Post telephone emergency numbers the child can use; practice when to use them.
10. Teach the child to tell telephone callers that the caregiver is busy, but never to say that the caregiver is not home.
11. Teach the child not to open the door to anyone.
12. Be specific about activities that are allowed and those that are not allowed.
13. Carefully survey your home for any hazards or dangerous temptations (ie, guns, motorcycle, ATV, swimming pool). Eliminate them, if possible, or ensure that rules about them are clear.
14. See if your community has a telephone friend program available for latchkey children.
15. A pet can relieve loneliness, but give the child clear guidelines about care of the pet during your absence.

children but may be better than the constant tension and turmoil that they have lived through in their home.

Children often feel responsible for the breakup and believe that it would not have occurred if they had just done the right thing or been good. On the other hand, children may blame one of the parents for deciding to end the marriage and thus causing the children grief and unhappiness. Children commonly feel unloved and, in a sense, feel that they too are being divorced. Counseling can help children to acknowledge and understand their anger and their need to blame one or the other of the parents. This process may take a considerable amount of time to resolve. Both parents should make every effort to eliminate the child's feeling of guilt and should avoid using the child as a spy or go-between with the estranged spouse. Parents must avoid trying to buy the affection of the children. This is especially true for the noncustodial parent, who must not shower the chil-

dren with special gifts, trips, and privileges when the children are visiting.

Children should be encouraged to ask questions about the separation and divorce. A child who does not ask questions may be afraid to ask for fear of retaliation by one of the parents. Children should be discouraged from thinking that they might be able to do something that would get

A Personal Glimpse

When I was 15, my dad told me that he and my mom were getting a divorce. I think he expected me to be sad or surprised, but really I was relieved. I hated living in a house with my parents fighting all the time or just not talking to each other. Also, I didn't think it was good for my younger brother.

Though I was happy that the era of fighting was over, the time after the divorce was difficult. Both my parents were very mean to one another, while trying to get me to take sides. I felt they were too concerned with their own lives. I was mad at them for the way they were acting and I didn't think they were being good parents. I figured that I could take care of myself and my brother better than they could; so I changed a lot. I had parties while I was babysitting, stayed out past curfew, skipped classes and studied less, and contradicted my parents' rules for my brother. I thought I was acting like an adult by making my own decisions and not caring about what my parents thought, but really I was acting more childish than ever before. The worst part was that I put myself and my brother in a lot of danger.

It would have been better for me to work with my parents than against them. I just didn't realize how hard it was for them; after all, I thought the divorce was a great idea. I wish they had confided in me. I think I would have understood. I also wish I had told them how I felt. I think they assumed I wasn't angry because I was okay with them getting a divorce.

Joelle, age 24

the parents back together again. They must be helped to recognize the finality of the divorce. Plans for the children should be made (eg, where and with whom the children will live, where they will go to school) and shared with the children as soon as possible. This can give the children a sense of security in their chaotic personal world. Each child's confidence and self-esteem must be strengthened through careful handling of the transition.

When a child of a divorce is hospitalized, the nurse must be certain to have clear information about who is the custodial parent, as well as who may visit or otherwise contact the child. The custodial parent's instructions and wishes should be honored.

The nurse may encourage the child to express feelings of fear and guilt. The nurse also can help the child understand that other children have divorced parents. The school nurse may function as an advocate for a counseling program in the school setting that brings together children of divorces. During counseling, children can voice their fears and concerns and begin to work through them with the help of an objective counselor in a protected environment. One of the most important aspects of such groups is the reassurance the children get that they are not alone in this crisis.

When the custodial parent begins to date and plans to remarry, the child may again have strong emotions that must be worked through. If the remarriage brings together a blended family of children from the previous marriages of both adults, the children may need extra support in accepting the new stepparent and stepsiblings. Adults who seek preventive counseling when planning to form a stepfamily have greater success than those who seek help only after problems are overwhelming.

Children react in various ways to the parent's new marriage, depending in part on age. The new marriage may introduce additional problems of a new home, new neighborhood, and new school that can cause anxiety for any child. Although children should not be permitted to veto the parent's choice of a new partner, every effort should be made to help them adjust to this new family member and view the change in a nonthreatening way.

THE HOMELESS FAMILY

A growing number of families are homeless in the United States. The causes of homelessness include job loss, loss of housing, drug addiction of adult caregivers, insufficient income, domestic turmoil, and separation or divorce. Single mothers with children make up an increasing number of these families. Many of these homeless single mothers and their families have multiple problems. In one study, homeless mothers in Los Angeles reported more than twice as many instances of abuse, drug use, and mental health problems as did those classified as housed poor.[7] In urban

areas, most homeless families are from minority groups, but in nonurban areas, the homeless families are primarily white.[8] Many of these families lived with relatives for a time before being reduced to living in a car, an empty building, a welfare hotel, or perhaps a cardboard box. These families sometimes seek temporary housing in a shelter for the homeless. They often move from one living situation to another, living in a shelter for the time allowed and then moving elsewhere, only to return after a while to repeat the cycle (Fig. 20-5).

Homelessness creates additional stresses for the family. Many homeless families have young children but have problems gaining entry into the health care system, even though these children are at high risk for developing an acute or chronic condition. Health care for these families commonly occurs as crisis intervention instead of the more effective preventive intervention. Pregnant homeless women receive little if any prenatal care, are poorly nourished, and bear low-birth weight infants, with their attendant problems. Most of the children of homeless families do not have adequate immunizations. Homeless children suffer from chronic illnesses at twice the rate of the general population.[8] These chronic conditions include anemia, heart disease, peripheral vascular disease, and neurologic disorders. Many homeless children have developmental delays, perform poorly when they attend school, and suffer from anxiety and depression in addition to having behavioral problems.

Many shelters available to the homeless are overcrowded, lack privacy (the bathroom facilities are used by many people), and have no personal bedding, no cribs for infants, and no facilities for cooking or refrigerating food. Because of limits to the length of stay, many families must move from one shelter to another. This adds to the prob-

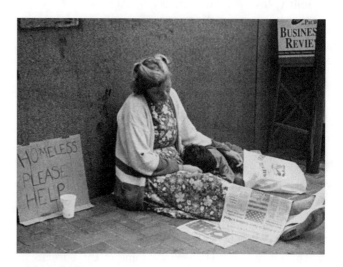

Figure 20-5
The homeless family has become a growing concern across the United States.

lems these families face, contributing to a lack of consistency in the services and programs available to them.

Nurses can set the tone of the interaction between the homeless family and the health care facility. It is important to establish an environment in which the caregiver feels respected and comfortable. Focusing initially on the positive factors in the caregiver's relationship with the children alleviates some of the caregiver's guilt and fear of being criticized. Make every effort to offer down-to-earth suggestions and help the family in the most practical manner.

On admission of the child to the health care facility, perform a complete admission assessment. Ask the caregiver about the family's living arrangements; such information will help in the care and planning for the child. During this interview, the nurse may become aware of problems of other family members that need attention. When giving assistance and guidance, be careful to supplement the family's functioning, not to take it over. For instance, tell the family how to go about getting a particular benefit, and be certain they have complete and accurate information, but do not do it for them. These families need to feel self-reliant and in control and need realistic solutions to their problems.

Outreach programs for the homeless have been established in many major cities. These programs conduct screening, treat acute illnesses, and help families contact local health care services when they are needed. Provide information to the family about any assistance that is available.

■ KEY POINTS

- Many stresses, such as job loss, a financial crisis, illness, injury, loss of home, and death, cause families to respond in a dysfunctional way.

- A growing number of families cannot handle these kinds of stresses.

- Child abuse can be physical, emotional, or sexual and is often complicated by the use of drugs and alcohol.

- The nurse must serve as an advocate for children in abusive homes.

- Older children often try to escape home situations they find unacceptable by running away, but they find life in the outside world even more traumatic.

- The caregivers of latchkey children must plan ahead to help the children accept the responsibilities they must assume when home alone.

- The nurse may help alleviate some of the burdens of divorce and homelessness on the family through counseling and education.

- The nurse must be sensitive to the underlying needs of

children in dysfunctional families and help by providing guidance for the whole family.

 CRITICAL THINKING

1. Maria, a pregnant teen, has been bragging about the "partying" she has been doing. Discuss your feelings about this. Explain what you can tell her about the use of alcohol during pregnancy and the symptoms of fetal alcohol syndrome.
2. Children react differently to living with a family caregiver who is addicted. What behaviors would cause you to be alert to a child with such a family problem?
3. Your neighbor, 17-year-old Holly, has an active 18-month-old toddler named Jason. You overhear Holly screaming at him and saying, "I'm going to beat you if you don't listen to me!" Describe your feelings about this. Discuss plans to help Holly diplomatically.
4. You are on duty in the emergency department when an infant is admitted with injuries that cause you to suspect abuse. The mother says her boyfriend was babysitting for her. State how you feel about this. Describe the observations you will make when assessing the infant. What are your plans to approach the mother?
5. You have an opportunity to talk to a youth group about the hazards of becoming a runaway. Explain some of the points you will make.
6. You have an 8-year-old daughter who must stay alone every day until you get home from work. How will you prepare her? What plans will you make?

REFERENCES

1. Ewing H. Care of women and children in the perinatal period. In Fleming MF, Barry KL, eds. Addictive disorders. St. Louis: Mosby–Year Book, 1992.
2. Kaltenback K. Finnegan LP. Neonatal abstinence syndrome: Pharmacotherapy and developmental outcome. Neurobehav Toxicol Teratol 8(4):353–355, 1986.
3. Brady JP, Posner M, Lang C, Rosati MJ. Risk and reality: The implications of prenatal exposure to alcohol and other drugs. The Education Development Center, Inc., 1994.
4. Wissow LS. Child maltreatment. In Oski FA, ed. Principles and practice of pediatrics. Philadelphia: JB Lippincott, 1994.
5. Walker C, Zangrillo P, Smith J. Parental drug abuse and African American children in foster care: Issues and study findings. Washington, DC: U.S. Department of Health and Human Services, National Black Child Development Institute, 1991.
6. Paradise JE. The medical evaluation of the sexually abused child. Pediatr Clin North Am 37(4):839–862, 1990.
7. Wood D, Valdez RB, Hayashi T, et al. Homeless and housed families in Los Angeles: A study comparing demographic, economic, and family function characteristics. Am J Public Health 80(9):104, 1990.
8. Weinreb LF, Bassuk EL. Health care of homeless families: A

growing challenge for family medicine. J Fam Pract 31(1): 74–80, 1990.

BIBLIOGRAPHY

Bassuk E, Rosenberg L. Psychosocial characteristics of homeless children and children with homes. Pediatrics 85(3):257–261, 1990.

Bresnahan K, Brooks C, Zuckerman B. Prenatal cocaine use: Impact on infants and mothers. Pediatr Nurs 17(2):123–129, 1991.

Coletti S. Maternal-child nursing. In Allen K. Nursing care of the addicted client. Philadelphia: Lippincott-Raven, 1996.

Culverwell M. Perinatal effects of cocaine. Childbirth Instr 1(1): 10–17, 1991.

D'Avanzo CE. Incest: Break the silence, break the cycle. RN 53(10):34–36, 1990.

Davidhizar R, Frank B. Understanding the physical and psychoso-cial stressors of the child who is homeless. Pediatr Nurs 18(6): 559–562, 1992.

Free T, Russell F, Mills B, et al. A descriptive study of infants and toddlers exposed prenatally to substance abuse. MCN 15(4): 245–249, 1990.

Jackson DB, Saunders RB. Child health nursing. Philadelphia: JB Lippincott, 1993.

Jurgrau A. How to spot child abuse. RN 53(10):26–33, 1990.

Kelley SJ, Walsh JH, Thompson K. Birth outcomes, health problems, and neglect with prenatal exposure to cocaine. Pediatr Nurs 17(2):130–136, 1991.

Malloy C. Children and poverty: America's future at risk. Pediatr Nurs 18(6):553–557, 1992.

Melnyk BM. Changes in parent–child relationships following divorce. Pediatr Nurs 17(4):337–341, 1991.

Pillitteri A. Maternal and child health nursing. Philadelphia: Lippincott-Raven, 1996.

Wong DL. Whaley and Wong's nursing care of infants and children, 5th ed. St. Louis: Mosby–Year Book, 1995.

Chapter 21

The Child With a Chronic Health Problem

COMMON PROBLEMS IN CHRONIC ILLNESS
EFFECTS OF CHRONIC ILLNESS ON THE FAMILY
Parents and Chronic Illness

The Child and Chronic Illness
Siblings and Chronic Illness
Nursing Process in Caring for a Child With a Chronic Illness

STUDENT OBJECTIVES

On completion of this chapter, the student will be able to:

1. Define the key terms.
2. Identify 10 conditions that cause chronic illness.
3. Identify 10 concerns that are common to many families of a child with a chronic illness.
4. Describe economic pressures that can overwhelm families of chronically ill children.
5. Discuss the importance of respite care.
6. Discuss the effect a developmental stage may have on the child's needs.
7. Identify positive and negative responses that well siblings may manifest in response to an ill sibling.
8. Describe how the nurse can help the family adjust to the child's condition.
9. Identify several ways the nurse may encourage self-care by the child.
10. Discuss general guidelines for preparing the family for home care of the child.

KEY TERMS

chronic illness   rejection
denial   respite care
gradual acceptance   stigma
overprotection

Chronic illness is a leading health problem in the United States. The numbers are growing as more infants and children survive prematurity, difficult births, congenital anomalies and illnesses that once were fatal, and accidents. Most children experience only brief, acute episodes of illness; however, a significant number are affected by chronic health problems. Diseases that cause chronic illness include congenital heart disease, cystic fibrosis, juvenile arthritis, asthma, hemophilia, muscular dystrophy, leukemia and other malignancies, spina bifida, and immunodeficiency syndromes. When a family member has a chronic illness, the entire family is affected in many ways. Chronic illness may affect the child's physical, psychosocial, and cognitive development. Because nurses are usually involved from the early stages of diagnosis, and because the child and family have ongoing, long-term needs, the nurse can play a vital role in helping the family adjust to the condition.

COMMON PROBLEMS IN CHRONIC ILLNESS

Chronic illness is a condition that interferes with daily functioning for more than 3 months in a year, causes hospitalization of more than 1 month in a year, or (at time of diagnosis) is likely to do either of these.[1] Specific chronic health problems of children were discussed in earlier chapters. Each requires individualized management based on the disease process and the ability of the patient and family to understand and comply with the treatment regimen. All chronic health problems, however, create some common difficulties for patients and families, and these are the focus of this chapter. Some of these concerns are:

- Financial concerns—paying for treatment, living expenses at a distant health care facility, caregiver's loss of job because of lost time
- Administration of treatments and medications at home
- Disruption of family life—vacations, family goals, careers
- Educational opportunities for the child
- Social isolation due to the child's condition
- Family adjustments due to the changing course of the disease

- Reaction of well siblings
- Stress among caregivers
- Guilt about and acceptance of the chronic condition
- Care of the child when family caregivers can no longer provide care.

EFFECTS OF CHRONIC ILLNESS ON THE FAMILY

The diagnosis of a chronic health problem causes a crisis in the family, whether it happens during the first few hours or days of the child's life or much later. How families cope with chronic illness varies greatly from one family to another, but they all face many of the same problems.

Parents and Chronic Illness

When family caregivers learn of the child's diagnosis, their first reaction may be shock, disbelief, and denial. These reactions may last for a varied amount of time, from days to months. The initial response may be one of mourning for the "perfect" child they lost, combined with guilt, blame, and rationalization. The caregivers may seek advice from other professionals and actually may go "shopping" for another physician. They may refuse to accept the diagnosis or refuse to talk about it, or they may delay seeking or agreeing to treatment. Gradually, they adjust to the diagnosis. They may enter a period of chronic sorrow in which they adapt to the child's state of chronic illness but do not necessarily accept it. They often waver between the stages and experience highs and lows of emotions as they care for the child and meet the challenges of daily life. Families who have a strong support system usually are better able to meet these challenges.

Economic pressures can become overwhelming to the families of chronically ill children. If the family does not have adequate health insurance, the costs of treatment may be enormous. Away-from-home living costs may become a problem if the child must go to a distant hospital for further diagnosis or treatment. To keep health insurance benefits, a family caregiver may feel tied to a job, which creates additional stress. The time required to take the child to medical appointments can be excessive and may cause an additional threat to job security because of the time lost from the job.

Families must make many adjustments to care for the chronically ill child. The family caregivers may have to learn to perform treatments and give medications. Family life is often disrupted. Vacations may be nonexistent, and the family may be limited in how they can spend their leisure time. Families may have difficulty finding babysitters and have little opportunity for a break in the routine. Some families become isolated from customary social activities because of the responsibilities of caring for their

COMMUNICATIONS BOX

The nurse is completing a home visit to see 14-year-old Anna, who has had a severe exacerbation of her cystic fibrosis. Her mother, Marie, cares for her. The nurse notices that Marie appears exhausted.

INEFFECTIVE COMMUNICATION

Nurse: Marie, you look exhausted. Are you getting enough sleep?
Marie: Oh, I'm OK.
Nurse: Well, you mustn't let yourself get overtired or you won't be able to take care of Anna.
Marie: I'll be all right. I can take care of her just fine.
Nurse: If you need help, I could see if I can find someone to help you out. You know you can't do everything yourself.
Marie: Really, I'll be OK. You just caught me at a bad time.
Nurse: Well, all right, but I worry about you.

The nurse's first comment put Marie on the defensive. Marie felt she had to defend herself and protest that she was doing everything she should to take care of her daughter. Unfortunately, the nurse did nothing to boost Marie's self-image, so Marie continued to defend herself. The nurse ended up without helping to solve the problem.

EFFECTIVE COMMUNICATION

Nurse: Marie, I know that caring for Anna is very wearing. Perhaps we can plan together to give you some respite from caring for her 24 hours a day.
Marie: Oh, I don't know. I'm doing all right, I think.
Nurse: You are doing a great job. However, I am concerned about the long term. I don't want you to run the risk of tiring yourself so much you won't be able to care for her.
Marie: Well, yes, but I am strong, I think I can handle it.
Nurse: Yes, I know you are strong and I have such admiration for the job you are doing. But let's just sit down and look at some ways we can plan together to ease things a little for you and perhaps give you some free time.
Marie: OK. I guess that sounds like a good idea.

By opening the subject with a positive, noncritical statement, the nurse begins to establish a good connection with Marie. Immediately Marie feels the nurse's recognition of her hard work. The nurse continues by telling her what a good job she is doing. By suggesting they work on solving the problem together the nurse gains Marie's cooperation.

child. **Respite care** (care of the ill child so that the caregivers can have a period of rest and refreshment) is often desperately needed but is not readily available in many communities. Families where both parents worked may have to forgo the second income so that one adult can stay home with the child.

As the child grows, concerns about education may become foremost among the caregivers' worries. These concerns include the availability of appropriate education, early learning opportunities, physical accessibility of the facilities, acceptance of the child by school personnel and classmates, mainstreaming versus segregated classes, availability and quality of homebound teaching, and general flexibility of the school's teachers and administrators. Few schools are prepared to accommodate treatments at school that would otherwise require the child to leave during the school day. Family caregivers often must become the child's advocate to preserve as much normalcy as possible in the child's educational experience.

As the child's condition changes, the family must make additional changes. All these stresses may strain the marriage, although the divorce rate does not seem to be affected by the presence of a chronically ill child in the family.[2] However, single parents have significant needs to which health care personnel must be especially sensitive.

The Child and Chronic Illness

The child with a chronic illness may face many problems that interfere with normal growth and development. These problems vary with the diagnosis and condition. The child's attitude toward the condition is a critical element in the long-term management and in the family's adjustment.

A Personal Glimpse

I am 16 years old and I was diagnosed with cystic fibrosis at birth. Every morning I wake up and have many things that I have to accomplish: taking a breathing treatment, having percussions done, and taking many pills. I guess it isn't so bad if you are used to doing it every day, but it is a bit annoying having the same routine all the time. I have been doing all of this for 16 years. I sometimes feel that I am very different from other people. My friends don't feel it is weird having me as a friend, but they know that I have this disease and they are afraid of what can happen to me. My friends don't treat me any different. I think that is the most important thing. It is good that I have friends who can care so much that they don't let it bother them.

I don't like it when I have to cough all the time; every one stares at me. When I am in school, at lunch I have to take pills before I eat. Everyone is always asking me why I am taking the pills. Even when I go to a friend's house, I have to take my medication and get my percussions done. My friends usually help out with the percussions.

A lot of times I feel very lonely because I am the only one in my family that has this disease. No one knows what I am feeling, and that sometimes makes me very lonely and afraid. I have a twin brother who really cares for me a lot. When anyone asks about my illness, he is usually the person to explain it to them. He has always been there for me when I needed him. When I have to go in the hospital, he gets my work for me. We are very close. I am glad to have a brother like him.

I am very lucky to have a family that cares for me and loves me like they do. They are always helping me when I need percussions done and they are very supportive. I don't know what I would do without their help. They all took care of me when I couldn't. They still do now. I owe them a lot of credit. I love them very much and always will.

Gretchen, age 16

For instance, the child who must be immobilized during school age while in the stage of industry versus inferiority cannot complete the tasks of industry, such as helping with household chores or working on special projects with siblings or peers.

The child's response to the chronic condition is influenced by the response of family caregivers. Several typical responses have been identified: **overprotection, rejection, denial,** and **gradual acceptance.** Overprotective caregivers try to protect the child at all costs, preventing the child from learning new skills by hovering, failing to use discipline, and using every means to prevent the child from experiencing any frustration. Rejecting caregivers distance themselves emotionally from the child; although they provide physical care, they tend to scold and correct the child continuously. Caregivers in denial behave as though the condition does not exist, encouraging the child to overcompensate for any disabilities. Caregivers who respond with gradual acceptance take a common-sense approach to the child's condition, helping the child to set realistic goals for self-care and independence and encouraging the child to achieve social and physical skills within his or her capability.

Children often perceive any illness as punishment for a bad thought or action. The child's perception of chronic illness is subject to the same magical thinking, depending on the child's developmental stage at the time of diagnosis. This perception is also influenced by the attitudes of parents and peers and by whether the dysfunctional body part is visible. Problems such as asthma, allergies, and epilepsy are difficult for children to understand because "what's wrong" is inside, not outside.

The child's family, peers, and school personnel make up the support system that can affect the child's adaptation. Sometimes the efforts necessary to meet the child's physical needs are so great that finding time and energy to meet the child's emotional needs can be difficult for members of the support team. The older child with a chronic illness also has developing sexual needs that should not be ignored but must be acknowledged and provided for.

Additional stresses continue to occur as the disease progresses. For instance, Hodgkin's disease can be successfully treated for a time with chemotherapy and radiation therapy, but that means adding the side effects of treatment (steroid-induced acne, edema, and alopecia) to the disease manifestations of night sweats, chronic fatigue, pruritus, and gastrointestinal bleeding. The child with Duchenne's muscular dystrophy gradually weakens, so that in adolescence he or she is wheelchair-bound when peers are actively involved in sports and exploring sexual relationships. These stresses can add up to more than one young person can cope with for long.

Discrimination continues to be present in the life of the chronically ill child and the family. Discrimination can occur in relationships among children; social exclusion of the chronically ill child is common. Physical barriers may present problems that families must struggle to help their child overcome. Sometimes hurtful discrimination is as simple as being stared at in public places.

Siblings and Chronic Illness

Some degree of sibling rivalry can be found in most families with healthy children, so it is not surprising that a child with a chronic health problem can seriously disrupt the lives of brothers and sisters. Much of the family caregivers' time, attention, and money is directed toward management of the ill child's problem. This can cause anger, resentment, and jealousy in the well siblings. The caregivers' failure to set limits for the ill child's behavior while maintaining discipline for the healthy siblings can cause further resentment. Some family caregivers unknowingly create feelings of guilt in the healthy children by overemphasizing the ill child's needs.

Siblings may feel **stigma** (embarrassment or shame) because of a brother or sister with a chronic illness, especially if the ill child has a physical disfigurement or apparent cognitive deficit. Siblings may choose not to tell others about the ill child or may be selective in whom they tell, choosing only persons they can trust. An older sibling is more likely to tell others than a younger one, perhaps because the older child tends to understand more about the illness and its effect.

Both positive and negative influences can be found in the behaviors of well siblings. Some siblings react with anger, hostility, jealousy, increased competition for attention, social withdrawal, and poor school performance. On the other hand, many siblings demonstrate positive behav-

Figure 21-1
A sister helps a ventilator-dependent sibling with dinner.

iors, such as caring and concern for the ill sibling, cooperating with family caregivers in helping care for the ill child, protecting the ill child from negative reaction of others, and including the ill child in activities with peers (Fig. 21-1).

How well siblings react to a chronically ill sibling may ultimately depend on how the family copes with stress and how its members feel about one another. Families that seem to adapt most successfully to the presence of a child with chronic illness are those in which the caregivers:

- Find time for special activities with the healthy children
- Explain the ill child's condition as simply as possible
- Involve the healthy siblings in the care of the ill child (according to their developmental ability)
- Set behavioral limits for all children in the family.

This is a delicate balance that is challenging and takes great effort and caring for a family to sustain, but the results are well worth it.

⚑⚐ Nursing Process in Caring for a Child ⚐⚑ With a Chronic Illness

ASSESSMENT

The assessment of the family and the child with a disability or chronic illness is an ongoing process. The assessment is reviewed and updated with each visit the child makes to the health care facility. Include the child in the assessment interview if he or she is old enough and able to participate. The child may have had many visits and treatments in the past that have left negative memories, so approach the child in a low-key, kind, gentle manner to gain cooperation. Unless the child is newly diagnosed, the family caregivers may have a good understanding of the condition. Assess this knowledge so that plans can be made to supplement it if needed.

During the assessment interview, determine how the family is coping with the child's condition and assess the family's strengths, weaknesses, and acceptance of the diagnosis. Identify the needs that change with the child's condition and include them in planning care. Also consider needs that change with the child's growth and development.

Adjust the physical assessment to correspond with the child's illness and current condition. Throughout the physical assessment, make every effort to gain the child's cooperation and explain what is being done in terms the child can understand. Offer praise for cooperating throughout the assessment to gain the child's (and the family caregivers') goodwill.

NURSING DIAGNOSES

The nursing diagnoses vary depending on the illness or disability, but certain developmental diagnoses are appropriate regardless of the medical diagnosis, such as:

- Altered Family Processes related to adjustment requirements for the child with chronic illness or disability

- Altered Growth and Development related to impaired ability to achieve developmental tasks or family caregivers' reactions to the child's condition

- Anxiety related to procedures, tests, or hospitalization

- Self Care Deficit related to limitations of illness or disability

- Anticipatory Grieving of family caregiver related to possible losses secondary to condition

- Risk for Social Isolation of the child or family related to the child's condition

- Health Seeking Behaviors by caregivers related to home care of the child

OUTCOME IDENTIFICATION AND PLANNING

Major goals for the chronically ill child are to accomplish growth and development milestones, perform self-care tasks, experience fewer feelings of social isolation and decreased anxiety. Goals for the caregiver or family are to improve their coping skills, alleviate their feelings of grief, anger, and guilt, and teach about the child's illness.

IMPLEMENTATION

HELPING THE FAMILY ADJUST TO THE CHILD'S CONDITION. The family's adjustment to the condition is assessed during the assessment interview. Adjustment may depend on how recently the child has been diagnosed. After determining the family's needs, provide an opportunity for the family members to express their feelings and anxieties. Help them explore any feelings of guilt or blame about the child's condition. Encourage them to express doubts they may have about their ability to cope with the child's future. Help the caregivers look realistically at their resources, and give them suggestions on ways to cope. Serve as a role model when caring for the child, expressing a positive attitude toward the child and the illness or disability.

Question the family to determine the resources and support systems available to them. Remind the family that these support systems may include immediate family members, extended family, friends, community services, and health care providers.

Encourage the caregivers to discuss the needs of the well siblings and their adjustment to the ill child's condition. Help the family meet the needs of the well siblings, and help the siblings feel comfortable with the ill child's problems and needs. Assist the family in setting reasonable expectations for all their children.

ENCOURAGING OPTIMAL GROWTH AND DEVELOPMENT. The family caregivers may become overprotective, preventing the ill child from exhibiting growth and development appropriate for his or her age and disability. Help the caregivers recognize the child's potential and set realistic growth and development goals. Consistent care by the same staff helps provide a sense of routine in which the child can be encouraged to have some control and perform age-appropriate tasks within the limitations of the disability. Set age-appropriate limits and enforce appropriate discipline. Accomplish this gradually, displaying a kind and caring attitude. Give the child choices within the limits of treatments and other aspects of required care. Encourage the child to dress when appropriate to reduce feelings of being an invalid. Encourage the child to learn about the condition. Introducing the child to other children with the same or a similar condition can help dispel feelings that he or she is the only person with such a condition. An older child or adolescent benefits from social interaction with peers with or without disabilities (Fig. 21-2). Encourage family caregivers to help the adolescent join in age-appropriate activities. The adolescent also may need some help in dressing or using makeup to improve his or her appearance and minimize any physical disability.

REDUCING ANXIETY ABOUT PROCEDURES AND TREATMENTS. Periodically, perhaps over a long period, the child may need to undergo procedures, tests, and treatments. The child may also be hospitalized frequently. Many

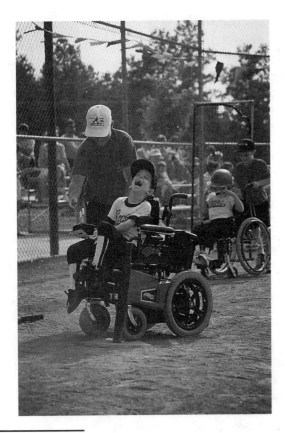

Figure 21-2
Volunteer buddies assist in Little League Challenger Handicapped Division.

of the procedures may be painful, or at least uncomfortable. Explain the tests, treatments, and procedures to the child ahead of time and encourage the child to ask questions. Acknowledge to the child that a particular procedure is painful and help the child plan ways to handle the pain. Advise family caregivers that they should also help the child prepare for hospitalization ahead of time whenever possible.

PROMOTING SELF-CARE.   To encourage the child to assist in self-care, devise aids to ease tasks. When appropriate, integrate play and toys into the care to help encourage cooperation. Praise the child genuinely and generously for tasks that are attempted, even if they are not totally completed. Do not expect the child to perform tasks beyond his or her capabilities. Make certain the child is well rested before any energy-taxing tasks are attempted. Use a chart or other visual aid with the tasks listed as a tool to help the child reach a desired goal. Stickers can record the child's progress. School-age children often respond well to contracts—for instance, when a set number of stickers are earned, a special privilege or other incentive is awarded. Remember that these tasks often are hard work for the child.

PREVENTING SOCIAL ISOLATION.   A child who requires constant or frequent attention often wears on the family caregivers. The family with no close extended family and few close friends may find getting away for rest and relaxation, even for an evening, almost impossible. Help the family caregivers find resources for respite care. Any caregiver, no matter how devoted, needs to have a break from everyday cares and concerns. Refer the family to social services, where they can get help. Sometimes a caregiver may feel that another person cannot care for the child adequately. Encourage this caregiver to express fears and anxieties about leaving the child. This helps the caregiver work through some of these anxieties and feel more confident about getting away for a period of rest.

The child may feel isolated from peers. When the child is hospitalized, consider arranging for contact with peers by phone, in writing, or through visits. Encourage regular school attendance as soon as the child is physically able. If the child is mainstreamed in a regular classroom, suggest that the caregiver make arrangements with the school for rest periods as needed. Ask the child about interests; these may give some clues about suitable after-school activities that will increase the child's interactions with peers. Make suggestions and confer with family caregivers to ensure that proposed plans are carried out. Listen carefully to the child during discussions about social activities to gain insight into his or her feelings about socialization.

AIDING CAREGIVERS' ACCEPTANCE OF THE CONDITION.   When anyone suffers a serious loss, a grief reaction occurs. This is true of family caregivers when they first learn that their child has a chronic or disabling illness: they must mourn the loss of their desired or "perfect" child. Encourage family caregivers to express these feelings and help them understand that this reaction is common and acceptable.

Denial is usually the first reaction that family caregivers have to the diagnosis. This is a time when they say, "How could this be?" or "Why my child?" Let them express their emotions, and respond in a nonjudgmental way. Staying with them and offering quiet, accepting support may be helpful. Statements such as, "It will seem better in time" are inappropriate. Acknowledge the caregivers' feelings as acceptable and reasonable.

During the next stage, guilt, listen to the caregivers express their feelings of guilt and remorse. Again, acknowledging their feelings is useful. Accept expressions of anger by family caregivers without viewing them as a personal attack. Using listening techniques that reflect the caregivers' feelings, such as "You sound very angry," is a helpful method of handling these emotions.

Grief reactions also may occur when the family caregivers are informed that their child is deteriorating or has had a setback. Although caregivers usually cycle through these reactions much more quickly at this time, the same methods are useful.

PLANNING FOR HOME CARE.   Home care planning begins when the child is admitted to the health care facility and continues until discharge. Focus plans for care at home on the continuing care, medications, and treatments the child will need. During a health care visit or hospitalization, include family caregivers when caring for the child so that they become comfortable with the care. Children are often sent home with sophisticated equipment and treatments; therefore, demonstrate the use of the equipment and treatments and give the family caregivers a chance to perform the treatments under guidance and supervision. A discussion of the home's facilities may be appropriate to help the family accommodate any special needs the child may have. Give the caregivers a list of community services and organizations they can turn to for help and support, including appropriate disease- or disability-specific organizations.

Teach the caregivers about growth and development guidelines so that they have a realistic concept of what to expect as the child develops. Throughout the child's stay, encourage caregivers to express their concerns to help solve whatever problems the family anticipates while caring for the child at home. Give the family the name and telephone number of a contact person they can call for support. Families face many hurdles while caring for a chronically ill child, but with the reassurance that help is just a telephone call away, they are more likely to feel that they can competently face the future.

Caring for a chronically ill child can be an overwhelming task and requires cooperation by all involved with the child and the family. Family caregivers deserve all the help they can get. (See Nursing Care Plan for the Chronically Ill Child and Family.)

Nursing Care Plan
for the Chronically Ill Child and Family

Billy is a 10-year-old who has Duchenne muscular dystrophy. His condition has worsened and he has recently begun to use a walker. He has gradually begun to need more assistance in his activities of daily living. He has a sister who is 8 years old and a 5-year-old brother. Both parents live at home.

NURSING DIAGNOSIS

Altered Family Processes related to adjustment to the child with chronic illness

GOAL: *Billy's family will adjust to his weakening condition.*

OUTCOME CRITERIA

• The family members express fears and anxieties about Billy's weakening condition.
• The family verbalizes a positive attitude to Billy about his adaptations to his growing weakness.
• Billy's mother expresses her feelings of guilt about his illness and deals with them positively.

Nursing Interventions	Rationale
Provide opportunities for family members to express feelings, including fears about his weakening.	The family may need encouragement to talk about some of their fears and anxieties.
Maintain a positive but realistic attitude about Billy's growing disabilities, both when providing care and when discussing the impact of Billy's illness on the family.	The nurse serves as a role model for the family; modeling a positive attitude will help family caregivers take the same approach.
Explore with Billy's mother her feelings of guilt.	The mother needs to resolve her feelings of guilt.
Provide the family with resources and support systems. Encourage them to talk with their younger children about their feelings concerning Billy's illness.	The family needs to use community resources and support systems to help them with the long-term needs of the entire family.

(continued)

Nursing Care Plan (Continued)
for the Chronically Ill Child and Family

NURSING DIAGNOSIS

Altered Growth and Development related to impaired ability to achieve developmental tasks and family caregivers' reactions to the child's condition

GOAL: *Optimal growth and development will be accomplished, within Billy's capabilities.*

OUTCOME CRITERIA

- Family sets realistic developmental goals for Billy.
- Family encourages Billy to reach his potential.
- Billy demonstrates a positive outlook about his achievements.

Nursing Interventions	Rationale
Discuss with Billy's family the effects of overprotectiveness on his development.	Many families react to a child's long-term illness by shielding the child from challenges that the child could cope with if allowed to do so.
Help Billy's family recognize his potential and help them set realistic goals; encourage them to set age-appropriate limits for activities, with appropriate discipline for violations.	Family caregivers may not know what to expect in terms of their child's development and may tend to overprotect the child, preventing him from reaching his potential; it is important to allow him to reach for his potential without overprotecting him.
Encourage Billy to carry out self-care appropriate for his age and stage of mobility; allow him to make as many choices as possible.	Billy will have a better feeling of control and self-worth; he will be encouraged to try new things and not to let his illness unnecessarily stop him.

NURSING DIAGNOSIS

Self Care Deficit related to limitations of illness

GOAL: *Self-care tasks will be performed.*

OUTCOME CRITERIA

- Billy participates in self-care as appropriate for his age and capabilities.
- Billy demonstrates evidence of using creative problem-solving techniques.

Nursing Interventions	Rationale
Generously praise any self-care Billy performs; carefully avoid expecting him to do tasks beyond his capabilities.	Positive reinforcement gives Billy self-confidence and pride in his accomplishments.
When Billy finds a task difficult to accomplish, assist him by devising aids to help him with the task rather than doing it for him.	Reinforces importance of self-care and independence; demonstrates creative problem-solving techniques, which Billy can use in the future.

NURSING DIAGNOSIS

Risk for Social Isolation related to the child's condition

GOAL: *Social interaction will be promoted.*

(continued)

Nursing Care Plan (Continued)
for the Chronically Ill Child and Family

OUTCOME CRITERIA
- Billy participates in activities with his peers.
- Billy's family finds adequate respite care for Billy.
- Billy's family gets away for a break with minimal anxieties.

Nursing Interventions	Rationale
Encourage the family to establish and maintain Billy's contacts with his peers. Advise the family that this may take advance planning and creative solutions for him to participate in activities such as team sports.	Billy needs to feel that he is part of the world in which his schoolmates and friends are involved; he needs activities to look forward to.
Help family caregivers find resources for respite care, making referrals to social services or other resources as necessary.	Family caregivers who periodically get away from the responsibilities of caring for the child will be re-energized and return with a refreshed spirit.
Encourage the family caregivers to express anxieties about leaving Billy with someone else.	Talking with the family about such fears helps them work through anxieties, dismiss unrealistic fears, and make specific plans for legitimate ones. This helps the family to have a more restful time when away.

NURSING DIAGNOSIS
Health Seeking Behaviors related to home care of a child with chronic illness

GOAL: *Family members will learn to care for Billy at home.*

OUTCOME CRITERIA
- Family members demonstrate ability to perform Billy's care and treatment.
- Family members make contact with support group and community services.

Nursing Interventions	Rationale
Explain and demonstrate any equipment used in Billy's care; demonstrate treatments or therapy the family will need to do at home; provide opportunities for practice under the guidance of a nurse or therapist.	Watching someone who knows how to perform a technique well and performing that technique yourself are very different matters. Practice and opportunities for questions are essential.
Provide the family with a list of community services and organizations to which they can turn for help and support; include the name and telephone number of a contact person at the health care facility whom the family can call with questions or concerns.	Knowing whom to contact and how to reach that person gives the family reassurance that help is close by and increases their self-confidence about being able to handle their child's care.

EVALUATION: GOALS AND OUTCOME CRITERIA

■ *Goal*: The family caregivers' anxieties and fears will be reduced.
Criteria: Family caregivers express feelings of guilt and fears and anxieties about the child's condition.

■ *Goal*: The family caregivers will acknowledge appropriate growth and development expectations.
Criteria: Family caregivers acknowledge the child's capabilities, encourage the child, and set realistic goals for the child.

■ *Goal*: The child will have reduced anxiety.

Criteria: The child's anxiety is minimized, as evidenced by cooperation with care and treatments.

- *Goal*: The child will become involved in self-care activities
  Criteria: The child participates in self-care as appropriate for age and capabilities.

- *Goal*: The family and the child will actively socialize with others.
  Criteria: The family and child use opportunities to socialize with others; the family seeks and finds adequate respite care for the child.

- *Goal*: The family will deal with their feelings of anger, grief, guilt, and loss.
  Criteria: Family caregivers receive support for their feelings while working toward accepting the child's condition.

- *Goal*: The family caregivers will actively participate in the child's home care.
  Criteria: Family caregivers ask pertinent questions, contact support groups and community agencies for help, and demonstrate their ability to perform care and treatments.

■ KEY POINTS

- Advances in medical technology have increased the number of families who must care for a child with a chronic illness or disability.

- Caring for such a child over a long period can create much stress in the family.

- Family caregivers often react with denial, guilt, and anger when they first realize they have a child with serious, long-term problems.

- Caregivers sometimes focus on the ill child, losing sight of the needs of the well siblings.

- Volunteer and community agencies provide support and guidance for families, often specific to the child's condition.

- Families must set realistic goals for all family members and use all the support systems available to them.

? CRITICAL THINKING

1. You are caring for 5-year-old Abby, a bright girl with cystic fibrosis. Her mother, Mattie, has been overprotective and has always done everything for her. Describe how you will involve Abby in self-care. Explain what you can say or do to help Mattie encourage Abby to do more of her own care.

2. Nine-year-old Tyson is angry. He tells you he hates his 6-year-old brother, Josh, who has Down syndrome. Relate how you would discuss this with Tyson. If you have the opportunity to talk to his family caregiver, what would you say?

3. Teena and José are the young parents of Nina, a 12-month-old with meningomyelocele (spina bifida). Nina must be catheterized at least four times a day and also has mobility problems. Explore some of the economic and other stresses that this young couple faces.

4. Cassie is a 16-year-old with cerebral palsy. She wants to go to the school prom, but her family caregivers are very resistant to the idea. Cassie pleads with you to talk to them. How will you approach this problem? What are your responses to Cassie and to her caregivers?

5. Eight-year-old Jason, a patient in your pediatric unit, is undergoing chemotherapy. He seems very lonely and sad, although his family visits him regularly. You decide he may need contact with children his own age. Describe plans you will make to provide contact with peers.

6. Using your local phone book, make a list of agencies to which you could refer families for assistance and support in the care of a chronically ill child.

REFERENCES

1. Hobbs N, Perrin JM, eds. Issues in the care of children with chronic illness. San Francisco: Jossey-Bass, 1985.
2. Longo OC, Bond L. Families of the handicapped child: Research and practice. Family Relat 33:57–65, 1984.

BIBLIOGRAPHY

Austin JK. Assessment of coping mechanisms used by parents and children with chronic illness. MCN 15(2):98–102, 1990.

Clements DB, Copeland LG, Loftus M. Critical times for families with a chronically ill child. Pediatr Nurs 16(2):157–161, 1990.

Clubb RL. Chronic sorrow: Adaptation patterns of parents with chronically ill children. Pediatr Nurs 17(5):461–466, 1991.

Crick NR, Ladd GW. Children's perceptions of their peer experiences: Attributions, loneliness, social anxiety, and social avoidance. Devel Psych 29:244–254, 1993.

Davis BD, Steele S. Case management for young children with special health care needs. Pediatr Nurs 17(1):15–19, 1991.

Gallo AM, Breitmayer BJ, Knafl KA, et al. Stigma in childhood chronic illness: A well sibling perspective. Pediatr Nurs 17(1): 21–25, 1991.

Selekman J. Pediatric rehabilitation: From concepts to practice. Pediatr Nurs 17(1):11–14, 1991.

Turner-Henson A, Hoaday B, Corser N, Ogletree G, Swan JH. The experiences of discrimination: Challenges for chronically ill children. Pediatr Nurs 20(6):571–577, 1994.

The Dying Child

STUDENT OBJECTIVES

On completion of this chapter, the student will be able to:

1. Describe the role of anticipatory grief in the grieving process.
2. Identify reasons why nurses may have difficulty working effectively with dying children.
3. Identify how a nurse can personally prepare to care for a dying child.
4. List the factors that affect the child's understanding of death.
5. Describe how a child's understanding of death changes at each developmental level.
6. State the importance of encouraging families to complete unfinished business.
7. Describe why a family may suffer excessive grief and guilt when a child dies suddenly.
8. Describe possible reactions in a child when a sibling dies.
9. Identify settings for caring for the dying child and the advantages and disadvantages of each.

KEY TERMS

anticipatory grief	thanatologist
hospice	unfinished business

The most difficult death to accept is the death of a child. We can accept that elderly patients have lived a full life and that life must end, but the life of a child still holds the hopes, dreams, and promises of the future. When a child's life ends early, whether abruptly as the result of an accident or after a prolonged illness, we ask ourselves, "Why? What's the justice of this?" Caring for a dying child and his or her family is stressful but can be extremely rewarding.

Caring for a family facing the death of their child calls on every personal and professional skill of the nurse. It means offering sensitive, gentle physical care and comfort measures for the child and continuing emotional support for the child, the family caregivers, and the siblings. This kind of caring demands an understanding of the nurse's own feelings about death and dying, knowledge of the grieving process that terminally ill patients and their families experience, and a willingness to become involved.

Like chronic illness, terminal illness creates a family crisis that can either destroy or strengthen the family as a unit and as individuals. Nurses and other health professionals who can offer knowledgeable, sensitive care to these families help make the remainder of the child's life more meaningful and the family's mourning experience more healing. Helping a family struggle through this crisis and emerge stronger and closer can yield deep satisfaction.

Diagnosis of a fatal illness initiates the grieving process in the child and the family: denial and isolation, anger, bargaining, depression and acute grief, and finally acceptance. Not every child or family will complete the process because each family, as well as each death, is personal and unique.

When death is expected, the family begins to mourn, a phenomenon called **anticipatory grief**. For some people, this shortens the period of acute grief and loss after the child's death. Unexpected death offers no chance for preparation, and grief may last longer and be more difficult to resolve.

Death is a tragic reality for thousands of children each year. Accidents are the leading cause of death in children between the ages of 1 and 14 years; cancer is the number one fatal disease in this age group. Nearly all these children leave behind at least one grieving family caregiver and perhaps brothers, sisters, and grandparents. Nurses who care for children and families must be prepared for encounters with the dying and the bereaved.

THE NURSE'S REACTION TO DEATH AND DYING

I am a student nurse. I am dying. I write this to you who are and will become nurses in the hope that by my sharing my feelings with you, you may someday be better able to help those who share my experience. . . . You slip in and out of my room, give me medications and check my blood pressure. Is it because I am a student nurse, myself, or just a human being, that I sense your fright? And your fears enhance mine. Why are you afraid? I am the one who is dying!

I know you feel insecure, don't know what to say, don't know what to do. But please believe me, if you care, you can't go wrong. Just admit that you care . . . Don't run away—wait—all I want to know is that there will be someone to hold my hand when I need it. . . . If only we could be honest, both admit our fears, touch one another. If you really care, would you lose so much of your valuable professionalism if you even cried with me? Just person to person? Then it might not be so hard to die—in a hospital—with friends close by.[1]

The feelings expressed by this young student nurse are not uncommon. Health care workers often are uncomfortable with dying patients, so they avoid them, afraid that the patients will ask questions they cannot or should not answer. These caregivers signal by their behavior that the patient should avoid the fact of his or her impending death and should keep up a show of bravery. In effect, they are asking the patient to meet their needs instead of trying to meet the patient's needs.

Death reminds us of our own mortality, a thought with which many of us are uncomfortable. The thought that someone even younger than we are is about to die makes us feel more vulnerable. Every nurse needs to examine his or her own feelings about death and the reason for these feelings. How have you reacted to the death of a friend or a family member? When growing up, was talking and thinking about death avoided because of your family's attitudes? Admitting that death is a part of life, and that patients should be helped to live each day to the fullest until death, is a step toward understanding and being able to communicate with those who are dying. A workshop, conference, or seminar in which one's own feelings about life and death are explored is useful in preparing the nurse to care for the dying child and family (Box 22-1).

Learning to care for the dying patient means talking with other professionals, sharing concerns, and comforting each other in stressful times. It means reading studies that have been done on death to discover how dying patients feel about their care, their illness, and their families and how they want to spend the rest of their lives. It also means being a sensitive, empathic, nonjudgmental listener to patients and families who need to express their feelings, even if they may not be able to express them to each other.

Box 22-1. *Questions to Cover in a Self-Examination About Death*

Some Considerations in the Resolution of Death and Dying

1. What was your first conscious memory of death? What were your feelings and reactions?
2. What is your most recent memory of death? How was it the same or different from your first memory?
3. What experience of death had the most effect on you? Why?

Get Comfortable and Imagine Now—

You have just been told you have 6 months to live. What is your *first* reaction to that news?

3 months later—What relationships might require you to tie up loose ends? What unfinished business do you have to deal with? You and your significant other are trying to cope with the news. What changes occur in your relationship?

1 month remains—What do you need to have happen in the remaining time? What hopes, dreams, and plans can or need to be fulfilled?

1 week remains—You are very weak and barely have enough energy to talk. You don't even want to look at yourself. Nausea and vomiting are constant companions. Write a letter to the one person you feel would be the most affected by your dying.

24 hours remain—You are dying. Breathing is difficult; you feel very hot inside; overwhelming fatigue is ever-present. How would you like to spend this last day?

These questions can be used in a group with a hospice or other facilitator. They can be used to help heighten your awareness of yourself: who you are, how you have gotten to where you are today, what you are doing with your life and why, how you would change the way you live, your feelings about death—in general, in relation to your friends and family, and in regard to your own death.

With permission from Ruth Anne Sieber, Hospice: The Bridge, Lewistown, PA.

 A Personal Glimpse

I sat in silence rocking the baby, reflecting upon life and death. And as I felt the small bundle of warmth stir within my arms, I realized that while life's essence had died within one it had been born anew within another, continuing and completing the cycle. And that there is never really death, only passing from this world into another; that the spiritual flame is never extinguished, only shared and passed on. And as I held the baby closer still I felt how young and innocent she was, how very much she had to experience and learn. And I felt her vulnerability as my own, realizing that the child in my arms was me, just as she was a symbol of all humanity—and the child within each one of us.

Karen Wapner, age 17 (written while working through her grief after the death of a very close friend)

with death. How the family deals with the death has a great impact on the child's understanding of death, but children usually do not have a realistic comprehension of the finality of death until they are nearing preadolescence. Although the dying child may be unable to understand death, the emotions of family caregivers and others alert the child that something is threatening his or her secure world. Dealing with the child's anxieties with openness and honesty restores the child's trust and comfort.

Developmental Stage

Infants and toddlers have little if any understanding of death. The toddler may fear separation from beloved caregivers but have no recognition of the fact that death is nearing and irreversible. A toddler may say, "Nana's gone bye-bye to be with God" or "Grampy went to heaven" and a few moments later ask to go visit the deceased person. This is an opportunity to explain to the child that Nana or Grampy is in a special place and cannot be visited, but the family has many memories of him or her that they will always treasure. The child should not be scolded for not understanding. Questions are best answered simply and honestly.

If the infant's or toddler's own death is approaching, family caregivers can be encouraged to stay with the child

Caring for the dying is usually a team effort that may involve a nurse, a physician, a chaplain, a social worker, a psychiatrist, a hospice nurse, or a **thanatologist** (a person trained especially to work with the dying and their families, sometimes a nurse), but often the nurse is the person who coordinates the care.

THE CHILD'S UNDERSTANDING OF DEATH

Stage of development, cognitive ability, and experiences influence children's understanding of death. The death of a pet or a family member may be a child's first experience to provide comfort, love, and security. Maintaining routines as much as possible helps give the toddler a greater sense of security. The egocentric thinking of preschool children contributes to a belief that they may have caused a person or pet to die by thinking angry thoughts. Magical thinking also plays an important part in the preschooler's beliefs about death. It is not unusual for a preschool child to insist on burying a dead pet or bird and then in a few hours, or a day or two, dig it up to see if it is still there (Fig. 22-1). This may be especially true if the child has been told that it will "go to heaven." Many preschoolers think of death as a kind of sleep, not understanding that the dead person will not wake up; they may fear going to sleep after the death of a close family member because they fear *they* may not wake up. Family caregivers must watch for this kind of reaction so that they can encourage children to talk about these fears and reassure them that they need not fear dying while sleeping. The child's feelings must be acknowledged as real, and the child must be helped to resolve them. The feelings must never be ridiculed.

A preschool child may view personal illness as punishment for thoughts or actions. Because preschoolers do not have an accurate concept of death, they fear separation from family caregivers. Caregivers can provide security and comfort by staying with the child as much as possible.

The child who is 6 or 7 years old is still in the magical thinking stage and continues to think of death in the same way as the preschool child. At about 8 or 9 years of age, children gain the concept that death is universal and irreversible. Around this age, death is personified—that is, it is given characteristics of a person and may be called the devil, God, a monster, or the bogeyman. Children of this age often believe they can protect themselves from death by running past a cemetery while holding their breath, keeping doors locked, staying out of dark rooms, staying away from funeral homes and dead people, and avoiding stepping on cracks in the sidewalk.

When faced with the prospect of their own death, school-age children usually are sad that they will be leaving their family and the people they love. They may be apprehensive about how they will manage when they no longer have their parents around to help them. Often, they view death as another new experience, like going to school, leaving for camp, or flying in an airplane for the first time. They may fear the loss of control that death represents to them, expressing this fear through vocal aggression. Family caregivers and nurses must recognize this as an expression of their fear and avoid scolding or disciplining them for this behavior. This is a time when the people close to the child can help him or her voice anxieties about the future and provide an outlet for these aggressive feelings. The presence of family members and maintenance of relatively normal routines help give the child a sense of security.

Adolescents have an adult understanding of death but feel that they are immortal—that is, death will happen to others but not to them. This belief contributes to adolescents' sometimes dangerous, life-threatening behavior. This denial of the possibility of serious personal danger may contribute to an adolescent's delay in reporting symptoms or seeking help. Diagnosis of a life-threatening or terminal illness creates a crisis for the adolescent. The adolescent must draw on cognitive functioning, past experiences, family support, and problem-solving ability. Depression, helplessness, anger, fear of pain, and hopelessness often are expressed by adolescents with a terminal illness, but they generally choose to concentrate on living as fully as possible for the time that they have.[2]

Adolescents may be upset by the results of treatments that make them feel weak and alter their appearance, such as alopecia, edema resulting from steroid therapy, and pallor. They may need assistance in presenting themselves as attractively as possible to their peers. Adolescents need opportunities to acknowledge their impending death and can be encouraged to express fears and anxieties and ask questions about death. Participating in their usual activities helps adolescents feel in control.

Experience With Death and Loss

Every death that touches the life of a child makes an impression that affects the way the child thinks about every other death, including his or her own. Attitudes of family

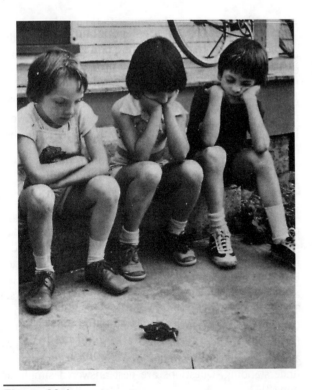

Figure 22-1
A funeral and burial for an animal facilitate respect for life as well as an emerging concept of death.

members are powerful influences. Family caregivers must be able to discuss death with children when a grandparent or other family member dies, even though the discussion may be painful. Otherwise, the child thinks that death is a forbidden topic, and avoiding the subject leaves immeasurable room for fantasy and distortion in the child's imagination.

Many books are available to help a child deal with loss and death. *A Balloon Story*, a simply produced 13-page coloring storybook by hospice nurse Ruth Anne Sieber, is an introduction to loss appropriate for the young child. This story of two children who go to a fair with their mothers is illustrated with large line drawings to color. The children each select and purchase a helium balloon, of which they are quite proud. Unfortunately, Nathan's balloon slips from his hand and floats away, forever. Nathan displays typical grief reactions of protest, anger, and finally acceptance (Fig. 22-2). Reading the story to a child provides the adult with the perfect opening to discuss loss. A small booklet for caregivers accompanies *A Balloon Story* and contains excellent guidelines for discussing death and loss with a child. *A Balloon Story* can be obtained from Hospice: The Bridge, Lewistown Hospital, Lewistown, PA 17044.

Another small booklet that is excellent to use with any

Figure 22-3
Drawings done by the fourth-grade students after a presentation about death that included a reading of *Water Bugs and Butterflies*. (A) In the s[t]ages of life we change. At the center of the drawing is a pond with three lily pads. The stems at the end represent plants that waterbugs crawl up on before turning into dragonflies. (B) Nobody lives forever. (Courtesy of Ruth Anne Sieber.)

Figure 22-2
Nathan cried and kept jumping and reaching after everyone else had given up. (Courtesy of Ruth Anne Sieber.)

age group is *Water Bugs and Dragonflies*. This story approaches life and death as stages of existence by illustrating that after a water bug turns into a dragonfly, he can no longer go back and tell the other curious water bugs what life is like in this beautiful new world to which he has gone. This story can serve as the foundation for further discussion about death (Fig. 22-3).

A number of books focus on the death of an animal or pet. Many of the stories deal with death as a result of old age. Several books have an accident as the cause of death. Most of the books are fiction, but several nonfiction ones are available for older children (Box 22-2). There is no discussion of one's own death in these books, which is consistent with the Western philosophy of handling death as something that happens to others but not to oneself.[3]

Box 22-2 *Books About Death for Children*

Book	Who Died	Cause of Death	Age Appropriate
Anderson L. *It's OK to Cry.* Chicago: Chicago Press, 1979	Uncle	Accident	5–11
Anderson L. *Death.* New York: First Book, 1980 (nonfiction)	Various	Various	11–15
Bradley B. *Endings: A Book About Death.* Reading, MA: Addison-Wesley, 1979 (nonfiction)	Various	Various	11–14
Brandenberg A. *The Two of Them.* New York: Greenwillow, 1979	Grandpa	Old age	5–12
Brown M. *The Dead Bird.* Reading, MA: Addison-Wesley, 1965	Bird	Unknown	3–12
Bunting E. *The Happy Funeral.* New York: Harper & Row, 1982	Grandpa	Old age	3–8
Buscaglia L. *The Fall of Freddie the Leaf.* Thorofare, NJ: Charles B. Slack, 1982	Leaf	Old age	All
Carrick C. *The Accident.* New York: Seabury, 1976	Dog	Accident	4–9
Clifton L. *Everett Anderson's Good-bye.* New York: Holt, Rinehart, & Winston, 1983	Parent	Unknown	3–9
Cohen M. *Jim's Dog Muffin.* New York: Greenwillow, 1984	Dog	Accident	3–7
Herriot J. *The Christmas Day Kitten.* New York: St. Martin's Press, 1976	Cat	Illness	All
Hurd E. *The Black Dog Who Went into the Woods.* New York: Harper & Row, 1980	Dog	Unknown	5–8
Kantrowitz M. *When Violet Died.* New York: Parents' Magazine Press, 1975	Bird	Old age	5–11
Keller H. *Good-bye Max.* New York: Greenwillow, 1987	Dog	Old age	3–7
Leshan E. *Learning to Say Good-bye.* New York: Macmillan, 1976	Parent	Various	10–13
Patterson K. *Bridge to Terabithia.* Santa Barbara, CA: Cornerstone, 1977	Friend	Accident	10–15
Pringle L. *Death is Natural.* New York: Four Winds, 1977 (nonfiction)	—	Old age	8–12
Rofes E. *The Kids' Book About Death and Dying.* Boston: Little Brown, 1985 (nonfiction)	Various	Various	11–15
Sanford D. *It Must Hurt a Lot.* Portland, OR: Multnomah, 1985	Dog	Accident	5–11
Simon N. *The Saddest Time.* Niles, IL: Albert Whitmont, 1986	Uncle	Illness	9–15
Smith D. *A Taste of Blackberries.* New York: Thomas Y. Crowall, 1973	Friend	Accident	9–14
Stein S. *About Dying.* New York: Walker & Company, 1974	Bird and grandpa	Old age	3–8
Stevens M. *When Grandpa Died.* Chicago: Chicago Press, 1979	Grandpa	Old age	5–9
Tobias T. *Petey.* New York: G.P. Putnam's Sons, 1978	Gerbil	Old age	4–8
Viorst J. *The Tenth Good Thing About Barney.* Atheneum, NY: Connecticut Printers, 1971	Cat	Unknown	5–14

Adapted from Bowden VR. Children's literature: The death experience. Pediatr Nurs 19(1):17–21, 1993.

Awareness of Impending Death

Children know when they are dying. They sense and fear what is going to happen even if they cannot identify it by name. Their play activities, artwork, dreams, and symbolic language demonstrate this knowledge.

Family caregivers who insist that a child not learn the truth about his or her illness place health care professionals at a disadvantage because they are not free to help the child deal with fears and concerns. If caregivers permit openness and honesty in communication with a dying child, the health care staff can meet the child's needs more effectively, dispel misunderstandings, and see that the child and the family are able to resolve any problems or **unfinished business**. Completing unfinished business may mean spending more time with the child, helping siblings understand the child's illness and impending death, and giving family members a chance to share their love with the child. Allowing openness does not mean that nurses and other personnel offer information not asked for by the child, but simply that the child be given the information desired, using words that the child can understand, in a gentle and straightforward manner. The truth can be kind as well as cruel. Honest, specific answers leave less room for misinterpretation and distortion.

Adolescents are usually sensitive to what is happening to them and may need the nurse to be an advocate for them if they have wishes they want to fulfill before dying. An adolescent may sense the nurse's willingness and ability to discuss feelings that he or she is uncomfortable discussing with family members. The nurse can talk with the adolescent and work with the family to help them understand the adolescent's desires and needs. The nurse can call on hospice workers, social or psychiatric services, or a member of the clergy to help the family express and resolve their concerns and recognize the adolescent's needs.

THE FAMILY'S REACTION TO DYING AND DEATH

Diagnosis of a potentially fatal disease, such as AIDS, cystic fibrosis, or cancer, sends feelings of shock, disbelief, and guilt through every family member. Anticipatory grief begins then and continues until remission or death occurs. When the disease is rapidly advancing, anticipatory grief may be short-lived as the child's death nears.

Family Caregivers

The family caregivers of children in the final stages of a terminal illness may have had to cope with many hospital admissions between periods at home. During this time, the family may be faced with decisions about the child's physical care as well as learning to live with a dying child (Fig. 22-4). As the child's condition deteriorates, the family can be encouraged to talk to their child about dying. This is a

Figure 22-4
Caregivers experience and deal with grief in many different ways. This mom finds comfort in spending quiet moments with her dying daughter.

task they may find very difficult. Support from a religious counselor, hospice nurse, or social service or psychiatric worker can help them through this difficult task. Family caregivers can be encouraged to provide as much normalcy as possible in the child's schedule. School attendance and special trips can be encouraged, within the child's capabilities and desires.

During this time, family caregivers may find themselves going through a grieving process of anger, depression, ambivalence, and bargaining over and over again. The caregivers may direct anger at the hospital staff, themselves (because of guilt), at each other, or at the child. Reassure the caregivers that this is a normal reaction, but avoid taking sides.

If the child improves enough to go home again, parents may find that they tend to be overprotective of the child. As in chronic illness, this overprotective attitude reinforces the child's sick behavior and dependency and is usually accompanied by a lack of discipline. Failure to set limits accentuates the child's feelings of being different and creates problems with siblings. The child learns to manipulate family members, only to find that this kind of behavior does not bring positive results when attempted with peers or health care personnel.

When the child has to return to the hospital because of increasing symptoms, family caregivers may experience all the stages of the grieving process again. The family members dread the child's approaching death and fear that the child will be in great pain or may die when they are not present. Nurses can help relieve these fears by keeping the family informed about the child's condition, making the child as comfortable as possible, and reassuring the family members that they will be summoned if death appears to be near.

When death comes, it is perfectly appropriate to share the family's grief, crying with them and then giving them privacy to express their sorrow. The nurse can stay with the family for awhile, remaining quietly supportive, with an attitude of a comforting listener. An appropriate comment may be, "I am so sorry" or "This is a very sad time." Keep the focus on the family's grief, and never share personal experiences of loss.[4]

The family may want to hold the child to say a final good-bye, and the nurse can encourage and assist them in this. Intravenous lines and other equipment can be removed to make holding the child easier. The family may be left alone during this time if they desire. The nurse must be sensitive to the family's needs and desires to provide them with comfort.

During anticipatory grief, the family of a child with a terminal illness has an opportunity to complete any unfinished business. This can help them prepare for the child's death. However, when a child dies suddenly and unexpectedly, the family has not had the opportunity to go through anticipatory grief. Such a family may have excessive guilt and remorse for something they felt they left unsaid or undone. Even if a child has had a traumatic death with disfigurement, the family must be given the opportunity to be with, see, and hold the child to help with closure of the child's life. The nurse can prepare the family for seeing the child, explaining why parts of the body may be covered. Viewing the child, even if severely mutilated, helps the family have a realistic view of the child and aids in the grief process.

The family may face a number of decisions that must be made rather quickly, especially when the death of the child was unexpected. Families of terminally ill children usually have made some plans for the child's death and may know exactly what they want done. However, when the child dies unexpectedly, decisions may be necessary concerning organ donation, funeral arrangements, and an autopsy. If the death has been the result of violence or is unexplained, an autopsy is required by law, but there may be other reasons that an autopsy is desired. Organ donation can be discussed with the family by the hospital's organ donor coordinator or other designated person. The family needs to be well informed and must be supported throughout these difficult decisions.

Grief for the death of a child is not limited in time but may continue for years. Sometimes, professional counseling is necessary to help family members work through grief. The support of others who have experienced the same sort of loss can be helpful. Two national organizations founded to offer support are the Candlelighters Childhood Cancer Foundation (1901 Pennsylvania Avenue, NW, Washington DC 20006; 202-659-5136) and Compassionate Friends (PO Box 3696, Oak Brook, IL 60522-3696; 708-990-0010). These organizations have many local chapters.

The Child

The dying child may have a decreased level of consciousness, but hearing remains intact. Family members at the bedside and health care personnel may need to be reminded to avoid saying anything that would not be said if the child were fully conscious. Gentle touching and caressing may provide comfort to the child. Excellent nursing care is required. Medications for pain are given intravenously because they are poorly absorbed from muscle due to poor circulation. Mucous membranes are kept clean, and petroleum jelly (Vaseline) can be applied to the lips to prevent drying and cracking. The conjunctiva of the eyes can be moistened with normal saline eye drops, such as Artificial Tears, if drying occurs. The skin is kept clean and dry, and the child is turned and positioned regularly to provide comfort and prevent skin breakdown. While caring for the child, the nurse should talk to the child and explain everything that is being done.

As death approaches, the internal body temperature increases; thus, dying patients seem to be unaware of cold, even though their skin feels cool. Explain this to family members so they do not think the child needs additional

covering. Just before death, the child who has remained conscious may become restless, followed by a time of peace and calm. The nurse and family members should be aware of these reactions and know that death is near.

Siblings

Just as in chronic illness, siblings resent the attention given to the ill child and are angry about the disruption in the family. Reaction varies according to the developmental age of the sibling and parental attitudes and actions. Younger children find it almost impossible to understand what is happening; it is difficult even for older children to grasp. Reaction to the illness and its accompanying stresses can cause classroom problems for school-age siblings; these may be incorrectly labeled as learning disabilities or behavioral disorders unless school personnel are aware of the family situation.

When the child dies, young siblings who are still prone to magical thinking may feel guilty, particularly if a strong degree of rivalry existed before the illness. These children need continued reassurance that they did not cause or help cause their sibling's death.

The decision of whether a sibling should attend funeral services for the child may be difficult. Although there has been little research, the current thinking among many health professionals supports the presence of the sibling. The sibling may be encouraged to leave a token of love and good-bye with the child—a drawing, a note, a toy, or another special memento. Siblings can visit the dead child in privacy when there are not a lot of other mourners present. Dealing with the realities of the brother's or sister's death openly is more likely to be of benefit than avoiding the issue and allowing the sibling to use his or her imagination about it (Box 22-3).

SETTINGS FOR CARE OF THE DYING CHILD

The family's response to and acceptance of a child's death can be greatly influenced by where the child dies. In a hospital, the child may receive the most professional care and the most technologically advanced treatment, but having a child in the hospital can contribute to family separation, a feeling of loss of control, and a sense of isolation. An increasing number of families are choosing to keep the child at home to die.

Hospice Care

In medieval times, a **hospice** was a refuge for travelers, not only those who traveled through the countryside but those who were leaving this life for another, the terminally ill. Hospices often were operated by religious orders and

Box 22-3. *Guidelines for Helping Children Cope with Death*

DO	DON'T
1. Know your own beliefs.	1. Praise stoicism (detached, unemotional behavior).
2. Begin where the child is.	2. Use euphemisms (mild expressions substituted for ones that might be offensive).
3. Be there.	
4. Confront reality.	
5. Encourage expression of feelings.	3. Be nonchalant.
6. Be truthful.	4. Glamorize death.
7. Include the child in family rituals.	5. Tell fairy tales or half-truths.
8. Encourage remembrance.	6. Close the door to questions.
9. Admit when you don't know the answer.	7. Be judgmental of feelings and behaviors.
10. Use touch to communicate.	8. Protect the child from exposure to experiences with death.
11. Start death education early, simply, using naturally occurring events.	9. Encourage forgetting the deceased.
12. Recognize symptoms of grief, and deal with the grief.	10. Encourage the child to be like the deceased.
13. Accept differing reactions to death.	

Courtesy of Alice Demi, President, Grief Education Institute, PO Box 623, Englewood, CO 80151.

became havens for the dying. The current hospice movement in health care began in England, when Dr. Cicely Saunders founded St. Christopher's Hospice in London in 1967. This institution has become the model for others in the United States and Canada, with emphasis on sensitive, humane care for the dying. Hospice principles of care include relief of pain, attention to the needs of the total person, and absence of heroic life-saving measures.

The first hospice in the United States was the New Haven Hospice in Connecticut. Many communities now have hospice programs that may or may not be affiliated with a hospital. Some programs offer a hospice setting to which patients go in terminal stages of illness; others provide support and guidance for the patient and family while the patient remains in the hospital or is cared for at home. Most of these hospice programs are established primarily for adult, and only about 200 of the estimated 1,700 accept children as patients.[5]

Children's Hospice International, founded in 1983, is an organization dedicated to hospice support of children. Through an individualized plan of care, Children's Hospice addresses the physical, developmental, psychological, social, and spiritual needs of children and families in a comprehensive and consistent way. It serves as a resource and advocacy center, providing education for parents and professionals. The organization conducts seminars and conferences, publishes training manuals, and supports a clearinghouse of information available through a national hotline (1-800-24-CHILD). Its Internet Web page (http://

www.chionline.com) provides information for adults and games, books, and an excellent list of Web sites for children.

Home Care

Caring for the dying patient, young or old, at home has become increasingly common in recent years. More families are choosing to keep their child at home during the terminal stage of illness. Factors that contribute to the decision to care for a child at home include:

- Concerns about cost, both for hospitalization and for the nonmedical expenses of the family's travel, housing, and food
- Stress from repeated family separations
- Loss of control over the care of the child and family life.

Families feel that the more loving, caring environment of the home draws the family closer and helps reduce the guilt that often is a part of bereavement. All members of the family can be involved to some extent in the child's care and in this way gain a feeling of usefulness. Family caregivers feel that they remain in control.

There are disadvantages, however. Costs that would have been covered by health insurance if the child were hospitalized may not be covered if the child is cared for at home. Caring for a dying child can be extremely difficult, both emotionally and physically. Not every family has someone who can carry out the procedures that may need to be performed regularly. In some instances, home nursing assistance is available, but this varies from community to community. Usually, the home care nurse visits several days a week and may be on call the rest of the time. In some communities, hospice nurses may provide the teaching and support that families need.

Deciding whether to care for a dying child at home is an extremely difficult decision for a family to make. Family members need support and guidance from health care personnel when they are trying to make the decision, after the decision is made, and even after the child dies.

Hospital Care

Dying in the hospital has limitations and advantages. Both the child and family may find support from others in the same situation. Family members may not have the physical or emotional strength to cope with total care of the child at home, but they can participate in care that is supported by the hospital staff. Hospital care is much more expensive, but this may not be important to some families, especially if they have health insurance. The hospital is still the culturally accepted place to die, and this is important to some persons. Patients and families who choose hospital care need to know that they have rights and can exert some control over what happens to them.

▶◣ *Nursing Process for the Dying Child* ◤◢

ASSESSMENT

The assessment of the terminally ill child and family is an ongoing process developed over a period of time. The assessment covers the developmental level of the child, the influence of cultural and spiritual concerns, the family's support system, present indications of grieving (ie, anticipatory grief), interactions among family members, and unfinished business. To understand the child's view of death, consider the child's previous experiences, developmental level, and cognitive ability.

NURSING DIAGNOSES

Nursing diagnoses for the dying child include those appropriate for the child's illness as well as the following, which are specific to the dying process:

- Pain related to illness and weakened condition

- Risk for Social Isolation related to terminal illness

- Anxiety related to condition and prognosis

- Risk for Ineffective Family Coping related to approaching death

- Powerlessness of family caregivers related to inability to control child's condition

OUTCOME IDENTIFICATION AND PLANNING

The goals that are set and the planning done to meet those goals depend on the stage of the illness, the child's and the family's acceptance of the illness, and their attitudes and beliefs about death and dying. Major goals for the child include minimizing pain, diminishing feelings of abandonment by peers and friends, and relieving anxiety about the future. Goals for the family include helping coping with the impending death and identifying and perform tasks that provide comfort to the child.

RELIEVING PAIN AND DISCOMFORT. The child may be in pain for many reasons, such as chemotherapy; nausea, vomiting, and gastrointestinal cramping; pressure caused by positioning; or constipation. Until the child is comfortable and relatively pain-free, all other nursing interventions are fruitless; pain becomes the primary focus of the child until relief is provided. Nursing measures to relieve pain may include positioning, using pillows as needed; changing linens; providing conscientious skin and mouth care; protecting skin surfaces from rubbing together; offering backrubs and massages; and administering antiemetics, analgesics, and stool softeners as appropriate.

PROVIDING APPROPRIATE DIVERSIONAL ACTIVITIES. Encourage the child's siblings and friends to maintain contact. Provide opportunities for peers to visit, write, or telephone as the child is able. Read to the child and engage in other activities that he or she is interested in and physically can tolerate. Encourage the child to make decisions, when possible, to foster a feeling of control. Explain all procedures and how they will affect the child. Provide the child with privacy, but do not neglect him or her. Provide ample periods of rest. Continue to talk to and tell the child what you are doing, even though the child may seem unresponsive.

EASING THE CHILD'S ANXIETY. Ask family caregivers about the child's understanding of death and previous experiences with death. Observe how the child exhibits fear, and ask family caregivers for any additional information. Encourage the child to use a doll, a pillow, or another special "warm fuzzy" for comfort. Use words such as "dead" or "dying" if appropriate in conversation, because this may give the child an opening to talk about death. Nighttime is especially frightening for children because they often think they will die at night. Provide company and comfort, and be alert for periods of wakefulness during which the child may need someone to talk to. Be honest and straightforward, and avoid injecting your beliefs into the conversation. If appropriate, read a book about death to the child to initiate conversation (although this should have been done much earlier in the child's care).

Nursing Care Plan
for the Dying Child and Family

Janelle is a 7-year-old who has a terminal illness. She is not expected to live more than a few more weeks. She has a brother who is 10 and a sister who is 4. A family member is with her continuously.

NURSING DIAGNOSIS

Pain related to illness and weakened condition

GOAL: *Janelle's pain will be relieved.*

OUTCOME CRITERIA

- Janelle has uninterrupted periods of quiet rest.
- Using a pain scale, Janelle indicates she experiences relief from pain.

Nursing Interventions	Rationale
Pain relief must be the primary focus of all nursing care until the child is comfortable.	Pain is the child's primary focus, and until it is relieved, all other nursing interventions are fruitless.
Administer pain relief medication, but also include such nursing measures as positioning, providing backrubs and massages, changing linens, providing conscientious skin and mouth care, and protecting skin surfaces from rubbing together to increase Janelle's comfort.	Each child's pain experience is unique, and it may vary from one time to another. Some measures may relieve pain in one situation but not another. Discover the measures that work most frequently for this child.

NURSING DIAGNOSIS

Risk for Social Isolation related to terminal illness

GOAL: *Social interactions will be promoted.*

OUTCOME CRITERIA

- Janelle engages in social interaction with her classmates and other peers.
- Family caregivers and others play games with or read to Janelle within her physical limitations.
- Caregivers talk with Janelle when giving care regardless of her apparent level of consciousness.

Nursing Interventions	Rationale
Encourage Janelle's siblings and peers (including school friends) to maintain contact; provide opportunities for such contact by arranging for convenient visiting hours, providing paper and pens for writing, and making a telephone available.	The child needs to feel that she is not cut off from everyone and everything. This helps relieve boredom and also diverts the child's attention from her condition.
Spend time with and talk to the child, even when you are not sure she is responsive.	Hearing is often the last sense to shut down; the child will feel reassured by your voice and presence.

(continued)

Nursing Care Plan (Continued)
for the Dying Child and Family

NURSING DIAGNOSIS

Anxiety related to condition and prognosis

GOAL: *The child's and the family's anxiety will be eased.*

OUTCOME CRITERIA

- Janelle talks to her family or the nurse about death.
- Janelle has a "warm fuzzy" close by.
- Janelle freely expresses her fears about dying, especially fears about nighttime.

Nursing Interventions	*Rationale*
Discuss with the family Janelle's understanding of death, and note how she exhibits fear. Use straightforward terminology when discussing death.	The child may or may not have discussed death with the family, and it is important for the nurse to respond to the child appropriately. The nurse is able at the same time to get a sense of how the family views the child's death and what sort of help they may need in discussing the topic with their child and each other.
Encourage Janelle to keep a favorite object or "warm fuzzy" for comfort and reassurance. Provide company and comfort, particularly at night. Keep a night light on to ease anxieties.	Many children think they will die at night; periods of wakefulness are common; if the child is left alone, fears may compound. A night light provides some sense of security.

NURSING DIAGNOSIS

Risk for Ineffective Family Coping related to the child's approaching death

GOAL: *The family will improve coping skills.*

OUTCOME CRITERIA

- Family caregivers express their feelings and anxieties.
- Family caregivers contact a spiritual advisor for support.
- Family caregivers identify signs in the child that indicate approaching death.

Nursing Interventions	*Rationale*
Encourage family caregivers to discuss their feelings about Janelle and to acknowledge their fears and emotions; reassure them their reactions are normal.	It may be very difficult for family members to talk about their child's death; they may feel they need to "keep up a brave front" for the child or siblings. However, it is important for them to acknowledge the death and begin to let out some of their emotions.
Help the family contact their spiritual advisor or a hospital chaplain, if they desire.	The support of a spiritual counselor, particularly one already known to the family, may be helpful.
Help the family recognize and acknowledge signs of Janelle's impending death. Help them talk with her siblings.	Acknowledging the impending signs of death helps the family caregivers to be realistic about the approaching death. They also may need support and guidance to know how to talk with the other children.

(continued)

Nursing Care Plan (Continued)
for the Dying Child and Family

| Make sure family caregivers are resting and eating adequately. | The family caregivers must avoid exhaustion; lack of sleep and inadequate nutrition will only make it harder for them to cope. |

NURSING DIAGNOSIS

Powerlessness of family caregivers related to inability to control child's condition

GOAL: *The family will participate in the child's care.*

OUTCOME CRITERIA

- Family caregivers provide comfort measures for Janelle.
- Family caregivers talk with Janelle and complete unfinished business with her.

Nursing Interventions	*Rationale*
Suggest specific care measures family members might perform to provide comfort for Janelle; encourage the family to carry out cultural practices if they desire.	Caregivers need to feel they are doing something to help their child; performing meaningful cultural customs helps the family express their feelings and provides a feeling of continuity.
Explain "unfinished business" to the family and encourage them to complete any unfinished business on their agenda.	Discussion of unfinished business provides another opportunity for family members to engage in meaningful activity with their child before the child's death.
Encourage family members to talk to talk to Janelle, even when she seems unresponsive.	The child may be able to hear voices, even when unable to respond; family caregivers will feel better when they can still communicate love and support.

HELPING THE FAMILY COPE. Family caregivers may need encouragement to discuss their feelings about the child. Emotions and fears must be acknowledged and caregivers reassured that their reactions are normal. The support of a member of the clergy may be helpful during this time. Help the family contact their own spiritual counselor, or offer to contact the hospital chaplain if the family desires. Encourage family caregivers to eat and rest properly so they will not become ill or exhausted themselves. Explain the child's condition to the family and answer any questions. The family can be reassured that everything is being done to keep the child as comfortable and pain-free as possible. Interpret signs of approaching death for the family.

If appropriate, ask the family about the siblings—what they know, how much they understand, and whether the family has discussed the approaching death. Offer to help the caregivers talk with siblings.

HELPING THE FAMILY FEEL INVOLVED IN THE CHILD'S CARE. Respond to the family's need to feel some control over the situation by suggesting specific measures they can perform to provide comfort for the child, such as positioning, moistening lips, and reading or telling

a favorite story. Encourage the caregivers to talk to the child, even if the child does not respond. Discourage whispered conversations in the room. Encourage and help the family to carry out cultural customs if they wish. Help the family complete any unfinished business on the agenda; this may include the need for the child to go home to die. Contact support persons, such as hospice workers or social services, to help complete unfinished business, if necessary. (See the Nursing Care Plan for the Dying Child and the Family.)

EVALUATION: GOALS AND OUTCOME CRITERIA

- *Goal*: The child will have minimal pain.
  Criteria: The child rests quietly and denies pain when asked.
- *Goal*: The child will have social interaction with others.
  Criteria: Within physical capabilities, the child engages in activities with peers and others.
- *Goal*: The child will learn to handle anxiety.
  Criteria: The child keeps a "warm fuzzy" close by for comfort and talks about death to the nurse or family.

The child is comforted when awake at night by the presence of someone to talk to.

- *Goal*: Family members will cope with the child's approaching death.
- *Criteria*: Family members express their feelings and identify signs that indicate approaching death.
- *Goal*: The siblings will be included in learning to cope with the child's death.
- *Criteria*: Siblings visit and show an understanding of the child's approaching death.
- *Goal*: Family members will be involved in child's care to decrease feelings of powerlessness.
  Criteria: Family members provide comfort measures for the child, talk to the child, and complete unfinished business with the child.

■ KEY POINTS

- A child's death affects health care personnel as well as the family. To work with dying patients effectively, health care personnel must work through their own feelings about death.
- The child's stage of development, cognitive ability, and experiences contribute to his or her understanding of death.
- The concept of death is greatly influenced by magical thinking before the age of 8 or 9 years.
- Adolescents have an attitude of immortality and may deny the possibility that they will die.
- The grieving process is a multistep process and does not follow a predictable schedule from one person to another.
- Family experiences vary with the length of the child's illness. With a chronic illness, the family experiences anticipatory grief, which gives them an opportunity to complete unfinished business and helps them resolve their grief when death occurs. However, if a child dies suddenly or unexpectedly, the family has not had that opportunity and may experience grief more profoundly.
- Hospital, home, and hospice care are all options during the terminal stage of the child's illness. Each has advantages and disadvantages.

? CRITICAL THINKING

1. The Jones family has an 8-year-old daughter with a terminal illness. Discuss the factors they need to consider when deciding if they wish to care for her at home.
2. The Joneses decide they cannot care for the child at home. Examine your feelings about this.

3. Describe your feelings about the story by the student nurse early in this chapter.
4. How does a preschooler typically respond to the death of a family caregiver? of a pet? Describe how you would help 4-year-old Chelsea handle the death of her pet hamster.
5. Survey your area to see if there a hospice available. Describe how it functions. Find out if it accepts children as patients and if there are any restrictions concerning children.
6. Fifteen-year-old Josh has a terminal illness and has been very rebellious. Explain what you believe to be contributing to his behavior. Describe some ways you would help him. Identify the developmental characteristics of adolescents that affect their view of death.

REFERENCES

1. Am J Nurs 70(2), 1970.
2. Peronne J. Adolescents with cancer: Are they at risk for suicide? Pediatr Nurs 19(1):22–25, 1993.
3. Bowden VR. Children's literature: The death experience. Pediatr Nurs 19(1):17–21, 1993.
4. Miles A. Caring for families when a child dies. Pediatr Nurs 16(4):346–347, 1990.
5. Armstrong-Dailey A. About our children. Am J Hospice Care 4(5):11–12, 1987.

BIBLIOGRAPHY

Castiglia PT, Harbin RE. Child health care: Process and practice. Philadelphia: JB Lippincott, 1992.
Consolvo CA. Jeff's last wish . . . A dying child wanted to go home to his rocking chair. Nursing 20(9):152, 1990.
Coody D. High expectations: Nurses who work with children who might die. Nurs Clin North Am 20(1):131–142, 1985.
Davies B, Eng B. Factors influencing nursing care of children who are terminally ill. Pediatr Nurs 19(1):9–14, 1993.
Grogan LB. Grief of an adolescent when a sibling dies. MCN 15(1):21–24, 1990.
Jackson DB, Saunders RB. Child health nursing. Philadelphia: JB Lippincott, 1993.
Pazola KJ, Gerber AK. Privileged communication: Talking with a dying adolescent. MCN 15(1):16–21, 1990.
Pillitteri A. Maternal and child health nursing, 2d ed. Philadelphia: Lippincott-Raven, 1996.
Rushton CH, Hogue EE, Billet CA, et al. End of life care for infants with AIDS: Ethical and legal issues. Pediatr Nurs 19(1):79–83, 1993.
Rushton CH, Hogue EE. When parents demand "everything." Pediatr Nurs 19(2):180–183, 1993.
Schuster CS, Ashburn SS. The process of human development, 3d ed. Philadelphia: JB Lippincott, 1992.
Stickney D. Water bugs and dragonflies. New York: Pilgrim Press, 1982.
Wong DL. Whaley and Wong's nursing care of infants and children, 5th ed. St. Louis: Mosby, 1995.

Glossary

abdominal paracentesis surgical puncture into the abdomen to drain fluid.

abuse misuse, excessive use, rough or bad treatment; used to refer to misuse of alcohol or drugs (substance abuse) and mistreatment of children or family members (child abuse, domestic abuse).

achylia absence of pancreatic enzymes in gastric secretions.

acid–base balance state of equilibrium between the acidity and the alkalinity of body fluids.

acrocyanosis cyanosis of the hands and feet seen periodically in the newborn.

actual nursing diagnoses diagnoses that identify existing health problems.

adenoids mass of lymphoid tissue in the nasal pharynx, extending from the roof of the nasal pharynx to the free edge of the soft palate.

adenopathy enlarged lymph glands.

alcohol abuse drinking sufficient alcoholic beverages to induce intoxication.

alcoholism chronic alcohol abuse.

allergen antigen that causes an allergic reaction.

allograft skin graft taken from a genetically different person for temporary coverage during burn healing; skin from a cadaver sometimes is used.

alopecia loss of hair.

amblyopia dimness of vision from disuse of the eye; sometimes called "lazy eye."

amenorrhea absence of menstruation.

amniocentesis analysis of amniotic fluid that reveals much about the fetus including sex, state of health, and maturity. A sample of amniotic fluid is withdrawn for early diagnosis of possible disorders, such as chromosomal abnormalities and blood disorders. The procedure is done by inserting a needle through the abdominal and uterine walls into the amniotic sac and withdrawing a small amount of fluid (10–20 mL) through a syringe.

amniotic sac strong translucent membrane that encloses the fetus suspended in amniotic fluid, the environment that provides protection for the developing child. This membrane is large and elastic enough to permit the fetus to move about and turn at will during most of its intrauterine life.

ankylosis immobility of a joint.

anorexia nervosa eating disorder characterized by loss of appetite due to emotional causes, usually excessive fear of becoming (or being) fat.

anthelmintic medication that expels intestinal worms; vermifuge.

anticipatory grief preparatory grieving that often helps the caregivers mourn the loss of their child when death actually comes.

antigen protein substance found on the surface of red blood cells capable of inducing a specific immune response and reacting with the products of that response.

antigen–antibody response response of the body to an antigen causing the formation of antibodies that protect the body from an invading antigen.

anuria absence of urine.

apnea temporary interruption of the breathing impulse.

archetypes predetermined patterns of human development, which according to Carl Jung, replace instinctive behavior of other animals; prototype.

areola darkened area around the nipple.

arthralgia painful joints.

ascites edema in the peritoneal cavity.

associative play being engaged in a common activity without any sense of belonging or fixed rules.

astigmatism error in refraction of light on the retina caused by unequal curvature in the cornea of the eye bending light rays in different directions, producing a blurred image.

ataxia lack of coordination caused by disturbances in the kinesthetic and balance senses.

atresia absence of a normal body opening or the abnormal closure of a body passage.

aura a sensation that signals an impending epileptic attack; may be visual, aromatic, or other sensation.

autistic totally self-centered and unable to relate to others, often exhibiting bizarre behaviors; autistic children can sometimes be destructive to themselves and others.

autograft skin taken from an individual's own body; it is the only kind of skin accepted permanently by recipient tissues, except for the skin of an identical twin.

autonomy ability to function in an independent manner.

autosomal recessive trait trait or condition that is not expressed unless both parents carry the gene for that trait.

autosomal dominant trait trait or condition appearing in a heterozygous person resulting from a dominant gene within a pair.

autosomes 22 pairs of chromosomes that are alike in the male and female; the sex chromosomes are not autosomes.

azotemia nitrogen-containing compounds in the blood.

Babinski reflex the flaring open of the infant's toes when the lateral plantar surface is stroked. Also called the plantar reflex, this reaction usually disappears by the end of the first year.

bilateral pertaining to both sides; eg, bilateral cleft lip involves both sides of the lip.

binocular vision normal vision that is maintained through the muscular coordination of eye movements of both eyes, so that a single vision results.

blended family both partners in a marriage bring children from a previous marriage into the household; his, hers, and theirs.

body surface area (BSA) most reliable formula to calculate dosages. Using a West nomogram, the child's weight is marked down on the right scale and the height is marked on the left scale. A straightedge is used to draw a line between the two marks. The point at which it crosses the column labeled SA (surface area) is the BSA expressed in square meters (m^2).

bonding development of a close emotional tie between the newborn and the parent or parents.

bottle mouth (nursing bottle) caries condition caused by the erosion of enamel on the infant's deciduous teeth caused by sugar from the formula or sweetened juice, which coats the teeth for long periods. This condition also can occur in infants who sleep with their mother and nurse intermittently throughout the night.

brachycephaly shortness of the head.

bulimia nervosa eating disorder characterized by episodes of binge eating followed by purging by self-induced vomiting or use of laxatives.

caput succedaneum edematous swelling of the soft tissues of the scalp caused by prolonged pressure of the occiput against the cervix during labor and delivery. The edema disappears within a few days.

carditis inflammation of the heart.

cataract development of opacity in the crystalline lens that prevents light rays from entering the eye.

cavernous hemangiomas congenital malformations that are subcutaneous collections of blood vessels with bluish overlying skin. Although these lesions are benign tumors, they may become so extensive as to interfere with the functions of the body part on which they appear.

celiac syndrome term used to designate the complex of malabsorptive disorders.

centromere portion of the chromosome by which the chromosome is attached to the spindle during cell division.

cephalhematoma collection of blood between the periosteum and the skull caused by excessive pressure on the head during birth.

chancre hard, red, painless primary lesion of syphilis at the point of entry of the spirochete.

chelating agent agent that binds with metal.

child neglect failing to provide adequate hygiene, health care, nutrition, love, nurturing, and supervision as needed for growth and development

child-life program program to make hospitalization less threatening for children and their parents. These programs are usually under the direction of a child-life specialist whose background is in psychology and early childhood development.

chordee chordlike anomaly that extends from the scrotum to the penis, pulling the penis downward in an arc.

chorea rapid, jerky involuntary movements that are continuous.

chromosomes threadlike structures that occur in pairs and carry genetic information.

chronic illness condition that interferes with daily functioning for more than 3 months in a year, causes hospitalization of more than 1 month in a year, or (at time of diagnosis) is likely to do either of these.

circumcision surgical removal of all or part of the foreskin (prepuce) of the penis.

classification ability to group objects by rank, grade, or class.

clonus rapid involuntary muscle contraction and relaxation.

clove hitch restraints restraints used to secure an arm or leg, most often when a child is receiving an intravenous infusion. The restraint is made of soft cloth formed in a figure eight.

co-dependent parent parent who supports, directly or indirectly, the other parent's addictive behavior.

cognitive development progressive change in the intellectual process, including perception, memory, and judgment.

colic recurrent paroxysmal bouts of abdominal pain that are fairly common among young infants and that usually disappear around the age of 3 months.

colostrum thin, yellowish, milky fluid secreted by the mother's breasts during pregnancy or just after delivery (before the secretion of milk).

comedo collection of keratin and sebum in the hair follicle; blackhead; whitehead.

communal family alternative family in which members share responsibility for homemaking and childrearing; all children are the collective responsibility of adult members.

conception occurs when a sperm cell reaches and penetrates an ovum.

conduction heat loss that occurs when the neonate's skin is in direct contact with a cooler solid object.

congenital hip dysplasia abnormal fetal development of the acetabulum that may or may not cause dislocation of the hip. If the malformed acetabulum permits dislocation, the head of the femur displaces upward and backward. May be difficult to recognize in early infancy.

congestive heart failure (CHF) result of impaired pumping capability of the heart. It may appear in the first year of life in infants with conditions such as large ventricular septal defects, coarctation of the aorta, and other defects that place an increased workload on the ventricles.

conjunctivitis acute inflammation of the conjunctiva that may be caused by a virus, bacteria, allergy, or foreign body.

conservation ability to recognize that change in shape does not necessarily mean change in amount or mass.

contracture fibrous scarring that forms over a movable body part that had been burned; this part of the healing process can cause serious deformities and limit movement.

convection heat loss similar to conduction but increased by moving air currents.

cooperative play children play with each other, as in team sports.

coryza runny nose.

cradle cap accumulation of oil and dirt that often forms on an infant's scalp; seborrheic dermatitis.

craniotabes softening of the occipital bones caused by a reduction of mineralization of the skull.

croup general term that typically includes symptoms of a barking cough, hoarseness, and inspiratory stridor.

currant jelly stools stools that consist of blood and mucus.

cyanotic heart disease congenital heart disease that causes right-to-left shunting of blood in the heart, resulting in a depletion of oxygen to such an extent that the oxygen saturation of the peripheral arterial blood is 85% or less. Defects that permit right-to-left shunting may occur at the atrial, ventricular, or aortic level.

dawdling wasting time; whiling away time; being idle.

débridement removal of necrotic tissue.

decentration ability to see several aspects of a problem at the same time and understand the relation of various parts to the whole situation.

deciduous teeth primary teeth that usually erupt between 6 and 8 months of age.

deliriants inhalants that contain chemicals whose fumes can produce confusion, disorientation, excitement, and hallucinations.

denial defense mechanism in which the existence of unpleasant actions or ideas is unconsciously repressed; in the grieving process, one of the stages many people go through; also, a type of response by caregivers when caring for chronically ill children in which the caregivers deny the existence of the condition and encourage the child to overcompensate for any disabilities.

dependence compulsive need to use a substance for its satisfying or pleasurable effects.

dependent nursing actions nursing actions that the nurse performs as a result of a physician's orders, such as administering analgesics for pain.

development progressive change in the child's maturation.

developmental tasks basic achievements associated with each stage of development; these tasks must be mastered to move on the next developmental stage. Developmental tasks must be completed successfully at each stage for a person to achieve maturity.

diabetic acidosis characterized by drowsiness, dry skin, flushed cheeks, cherry-red lips, and acetone breath with a fruity smell as a result of excessive ketones in the blood in uncontrolled diabetes.

differentiation changes in the dividing cells, creating specialized tissues necessary to form an organized, coordinated, unique individual.

diplopia double vision.

discipline to train or instruct to produce a particular behavior pattern, especially moral or mental improvement, and self-control.

dominant gene gene that is expressed in only one of a chromosomal pair.

ductus arteriosus prenatal blood vessel between the pulmonary artery and the aorta that closes functionally within the first 3 or 4 days of life.

ductus venosus prenatal blood vessel between the umbilical vein and the inferior vena cava; does not achieve complete closure until the end of the second month of life.

dysarthria poor speech articulation.

dysfunctional family family that cannot resolve routine stresses in a positive, socially acceptable manner.

dysmenorrhea painful menstruation.

dysphagia difficulty in swallowing.

early adolescence begins at about age 10 in girls and about age 12 in boys with a dramatic growth spurt that signals the advent of puberty; preadolescence; pubescence.

echolalia "parrot speech" typical of autistic children; they echo words they hear, such as a television commercial, but do not appear to understand the words.

ego in psychoanalytic theory, the conscious self that controls the pleasure principle of the id by delaying the instincts until an appropriate time.

egocentric concerned only with one's own activities or needs; unable to put oneself in another's place or to see another's point of view.

elbow restraints restraints made of muslin with two layers. Pockets wide enough to fit tongue depressors are placed vertically along the width of the fabric. The restraints are wrapped around the arm to prevent the infant from bending the arm.

elderly primigravida woman becoming pregnant for the first time after the age of 35 years.

electrolytes chemical compounds (minerals) that break down into ions when placed in water.

embryo product of conception from the second to the eighth week of pregnancy.

emetic agent that causes vomiting.

en face position establishment of eye contact in the same plane between the caregiver and infant; extremely important to parent–infant bonding. Also called mutual gazing.

encephalopathy degenerative disease of the brain.

encopresis chronic involuntary fecal soiling with no medical cause.

enteric precautions procedures issued by the Centers for Disease Control required in the care of children with gastroenteritis to prevent the spread of possibly infectious organisms to other pediatric patients.

enuresis involuntary urination, especially at night; bed-wetting beyond the usual age of control.

epiphyses growth centers at the end of long bones and at the wrists.

epistaxis nosebleed.

erythema toxicum fine rash of the newborn that may appear over the trunk, back, abdomen, and buttocks. It appears about 24 hours after birth and disappears in several days.

erythroblastosis fetalis hemolytic disease of the newborn in which maternal anti-Rh antibodies in the infant's system destroy the infant's Rh-containing red blood cells, producing severe anemia and hyperbilirubinemia.

eschar hard crust or scab.

esotropia eye deviation toward the other eye.

evaporation heat loss through conversion of a liquid to a vapor.

exotropia eye deviation away from the other eye.

extended family consists of one or more nuclear families plus other relatives, often crossing generations to include grandparents, aunts, uncles, and cousins. The needs of individual members are subordinate to the needs of the group, and the children are considered an economic asset.

external hordeolum purulent infection of the follicle of an eyelash, generally caused by *Staphylococcus aureus.* Localized swelling, tenderness, and pain are present with a reddened lid edge; a stye.

extracellular fluid fluid situated outside a cell or cells.

extravasation escape of fluid into surrounding tissue.

extrusion reflex infant's way of taking food by thrusting the tongue forward as if to suck, which has the effect of pushing solid food out of the mouth.

febrile seizure seizure occurring in infants and young children commonly associated with a fever of 102° to 106°F (38.9°–41.1°C).

fertilization process by which the male's sperm unites with the female's ovum.

fetal alcohol syndrome (FAS) symptoms seen in an infant born to a woman who abused alcohol during pregnancy, including shorter stature, lower birth weight, possible microcephaly, facial deformities, hearing disorders, poor coordination, minor joint and limb abnormalities, heart defects, delayed development, and mental retardation.

fetus term for the organism after it has reached the eighth week of life and acquires a human likeness.

fiberoptic blanket specialized pad with illuminating plastic fibers used to break down bilirubin in an infant's blood. The blanket is covered with a disposable protective cover that disperses therapeutic light when wrapped around the infant; an alternative type of phototherapy.

fontanelle "soft spot" covered by a tough membrane at the junctures of the six bones of a newborn's skull. At birth two fontanelles can be detected—the anterior fontanelle at the junction of the frontal and parietal bones and the posterior fontanelle at the junction of the parietal and occipital bones. They are ossified (filled in by bone) during the normal growth process.

foramen ovale opening between the left and right atria of the fetal heart that closes with the first breath.

forceps marks noticeable marks on the infant's face that may occur if delivery was assisted with forceps; usually disappear within a day or two.

gag reflex reaction to any stimulation of the posterior pharynx by food, suction, or the passage of a tube that causes elevation of the soft palate and a strong involuntary effort to vomit. Continues throughout life.

galactosemia recessive hereditary metabolic disorder in which the enzyme necessary for converting galactose into glucose is missing. The infants generally appear normal at birth but experience difficulties after the ingestion of milk.

gastroenteritis infectious diarrhea caused by infectious organisms, including salmonella, *Escherichia coli,* dysentery bacilli, and various viruses, most notably rotaviruses.

gastrostomy tube tube surgically inserted through the abdominal wall into the stomach under general anesthesia. Used in children who have obstructions or surgical repairs in the mouth, pharynx, esophagus, or cardiac sphincter of the stomach or who are respirator-dependent.

gavage feeding nourishment provided directly through a tube passed into the stomach.

genes units threaded along chromosomes that carry genetic instructions from one generation to another. Like chromosomes, genes also occur in pairs. There are thousands of genes in the chromosomes of each cell nucleus.

genetic counseling study of the family history and tissue analysis of both partners to determine chromosome patterns for couples concerned about transmitting a specific disease to their unborn children.

genetic code blueprint for the development of the individual organism.

genotype each person's unique set of genes.

gestation period of development from fertilization to birth; the length in time of a pregnancy.

goniotomy surgical opening into Schlemm's canal that allows drainage of aqueous humor; performed to relieve intraocular pressure in glaucoma.

gradual acceptance type of response by caregivers when caring for chronically ill children in which caregivers adopt a common-sense approach to the child's condition, encouraging the child to function within his or her capabilities.

granulocytes type of white blood cell; divided into eosinophils, basophils, and neutrophils.

growth result of cell division and marked by an increase in size and weight; physical increase in size and appearance of the body caused by increasing numbers of new cells.

gynecomastia excessive growth of the mammary glands in the male.

halo traction metal ring attached to the skull that is added to a body cast using stainless steel pins inserted into the skull and into the femurs or iliac wings.

health maintenance organizations (HMOs) professional groups of physicians, laboratory service personnel, nurse practitioners, nurses, and consultants who care for the health of a family on a continuing basis and are geared to health care and disease prevention. The family pays a set fee for total care; any necessary hospitalization is covered by that fee. The emphasis is on health and prevention.

hemarthrosis bleeding into the joints.

hemolysis destruction of red blood cells with the release of hemoglobin into the plasma.

hernia abnormal protrusion of part of an organ through a weak spot or other abnormal opening in a body wall.

heterograft graft of tissue obtained from an animal; for burn patients, pig skin (porcine) is often used.

heterosexual relationship intimate relationship of two people of the opposite sex.

heterozygous term used to describe a particular trait of an individual when each member of a pair of genes carries different instructions for that trait.

hierarchical arrangement grouping by some common system, such as rank, grade, or class.

high-risk nursing diagnoses category of diagnoses that identify health problems to which the patient is especially vulnerable.

hirsutism abnormal body and facial hair growth.

homeostasis uniform state; signifies biologically the dynamic equilibrium of the healthy organism.

homosexual relationship intimate relationship of two people of the same sex.

homozygous term used to describe a particular trait of an individual when any two members of a pair of genes carry the same genetic instructions for that trait.

hospice provides comforting and supportive care to terminally ill patients and their families. There are few hospice programs for children in the United States.

hyaline membrane disease also known as respiratory distress syndrome (RDS); occurs due to immature lungs, which lack sufficient surfactant to decrease the surface tension of the alveoli; affects about half of all preterm newborns.

hydrops fetalis excessive edema, marked anemia, jaundice, and enlargement of the liver and spleen resulting from erythroblastosis fetalis.

hydrotherapy use of water in a treatment.

hyperalimentation also called total parenteral nutrition (TPN); administration of dextrose, lipids, amino acids, electrolytes, vitamins, minerals, and trace elements into the circulatory system to meet the nutritional needs of the child whose needs cannot be met through the gastrointestinal tract.

hyperlipidemia increase in the level of cholesterol in the blood.

hyperopia refractive condition in which the person can see objects better at a distance; farsightedness.

hyperpnea increase in depth and rate of breathing.

hyperthermia overheating.

hypocholia diminished flow of pancreatic enzymes.

hyposensitization immunization therapy by injection; immunotherapy.

hypothermia low body temperature; may be a symptoms of a disease or dysfunction of the temperature-regulating mechanism of the body, or it may be deliberately induced, such as during open-heart surgery, to reduce oxygen needs and provide a longer time for the surgeon to complete the operation without brain damage. When caring for the newborn, it is important to remember that heat loss can lead to hypothermia because of the infant's immature temperature-regulating system.

hypovolemia decreased volume of circulating plasma.

id in psychoanalytic theory, part of the personality that controls physical needs and instincts of the body; dominated by the pleasure principle.

imperforate anus congenital disorder in which the rectal pouch ends blindly above the anus and there is no anal orifice.

impunity belief, common among adolescents, that nothing can hurt them.

incest sexually arousing physical contact between family members not married to each other.

independent nursing actions nursing actions that may be performed based on the nurse's own clinical judgment.

induration hardness.

inhalant substance that may be taken into the body through inhaling; substance whose volatile vapors can be abused.

insulin reaction excessively low blood sugar caused by insulin overload, resulting in too rapid metabolism of the body's glucose; insulin shock; hypoglycemia.

intercurrent infection infection that occurs during the course of an already existing disease.

interdependent nursing actions nursing actions that the nurse must work with other health team members to accomplish, such as meal planning with a dietary therapist and teaching breathing exercises with a respiratory therapist.

interstitial fluid also called intracellular or tissue fluid; has a composition similar to plasma but contains almost no protein. This reservoir of fluid outside the body cells decreases or increases easily in response to disease.

interstitial keratitis inflammation of the cornea, often caused by congenital syphilis and usually accompanied by lacrimation, photophobia, and opacity of the lens; may lead to blindness.

intracellular fluid fluid contained within the cell membranes; constitutes about two thirds of the total body fluids.

intrathecal administration injection into the cerebrospinal fluid by lumbar puncture.

intravascular fluid fluid situated within the blood vessels or blood plasma.

invagination telescoping; infolding of one part of a structure into another.

karyotype chromosomal constitution of the cell nucleus; the photomicrograph of chromosomes used to locate malformations and translocations.

kernicterus severe brain damage as a result of excessive bilirubin levels.

Kussmaul breathing abnormal increase in the depth and rate of the respiratory movements.

kwashiorkor syndrome occurring in infants and young children soon after weaning, resulting from severe deficiency of protein. Symptoms include a swollen abdomen, retarded growth with muscle wasting, edema, gastrointestinal changes, thin dry hair with patchy alopecia, apathy, and irritability.

kyphoscoliosis backward and lateral curvature of the spine; hunchback.

lacrimation secretion of tears.

lactose a sugar found in milk that, when hydrolyzed, yields glucose and galactose.

lactose intolerance inability to digest lactose because of an inborn deficiency of the enzyme lactase.

lanugo fine, downy hair that covers the skin of the fetus.

latchkey child child who comes home to an empty house after school each day because the family caregivers are at work.

lecithin major component of surfactant.

leukemia uncontrolled reproduction of deformed white blood cells.

leukopenia leukocyte count less than 5,000 mm^3.

libido sexual drive.

lordosis forward curvature of the lumbar spine; swayback.

lymphoblast lymphocyte that has been changed by antigenic stimulation to a structurally immature lymphocyte.

lymphocytes single-nucleus, nonphagocytic leukocytes that are instrumental in the body's immune response.

magical thinking child's belief that thoughts are powerful and can cause something to happen (eg, illness or death of a loved one occurs because the child wished it in a moment of anger).

marasmus deficiency in calories as well as protein. The child suffers growth retardation and wasting of subcutaneous fat and muscle.

meconium first stools of the newborn; a sticky, greenish-black substance composed of bile, mucus, cellular waste, intestinal secretions, fat, hair, and other materials swallowed during fetal life, together with amniotic fluid.

menarche beginning of menstruation.

metered-dose inhaler hand-held plastic device that delivers a premeasured dose of medicine.

microcephaly small head.

micrognathia abnormal smallness of the lower jaw.

milia pearly white cysts usually seen over the bridge of the nose, chin, and cheeks of a newborn. They are usually retention cysts of sebaceous glands or hair follicles and disappear within a few weeks without treatment.

mittelschmerz pain experienced midcycle in the menstrual cycle, at the time of ovulation.

mongolian spots areas of bluish-black pigmentation resembling bruises. Most often seen over the sacral or gluteal regions of infants of African, Mediterranean, Native American, or Asian descent, they usually fade within 1 or 2 years.

monocytes 5% to 10% of white blood cells that defend the body against infection.

Moro reflex abduction of the arms and legs and flexion of the elbows in response to a sudden loud noise, jarring, or abrupt change in equilibrium: fingers flare, except the forefinger and thumb, which are clenched to form a C-shape. Occurs in the normal newborn up to the end of the fourth and fifth month.

mother–baby nursing cross-education of postpartum and nursery nurses, so that one nurse takes care of both mother and infant. The infant's bassinet is kept beside the mother, who helps care for her newborn while being carefully guided and taught by the nurse.

mummy restraint used to restrain an infant or small child during procedures that involve only the head or neck.

mutation fundamental change that takes place in the structure of a gene, resulting in the transmission of a trait different from that normally carried by that particular gene.

mutual gazing see *en face position*.

myopia ability to see objects clearly at close range but not at a distance; nearsightedness.

myringotomy incision of the eardrum performed to establish drainage and to insert tiny tubes into the tympanic membrane to facilitate drainage of serous or purulent fluid in the middle ear.

nebulizer tube attached to a wall unit or cylinder that delivers moist air via a face mask.

necrotizing enterocolitis (NEC) acute inflammatory disease of the intestine that occurs most often in small preterm infants; necrotic patches develop interfering with digestion, and can result in perforation and peritonitis.

negativism opposition to suggestion or advice; associated with the toddler age group because the toddler, in search of autonomy, frequently responds "no" to almost everything.

neonatal abstinence syndrome (NAS) symptoms seen in the newborn of the woman who has abused substances during pregnancy; withdrawal symptoms.

neonate term used to describe a newborn in the first 28 days of life.

noncommunicative language egocentric speech exhibited by children who talk to themselves, toys, or pets without any purpose other than the pleasure of using words.

nuchal rigidity stiff neck.

nuclear family family structure that consists of only the father, the mother, and the children living in one household.

nursing process proven form of problem solving based on the scientific method. The nursing process consists of five components: assessment, nursing diagnosis, planning, implementation, and evaluation.

obesity excessive accumulation of fat that increases body weight by 20% or more over ideal weight.

objective data in the nursing assessment, the data gained by direct observation by the nurse.

oliguria decreased production of urine, especially in relation to fluid intake.

onlooker play interest in the observation of an activity without participation.

opisthotonos arching of the back so that the head and the heels are bent backward and the body is forward.

orchiopexy surgical procedure used to bring an undescended testis down into the scrotum and anchor it there.

organogenesis process by which cells differentiate into major organ systems; commences shortly after conception and is almost completed by the end of the eighth week.

orthoptics therapeutic exercises to improve the quality of vision.

overprotection type of response by caregivers when caring for chronically ill children in which the caregivers protect the child at all costs, prevent the child from achieving new skills by hovering, avoid the use of discipline, and use every means to prevent the child from suffering any frustration.

overriding aorta in tetralogy of Fallot; the aorta shifts to the right over the opening in the ventricular septum so that blood from both the right and left ventricles is pumped into the aorta.

overweight more than 10% over ideal weight.

palmar grasp reflex phenomenon that results as pressure on the palms of the hands or soles of the feet near the base of the digits causes flexion of hands or toes.

palpebral fissures opening between the eyes.

papoose board commercial restraint board for use with toddlers or preschool-age children that uses canvas strips to secure the child's body and extremities. One extremity can be released to allow treatment to be performed on that extremity.

parallel play one child plays alongside another child or children involved in the same type of activity, but they do not interact with each other.

patient-controlled analgesia (PCA) programmed intravenous infusion of narcotic analgesia that the patient can control, within set limits.

pediatric nurse practitioner (PNP) professional nurse prepared at the postbaccalaureate level to give primary health care to children and families; these nurses use pediatricians or family physicians as consultants but offer day-to-day assessment and care.

pedodontist dentist who specializes in the care and treatment of children's teeth.

petechiae small bluish-purple spots caused by tiny broken capillaries; pinpoint hemorrhages beneath the skin.

phenylketonuria (PKU) recessive hereditary defect of metabolism that results in a congenital disease due to a defect in the enzyme that normally changes the essential amino acid, phenylalanine, into tyrosine. If untreated, PKU results in severe mental retardation.

philtrum vertical groove in the middle of the upper lip.

phimosis adherence of the foreskin to the glans penis.

photophobia intolerance to light.

photosensitivity sensitivity to sunlight.

phototherapy exposure of newborns to fluorescent lights to prevent the bilirubin concentration from reaching dangerous levels.

physiologic jaundice icterus neonatorum; jaundice that occurs in a large number of newborns but has no medical significance; result of the breakdown of fetal red blood cells.

pica compulsive eating of nonfood substances.

placenta organ linking the fetus to the mother; performs four functions for the developing fetus: respiration, nutrition, excretion, and protection; also called afterbirth.

play therapy technical of psychoanalysis that psychiatrists or psychiatric nurse clinicians use to uncover a disturbed child's underlying thoughts, feelings, and motivations to help understand them better.

polyarthritis inflammation of several joints.

polydipsia abnormal thirst.

polyphagia increased food consumption.

polyuria dramatic increase in urinary output, often with enuresis.

postterm (postmature) infant one born after completion of the 42nd week of gestation, regardless of birth weight.

premenstrual syndrome (PMS) symptoms in the period before menstruation, including edema (resulting in weight gain), headache, increased anxiety, mild depression, or mood swings; premenstrual tension.

preterm (premature) infant any infant of less than 37 weeks' gestation.

priapism prolonged, abnormal erection of the penis.

primary nursing system whereby one nurse plans the total care for a child and directs the efforts of nurses on the other shifts.

pruritus itching.

pseudomenses false menstruation; a slight red-tinged vaginal discharge in female infants resulting from a decline in the hormonal level after birth compared with the higher concentration in the maternal hormone environment before birth.

pseudostrabismus the cross-eyed look found in infants due to incomplete development of the nerves and muscles that control focusing and coordination; begins to disappear in the sixth month.

puberty period during which secondary sexual characteristics begin to develop and reproductive maturity is attained.

pulmonary stenosis narrowing of the opening between the right ventricle and the pulmonary artery, decreasing the flow of blood to the lungs.

pulse oximeter photoelectric device used to measure oxygen saturation in an artery. Can be attached to a finger, toe, or the heel of an infant.

punishment penalty given for wrongdoing.

purpura hemorrhages into the skin or mucous membranes.

purpuric rash rash consisting of ecchymoses (bruises) and petechiae caused by bleeding under the skin.

radiation in heat loss, it is the transfer of body heat to cooler solid objects that are not in direct contact with the infant.

recessive gene gene carrying different information for a trait within a pair that is not expressed (eg, blue eyes versus brown eyes). A recessive gene is detectable only when present on both chromosomes.

refraction the way light rays bend as they pass through the lens of the eye to the retina.

regurgitation spitting up of small quantities of milk; occurs rather easily in the young infant.

rejection type of response by caregivers when caring for chronically ill children in which the caregivers distance themselves emotionally from the child and, although they provide physical care, tend to scold and correct the child continuously.

respiratory distress syndrome (RDS) see *hyaline membrane disease.*

respite care care of the child by someone other than the usual caregiver so that the caregiver can get temporary relief and rest.

retinopathy of prematurity (ROP) overgrowth of blood vessels of the eye caused by constriction of the capillaries of the retina due to high blood concentration of oxygen.

retrolental fibroplasia (RLF) the final stage of ROP in which scarring occurs, resulting in retinal detachment and blindness.

reversibility ability to think in either direction.

RhoGAM commercial preparation of Rh_o (D antigen) immune globulin given to nonsensitized Rh-negative mothers.

right ventricular hypertrophy increase in thickness of the myocardium of the right ventricle.

ritualism practice employed by the young child to help develop security; consists of following a certain routine, making rituals of simple tasks.

rooming-in arrangement in which the health care facility permits a family caregiver to stay with a child; a cot or sleeping chair is provided for the caregiver.

rooting reflex infant's response of turning the head when the cheek is stroked toward the stroked side.

rumination voluntary regurgitation.

runaway child child who is absent from home for overnight or longer without the permission of the caregiver.

school phobia fear of child resulting in dread of a school situation or fear of leaving home; can be a combination of both.

scoliosis lateral curvature of the spine.

sebum oily secretion of the sebaceous glands.

seizure series of involuntary contractions of voluntary muscles; convulsion.

sex chromosomes one pair of chromosomes that differ in the male and the female.

sexual assault sexual contact made by someone who is not functioning in the role of caretaker of the child.

sexual abuse sexual contact between a child and someone in a caretaking position, such as a parent, babysitter, or teacher.

single-parent family household headed by one adult of either sex; there may be one or more children in the family.

skeletal traction pull exerted directly on skeletal structures by means of pins, wire, tongs, or another device surgically inserted through the bone.

skin traction pull on tape, rubber, or plastic materials attached to the skin that indirectly exerts pull on the musculoskeletal system.

small for gestation age (SGA) expression used to signify term infants of low birth weight.

smegma the cheeselike secretion of the sebaceous glands found under the foreskin.

socialization process by which a child learns the rules of the society and culture in which the family lives; its language, values, ethics, and acceptable behaviors.

soft neurologic signs signs of clumsiness or poor coordination that may be appropriate for a younger child.

solitary independent play playing apart from others without making an effort to be part of the group or their activity.

spina bifida failure of the posterior lamina of the vertebrae to close, leaving an opening through which the spinal meninges and spinal cord may protrude.

startle reflex follows any loud noise; similar to the Moro reflex, but the hands remain clenched; this reflex is never lost.

steatorrhea fatty stools.

step reflex also called the dance reflex; tendency of infants to make stepping movements when held upright.

stepfamily consists of custodial parent, children, and a new spouse.

stigma negative perception of a person because he or she is believed to be different from the general population; may cause embarrassment or shame by the person being stigmatized.

strabismus failure of the two eyes to direct their gaze at the same object simultaneously; squint; crossed eyes.

striae stretch marks.

stridor shrill, harsh respiratory sound, usually on inspiration.

subjective data in the nursing assessment, data spoken by the child or family.

sublimation process of directing a desire or impulse into more acceptable behaviors.

sucking reflex infant's response of strong, vigorous sucking when a nipple, finger, or tongue blade is put in his or her mouth.

superego in psychoanalytic theory, the conscience or parental value system; acts primarily as a monitor over the ego.

supernumerary excessive in number (eg, more than the usual number of teeth).

surfactant surface-active agent produced in the alveoli of the lungs that reduces surface tension inside the alveoli and bronchioles, preventing collapse and allowing free air exchange.

suture narrow band of connective tissue that divides the six nonunited bones of a newborn's skull.

swaddling wrapping securely in a small blanket.

sympathetic ophthalmia inflammatory reaction of the uninjured eye; symptoms can include photophobia, lacrimation, and some dimness of vision.

synovitis inflammation of a joint, most commonly the hip in children.

talipes equinovarus clubfoot with plantar flexion.

temper tantrum behavior in children that springs from frustrations caused by their urge for independence; a violent display of temper. The child reacts with enthusiastic rebellion against the wishes of the caregiver.

teratogens from the Greek *terato,* meaning monster, and *genesis,* meaning birth, an agent or influence that causes a defect or disruption in the prenatal growth process. The effect of a teratogen depends on when it enters the fetal system and the stage of differentiation of the organs or organ systems at that time. Generally, the fetus is most vulnerable to teratogens during the first trimester.

term infant infant born between the beginning of the 38th week and the end of the 42nd week of gestation, regardless of birth weight.

thanatologist person trained especially to work with the dying and their families, sometimes a nurse.

therapeutic play play technique that may be used by play therapists, nurses, child-life specialists, or trained volunteers.

thermoregulation regulation of temperature.

throwaway child child (often a teenager) who has been forced to leave home and is not wanted back by the adults in the home.

tinea ringworm.

tissue perfusion circulation of blood through the capillaries carrying nutrients and oxygen to the cells.

tolerance in substance abuse, ability of body tissues to endure and adapt to continued or increased use of a substance.

tonic neck reflex also called the fencing reflex; seen when the infant lies on the back, with the head turned to one side and the arm and leg on that side extended, the opposite arm flexed as if in a fencing position.

tonsils two oval masses attached to the side walls of the back of the mouth between the anterior and posterior pillars (folds of mucous membranes at the side of the passage from the mouth to the pharynx).

total parenteral nutrition (TPN) often called hyperalimentation; the administration of dextrose, lipids, amino acids, electrolytes, vitamins, minerals, and trace elements into the circulatory system to meet the nutritional needs of the child whose needs cannot be met through the gastrointestinal tract.

traction force applied to an extremity or other part of the body to maintain proper alignment and facilitate healing of a fractured bone or dislocated joint.

trimester period of 3 months; pregnancy is divided in three trimesters.

tympanic membrane sensor device used to determine the temperature of the tympanic membrane by rapidly sensing infrared radiation from the membrane. The tympanic thermometer offers the advantage of recording the temperature rapidly with little disturbance to the child.

umbilical cord connects the fetus to the placenta; contains one vein and two arteries that carry blood between the fetus and the placenta.

unfinished business completing matters that will help ease the death of a loved one; saying the unsaid and doing the undone acts of love and caring that may seem difficult to express; recognizing time is limited and filling that time with the important issues that need to be taken care of.

unilateral one side (eg, in cleft lip, only one side of the lip is cleft).

unoccupied behavior daydreaming, fingering clothing or a toy without any apparent purpose.

urticaria hives.

vaginitis inflammation of the vagina.

vascular nevus commonly known as a strawberry mark, a slightly raised, bright-red collection of hypertrophied skin capillaries that does not blanch completely on pressure.

ventricular septal defect abnormal opening in the septum of the heart between the ventricles, allowing blood to pass directly from the left to the right side of the heart. The most common intracardiac defect.

ventriculoatrial shunting plastic tubing implanted into the cerebral ventricle passing under the skin to the cardiac atrium, providing drainage for excessive cerebrospinal fluid.

ventriculoperitoneal shunting plastic tubing implanted into the cerebral ventricle passing under the skin to the peritoneal cavity, providing drainage for excessive cerebrospinal fluid. Excessive tubing can be inserted to accommodate the child's growth.

vernix caseosa greasy, cheeselike substance that protects the skin during fetal life; consists of sebum and desquamated epithelial cells.

viability ability to maintain life after birth; the age of viability is the earliest gestational age at which a fetus can survive outside the uterine environment.

wellness nursing diagnoses diagnoses that identify the potential of an individual, family, or community to move to a higher level of wellness.

West nomogram graph with several scales arranged so that when two values are known, the third can be plotted by drawing a line with a straightedge; commonly used to calculate BSA.

wheezing sound of expired air being pushed through obstructed bronchioles.

withdrawal symptoms in substance abuse, physical and psychological symptoms that occur when the drug is no longer being used.

zygote fertilized ovum.

Resources for Families and Caretakers of Children

American Anorexia/Bulemia Association, Inc.
425 E. 61st St.
New York, NY 10021
212-891-8686

**Association for Children and Adults with Learning
  Disabilities**
4156 Library Road
Pittsburgh, PA 15234
412-341-1515

American Cleft Palate Association
1218 Grandview Ave.
Pittsburgh, PA 15211
800-24-CLEFT (800-242-5338)

Association for the Care of Children's Health
7910 Woodmont Ave., Ste. 300
Bethesda, MD 20814
301-654-6549

Association of Retarded Citizens of the United States
PO Box 6109
Arlington, TX 76005
817-640-0204

Autism Society of America
8601 Georgia Av., Ste. 503
Silver Springs, MD 20910
301-565-0433

Candlelighter's Childhood Cancer Foundation
7910 Woodmont Ave., Ste. 460
Bethesda, MD 20814
800-366-2223

Children's Hospice International
700 Princess St., Ste. 3
Alexandria, VA 22314
800-24-CHILD (800-242-4453)

Clearinghouse for Disability Information
Room 3132, Switzer Building, C St. S.W.
Washington, DC 20202
202-732-1250

Compassionate Friends
PO Box 3696
Oak Brook, IL 60522-3696
708-990-0010

John T. Tracey Clinic
806 West Adams Blvd.
Los Angeles, CA 90007
213-748-5481

Leukemia Society of America
600 Third Ave.
New York, NY 10016
212-573-8484
800-955-4572

March of Dimes Birth Defect Foundation
1275 Mamaroneck Ave.
White Plains, NY 10605
914-428-7100

**National Association of Anorexia Nervosa and
  Associated Disorders, Inc. (ANAD)**
PO Box 7
Highland Park, IL 60035
708-831-3438

National Childhood Grief Institute
6200 Colonial Way
Minneapolis, MN 55436
616-920-0737

National Clearinghouse for Alcohol and Drug Abuse Information
PO Box 2345
Rockville, MD 20852
800-729-6686

National Down Syndrome Society
666 Broadway, Ste. 810
New York, NY 10012
800-221-4602

National Easter Seal Society
2023 West Ogden Ave.
Chicago, IL 60612
312-243-8400

National Fragile X Foundation
1441 York St., Ste. 215
Denver, CO 80206
800-688-8765
313-333-6155

National Hospice Organization
1901 N. Moore St., Ste. 901
Arlington, VA 22209
800-658-8898

National Hydrocephalus Foundation
Route One, River Road, Box 210A
Joliet, IL 60436
815-467-6548

National Self-Help Clearinghouse (families of chronically ill)
CUNY Graduate Center
33 W. 42nd St., Room 620 N
New York, NY 10036
212-642-2944

National Sudden Infant Death Syndrome Foundation
10500 Little Patuxent Parkway, Ste. 420
Columbia, MD 21044
800-221-5105

Parents Anonymous
7120 Franklin Ave.
Los Angeles, CA 90046
800-421-0353

Parents of Down Syndrome Children
11600 Nebel St.
Rockville, MD 20852
301-984-5792

Special Olympics
1350 New York Ave. N.W. Ste. 500
Washington, DC 20005-4709
202-628-3630

Spina Bifida Association of America
1700 Rockville Pike, Ste. 540
Rockville, MD 20852
800-621-5141

Stop Teenage Addiction to Tobacco (STAT)
511 E. Columbus Ave.
Springfield, MA 01115
413-732-STAT (413-732-7828)

Sudden Infant Death Syndrome Clearinghouse
8201 Greensboro Drive, Ste. 600
McLean, VA 22102
703-821-8955

Tourette Syndrome Association
4240 Belle Blvd.
Bayside, NY 11361
718-224-2999

Youth Suicide National Center
1825 I St., N.W.
Washington, DC 20006
202-429-0190

Growth Charts

Median Heights and Weights (United States)

Age	Weight		Height	
(years)	(kg)	(lb)	(cm)	(inches)
Infants				
0.0–0.5	6	13	60	24
0.5–1.0	9	20	71	28
Children				
1–3	13	29	90	35
4–6	20	44	112	44
7–10	28	62	132	52
Males				
11–14	45	99	157	62
15–18	66	145	176	69
19–24	72	160	177	70
25–50	79	174	176	70
51 +	77	170	173	68
Females				
11–14	46	101	157	62
15–18	55	120	163	64
19–24	58	128	164	65
25–50	63	138	163	64
51 +	65	143	160	63

BOYS: BIRTH TO 36 MON
PHYSICAL GROWTH
NCHS PERCENTILES*

NAME_____   RECORD #_____

Ross
Growth &
Development
Program

*Adapted from: Hamill PVV, Drizd TA, Johnson CL, Reed RB, Roche AF, Moore WM. Physical growth: National Center for Health Statistics percentiles. AM J CLIN NUTR 32:607-629, 1979. Data from the Fels Research Institute, Wright State University School of Medicine, Yellow Springs, Ohio.

c 1982 ROSS LABORATORIES

BOYS: BIRTH TO 36 MONTHS
PHYSICAL GROWTH
NCHS PERCENTILES*

NAME _____   RECORD # _____

*Adapted from Hamill PVV, Drizd TA, Johnson CL, Reed RB,
Roche AF, Moore WM. Physical growth: National Center for Health
Statistics percentiles. AM J CLIN NUTR 32:607-629, 1979. Data
from the Fels Research Institute, Wright State University School of
Medicine, Yellow Springs, Ohio.

© 1982 ROSS LABORATORIES

DATE	AGE	LENGTH	WEIGHT	HEAD CIRC.	COMMENT

GIRLS: BIRTH TO 36 MO......
PHYSICAL GROWTH
NCHS PERCENTILES*

NAME_____   RECORD #_____

GIRLS: BIRTH TO 36 MONTHS
PHYSICAL GROWTH
NCHS PERCENTILES*

NAME _____   RECORD # _____

*Adapted from Hamill PVV, Drizd TA, Johnson CL, Reed RB, Roche AF, Moore WM. Physical growth: National Center for Health Statistics percentiles. AM J CLIN NUTR 32 607-629, 1979. Data from the Fels Research Institute, Wright State University School of Medicine, Yellow Springs, Ohio

© 1982 ROSS LABORATORIES

DATE	AGE	LENGTH	WEIGHT	HEAD CIRC	COMMENT

BOYS: 2 TO 18 YEARS
PHYSICAL GROWTH
NCHS PERCENTILES*

NAME_____ RECORD #_____

*Adapted from: Hamill PVV, Drizd TA, Johnson CL, Reed RB,
Roche AF, Moore WM: Physical growth: National Center for Health
Statistics percentiles. AM J CLIN NUTR 32:607-629, 1979. Data
from the National Center for Health Statistics (NCHS) Hyattsville,
Maryland.
Ⓒ 1982 ROSS LABORATORIES

Ross
Growth &
Development
Program

GIRLS: 2 TO 18 YEAR
PHYSICAL GROWTH
NCHS PERCENTILES*

NAME_____ RECORD #_____

*Adapted from: Hamill PVV, Drizd TA, Johnson CL, Reed RB, Roche AF, Moore WM. Physical growth: National Center for Health Statistics percentiles. AM J CLIN NUTR 32:607-629, 1979. Data from the National Center for Health Statistics (NCHS) Hyattsville, Maryland.

© 1982 ROSS LABORATORIES

Pulse, Respiration, and Blood Pressure Values for Children

Normal Pulse Ranges in Children

Age	Normal Range	Average
0–24 hours	70–170 bpm	120 bpm
1–7 days	100–180 bpm	140 bpm
1 month	110–188 bpm	160 bpm
1 month–1 year	80–180 bpm	120–130 bpm
2 years	80–140 bpm	110 bpm
4 years	80–120 bpm	100 bpm
6 years	70–115 bpm	100 bpm
10 years	70–110 bpm	90 bpm
12–14 years	60–110 bpm	85–90 bpm
14–18 years	50–95 bpm	70–75 bpm

bpm, beats per minute.
From Skale N. Manual of Pediatric Nursing Procedures. Philadelphia: JB Lippincott, 1992, p. 35.

Normal Blood Pressure Ranges

Age	Systolic (mm Hg)	Diastolic (mm Hg)
Newborn–12 hr (less than 1000 g)	39–59	16–36
Newborn–12 hr (3000 g)	50–70	24–45
Newborn–96 hr (3000 g)	60–90	20–60
Infant	74–100	50–70
Toddler	80–112	50–80
Preschooler	82–110	50–78
School-age	84–120	54–80
Adolescent	94–140	62–88

From Skale N. Manual of Pediatric Nursing Procedures. Philadelphia: JB Lippincott, 1992, p. 46.

Variations in Respirations with Age

Age	Rate per Minute
Newborn	40–90
1 year	20–40
2 years	20–30
3 years	20–30
5 years	20–25
10 years	17–22
15 years	15–20
20 years	15–20

Lowrey GH. Growth and Development of Children, 6th ed.
Copyright © 1973 by Year Book Medical Publishers, Inc., Chicago.
Used by permission.

Conversion Charts

Conversion of Pounds to Kilograms

Pounds	0	1	2	3	4	5	6	7	8	9
0	—	0.45	0.90	1.36	1.81	2.26	2.72	3.17	3.62	4.08
10	4.53	4.98	5.44	5.89	6.35	6.80	7.25	7.71	8.16	8.61
20	9.07	9.52	9.97	10.43	10.88	11.34	11.79	12.24	12.70	13.15
30	13.60	14.06	14.51	14.96	15.42	15.87	16.32	16.78	17.23	17.69
40	18.14	18.59	19.05	19.50	19.95	20.41	20.86	21.31	21.77	22.22
50	22.68	23.13	23.58	24.04	24.49	24.94	25.40	25.85	26.30	26.76
60	27.21	27.66	28.12	28.57	29.03	29.48	29.93	30.39	30.84	31.29
70	31.75	32.20	32.65	33.11	33.56	34.02	34.47	34.92	35.38	35.83
80	36.28	36.74	37.19	37.64	38.10	38.55	39.00	39.46	39.91	40.37
90	40.82	41.27	41.73	42.18	42.63	43.09	43.54	43.99	44.45	44.90
100	45.36	45.81	46.26	46.72	47.17	47.62	48.08	48.53	48.98	49.44
110	49.89	50.34	50.80	51.25	51.71	52.16	52.61	53.07	53.52	53.97
120	54.43	54.88	55.33	55.79	56.24	56.70	57.15	57.60	58.06	58.51
130	58.96	59.42	59.87	60.32	60.78	61.23	61.68	62.14	62.59	63.05
140	63.50	63.95	64.41	64.86	65.31	65.77	66.22	66.67	67.13	67.58
150	68.04	68.49	68.94	69.40	69.85	70.30	70.76	71.21	71.66	72.12
160	72.57	73.02	73.48	73.93	74.39	74.84	75.29	75.75	76.20	76.65
170	77.11	77.56	78.01	78.47	78.92	79.38	79.83	80.28	80.74	81.19
180	81.64	82.10	82.55	83.00	83.46	83.91	84.36	84.82	85.27	85.73
190	86.18	86.68	87.09	87.54	87.99	88.45	88.90	89.35	89.81	90.26
200	90.72	91.17	91.62	92.08	92.53	92.98	93.44	93.89	94.34	94.80

Conversion of Fahreheit to Celsius

Celsius	Fahrenheit	Celsius	Fahrenheit	Celsius	Fahrenheit
34.0	93.2	37.0	98.6	40.0	104.0
34.2	93.6	37.2	99.0	40.2	104.4
34.4	93.9	37.4	99.3	40.4	104.7
34.6	94.3	37.6	99.7	40.6	105.2
34.8	94.6	37.8	100.0	40.8	105.4
35.0	95.0	38.0	100.4	41.0	105.9
35.2	95.4	38.2	100.8	41.2	106.1
35.4	95.7	38.4	101.1	42.4	106.5
35.6	96.1	38.6	101.5	41.6	106.8
35.8	96.4	38.8	101.8	41.8	107.2
36.0	96.8	39.0	102.2	42.0	107.6
36.2	97.2	39.2	102.6	42.2	108.0
36.4	97.5	39.4	102.9	42.4	108.3
36.6	97.9	39.6	103.3	42.6	108.7
36.8	98.2	39.8	103.6	42.8	109.0
				43.0	109.4

$$(°C) \times (9/5) + 32 = °F.$$
$$(°F - 32) \times (5/9) = °C.$$

Appendix E

Good Sources of Essential Nutrients

Protein	Vitamin A	Vitamin B			Vitamin C	Vitamin D	Minerals		
		Thiamine	Riboflavin	Niacin			Calcium	Iron	Iodine
Meat, poultry, fish, milk products and eggs. Whole wheat grains, nuts, peanut butter, legumes are also good sources of protein, but need to be supplemented by some animal protein, such as meat, eggs, milk, cheese, cottage cheese or yogurt.	Green leafy vegetables, deep yellow vegetables and fruits, whole milk or whole milk products, egg yolk.	Meat, fish, poultry, eggs, whole grain, legumes, potatoes, green leafy vegetables.	Milk (best source), meat, egg yolk, green vegetables.	Meat, fish, poultry, peanut butter, wheat germ, brewer's yeast. Although the amount in milk is small, children whose intake of milk is adequate do not develop pellagra.	Citrus fruits and tomatoes, fresh or frozen citrus fruit juices, strawberries, cantaloupe. Breast milk is an adequate source of vitamin C for young infants only if the mother's diet contains sufficient vitamin C.	Sunlight, fish liver oils, fortified milk and synthetic vitamin D.	Milk and milk products, squash, sweet potatoes, raisins, rhubarb, well-cooked dried beans, turnip greens, Swiss chard, mustard greens.	Green leafy vegetables, liver, meats and eggs, dried fruits, whole grain or enriched bread and cereals.	Seafoods, plants grown on soil near the sea, iodized salt.

Standard Precautions

Use Standard Precautions, or the equivalent, for the care of all patients. *Category IB**

A. Handwashing
  (1) Wash hands after touching blood, body fluids, secretions, excretions, and contaminated items, whether or not gloves are worn. Wash hands immediately after gloves are removed, between patient contacts, and when otherwise indicated to avoid transfer of microorganisms to other patients or environments. It may be necessary to wash hands between tasks and procedures on the same patient to prevent cross-contamination of different body sites. *Category IB*
  (2) Use a plain (nonantimicrobial) soap for routine handwashing. *Category IB*
  (3) Use an antimicrobial agent or a waterless antiseptic agent for specific circumstances (eg, control of outbreaks or hyperendemic infections), as defined by the infection control program. *Category IB* (see Contact Precautions for additional recommendations on using antimicrobial and antiseptic agents.)
B. Gloves
  Wear gloves (clean, nonsterile gloves are adequate) when touching blood, body fluids, secretions, excretions, and contaminated items. Put on clean gloves just before touching mucous membranes and nonintact skin. Change gloves between tasks and procedures on the same patient after contact with material that may contain a high concentration of microorganisms. Remove gloves promptly after use, before touching noncontaminated items and environmental surfaces, and before going to another patient, and wash hands imme-

diately to avoid transfer of microorganisms to other patients or environments. *Category IB.*
C. Mask, Eye Protection, Face Shield
  Wear a mask and eye protection or a face shield to protect mucous membranes of the eyes, nose, and mouth during procedures and patient-care activities that are likely to generate splashes or sprays of blood, body fluids, secretions, and excretions. *Category IB*
D. Gown
  Wear a gown (a clean, nonsterile gown is adequate) to protect skin and to prevent soiling of clothing during procedures and patient-care activities that are likely to generate splashes or sprays of blood, body fluids, secretions, or excretions. Select a gown that is appropriate for the activity and amount of fluid likely to be encountered. Remove a soiled gown as promptly as possible, and wash hands to avoid transfer of microorganisms to other patients or environments. *Category IB*
E. Patient-Care Equipment
  Handle used patient-care equipment soiled with blood, body fluids, secretions, and excretions in a manner that prevents skin and mucous membrane exposures, contamination of clothing, and transfer of microorganisms to other patients and environments. Ensure that reusable equipment is not used for the care of another patient until it has been cleaned and reprocessed appropriately. Ensure that single-use items are discarded properly. *Category IB*
F. Environmental Control
  Ensure that the hospital has adequate procedures for the routine care, cleaning, and disinfection of environmental surfaces, beds, bedrails, bedside equipment, and other frequently touched surfaces, and ensure that these procedures are being followed. *Category IB*
G. Linen
  Handle, transport, and process used linen soiled with blood, body fluids, secretions, and excretions in a manner that prevents skin and mucous membrane exposures and contamination of clothing, and that avoids transfer of microorganisms to other patients and environments. *Category IB*

---

* *Category IB.* Strongly recommended for all hospitals and reviewed as effective by experts in the field and a consensus of HIC-PAC based on strong rationale and suggestive evidence, even though definitive scientific studies have not been done.
  (From Guideline for isolation precautions in hospitals developed by the Centers for Disease Control and Prevention and the Hospital Infection Control Practices Advisory Committee (HICPAC), January 1996.)

H. Occupational Health and Bloodborne Pathogens
 (1) Take care to prevent injuries when using needles, scalpels, and other sharp instruments or devices; when handling sharp instruments after procedures; when cleaning used instruments; and when disposing of used needles. Never recap used needles, or otherwise manipulate them using both hands, or use any other technique that involves directing the point of a needle toward any part of the body; rather, use either a one-handed "scoop" technique or a mechanical device designed for holding the needle sheath. Do not remove used needles from disposable syringes by hand, and do not bend, break, or otherwise manipulate used needles by hand. Place used disposable syringes and needles, scalpel blades, and other sharp items in appropriate puncture-resistant containers, which are located as close as practical to the area in which the items were used, and place reusable syringes and needles in a puncture-resistant container for transport to the processing area. *Category IB*
 (2) Use mouthpieces, resuscitation bags, or other ventilation devices as an alternative to mouth-to-mouth resuscitation methods in areas where the need for resuscitation is predictable. *Category IB*

I. Patient Placement
 Place a patient who contaminates the environment or who does not (or cannot be expected to) assist in maintaining appropriate hygiene or environmental control in a private room. If a private room is not available, consult with infection control professionals regarding patient placement or other alternatives. *Category IB*

Photo Credit List

Figure 1-8: © Kathy Sloane
Figure 1-7: © B. Proud
Figure 2-1: Photo by C. Shea
Figure 2-2: © B. Proud; courtesy of Wayne Memorial Hospital/ Honesdale, PA
Figure 2-3: Photo by D. DiPalma
Figure 3-2: ©B Proud; courtesy of Wayne Memorial Hospital/ Honesdale, PA
Figure 3-3: © B. Proud; courtesy of Wayne Memorial Hospital/ Honesdale, PA
Figure 3-6: © B. Proud; courtesy of Wayne Memorial Hospital/ Honesdale, PA
Figure 3-7: Courtesy of Lewistown Hospital, Lewiston, PA
Figure 3-9: © B. Proud; courtesy of Wayne Memorial Hospital/ Honesdale, PA
Figure 3-10: Courtesy of Abbott Laboratories/Chicago, IL
Figure 3-11: ©B. Proud; courtesy of Wayne Memorial Hospital, Honesdale, PA
Figure 3-12B: ©B. Proud; courtesy of Wayne Memorial Hospital/ Honesdale, PA
Figure 3-16: ©B. Proud; courtesy of Wayne Memorial Hospital/ Honesdale, PA
Figure 3-18: ©B. Proud; courtesy of Wayne Memorial Hospital/ Honesdale, PA
Figure 4-1: Courtesy of the Department of Medical Photography/ Children's Hospital, Buffalo NY
Figure 4-2: ©B. Proud; courtesy of Wayne Memorial Hospital/ Honesdale, PA
Figure 4-3: ©B. Proud; courtesy of Wayne Memorial Hospital/ Honesdale, PA
Figure 4-7: ©Kathy Sloane; courtesy of Children's Hospital/Oakland, CA
Figure 4-10: ©B. Proud; courtesy of Wayne Memorial Hospital/ Honesdale, PA
Figure 5-2: Photo by B. Ainsworth
Figure 5-3: Photo by D. DiPalma
Figure 6-5: Courtesy of Dr. Kurt Hirschhorn
Figure 6-6: Courtesy of Dr. Kurt Hirschhorn
Figure 6-11: ©B. Proud; courtesy of Wayne Memorial Hospital/ Honesdale, PA
Figure 7-1: ©Kathy Sloane
Figure 7-6: Photo by Keith Cotton
Figure 7-7: Courtesy of Mead Johnson Laboratories/Evansville, IN
Figure 7-8: Courtesy of Mead Johnson Laboratories/Evansville, IN
Figure 7-9: Courtesy of the Department of Medical Photography/ Children's Hospital, Buffalo, NY
Figure 7-10: Courtesy of the Department of Medical Photography/ Children's Hospital, Buffalo, NY
Figure 7-12: ©Kathy Sloane
Figure 7-14: ©Kathy Sloane
Figure 7-15: ©Kathy Sloane
Figure 7-16: ©B. Proud; courtesy of Wayne Memorial Hospital/ Honesdale, PA

Figure 7-17: Photo by Imaginique Productions
Figure 7-18: ©B. Proud; courtesy of Wayne Memorial Hospital/ Honesdale, PA
Figure 7-19: Photo by Keith Cotton
Figure 7-21: ©B. Proud; courtesy of Wayne Memorial Hospital/ Honesdale, PA
Figure 8-3: Courtesy of Mead Johnson Laboratories/Evansville, IN
Figure 8-5: Courtesy of Mead Johnson Laboratories/Evansville, IN
Figure 8-7: Photo by Marcia Lieberman
Figure 8-8: © A. Haupt/Photo Researchers
Figure 8-9: © Gates Rhodes
Figure 9-1: From Pillitteri A. An introduction to clinical embryology/Chicago: Year Book, 1974
Figure 9-8: Courtesy of Dr. Mark Ravitch
Figure 10-3A: © B. Proud; courtesy of Wayne Memorial Hospital/ Honesdale, PA
Figure 10-3B: © B. Proud; courtesy of Wayne Memorial Hospital/ Honesdale, PA
Figure 10-3C: © B. Proud; courtesy of Wayne Memorial Hospital/ Honesdale, PA
Figure 10-3D: © B. Proud; courtesy of Wayne Memorial Hospital/ Honesdale, PA
Figure 10-3E: © B. Proud; courtesy of Wayne Memorial Hospital/ Honesdale, PA
Figure 10-4A: © Caroline Brown
Figure 10-4B: ©Kathy Sloane
Figure 10-6: Courtesy of the Department of Medical Photography, Children's Hospital/Buffalo NY
Figure 10-8: © B. Proud
Figure 11-9: © B. Proud; courtesy of Wayne Memorial Hospital/ Honesdale, PA
figure 11-10: Courtesy of Life Watch Systems, 1050 St., Suite 900, Denver, CO
Figure 12-1: © B. Proud; courtesy of Wayne Memorial Hospital/ Honesdale, PA
Figure 12-2: © B. Proud; courtesy of Wayne Memorial Hospital/ Honesdale, PA
Figure 12-5: © B. Proud; courtesy of Wayne Memorial Hospital/ Honesdale, PA
Figure 12-6: Photo by D. DiPalma
Figure 13-2: © B. Proud; courtesy of Wayne Memorial Hospital/ Honesdale, PA
Figure 14-1: © B. Proud; courtesy of Wayne Memorial Hospital/ Honesdale, PA
Figure 14-2: Courtesy of Janet Weber
Figure 14-3: Photo by D. DiPalma
Figure 14-4: © B. Proud; courtesy of Wayne Memorial Hospital/ Honesdale, PA
Figure 15-1: Courtesy of the John Tracy Clinic/Los Angeles, CA
Figure 15-2: Courtesy of the John Tracy Clinic/Los Angeles, CA
Figure 15-3: National Society to Prevent Blindness/New York, NY

Figure 15-4: Courtesy of the Perkins School for the Blind/Watertown, MA

Figure 15-5: Courtesy of the Perkins School for the Blind/Watertown, MA

Figure 15-6: © B. Proud; courtesy of Wayne Memorial Hospital/Honesdale, PA

Figure 15-8: © B. Proud; courtesy of Wayne Memorial Hospital/Honesdale, PA

Figure 15-11: Courtesy of the Department of Medical Photography, Children's Hospital/Buffalo, NY

Figure 16-2: Courtesy of S. Robbins

Figure 16-3. Photo by Elizabeth McKinney Chmiel

Figure 16-4: Photo by D. DiPalma

Figure 16-5A: © B. Proud

Figure 16-5B: © B. Proud

Figure 16-7: Photo by D. DiPalma

Figure 16-8: Courtesy of J Nurs Care, Westport, CT

Figure 17-1: Courtesy of the Upjohn Company/Kalamazoo, MI & MB Marks, MD/Miami, FL

Figure 17-2: Photo by Marcia Lieberman

Figure 17-4A: © B. Proud; courtesy of Wayne Memorial Hospital/Honesdale, PA

Figure 17-4B: © B. Proud; courtesy of Wayne Memorial Hospital/Honesdale, PA

Figure 17-7: From O'Connor BJ, Scoliosis: Classification and diagnosis in pediatric orthopedics. ONAJ 3:84, 1976

Figure 17-9: Courtesy of JH Moe, MD

Figure 17-7: Courtesy of the Centers for Disease Control and Prevention/Atlanta, GA

Figure 17-11: From Brady MII. Lifelong care of the child with Duchene muscular dystrophy. Am J Matern Child Health 4: 227–230, 1979

Figure 18-1: © B. Proud; courtesy of Wayne Memorial Hospital/Honesdale, PA

Figure 18-2: Photo by D. DiPalma

Figure 18-3: © Kathy Sloane

Figure 18-5: © B. Proud; courtesy of Wayne Memorial Hospital/Honesdale, PA

Figure 19-1: © B. Proud; courtesy of Wayne Memorial Hospital/Honesdale, PA

Figure 19-4: © B. Proud; courtesy of Wayne Memorial Hospital/Honesdale, PA

Figure 20-4: Photo by D. DiPalma

Figure 20-5: © Kathy Sloane

Figure 21-1: Courtesy of the Department of Medical Photography, Children's Hospital/Buffalo, NY

Figure 21-2: © Phyllis Picardi/Stock Boston

Figure 22-4: © Kathy Sloane

Index

References with "t" denote tables; "f" denote figures; "b" denote boxes

A

abdominal paracentesis, 332
ABO incompatibility, 141
absence seizures, 352
abuse
   emotional, 445–446
   physical, 444–445, 445f
   sexual, 446
accidents, prevention of
   in adolescent, 405
   burns. *see* burns
   drowning, 255, 277–278
   head injuries, 290
   in infant, 198
   motor vehicle accidents, 254–255
   in preschool child, 300–301
   in school-age child, 345, 347
   in toddler, 254. *see also specific*
      accident
   toxic substances ingestions. *see* toxic
      substances, ingestion of
Accutane. *see* isotretinoin
acetaminophen, 275t
acetylsalicylic acid, 275t
achylia, 268
acid–base balance
   defects in. *see* acidosis; alkalosis
   definition of, 48
acidosis, 48
acne vulgaris, 417–418
acquired immunodeficiency syndrome
      (AIDS). *see also* human
      immunodeficiency virus
   in adolescent, 423–424
   characteristics of, 422t
   nursing process, 424–426, 428
acrocyanosis, 106
actual nursing diagnoses, 12
acute bronchiolitis, 224–225
acute glomerulonephritis, 333t, 333–334
acute interstitial pneumonia. *see* acute
      bronchiolitis
acute laryngotracheobronchitis, 265
acute leukemia
   clinical manifestations, 323–324
   description of, 323
   diagnosis, 324
   nursing process for, 324–326
   pathophysiology, 323
   treatment, 324

acute lymphatic leukemia (ALL), 323
acute myeloid leukemia (AML), 323
acute nasopharyngitis, 223
addicted mother, 142
adenoids, 321
admissions, to pediatric hospital
   emergency, 58–59
   interview, 59, 60f–61f
   physical assessment, 59, 62
   planned, 58
adolescence
   developmental tasks, 395t
   early. *see* preadolescence
   time span, 394
adolescent
   accident prevention, 405
   acne vulgaris, 417–418
   alcohol abuse, 432–433
   amphetamines use, 434
   anorexia nervosa, 409–410, 410–411
   body image, 397
   breast self-examination, 401, 402f
   bulimia nervosa, 411–412
   cocaine abuse, 433–434
   communicating with, 16
   current health status of, 8–9
   dental checkups, 400
   diabetes mellitus in, 371
   eating disorders, 409–417
   family teaching tips, 401
   food guide pyramid for, 399f
   growth charts, 496–497
   in health care facility, 405–406
   health education and counseling,
      401–404
   health problems of, 409–437
   health promotion and maintenance,
      398–405
   highest risks for injury, 8
   hospitalization of, 405–406
   hospital play program for, 67–68
   hypnotics use, 434
   infectious diseases, 419–420
   infectious mononucleosis, 419
   marijuana abuse, 433
   masturbation, 401
   medication administration, 41t
   menstrual disorders, 418–419
   mental health, 404
   mortality causes, 405, 405f–406f
   narcotics, 434

   nutrition, 397–398, 398t
   obesity, 409–410
   pelvic examinations, 400
   personality development, 396–397
   physical development, 396
   pregnancy, 428–431
   psychedelic drug use, 434
   psychosocial development, 396
   routine checkups, 399–400
   sexually transmitted diseases,
      420–421, 422t, 423–424
   sexual responsibility, 401, 403
   skin disorders, 417–418
   steroids use, 434
   substance abuse, 403–404, 431, 432t
   suicide, 435
   testicular self-examination, 401, 403f
   tobacco abuse, 433
   tuberculosis in, 419–420
   understanding of death, 468
   vaginitis in, 420, 421t
   violence incidents, 405
aggression
   observation of, 15
   in preschool child, 297
airway clearance, cystic fibrosis, 271
akinetic seizures, 352
alcohol, teratogenic effects of, 93, 142
alcohol abuse
   by adolescent, 432–433
   information resources for, 443t
Alcoholics Anonymous (AA), 433
alcoholism, 432
alkalosis, 48
allergen, 354
allergic reactions
   allergic rhinitis, 354f, 354–355
   asthma, 355–360
   description of, 354
   plants, 389
allergic rhinitis, 354f, 354–355
allergic salute, 354, 354f
allergies, food
   common sources, 206t
   in eczema, 239
   lactose intolerance, 206
   milk, 206
allograft, 284
alopecia, 325
alphafetoprotein levels, spina bifida
      diagnosis using, 156